Amyotrophic Lateral Sclerosis

Amyotrophic Lateral Sclerosis

Edited by **Lisa Rowe**

hayle medical

New York

Published by Hayle Medical,
30 West, 37th Street, Suite 612,
New York, NY 10018, USA
www.haylemedical.com

Amyotrophic Lateral Sclerosis
Edited by Lisa Rowe

International Standard Book Number: 978-1-63241-040-5 (Hardback)

Printed in China.

Contents

Preface

Though ample amount of research; both pre-clinical and clinical, has been conducted during the past few years, Amyotrophic Lateral Sclerosis (ALS) continues to be one of the mysterious diseases of 21st century. Significant attempts have been made for the progress of pathophysiological models and understanding the underlying pathology, and with new instruments in genetics and transgenic techniques, the goal of finding a durable cure has come into scope. On the contrary, most pharmacological trials have remained unsuccessful in depicting an advantage for ALS patients. In this book, readers will find a compilation of state-of-the-art examination of etiology, epidemiology, and pathophysiology of ALS, including the advantages and pitfalls in experimental models of Amyotrophic Lateral Sclerosis.

This book is a result of research of several months to collate the most relevant data in the field.

When I was approached with the idea of this book and the proposal to edit it, I was overwhelmed. It gave me an opportunity to reach out to all those who share a common interest with me in this field. I had 3 main parameters for editing this text:

1. Accuracy - The data and information provided in this book should be up-to-date and valuable to the readers.
2. Structure - The data must be presented in a structured format for easy understanding and better grasping of the readers.
3. Universal Approach - This book not only targets students but also experts and innovators in the field, thus my aim was to present topics which are of use to all.

Thus, it took me a couple of months to finish the editing of this book.

I would like to make a special mention of my publisher who considered me worthy of this opportunity and also supported me throughout the editing process. I would also like to thank the editing team at the back-end who extended their help whenever required.

Editor

Part 1

Pathophysiology and Methodology

1

Amyotrophic Lateral Sclerosis: An Introduction to Treatment and Trials

Martin H. Maurer
Dept. of Physiology and Pathophysiology, University of Heidelberg
Germany

1. Introduction

There are several synonyms for Amyotrophic Lateral Sclerosis (ALS) which include Motor Neuron Disease (MND), Charcot's disease, and Lou Gehrig's disease. The latter is named after the American baseball professional Lou Gehrig, who died of ALS in the 1940s (Miller, 2011).
The symptoms of motor neuron disease (MND) have first been described by several neurologists by the mid-19th century. The French neurologist Charcot defined the nosological entity "amyotrophic lateral sclerosis" (ALS) some years later (historic aspects of ALS are reviewed in (Eisen, 2007; Mitsumoto et al., 2006; Oliveira & Pereira, 2009; Rowland, 2001; Wijesekera & Leigh, 2009)).
In the present understanding, MND comprehends a spectrum of different neurodegenerative syndromes which show a common neuropathology, i. e. the progressive degeneration of motor neurons.
These syndromes include the "classical" ALS, progressive bulbar palsy (PBP), progressive muscular atrophy (PMA), primary lateral sclerosis (PLS), flail arm syndrome (Vulpian-Bernhardt syndrome), flail leg syndrome, and ALS with multi-system involvement (e.g., Fronto-Temporal Dementia, FTD) (**Fig. 1**) (reviewed in Lillo & Hodges, 2009; Silani et al., 2011).

2. Diagnostic criteria

2.1 Clinical features

The diagnosis of ALS is based on a catalogue of criteria specified by the World Federation of Neurology (www.wfneurology.org). These criteria are known as the "El Escorial" criteria, named after the Spanish historic site El Escorial. The original criteria of 1994 (Brooks, 1994; Mitsumoto, 1997) have been revised in 1998 (Brooks et al., 2000; Ross et al., 1998), which are known as the "Airlie House" criteria, named after the conference site at Warrenton, VA, U.S.A. In 2006, a consensus conference at Awaji-shima defined criteria of electromyographic and nerve conduction measurements for the diagnosis of ALS (de Carvalho et al., 2008).
The clinical features comprehend the presence of (i) lower motorneuron (LMN) signs such as the loss of muscle strength, muscular atrophy, fasciculations, hyporeflexia, hypotonicity or flaccidity, or muscle cramps, in at least two limbs; (ii) upper motorneuron (UMN) signs such as extensor plantar responses, spasticity, or pathologic hyperreflexia, in at least one region (bulbar, cervical, or lumbosacral), and (iii) the progression of the disease defined as increasing symptomatic impairment by history in the same region or new regions (Ferguson & Elman, 2007).

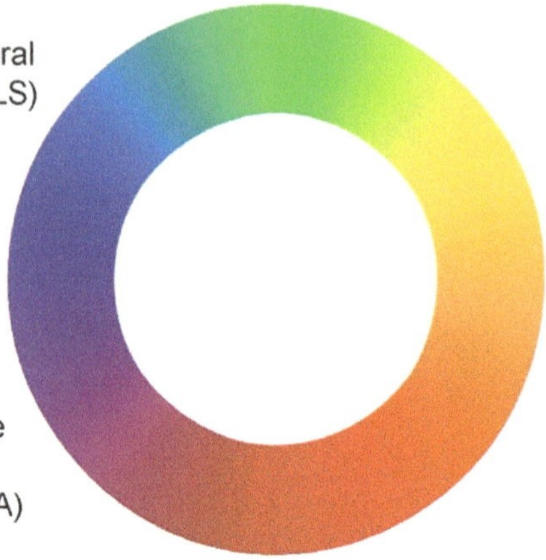

Fig. 1. Spectrum of motor neuron disease (MND). Currently, the understanding of MND comprehends a variety of neurodegenerative syndromes with progressive degeneration of motor neurons.

Neuropathological findings defining the MND spectrum are, on the cellular level, the progressive degeneration of upper and/or lower motor neurons, respectively, and on the molecular level, the presence of intraneuronal inclusion bodies which are immunopositive for ubiquitin-(Ub) and the 43 kB TAR DNA-binding protein (TDP-43) (reviewed in Colombrita et al., 2011; Geser et al., 2010), named Bunina, or Hirano, inclusion bodies (Rowland, 2009).

Moreover, sensory signs (except those attributable to aging), neurogenic sphincter abnormalities, other progredient diseases of the central nervous system (CNS) or peripheral nervous system (PNS) must be absent. Additionally, ALS-like syndromes must be ruled out. These include myelopathy, structural lesions of the spinal cord, multifocal motor neuropathy, hyperthyroidism, hyperparathyroidism, hematologic malignancy associated with monoclonal gammopathy, lead poisoning, a history of radiation to the CNS, and hexosaminidase A deficiency in patients younger than 30 years of age.

The revised criteria defined a certain probability level for the diagnostic criteria (Brooks et al., 2000), which have been questioned by the later electrophysiological consensus (de Carvalho et al., 2008; Sathasivam, 2010).

At present, a consensus conference has defined morphological markers by MRI, which may lead to a biomarker for ALS diagnosis (Kiernan et al., 2011; Turner et al.).

2.2 Neuropsychiatry of ALS

Only in recent years, psychiatric and behavioural symptoms of ALS patients came into the focus of interest. It has become clear that psychiatric symptoms are not only secondary phenomena of a disabilitating disease, but are also inherent and specific in ALS. On the other hand, the etiopathological connections remain unknown.

With regard to the diagnoses and prevalence of these in ALS patients, there are only few data available, which are summarized in **Table 1**.

Psychiatric Diagnosis	Prevalence (percentages, rounded) and reference
Depression	30(Atassi et al., 2011; Lillo et al., 2011); 15 (Ferentinos et al., 2011); 10 (Kurt et al., 2007)
Dementia	10 (Lillo et al., 2011)
Stereotypical behavior	20 (Lillo et al., 2011)
Reduction in motivation	80 (Lillo et al., 2011)
Apathy	40 (Lillo et al., 2011)
Cognitive impairment	50 (Woolley & Jonathan, 2008)
Sleep disturbances	Unknown (Hetta & Jansson, 1997)
Fatigue	Unknown
Psychosis	Unknown

Table 1. Common psychiatric symptoms and diagnoses reported in ALS patients.

In the following paragraphs, I will shortly describe the major psychiatric abnormalities in ALS patients and current findings.

2.2.1 Dementia

In the concept of a "continuum" of TDP-43 proteinopathies (Geser et al., 2009), ALS is classified together with fronto-temporal dementia (Giordana et al., 2011; Lillo & Hodges, 2009; Nakano, 2000; Woolley & Jonathan, 2008; Yoshida, 2004; Zago et al., 2011). This has also been shown on the morphological level (Tsujimoto et al., 2011).

Another pathophysiological pathway discussed in the pathogenesis of FTD is the progranulin pathway (Sleegers et al., 2010).

Cognitive impairment and frontal lobe dysfunction is seen in about 40-60% of ALS patients (Abrahams et al., 1996; Evdokimidis et al., 2002; Witgert et al., 2009).

2.2.2 Sleep

In the current understanding, it is difficult to distinguish whether psychiatric abnormalities in ALS patients are integral part of the CNS disease, or if they are a secondary phenomenon. For example, sleep disturbances are a common problem in ALS patients, but besides anxiety, they may also result from reduced mobility, muscle cramps, or swallowing problems (Hetta & Jansson, 1997).

2.2.3 Fatigue

Fatigue is also a common problem in ALS patients, which does not describe physical exhaustion, but a pathological state of mind (Jackson & Bryan, 1998; Lou, 2008).

2.2.4 Depression and anxiety

The patients know about the devastating nature of ALS with only a short survival time remaining at the point of time at diagnosis, with a deteriorating quality of life, and without a pharmacological treatment option towards "healing". Therefore, a high prevalence of depression and anxiety in ALS patients would be expected. On the other hand, prevalence rates for depression in ALS patients range from 0-44% in the literature, whereas structured interviewing according to DSM-IV criteria reveals rates of 9-11% (Averill et al., 2007; Ferentinos et al., 2011; Kurt et al., 2007). Prevalence rates for anxiety in ALS have been reported with 0-30% (Kurt et al., 2007). Interestingly, the rate of depression and anxiety is not as high as expected (Huey et al., 2010; McLeod & Clarke, 2007; Norris et al., 2010), which means that the quality of life addressed by an individual is not dependent on the remaining lifetime.

2.2.5 Psychosis

The association of schizophrenia with ALS has been reported (Enns et al., 1993; Howland, 1990; Yase et al., 1972), but the pathophysiological interrelation remains unknown. There have been reports on a familial association (Burnstein, 1981).

3. Measuring the disease

The use of ALS assessment techniques such as rating scales is to monitor disease progression , to make outcome parameters in clinical trials comparable; and to predict efficacy of therapeutic strategies (Cudkowicz et al., 2004).
Typical ALS assessment techniques comprehend (i) global scales which are based on clinical observation, (ii) measuring of the muscular strength, (iii) electrophysiological testing, and (iv) the assessment of the quality of life.

3.1 Clinical assessment scales

Global scales subsume (i) scores based on subjective or historic data, such as the ALS functional rating scale (ALSFRS) (Cedarbaum & Stambler, 1997; The ALS CNTF treatment study (ACTS) phase I-II Study Group, 1996), and the ALS severity scale (ALSSS) (Hillel et al., 1989), (ii) scores based on clinical tests such as the Norris scale (Norris et al., 1974), or the Appel scale (Appel et al., 1987), and (iii) scales used both for ALS and other diseases such as the Schwab and England global rating scale (Schwab & England, 1969), or the modified Ashworth spasticity scale (Bohannon & Smith, 1987).

3.2 Muscular function testing

Measuring of the muscular strength includes quantitative tests, maximum voluntary isometric contraction, handheld dynamometry, Jamar grip strength, manual muscle testing. Moreover, the spirometric measurement of the forced vital capacity and maximum voluntary ventilation can also be included in muscle tests.

3.3 Electrophysiological measurements

Electrophysiological testing includes compound muscle action potentials (CMAPs) and motor unit number estimate (MUNE) (Shefner et al., 2011) or the motor unit number index (MUNIX) (Nandedkar et al., 2010; Neuwirth et al., 2011).

A consensus conference has defined electrophysiological criteria for the diagnosis of ALS (de Carvalho et al., 2008).

3.4 Assessment of the quality of life

The quality of life is assessed by questionnaires such as the Short form - 36 (SF-36), Short form - 12 (SF-12), ALSQ-40, or the Sickness Impact Profile (reviewed in Epton et al., 2009; McGuire et al., 1997; Williams et al., 2008).

4. The pathophysiological rationale for therapeutic interventions

4.1 Pathophysiology of motor neuron degeneration in ALS

Pathophysiological mechanisms involved in ALS include (reviewed in Mitsumoto et al., 2006; Wijesekera & Leigh, 2009):

- genetic factors (reviewed in Pasinelli & Brown, 2006; Robberecht, 2002; Ticozzi et al., 2011),
- excitotoxicity (reviewed in Bogaert et al., 2011; Foran & Trotti, 2009),
- oxidative stress (reviewed in Kaur & Ling, 2008; Orrell et al., 2008),
- mitochondrial and SOD1 dysfunction (reviewed in Benatar, 2007; Shi et al., 2010; Valentine et al., 2005),
- impaired axonal transport (reviewed in Costa et al., 2010),
- apoptosis and cell death (reviewed in Sathasivam et al., 2001),
- neurofilament and protein aggregation such as TDP-43 proteinopathies (reviewed in Geser et al., 2010; Worrall et al., 2000),
- neuro-inflammation (reviewed in Graber & Dhib-Jalbut, 2009; Holmoy, 2008; Lipton et al., 2007; Weydt & Moller, 2005), and
- the lack or dysfunction of neurotrophic factors (reviewed in Maurer et al., 2008; Siciliano et al., 2010; Traynor et al., 2006).

These pathophysiological mechanisms all end in motor neuron degeneration as the final pathway in disease progression (reviewed in Bruijn et al., 2004; Carlesi et al., 2011; Thatte & Dahanukar, 1997).

To address the genetic influence in ALS, two databases have been established. The ALSoD database (alsod.iop.kcl.ac.uk) contains detailed information about genes involved in ALS pathophysiology, and the ALSGene database lists genetic association studies (www.alsgene.org) (Lill et al., 2011).

4.2 Pathophysiological considerations in the planning of ALS treatment strategies

Most pre-clinical trials in ALS research started with the pathophysiological model of the disease. In counteracting the pathophysiology of the disease, motor neuron survival and stabilization of motor neuron function is increased (reviewed in Bedlack et al., 2007; Carlesi et al., 2011; Fornai et al., 2011; Ilieva et al., 2009; Pradat et al., 2010; Silani et al., 2011).

Current strategies for treatment concepts reach for counteracting the individual pathophysiological actors. They including the following groups of agents:

- Anti-excitotoxicitory drugs. Excitotoxicity is mainly modulated by the release of glutamate and contributes to an acute toxicity. Typical molecules involved are the NMDA and AMPA receptors and the glial glutamate transporter Excitatory amino-acid transporters type-2 (EAAT2), which is regulating most of the extracellular glutamate concentration.

- Anti-aggregation drugs. Cellular aggregates of proteins, such as the Bunina bodies, occur in the neuronal somata of ALS patients. The prevention of these cellular aggregates may also increase the survival of motor neurons. The subcellular component involved in the degradation of aggregates is the endoplasmic reticulum (ER). Defects in ER function may contribute to the formation of the protein aggregates, as well as the inhibition of the proteasome.
- Suppliers of cellular energy. In ALS, mitochondrial dysfunction contributes to the cellular energy loss. Thus the prevention of neuronal energy depletion may increase and prolong neuronal survival.
- Anti-oxidants. The generation of reactive oxygen species (ROS), such as H_2O_2, can produce major damage to the neuron. Thus specialized cellular systems exist in the cell to prevent oxidative damage. One of these systems include [Cu,Zn]-superoxide dismutase-1 (SOD1), of which mutations in humans can induce ALS.
- SOD1 reduction techniques. The clearance of the mutated and dysfunctional SOD1 protein may also positively influence motor neuron survival.
- Inducers of intraaxonal transport. Molecules that signal damage in the bouton terminal are transported to the neuronal soma. In ALS, this transport is retricted, thus the damage information reaches the peri-nuclear area only delayed.
- Drugs supporting nerve-muscle transmission. Defects in the transmission at the neuromuscular junction may contribute to disease progress.
- Stabilizers of the neuro-vascular unit. The loss of proteins at the tight junctions may disrupt the neuro-vascular unit. Thus molecules stabilizing the tight junctions may ameliorate the supply of neurons with substrates.
- Anti-inflammatory compounds. Neuroinflammation plays a role in the chronic detrimental processes occurring in the immediate microenvironment of the neuron.
- Neuroprotectants. Since neurodegeneration is the general mechanism in ALS progression, neuroprotective drugs may prevent or slow down neuronal break-down.
- Anti-apoptotic compounds. Cell death is the ultimate reason in the apoptotic cascade. Thus compounds preventing cell death may contribute to increased survival of motor neurons.
- Growth factors. Growth factors such as G-CSF, VEGF, GDNF and others can both stimulate the growth of novel neurons (neurogenesis) and the repair of damaged neurons (neuroregeneration).
- Various techniques whereby muscles can be strengthened even in an environment where motor neurons are degenerating, thus maintaining motor function.
- Gene therapy. In these approaches, the expression of endogenous proteins, such as growth factors, are used to increase
- Stem cell therapies. The transplantation of various sources, such as bone-marrow derived stem cells (BMSC), mesenchymal stem cells (MSC), or neuronal stem cells (NSC), may support the microenvironment and thus the survival of motor neurons, or supply new motor neurons by replacing apoptotic cells.

5. Clinical trials in ALS

5.1 Programmed failure in clinical trials for ALS?

In the typical process of drug development, preclinical data such as biochemical assays, cellular assays, and rodent models for the disease, lead to positive results with regard to predefined outcome parameters, for example, the increase in muscle strength, or survival time. For all of the drugs listed in the next section, promising preclinical data have been provided and published (for review, see (Ludolph & Sperfeld, 2005)). But why did the majority of the clinical trials fail, when preclinical data have been so promising?

Three major points came to my notice, when reviewing the literature: First, the animal models (mouse, rat, drosophila etc.) may either not sufficiently reflect the human pathology, or the animal pathology does not reflect human conditions (discussed in Green, 2002; Kiernan et al., 2011; Scott et al., 2008). Second, "ALS" is a clinical but not a pathophysiological entity. Thus, the inter-personal variability between patients is too big, and the inclusion criteria are too broad. Third, the design of the clinical trials may be insufficient (Aggarwal & Cudkowicz, 2008; Fornai et al., 2011; Kiernan et al., 2011; Maragakis, 2009), including:

- the number of subjects is too small,
- the time for follow-up is too short,
- the power of the study is calculated too low,
- the inclusion criteria are too broad,
- the outcome measures are not well-defined and comparable, or insufficient.

In future clinical trials, these issues should be discussed and included into the design of clinical ALS trials (Borasio, 1997).

5.2 Consensus guidelines for ALS trials

Therefore, a round table has been established to agree on minimal criteria for a "good" clinical trial (Miller et al., 1999). Of note, there have been substantial efforts also in other diseases such as stroke research to agree on clinical and pre-clinical guidelines for research, such as the "Stroke Therapy Academic Industry Roundtable (STAIR)" (STAIR - Stroke Treatment Academic Industry Roundtable, 2006).

In the following paragraphs, I will shortly summarize the consensus guidelines for ALS trial. The prerequisite for any ALS trial should be a substantial diagnosis according to the criteria defined by the World Federation of Neurology (see above). Moreover, the inclusion criteria should be handled strictly, including that both sporadic and familial ALS can be entered into the trial. The age of the patients should be limited between 18 and 85 years of age. Symptoms should show a disease progression within the first six months after onset, but not more than five years. Additionally, also exclusion criteria have been defined, for example, the patients should not show sensory abnormalities, dementia, other neurological diseases, they should not suffer from any uncompensated medical illness, substance abuse, or psychiatric illness. Of note, the patients should not be taking any other investigational drug.

The endpoints of the trial must be defined in advance, for example, survival time, muscle strength, or ventilator dependence are common endpoints. All trials should include a control group.

The quality of life should be assessed in every efficacy trial. The statistical analysis must be sound and planned with sufficient power. Any co-medication must be carefully re-considered.

Since there has been an early release of information about the efficacy in clinical ALS trials, which had to be revoked after thorough analysis, any information with regard to the efficacy of an investigational drug should only be released when peer-reviewed publication is at least imminent (with the exception of scientific meetings). The investigator is responsible for any conflict of interest.

The design of ALS trials should comprehend three phases (Brooks, 1997). In phase I, toxicity and pharmacokinetics is tested. In phase II (pilot, exploratory, or screening trials) information is gathered about dose finding, preliminary efficacy, and further safety observations. In phase III, definitive efficacy and safety is evaluated. Phase I trials should incorporate a placebo control group and the follow-up should be at least six months. Phase II trials may use placebo controls, historic controls, or a crossover design. If the prospective therapeutic value aims at improvement of signs and symptoms, such as increased muscle strength or ameliorated function, the follow-up should be at least six months, whereas trials aiming at stabilization or slowing of deterioration should observe the patients' condition for at least 12 months (Bedlack, 2010). All phase III trials should be placebo-controlled. The endpoints should include at least the survival time, assessment of strength measured by maximum voluntary isometric contraction, pulmonary function, and functional performance by the ALS rating scale. Of course, an independent data and safety monitoring board should be established.

Of note, since survival times are rather short, many patients feel desperate and take unapproved medication out of the reach of a clinical trial. By establishing these consensus guidelines, this potentially dangerous drug use may be reduced (Ross, 2009).

5.3 Overview over drug candidates in clinical ALS trials

In the following "inventory" of clinical trials in ALS, I will give an overview over drug candidates used in ALS trials. I have included all interventional clinical trials registered at Clinicaltrials.gov (http://clinicaltrials.gov/). Information on these trials can be obtained by accessing the website http://ClinicalTrials.gov/show/NCTxxx, where xxx stands for the registration number shown below.

Since there have been various clinical trials in the era before Clinicaltrials.gov required registration, and before a consensus conference established criteria for ALS trials (Miller et al., 1999), I have included some information on earlier trials. On the other hand, I excluded case reports, trials with nutritional supplements, and non-pharmacological therapeutic procedures such as plasma exchange, whole-body irridation, hyperbaric oxygenation, balneotherapy, cervico-dorsal electroshock therapy, adrenal cortex injection or stem cell injection, even when the stem cells are used as vehicles and vectors for the expression of biologicals.

Of note, this inventory is neither comprehensive, nor does it contain all available references due to space restriction. It is mainly based on a selective literature search in the PubMed database, and summarizes recent reviews in the field (Carlesi et al., 2011; Miller et al., 2005; Siciliano et al., 2010; Zinman & Cudkowicz, 2011; Zoccolella et al., 2009).

5.3.1 N-acetylcysteine

The anti-oxidant N-acetylcysteine did not show efficacy in a phase II clinical trial (Louwerse et al., 1995).

5.3.2 AEOL-10150

AEOL-10150 is a metalloporphyrin scavenging reactive oxygen species (ROS) (Orrell, 2006). It has been tested for safety and tolerability in three phase I trials, but further development has been halted.

5.3.3 Amantadine (1-adamantylamine, 1-aminoadamantane)

Amantadine shows a weak NMDA receptor antagonism and anti-cholinergic effects. In a cross-over study with guanidine, no benefits for ALS patients have been described (Munsat et al., 1981).

5.3.4 Anakinra

Anakinra is a recombinant antibody directed against the interleukin-1 receptor (IL-1R). IL-1 is involved in sustaining the neuroinflammatory process. Treatment with anakinra in the G93A-SOD1 transgenic mouse model of ALS extended the lifespan of the animals and decreased neuroinflammation (Meissner et al., 2010). Thus blocking of the IL-1R may be a potential target in decreasing the speed of ALS progression (van der Meer & Simon, 2010). Currently, a phase II study (NCT01277315), designed as a riluzole add-on study, investigates the safety and tolerability of anakinra in ALS.

5.3.5 Antioxidants

In a systematic review, no evidence for a benefit of anti-oxidant treatment with regard to survival, neither alone, nor in combination, has been described (Orrell et al., 2008). The antioxidants administered in ALS patients included vitamin E, acetylcysteine, L-methionine, and selenium.

5.3.6 Arimoclomol (BRX-220)

The small molecule arimoclomol is a co-inducer of heat-shock proteins (Phukan, 2010), namely of HSP70 (Brown, 2007). Thus it may be used to increase endogenous cellular protein repair and to prevent misfolding, or aggregation, of proteins by activating molecular chaperones (Kalmar & Greensmith, 2009).

Arimoclomol was tested in two phase II studies to evaluate safety and efficacy in ALS patients (NCT00561366) and to find a dose range and to determine pharmacokinetic parameters (NCT00244244) (Cudkowicz et al., 2008; Lanka et al., 2009).

Currently, arimoclomol is tested in a phase II/III trial in patients with SOD1-positive fALS (NCT00706147).

5.3.7 Arundic acid (ONO-2506)

Arundic acid is an enantiomeric, three carbon atom homolog of valproic acid, with anti-inflammatory and anti-glutamatergic effects (de Paulis, 2003).

It was tested in two phase II studies, designed as riluzole add-on, in clinical ALS trials for long-term safety (NCT00694941) and safety and efficacy (NCT00403104). The original evaluation of the trials did not show statistically significant differences between groups, but the subgroup analysis showed a possible positive effect for patients in early stages, namely within 14 months after onset of symptoms. On the other hand, patients with longer disease onset showed negative outcome (Thomas Meyer, 2005).

5.3.8 AVP-923 (Zenvia)

AVP-923 is a combinational formulation containing dextromethorphan hydrobromide, which is an NMDA antagonist and sigma-1 receptor agonist, and quinidine sulphate, which inhibits the cytochrome P450 2D6 (CYP2D6) enzyme. Dextromethorphan hydrobromide shows a high first pass metabolism in the liver, where it is metabolized by CYP2D6. Thus the addition of quinidine sulphate increases the bioavailability of dextromethorphan hydrobromide (Olney & Rosen, 2010).

AVP-923 was tested in two phase III trials in ALS patients with pseudobulbar affect (PBA), which is characterized by emotional dysregulation, such as uncontrollable outbursts of laughing or crying that are inappropriate to the emotions being experienced (Garnock-Jones, 2011; Olney & Rosen, 2010). The study showed that AVP-923 ameliorates symptoms of PBA in ALS patients and improved quality of life and quality of relationships (Brooks et al., 2004).

5.3.9 Azathioprine

The immunosuppressant azathioprine in combination with prednisolone did not show a benefit in ALS patients (Werdelin et al., 1990).

5.3.10 Brain-derived neurotrophic factor (BDNF)

The neuroprotective growth factor BDNF has been evaluated in a phase I/II clinical trial which reported a trend for prolonged survival after subcutaneous infusion (The BDNF Study Group & Bradley, 1995), a result which could not be reproduced in the subsequent phase III clinical trial (The BDNF Study Group (Phase III), 1999). The intrathecal administration was safe and well-tolerated (Ochs et al., 2000).

5.3.11 Branched-chain amino acids (BCAA)

The branched-chain amino acids comprehend leucine, isoleucine, and valine.

In clinical trials, branched chain amino acids did not show a beneficial effect in ALS patients (Tandan et al., 1996).

5.3.12 Bromocriptine

The dopamine agonist bromocriptine did not show a benefit in ALS patients (Szulc-Kuberska et al., 1990).

5.3.13 Buspirone

The anxiolytic agent buspirone did not show a benefit in ALS patients (The ALS Association, 2010).

5.3.14 Ceftriaxone

Ceftriaxone is a ß-lactam antibiotic which also shows anti-oxidant and anti-excitotoxity effects (Traynor et al., 2006).

Currently, ceftriaxone is evaluated in a phase III clinical trial in patients with ALS (NCT00349622).

5.3.15 Celecoxib

Celecoxib is an inhibitor of cyclooxygenase-2 (COX-2), an enzyme which promotes inflammation by releasing of inflammatory substances, such as prostaglandin E(2) (PGE2).

The rationale of celecoxib treatment is the reduction of PGE2 in the cerebrospinal fluid (CSF), thus preventing neuroinflammation and neuronal loss.
In a phase II clinical trial (NCT00355576), celecoxib did not show a beneficial effect on the decline in muscle strength, motor unit number estimates, vital capacity, ALS Functional Rating Scale-Revised, and overall survival (Cudkowicz et al., 2006). Moreover, PGE2 levels in the CSF were not elevated at baseline and did not decline during treatment (Cudkowicz et al., 2006). In this trial, celecoxib was combined with creatinine and/or minocycline (Gordon et al., 2008).

5.3.16 Ciclosporine A

The immunosuppressant cyclosporine A did not show a benefit in ALS patients (Appel et al., 1988).

5.3.17 Ciliary neurotrophic factor (CNTF)

CNTF is a neurotrophic factor with neuroprotective properties.
It has been tested in two clinical trials finding no effect on disease progression (ALS CNTF Treatment Study Group, 1996; Miller et al., 1996), but an increased trend of adverse effects (Miller et al., 1996).

5.3.18 Cistanche total glycosides (CTGs)

The glycosidic extract of the plant *Cistanche spp.* has a long tradition in its medicinally use in Traditional Chinese Medicine (TCM). It has been described as a neuroprotective agent in a mouse model of Parkinson's Disease (PD) (Li et al., 2008). Currently, Cistanche Total Glycosides are investigated in a phase II trial (NCT00753571). Of note, the CTGs are the only agents in registered ALS trials without a defined chemical composition, which may impose problems in future comparability to other medications and effectiveness of different preparations.

5.3.19 CK-2017357

With regard to the loss of skeletal muscle strength, the substituted urea derivative CK-2017357 is claimed to activate the muscle protein troponin in fast skeletal muscle fibres. A proposed mode-of-action is sensitizing the sarcomere to calcium, thus the neuro-muscular transmission is amplified, thus muscle power increases and the time to musclular fatigue is delayed (von Haehling et al., 2010).
A phase IIa study (NCT01089010) was completed in 2010 and showed a trend towards short-term improvements in grip-strength and respiration parameters.

5.3.20 Coenzyme Q10

Coenzyme Q10 has been proposed to inhibit neurodegeneration. In a phase II clinical trial, it was well tolerated and safe (Ferrante et al., 2005), but showed no efficacy in a phase II futility trial (NCT00243932) (Kaufmann et al., 2009; Levy et al., 2006).

5.3.21 Creatine

Creatine acts as anti-oxidant and is a mitochondrial co-factor.
It has been evaluated in several phase II clinical trials (NCT00070993, NCT00005674, NCT00005766) which reported no beneficial effect in ALS patients (Groeneveld et al., 2003; Shefner et al., 2004), as well as a phase III clinical trial (NCT00069186) (Rosenfeld et al., 2008).

Creatine supplementation temporarily increased maximal isometric power in ALS patients (Mazzini et al., 2001).
In a phase I dose-escalation trial, creatine concentrations in the brain increased after oral administration (Atassi et al., 2010).
Currently, creatine is evaluated in a phase II clinical trial (NCT01257581) in combination with tamoxifen in ALS patients.

5.3.22 Cyclophosphamide

The immunosuppressant cyclophosphamide showed only a temporary amelioration of symptoms in ALS patients without a long-term benefit (Gourie-Devi et al., 1997).

5.3.23 Dexpramipexole (R-(+) pramipexole; RPPX; KNS-760704)

Dexpramipexole is a synthetic amino-benzothiazole and the (+)-enantiomer of pramipexole which has dopaminergic activity and is a mitochondrial neuroprotectant by scavenging reactive oxygen and nitrogen species (RONS) (Cheah & Kiernan, 2010; Gribkoff & Bozik, 2008).
In earlier studies, RPPX reduced oxidative stress in sporadic ALS patients (Pattee et al., 2003). RPPX has been found to be safe and tolerable (Bozik et al., 2010; Wang et al., 2008), but did not change ALSFRS-R (NCT00140218, NCT00600873, NCT00596115, NCT00647296) (Wang et al., 2008). In the open-label extension protocol, RPPX caused a non-significant reduction in the slope of decline in the ALSFRS-R score (NCT00931944) (Wang et al., 2008).
RPPX is currently evaluated in a phase III study (NCT01281189) in ALS patients.

5.3.24 3,4-Diaminopyridine (DAP)

The potassium channel blocker DAP did not show a benefit in ALS patients (Aisen et al., 1996; Aisen et al., 1995). Currently, the drug is re-evaluated after a phase I safety study (Bertorini et al., 2011).

5.3.25 Dronabinol

Dronabinol is a synthetic Δ9-tetrahydrocannabinol (Delta-9-THC, Δ9-THC, THC).
It has been tested in a phase II study (NCT00812851) in ALS patients suffering from muscular cramps, where no subjective improvement of cramp intensity has been seen (Weber et al., 2010).

5.3.26 Edaravone (MCI-186; NSC 2629)

Edavarone is an anti-oxidant free radical scavenger (Takahashi, 2009).
It has been tested in several phase II/III clinical trials (NCT00330681, NCT00415519, NCT00424463) for safety and efficacy. A phase II study found a possible delay in the progression of functional motor symptoms in ALS patients (Yoshino & Kimura, 2006).

5.3.27 Erythropoietin (EPO)

EPO is a hematopoietic growth factor with neuroprotective properties (Maurer et al., 2008). Moreover, EPO exhibited anti-inflammatory and anti-apoptotic effects.
It has been evaluated in a phase II trial, finding no effects on survival and functional outcome (Lauria et al., 2009).

5.3.28 Escitalopram

Escitalopram is a selective serotonin reuptake inhibitor (SSRI) and used clinically as an antidepressant.

It has been tested in a phase III clinical trial (NCT00965497) for the improvement of depressive symptoms and the quality of life in ALS patients.

5.3.29 Gabapentin

Gabapentin is an anti-convulsant with anti-glutamatergic effects, which have been proposed to slow down neuronal pathology (Welty et al., 1995).

It has been tested in a phase II trial finding a smaller slope in arm strength decrase (Miller et al., 1996), but a subsequent phase III trial has not shown beneficial effects of (Miller et al., 2001). No effects on neuronal integrity have been found in an MR spectroscopy study (Kalra et al., 2003).

5.3.30 Gangliosides

Gangliosides are derivatives of sialylated glycosphingolipids containing one to five sialic acids at various anomeric linkage sites to the core glycan. They modulate the effect of nerve growth factor and activate protein kinase (DeFelice & Ellenberg, 1984; Rapport, 1990).

Gangliosides have been tested in several clinical trials without benefit for ALS patients (Bradley et al., 1984; Harrington et al., 1984; Lacomblez et al., 1989).

5.3.31 Glatiramer acetate

Glatiramer acetate is a random polymer composed of four amino acids that are found in myelin basic protein (MBP). It has been proposed that it inhibits neuroinflammation, stimulates anti-glutamatergic growth factor effects.

In a phase II clinical trial (NCT00326625), glatiramer acetate has not shown any beneficial effect in ALS patients (Meininger et al., 2009).

5.3.32 Granulocyte colony stimulating Factor (G-CSF; AX200)

G-CSF is a hematopoietic growth and maturation factor with neuroprotective and neuroregenerative effects (reviewed in Maurer et al., 2008).

G-CSF has been evaluated in a phase II study (NCT00298597) in ALS patients, finding no differences with regard to functional outcome between study groups, but slowing the progression of white matter tract destruction (Duning et al., 2011). In a second phase II trial (NCT00397423), the authors reported preliminary data on 13 patients with slower disease progression (Zhang et al., 2009). Another clinical trial did not report statistically significant differences between study and control group (Nefussy et al.), but a trend towards slowing down disease progression.

5.3.33 Growth hormone (GH, Somatropin)

Human growth hormone (hGH) stimulates the production and release of insulin-like growth factor I (IGF-1) which induces cell proliferation and differentiation (Rosenbloom, 2009).

GH has evaluated in a phase II trial (NCT00635960) with no effects on disease progression (Sacca et al., 2011).

5.3.34 GSK1223249

GSK1223249 is a humanised monoclonal antibody which counteracts the inhibition of neurite outgrowth by Nogo-A. Currently, GSK1223249 is evaluated in a phase I study (NCT00875446) for safety in ALS patients.

5.3.35 Guanidine

In a clinical trial, guanidine caused severe side effects such as acute paralysis (Norris et al., 1974; Norris et al., 1974). In a cross-over study with amantadine, no benefits for ALS patients have been described (Munsat et al., 1981).

5.3.36 Indinavir

The antiviral drug indinavir did not show a benefit in ALS patients (Scelsa et al., 2005).

5.3.37 Insulin-like growth factor-1 (IGF-1)

IGF-1 is a growth factor stimulated by the human growth hormone (hGH). It induces cell proliferation and differentiation (Rosenbloom, 2009).

Whereas a first trial of IGF-1 in ALS patients reported a slower disease progression of functional impairment and a higher quality of life score (Lai et al., 1997), a subsequent study did not find beneficial effects after 9 months of treatment (Borasio et al., 1998). A phase III clinical trial (NCT00035815) found no beneficial effects after 2 years of treatment in ALS patients (Sorenson et al., 2008).

5.3.38 Interferon

The immunomodulators interferon-alpha (Dalakas et al., 1986; Mora et al., 1986) and interferon-beta (Beghi et al., 2000; Bouche et al., 1986) did not show a benefit in ALS patients.

5.3.39 ISIS 333611 (ISIS-SOD1$_{Rx}$)

ISIS 333611 is an antisense oligonucleotide inhibitor of Cu/Zn superoxide dismutase (SOD1) (Smith et al., 2006). Currently, a phase I (NCT01041222) investigates the safety, tolerability, and activity familial ALS caused by SOD1 gene mutations.

5.3.40 Isoprinosine

The antiviral drug isoprinosine did not show a benefit in ALS patients (Fareed & Tyler, 1971; Percy et al., 1971).

5.3.41 Lamotrigine

Lamotrigine is an anti-epileptic drug with anti-excitotocicity effects. It has been tested in two clinical trials (Eisen et al., 1993; Ryberg et al., 2003) showing no effects on disease progression.

5.3.42 Lecithin

The term lecithin describes a group compounds consisting of phosphoric acid, choline, fatty acids, glycerol, glycolipids, triglycerides, and phospholipids. Typical members comprehend phosphatidylcholine, phosphatidylethanolamine, and phosphatidylinositol.

In a clinical trial, lecithin did not show a benefit in ALS patients (Kelemen et al., 1982).

5.3.43 Leuprorelin (Leuprolide)
Leuprorelin is a is a nonapeptide and a GnRH analog.
It has been tested in a phase II study in combination with testosterone (NCT00004771), the results are awaited.

5.3.44 Levamisole
Levamisole is a synthetic imidazothiazole derivative with anti-helmintic and immunomodulatory effects. In a clinical trial, no beneficial effects have been seen for ALS patients (Olarte & Shafer, 1985).

5.3.45 Lithium
Lithium has been described as inductor of autophagy and anti-oxidant. Clinically, it is used as mood stabilizer.
In a phase II study (EudraCT), lithium did not show efficacy with regard to survival and keeping of patient autonomy (Chio et al.).
In another phase II study, lithium was reported to delay disease progression (Fornai et al., 2008), but in a follow-up, riluzole add-on phase II study (NCT00818389), lithium has been proven to be safe and well tolerated in ALS patients, but did not slow disease progression (Aggarwal et al.). Due to these findings, two other studies of lithium are currently not recruiting patients (NCT00925847, NCT00790582).

5.3.46 Memantine
Memantine non-competitive antagonist at the NMDA and AMPA glutamate receptors with low affinity.
In two phase II/III clinical trials (NCT01020331, NCT00409721), memantine was safe and tolerated, but no efficacy has been found in ALS patients (de Carvalho et al., 2010).

5.3.47 Methylcobalamin (E0302, mecobalamin)
Methylcobalamin is an analog of vitamin B12, which reduces the concentration of homocystein, an excitatory amino acid which showed toxic effects on motor neurons by inducing apoptosis.
ALS patients treated with high doses of methylcobalamin (MeCbl) showed an increase in compound muscle action potential amplitudes (CMAPs) after 4 weeks of treatment (Kaji et al., 1998). It increased the decline in ALS patients with regard to becoming respirator-bound (Izumi & Kaji, 2007).
Methylcobalamin is currently evaluated in two phase III studies (NCT00445172, NCT00444613) in ALS patients

5.3.48 Minocycline
Minocycline has been described as anti-apoptotic and anti-inflammatory.
In a phase III study (NCT00047723), minocycline showed harmful effects of minocycline in ALS patients (Gordon et al., 2007).

5.3.49 Modafinil
Modafinil is a psychostimulant clinically used for the treatment of narcolepsy and other sleep disorders.

It is currently evaluated in a phase IV study (NCT00614926) for the treatment of fatigue in ALS patients.

5.3.50 Naloxone

The μ opioid receptor antagonist naloxone did not show a benefit in ALS patients (Silani et al., 1983).

5.3.51 Neostigmine

The cholinesterase inhibitor did not show a benefit in ALS patients (Aquilonius et al., 1986).

5.3.52 Nimodipine

The calcium channel antagonist nimodipine showed no beneficial effect in a clinical trail in ALS patients (Miller et al., 1996).

5.3.53 NP001

NP001 is a small molecule regulator of macrophage activation, which aims at restoring the neuroprotective state of macrophages, reducing inflammation, and normalizing the neuronal microenvironment.

NP001 has been tested in a phase I trial (NCT01091142) for safety and tolerability. It is currently evaluated in a subsequent phase II clinical trial (NCT01281631).

5.3.54 Olanzapine

Olanzapine is an atypic neuroleptic drug used in psychiatry for the treatment of schizophrenia and other psychoses. One of its effects is also weight gain. In ALS patients, an involuntary weight loss of more than 10 percent of the original body weight correlates with an increased mortality. Thus treatment with olanzapine might increase the body weight, or, at least, keep it constant.

Currently, olanzapine is evaluated in a phase II/III study (NCT00876772) in ALS patients.

5.3.55 Olesoxime (TRO19622)

Olesoxime is a neuroprotective agent with a cholesterol-like structure which is thought to act at the mitochondrial membrane (Bordet et al., 2010; Martin, 2010).

Currently, olesoxime is evaluated in a phase II/III trial (NCT00868166) as add-on to riluzole and a phase II/III safety extension study (NCT01285583).

5.3.56 Penicillamine

The metal ion chelating agent penicillamine did not show a benefit in ALS patients (Conradi et al., 1982).

5.3.57 Pentoxifylline

Pentoxifylline is an anti-apoptotic drug. It has been tested in a riluzole add-on phase II clinical trial, which did not show efficacy, but increased mortality (Meininger et al., 2006).

5.3.58 Phthalazine

The inhibitor of cyclic adenosine monophosphate (cAMP) phosphodiesterase and cyclic guanine monophosphate (cGMP) phosphodiesterase phthalazinol did not show a benefit in ALS patients (Engel & Brooks, 1980).

5.3.59 Physostigmine

The acetylcholine esterase inhibitor physostigmine did not show a benefit in ALS patients (Norris et al., 1993).

5.3.60 Pioglitazone

Pioglitazone activates the nuclear receptor peroxisome proliferator-activated receptor gamma (PPAR-γ) (Gillies & Dunn, 2000; Kiaei, 2008). It has been used as anti-diabetic drug in diabetes type 2.

In phase II clinical trial (NCT00690118), pioglitazone was found to be save and well-tolerated, but showed no effect on ALS disease progression (Ludolph et al., 2010).

In a riluzole add-on phase II study (NCT00919555), pioglitazone is currently evaluated in combination with tretinoin.

5.3.61 Prednisolone

The immunosuppressant prednisolone in combination with azathioprine did not show a benefit in ALS patients (Werdelin et al., 1990).

5.3.62 Pyrimethamine

The anti-malaria drug pyrimethamine was found to reduce SOD1 levels in vitro and in vivo in rodents as well as in humans (Lange, 2008).

Pyrimethamine is currently evaluated in a phase I/II trial (NCT01083667) for tolerability, safety, and efficacy in familial ALS.

5.3.63 Rasagiline

Rasagiline is a monoamine oxidase type B inhibitor with neuroprotective effects.

Rasagiline is currently evaluated in a phase II clinical trial (NCT01232738).

5.3.64 Riluzole

Riluzole is an anti-glutamatergic drug (Cheah et al., 2010; R.G. Miller et al., 2007).

In two clinical trials, riluzole showed a moderate increase of about two months in survival after 21 and 18 months of treatment, respectively (Bensimon et al., 1994; Lacomblez et al., 1996). An open-label phase IV study (NCT00542412) found a longer survival in riluzole-treated patients of 92 days in median.

In subsequent population-based trials, older patients and patients with bulbar-onset had the biggest beneficial effect of riluzole, but the effects were transient and lost after longer periods of observation (Traynor et al., 2003; Zoccolella et al., 2007).

5.3.65 SB-509

SB-509 is an engeineered zinc finger protein which up-regulates the transcription of the pro-angiogenic vascular entothelial growth factor A (VEGF-A) (Liu et al., 2001), which is also neuroprotective and neuroregenerative (Maurer et al., 2008)

SB-509 is currently evaluated in a phase II clinical trial (NCT00748501).

5.3.66 Selegiline

The anti-depressant drug selegiline is an inhibitor of monoamino oxidase B.
It has been tested in several clinical trials without benefit for ALS patients (Jossan et al., 1994; Lange et al., 1998; Mazzini et al., 1994).

5.3.67 Snake venom

Modified snake venom as neurotoxin did not show a benefit in ALS patients (Rivera et al., 1980).

5.3.68 Sodium phenylbutyrate

Sodium phenylbutyrate acts as a histone deacetylase inhibitor, therefore it improves transcription and stimulates post-transcriptional pathways.
In a phase II study (NCT00107770), sodium phenylbutyrate was safe and well tolerated (Cudkowicz et al., 2009).

5.3.69 Sodium valproate

Valproic acid (VPA) is a histone deacetylase inhibitor that showed antioxidative and antiapoptotic properties and reduced glutamate toxicity. It is used as antiepileptic drug.
In a phase II clinical trial (NCT00136110), VPA has been found safe but not effective with regard to survival and disease progression (Piepers et al., 2009).

5.3.70 Talampanel (GYKI 53405)

Talampanel is a derivated benzodiazepine which is a non-competitive antagonist at the AMPA glutamate receptor.
It has been evaluated in a phase II trial (NCT00982150) which showed safety and tolerability (Pascuzzi et al., 2010), whereas a subsequent phase II study (NCT00696332) did not show efficacy in ALS patients (reviewed in Carlesi et al., 2011).

5.3.71 Tamoxifen

The selective estrogen receptor modulator tamoxifen is an inhibitor of protein kinase C, which is a mediator in neuroinflammation.
It has been evaluated in a phase II study (NCT00214110) in ALS patients (Brooks et al., 2005) and was recommended for a phase III trial (mentioned in Traynor et al., 2006).
Currently, tamoxifen is evaluated in a phase II clinical trial (NCT01257581) in combination with creatine in ALS patients.

5.3.72 Tauroursodeoxycholic acid (TUDCA)

In preclinical data, tauroursodeoxycholic acid (TUDCA) has been found to be neuroprotective, antioxidative, and antiapoptotic in rat models of neurodegenerative diseases such as stroke (Rodrigues et al., 2002) and Huntington's disease (Keene et al., 2002).
TUDCA is currently evaluated in a phase II study (NCT00877604) for safety and efficacy.

5.3.73 TCH346

TCH 346 showed neuroprotective effects by binding glyceraldehydes-3-phosphate dehydrogenase (GAPDH) (Mück-Seler & Pivac, 2000).
It has been evaluated in three phase II studies (NCT00230074, NCT00072709, NCT00036413), where it showed no beneficial effects in ALS (R. Miller et al., 2007).

5.3.74 Testosterone

The sexual hormone testosterone has been tested in a phase II study in combination with leuprolide (NCT00004771), the results are awaited.

5.3.75 Tetrahydroaminoacridine (Tacrine, THA)

The reversible inhibitor of cholinesterase THA did not show a benefit in ALS patients (Askmark et al., 1990).

5.3.76 Thalidomide

Thalidomide is a small molecule which has been used as a sedative drug in the 1950s-1960s. Due to its teratogenic and neuropathic adverse effects, its use was discontinued until the 1990s, when thalidomide was introduced in oncology for its anti-angiogenic effects.
With regard to clinical trials in ALS, thalidomide was tested in a phase II clinical trial (NCT00140452) (Stommel et al., 2009), with no improvement in the ALS Functional Rating Scale (ALSFRS) and pulmonary function testing (PFT) curves after nine months of thalidomide treatment. Moreover, thalidomide showed severe side effects, and did not affect anti-inflammatory cytokine levels.
A second phase II clinical trial (NCT00231140) was terminated after severe adverse effects (Thomas Meyer, 2005).

5.3.77 L-Threonine

The hydroxylated essential amino acid L-threonine did not show a benefit in ALS patients (Blin et al., 1992; Tandan et al., 1996).

5.3.78 Thyreotropin releasing hormone (TRH, Protirelin)

TRH has been tested in a larger number of clinical trials, but none of them showed a benefit in ALS patients (Brooke et al., 1986; Brooks et al., 1987; Caroscio et al., 1986; Congia et al., 1991; Hawley et al., 1987; Imoto et al., 1984; Klimek et al., 1989; Klimek et al., 1988; Miller & Warnick, 1989; Mitsumoto et al., 1986; Munsat et al., 1992; Patrignani et al., 1992; Serratrice et al., 1985; Stober et al., 1985; Thielen et al., 1987; Yamane et al., 1986).

5.3.79 Tilorone

The antiviral drug tilorone did not show a benefit in ALS patients (Olson et al., 1978).

5.3.80 Tocopherol (Vitamin E)

The anti-oxidant tocopherol has been evaluated in two phase II clinical trials, where tocopherol has been as add-on medication to riluzole in ALS patients. Both studies reported safe and well-tolerated drug administration, but no beneficial effect for ALS patients (Desnuelle et al., 2001; Graf et al., 2005). In a retrospective case-control study, high dosage of tocopherol decreased the risk of developing ALS (Veldink et al., 2007).

5.3.81 Topiramate

Topiramate is an anti-convulsant with anti-glutamatergic effects. It has been tested in a clinical trial without benefit for ALS patients, but with an increased rate of life-threatening side effects (Cudkowicz et al., 2003).

5.3.82 Transfer factor

The antiviral agent transfer factor did not show a benefit in ALS patients (Jonas et al., 1979; Olarte et al., 1979).

5.3.83 Tretinoin (all-*trans* retinoic acid)

Tretinoin is the all-trans form of retinoic acid. It has various effects in the nervous system, including neuroprotection and neuroregeneration (for review, see (Lee et al., 2009)).
In a riluzole add-on phase II study (NCT00919555), tretinoin is currently evaluated in combination with pioglitazone.

5.3.84 Trypan blue and trypan red

The antimicrobial agents trypan blue and trypan red did not show a beneficial effect in ALS patients (Montanari & Pessina, 1955; Schwob & Bonduelle, 1952).

5.3.85 Vascular endothelial growth factor (VEGF, sNN0029)

VEGF is a neuroprotectice and angiogenic growth factor (Maurer et al., 2008). It is currently tested in a phase I/II clinical trial (NCT00800501) for safety and tolerability. Of note, VEGF must be administered into the CSF.

5.3.86 Verapamil

The calcium channel antagonist verapamil showed no beneficial effect in a clinical trail in ALS patients (Miller et al., 1996).

5.3.87 Xaliproden (SR57746)

The 5HT1R agonist xaliproden is neurotrophic and neuroprotective. It has been evaluated in phase II/III trials, which showed modest effects on vital capacity, but not on survival of ALS patients (Lacomblez et al., 2004; Meininger et al., 2004).

5.3.88 YAM80

There is no drug information available for YAM80 searching literature and chemical databases. YAM80 is evaluated in a phase II study (NCT00886977) for safety and efficacy in ALS patients.

5.3.89 Zidovudine

The antiviral drug zidovudine did not show a benefit in ALS patients (Westarp et al., 1993).

5.3.90 Preclinical agents

The following agents have shown promising results in preclinical assessment, but no clinical trials have been conducted:
Azathioprine, glycine, the tripeptide zVAD-fmk, AM-1241, celastrol, dantrolene, nordihydroguaiaretic acid, RO-28-2653, L-arginine, 5-hydroxytryptophan, N-acetylated alpha-linked acidic dipeptidase, mechano-growth factor (MGF), hepatocyte growth factor (HGF), glial-derived neurotrophic factor (GDNF), promethazine and other anti-histaminergic drugs, calcium disodium EDTA, toluloxy propane, ammonium tetramolybdate (for details, see (Mitsumoto, 2009; Zoccolella et al., 2007)), and cannabis (Carter et al., 2010).

5.3.91 "Alternative" therapeutic approaches

Since most clinical trials in ALS did not show a benefit for ALS patients, a number of "alternative" or off-label cures have been propagated. Besides severe ethical issues, these treatments are of experimental nature, but not in the sense of a registered trial.

Some ALS patients who are desperately looking for a relief, tend to participate in these treatments, although they have to pay large amounts of money by themselves, and no proven, or replicable outcome has been reported in a peer-reviewed journal.

To evaluate some of these treatments, the ALSUntangled group (www.alsuntangled.com), which is based on social networking of patients, clinicians, and scientists (Bedlack & Hardiman, 2009), reports sporadically on these treatments (see homepage for open and completed investigations).

6. Outlook

ALS remains a mysterious disease with a limited life expectancy and a deteriorating condition, although efforts in basic and clinical research brought some light in the understanding of pathophysiological aspects of MND.

With dozens of failed neuropharmacological trials in ALS, the current concept of the design of clinical trials in ALS patients must be reevaluated, as well as the pre-clinical models.

Future research may concentrate on the definition of ALS, maybe by the use of biomarkers, and on translational aspects, that is, how to transfer pre-clinical results into successful clinical treatment.

7. Abbreviations

ALS, amyotrophic lateral sclerosis
ALSFRS, ALS functional rating scale
ALSSS, ALS severity scale
CNS, central nervous system
FTD, Fronto-Temporal Dementia
LMN, lower motor neuron
MND, motor neuron disease
PBP, progressive bulbar palsy
PLS, primary lateral sclerosis
PMA, progressive muscular atrophy
ROS, Reactive oxygen species
SOD1, [Zn, Cu] Superoxide dismutase type 1
UMN, upper motor neuron

8. Acknowledgments

The author has been supported by grants of the European Union within the Framework Program 7, the Germany Ministry of Research and Education (BMBF) within the National Genome Research Network NGFN-2, the German Research Foundation DFG, the intramural program of the Medical Faculty of the University of Heidelberg, the Steuben-Schurz Society, and the Estate of Friedrich Fischer.

9. References

Abrahams, S., Goldstein, L.H., Kew, J.J., Brooks, D.J., Lloyd, C.M., Frith, C.D. & Leigh, P.N. (1996). Frontal lobe dysfunction in amyotrophic lateral sclerosis. A PET study. *Brain*, Vol. 119, No. Pt 6, pp. 2105-2120.

Aggarwal, S. & Cudkowicz, M. (2008). ALS drug development: reflections from the past and a way forward. *Neurotherapeutics*, Vol. 5, No. 4, pp. 516-527.

Aggarwal, S.P., Zinman, L., Simpson, E., McKinley, J., Jackson, K.E., Pinto, H., Kaufman, P., Conwit, R.A., Schoenfeld, D., Shefner, J. & Cudkowicz, M. (2010). Safety and efficacy of lithium in combination with riluzole for treatment of amyotrophic lateral sclerosis: a randomised, double-blind, placebo-controlled trial. *Lancet Neurol*, Vol. 9, No. 5, pp. 481-488.

Aisen, M.L., Sevilla, D., Edelstein, L. & Blass, J. (1996). A double-blind placebo-controlled study of 3,4-diaminopyridine in amytrophic lateral sclerosis patients on a rehabilitation unit. *J Neurol Sci*, Vol. 138, No. 1-2, pp. 93-96.

Aisen, M.L., Sevilla, D., Gibson, G., Kutt, H., Blau, A., Edelstein, L., Hatch, J. & Blass, J. (1995). 3,4-diaminopyridine as a treatment for amyotrophic lateral sclerosis. *J Neurol Sci*, Vol. 129, No. 1, pp. 21-24.

ALS CNTF Treatment Study Group. (1996). A double-blind placebo-controlled clinical trial of subcutaneous recombinant human ciliary neurotrophic factor (rHCNTF) in amyotrophic lateral sclerosis. . *Neurology*, Vol. 46, No. 5, pp. 1244-1249.

Appel, S.H., Stewart, S.S., Appel, V., Harati, Y., Mietlowski, W., Weiss, W. & Belendiuk, G.W. (1988). A double-blind study of the effectiveness of cyclosporine in amyotrophic lateral sclerosis. *Arch Neurol*, Vol. 45, No. 4, pp. 381-386.

Appel, V., Stewart, S.S., Smith, G. & Appel, S.H. (1987). A rating scale for amyotrophic lateral sclerosis: description and preliminary experience. *Ann Neurol*, Vol. 22, No. 3, pp. 328-333.

Aquilonius, S.M., Askmark, H., Eckernas, S.A., Gillberg, P.G., Hilton-Brown, P., Rydin, E. & Stalberg, E. (1986). Cholinesterase inhibitors lack therapeutic effect in amyotrophic lateral sclerosis. A controlled study of physostigmine versus neostigmine. *Acta Neurol Scand*, Vol. 73, No. 6, pp. 628-632.

Askmark, H., Aquilonius, S.M., Gillberg, P.G., Hartvig, P., Hilton-Brown, P., Lindstrom, B., Nilsson, D., Stalberg, E. & Winkler, T. (1990). Functional and pharmacokinetic studies of tetrahydroaminoacridine in patients with amyotrophic lateral sclerosis. *Acta Neurol Scand*, Vol. 82, No. 4, pp. 253-258.

Atassi, N., Cook, A., Pineda, C.M., Yerramilli-Rao, P., Pulley, D. & Cudkowicz, M. (2011). Depression in amyotrophic lateral sclerosis. *Amyotroph Lateral Scler*, Vol. 12, No. 2, pp. 109-112.

Atassi, N., Ratai, E.M., Greenblatt, D.J., Pulley, D., Zhao, Y., Bombardier, J., Wallace, S., Eckenrode, J., Cudkowicz, M. & Dibernardo, A. (2010). A phase I, pharmacokinetic, dosage escalation study of creatine monohydrate in subjects with amyotrophic lateral sclerosis. *Amyotroph Lateral Scler*, Vol. 11, No. 6, pp. 508-513.

Averill, A.J., Kasarskis, E.J. & Segerstrom, S.C. (2007). Psychological health in patients with amyotrophic lateral sclerosis. *Amyotroph Lateral Scler*, Vol. 8, No. 4, pp. 243-254.

Bedlack, R. & Hardiman, O. (2009). ALSUntangled (ALSU): a scientific approach to off-label treatment options for people with ALS using tweets and twitters. *Amyotroph Lateral Scler*, Vol. 10, No. 3, pp. 129-130.

Bedlack, R.S. (2010). Amyotrophic lateral sclerosis: current practice and future treatments. *Curr Opin Neurol*, Vol. 23, No. 5, pp. 524-529.

Bedlack, R.S., Traynor, B.J. & Cudkowicz, M.E. (2007). Emerging disease-modifying therapies for the treatment of motor neuron disease/amyotropic lateral sclerosis. *Expert Opin Emerg Drugs*, Vol. 12, No. 2, pp. 229-252.

Beghi, E., Chio, A., Inghilleri, M., Mazzini, L., Micheli, A., Mora, G., Poloni, M., Riva, R., Serlenga, L., Testa, D. & Tonali, P. (2000). A randomized controlled trial of recombinant interferon beta-1a in ALS. Italian Amyotrophic Lateral Sclerosis Study Group. *Neurology*, Vol. 54, No. 2, pp. 469-474.

Benatar, M. (2007). Lost in translation: treatment trials in the SOD1 mouse and in human ALS. *Neurobiol Dis*, Vol. 26, No. 1, pp. 1-13.

Bensimon, G., Lacomblez, L. & Meininger, V. (1994). A controlled trial of riluzole in amyotrophic lateral sclerosis. ALS/Riluzole Study Group. *N Engl J Med*, Vol. 330, No. 9, pp. 585-591.

Bertorini, T.E., Rashed, H., Zeno, M., Tolley, E.A., Igarashi, M. & Li, Y.D. (2011). Effects of 3-4 diaminopyridine (DAP) in motor neuron diseases. *J Clin Neuromuscul Dis*, Vol. 12, No. 3, pp. 129-137.

Blin, O., Pouget, J., Aubrespy, G., Guelton, C., Crevat, A. & Serratrice, G. (1992). A double-blind placebo-controlled trial of L-threonine in amyotrophic lateral sclerosis. *J Neurol*, Vol. 239, No. 2, pp. 79-81.

Bogaert, E., d'Ydewalle, C. & Van Den Bosch, L. (2011). Amyotrophic lateral sclerosis and excitotoxicity: from pathological mechanism to therapeutic target. *CNS Neurol Disord Drug Targets*, Vol. 9, No. 3, pp. 297-304.

Bohannon, R.W. & Smith, M.B. (1987). Interrater reliability of a modified Ashworth scale of muscle spasticity. *Phys Ther*, Vol. 67, No. 2, pp. 206-207.

Borasio, G.D. (1997). Amyotrophic lateral sclerosis: lessons in trial design from recent trials. *J Neurol Sci*, Vol. 152 Suppl 1, No. 1, pp. S23-28.

Borasio, G.D., Robberecht, W., Leigh, P.N., Emile, J., Guiloff, R.J., Jerusalem, F., Silani, V., Vos, P.E., Wokke, J.H. & Dobbins, T. (1998). A placebo-controlled trial of insulin-like growth factor-I in amyotrophic lateral sclerosis. European ALS/IGF-I Study Group. *Neurology*, Vol. 51, No. 2, pp. 583-586.

Bordet, T., Berna, P., Abitbol, J.-L. & Pruss, R.M. (2010). Olesoxime (TRO19622): A Novel Mitochondrial-Targeted Neuroprotective Compound. *Pharmaceuticals*, Vol. 3, No. 2, pp. 345-368.

Bouche, P., Hanin, B. & Castaigne, P. (1986). Effects of intrathecal interferon therapy in amyotrophic lateral sclerosis. *Neurology*, Vol. 36, No. 5, pp. 735-736.

Bozik, M.E., Mather, J.L., Kramer, W.G., Gribkoff, V.K. & Ingersoll, E.W. (2010). Safety, Tolerability, and Pharmacokinetics of KNS-760704 (Dexpramipexole) in Healthy Adult Subjects. *J Clin Pharmacol*.

Bradley, W.G., Hedlund, W., Cooper, C., Desousa, G.J., Gabbai, A., Mora, J.S., Munsat, T.L. & Scheife, R. (1984). A double-blind controlled trial of bovine brain gangliosides in amyotrophic lateral sclerosis. *Neurology*, Vol. 34, No. 8, pp. 1079-1082.

Brooke, M.H., Florence, J.M., Heller, S.L., Kaiser, K.K., Phillips, D., Gruber, A., Babcock, D. & Miller, J.P. (1986). Controlled trial of thyrotropin releasing hormone in amyotrophic lateral sclerosis. *Neurology*, Vol. 36, No. 2, pp. 146-151.

Brooks, B., Sanjak, M., Roelke, K. & al., e. (2005). Phase 2B randomized dose ranging clinical trial of tamoxifen, a selective estrogen receptor modulator [SERM], in ALS:

sensitivity analyses of discordance between survival and functional outcomes with long-term follow-up. *Amyotroph Lateral Scler Other Motor Neuron Disord*, Vol. 6, No. Suppl 1, pp. 118.

Brooks, B.R. (1994). El Escorial World Federation of Neurology criteria for the diagnosis of amyotrophic lateral sclerosis. Subcommittee on Motor Neuron Diseases/Amyotrophic Lateral Sclerosis of the World Federation of Neurology Research Group on Neuromuscular Diseases and the El Escorial "Clinical limits of amyotrophic lateral sclerosis" workshop contributors. *J Neurol Sci*, Vol. 124 Suppl, pp. 96-107.

Brooks, B.R. (1997). Clinical evaluation of ALS drugs. *Neurology*, Vol. 48, No. Suppl 4, pp. S23-S27.

Brooks, B.R., Miller, R.G., Swash, M. & Munsat, T.L. (2000). El Escorial revisited: revised criteria for the diagnosis of amyotrophic lateral sclerosis. *Amyotroph Lateral Scler Other Motor Neuron Disord*, Vol. 1, No. 5, pp. 293-299.

Brooks, B.R., Sufit, R.L., Montgomery, G.K., Beaulieu, D.A. & Erickson, L.M. (1987). Intravenous thyrotropin-releasing hormone in patients with amyotrophic lateral sclerosis. Dose-response and randomized concurrent placebo-controlled pilot studies. *Neurol Clin*, Vol. 5, No. 1, pp. 143-158.

Brooks, B.R., Thisted, R.A., Appel, S.H., Bradley, W.G., Olney, R.K., Berg, J.E., Pope, L.E. & Smith, R.A. (2004). Treatment of pseudobulbar affect in ALS with dextromethorphan/quinidine: a randomized trial. *Neurology*, Vol. 63, No. 8, pp. 1364-1370.

Brown, I.R. (2007). Heat shock proteins and protection of the nervous system. *Ann N Y Acad Sci*, Vol. 1113, pp. 147-158.

Bruijn, L.I., Miller, T.M. & Cleveland, D.W. (2004). Unraveling the mechanisms involved in motor neuron degeneration in ALS. *Annu Rev Neurosci*, Vol. 27, pp. 723-749.

Burnstein, M.H. (1981). Familial amyotrophic lateral sclerosis, dementia, and psychosis. *Psychosomatics*, Vol. 22, No. 2, pp. 151-157.

Carlesi, C., Pasquali, L., Piazza, S., Lo Gerfo, A., Caldarazzo Ienco, E., Alessi, R., Fornai, F. & Siciliano, G. (2011). Strategies for clinical approach to neurodegeneration in amyotrophic lateral sclerosis. *Arch Ital Biol*, Vol. 149, No. 1, pp. 151-167.

Caroscio, J.T., Cohen, J.A., Zawodniak, J., Takai, V., Shapiro, A., Blaustein, S., Mulvihill, M.N., Loucas, S.P., Gudesblatt, M., Rube, D. & et al. (1986). A double-blind, placebo-controlled trial of TRH in amyotrophic lateral sclerosis. *Neurology*, Vol. 36, No. 2, pp. 141-145.

Carter, G.T., Abood, M.E., Aggarwal, S.K. & Weiss, M.D. (2010). Cannabis and amyotrophic lateral sclerosis: hypothetical and practical applications, and a call for clinical trials. *Am J Hosp Palliat Care*, Vol. 27, No. 5, pp. 347-356.

Cedarbaum, J.M. & Stambler, N. (1997). Performance of the Amyotrophic Lateral Sclerosis Functional Rating Scale (ALSFRS) in multicenter clinical trials. *J Neurol Sci*, Vol. 152 Suppl 1, pp. S1-9.

Cheah, B.C. & Kiernan, M.C. (2010). Dexpramipexole, the R(+) enantiomer of pramipexole, for the potential treatment of amyotrophic lateral sclerosis. *IDrugs*, Vol. 13, No. 12, pp. 911-920.

Cheah, B.C., Vucic, S., Krishnan, A.V. & Kiernan, M.C. (2010). Riluzole, neuroprotection and amyotrophic lateral sclerosis. *Curr Med Chem*, Vol. 17, No. 18, pp. 1942-1199.

Chio, A., Borghero, G., Calvo, A., Capasso, M., Caponnetto, C., Corbo, M., Giannini, F., Logroscino, G., Mandrioli, J., Marcello, N., Mazzini, L., Moglia, C., Monsurro, M.R., Mora, G., Patti, F., Perini, M., Pietrini, V., Pisano, F., Pupillo, E., Sabatelli, M., Salvi, F., Silani, V., Simone, I.L., Soraru, G., Tola, M.R., Volanti, P. & Beghi, E. (2010). Lithium carbonate in amyotrophic lateral sclerosis: lack of efficacy in a dose-finding trial. *Neurology*, Vol. 75, No. 7, pp. 619-625.

Colombrita, C., Onesto, E., Tiloca, C., Ticozzi, N., Silani, V. & Ratti, A. (2011). RNA-binding proteins and RNA metabolism: a new scenario in the pathogenesis of Amyotrophic lateral sclerosis. *Arch Ital Biol*, Vol. 149, No. 1, pp. 83-99.

Congia, S., Tronci, S., Ledda, M., Porcella, A. & Coppola, G. (1991). Low doses of TRH in amyotrophic lateral sclerosis and in other neurological diseases. *Ital J Neurol Sci*, Vol. 12, No. 2, pp. 193-198.

Conradi, S., Ronnevi, L.O., Nise, G. & Vesterberg, O. (1982). Long-time penicillamine-treatment in amyotrophic lateral sclerosis with parallel determination of lead in blood, plasma and urine. *Acta Neurol Scand*, Vol. 65, No. 3, pp. 203-211.

Costa, J., Gomes, C. & de Carvalho, M. (2010). Diagnosis, pathogenesis and therapeutic targets in amyotrophic lateral sclerosis. *CNS Neurol Disord Drug Targets*, Vol. 9, No. 6, pp. 764-778.

Cudkowicz, M., Qureshi, M. & Shefner, J. (2004). Measures and markers in amyotrophic lateral sclerosis. *NeuroRx*, Vol. 1, No. 2, pp. 273-283.

Cudkowicz, M.E., Andres, P.L., Macdonald, S.A., Bedlack, R.S., Choudry, R., Brown, R.H., Jr., Zhang, H., Schoenfeld, D.A., Shefner, J., Matson, S., Matson, W.R. & Ferrante, R.J. (2009). Phase 2 study of sodium phenylbutyrate in ALS. *Amyotroph Lateral Scler*, Vol. 10, No. 2, pp. 99-106.

Cudkowicz, M.E., Shefner, J.M., Schoenfeld, D.A., Brown, R.H., Jr., Johnson, H., Qureshi, M., Jacobs, M., Rothstein, J.D., Appel, S.H., Pascuzzi, R.M., Heiman-Patterson, T.D., Donofrio, P.D., David, W.S., Russell, J.A., Tandan, R., Pioro, E.P., Felice, K.J., Rosenfeld, J., Mandler, R.N., Sachs, G.M., Bradley, W.G., Raynor, E.M., Baquis, G.D., Belsh, J.M., Novella, S., Goldstein, J. & Hulihan, J. (2003). A randomized, placebo-controlled trial of topiramate in amyotrophic lateral sclerosis. *Neurology*, Vol. 61, No. 4, pp. 456-464.

Cudkowicz, M.E., Shefner, J.M., Schoenfeld, D.A., Zhang, H., Andreasson, K.I., Rothstein, J.D. & Drachman, D.B. (2006). Trial of celecoxib in amyotrophic lateral sclerosis. *Ann Neurol*, Vol. 60, No. 1, pp. 22-31.

Cudkowicz, M.E., Shefner, J.M., Simpson, E., Grasso, D., Yu, H., Zhang, H., Shui, A., Schoenfeld, D., Brown, R.H., Wieland, S. & Barber, J.R. (2008). Arimoclomol at dosages up to 300 mg/day is well tolerated and safe in amyotrophic lateral sclerosis. *Muscle Nerve*, Vol. 38, No. 1, pp. 837-844.

Dalakas, M.C., Aksamit, A.J., Madden, D.L. & Sever, J.L. (1986). Administration of recombinant human leukocyte alpha 2-interferon in patients with amyotrophic lateral sclerosis. *Arch Neurol*, Vol. 43, No. 9, pp. 933-935.

de Carvalho, M., Dengler, R., Eisen, A., England, J.D., Kaji, R., Kimura, J., Mills, K., Mitsumoto, H., Nodera, H., Shefner, J. & Swash, M. (2008). Electrodiagnostic criteria for diagnosis of ALS. *Clin Neurophysiol*, Vol. 119, No. 3, pp. 497-503.

de Carvalho, M., Pinto, S., Costa, J., Evangelista, T., Ohana, B. & Pinto, A. (2010). A randomized, placebo-controlled trial of memantine for functional disability in amyotrophic lateral sclerosis. *Amyotroph Lateral Scler*, Vol. 11, No. 5, pp. 456-460.

de Paulis, T. (2003). ONO-2506. Ono. *Curr Opin Investig Drugs*, Vol. 4, No. 7, pp. 863-867.
DeFelice, S.L. & Ellenberg, M. (1984). Gangliosides--clinical overview. *Adv Exp Med Biol*, Vol. 174, pp. 625-628.
Desnuelle, C., Dib, M., Garrel, C. & Favier, A. (2001). A double-blind, placebo-controlled randomized clinical trial of alpha-tocopherol (vitamin E) in the treatment of amyotrophic lateral sclerosis. ALS riluzole-tocopherol Study Group. *Amyotroph Lateral Scler Other Motor Neuron Disord*, Vol. 2, No. 1, pp. 9-18.
Duning, T., Schiffbauer, H., Warnecke, T., Mohammadi, S., Floel, A., Kolpatzik, K., Kugel, H., Schneider, A., Knecht, S., Deppe, M. & Schabitz, W.R. (2011). G-CSF prevents the progression of structural disintegration of white matter tracts in amyotrophic lateral sclerosis: a pilot trial. *PLoS One*, Vol. 6, No. 3, pp. e17770.
Eisen, A., Stewart, H., Schulzer, M. & Cameron, D. (1993). Anti-glutamate therapy in amyotrophic lateral sclerosis: a trial using lamotrigine. *Can J Neurol Sci*, Vol. 20, No. 4, pp. 297-301.
Eisen, A.A. (2007). Historical aspects of motor neuron diseases, In: *Handbook of Clinical Neurology Motor Neuron Disorders and Related Diseases*, Eisen, A.A. & Shaw, P.J. (Eds.), pp. 1-11, Elsevier B.V., Amsterdam.
Engel, W.K. & Brooks, B.R. (1980). Phthalazinol, thrombocytopenia, and amyotrophic lateral sclerosis. *Arch Neurol*, Vol. 37, No. 5, pp. 320.
Enns, M.W., Barakat, S.M. & Brown, J.H. (1993). Amyotrophic lateral sclerosis presenting with psychosis. *Psychosomatics*, Vol. 34, No. 5, pp. 453-455.
Epton, J., Harris, R. & Jenkinson, C. (2009). Quality of life in amyotrophic lateral sclerosis/motor neuron disease: a structured review. *Amyotroph Lateral Scler*, Vol. 10, No. 1, pp. 15-26.
Evdokimidis, I., Constantinidis, T.S., Gourtzelidis, P., Smyrnis, N., Zalonis, I., Zis, P.V., Andreadou, E. & Papageorgiou, C. (2002). Frontal lobe dysfunction in amyotrophic lateral sclerosis. *J Neurol Sci*, Vol. 195, No. 1, pp. 25-33.
Fareed, G.C. & Tyler, H.R. (1971). The use of isoprinosine in patients with amyotrophic lateral sclerosis. *Neurology*, Vol. 21, No. 9, pp. 937-940.
Ferentinos, P., Paparrigopoulos, T., Rentzos, M., Zouvelou, V., Alexakis, T. & Evdokimidis, I. (2011). Prevalence of major depression in ALS: Comparison of a semi-structured interview and four self-report measures. *Amyotroph Lateral Scler*, Vol. 12, No. 4, pp. 297-302.
Ferguson, T.A. & Elman, L.B. (2007). Clinical presentation and diagnosis of Amyotrophic Lateral Sclerosis. *NeuroRehabilitation*, Vol. 22, pp. 409-416.
Ferrante, K.L., Shefner, J., Zhang, H., Betensky, R., O'Brien, M., Yu, H., Fantasia, M., Taft, J., Beal, M.F., Traynor, B., Newhall, K., Donofrio, P., Caress, J., Ashburn, C., Freiberg, B., O'Neill, C., Paladenech, C., Walker, T., Pestronk, A., Abrams, B., Florence, J., Renna, R., Schierbecker, J., Malkus, B. & Cudkowicz, M. (2005). Tolerance of high-dose (3,000 mg/day) coenzyme Q10 in ALS. *Neurology*, Vol. 65, No. 1, pp. 1834-1836.
Foran, E. & Trotti, D. (2009). Glutamate transporters and the excitotoxic path to motor neuron degeneration in amyotrophic lateral sclerosis. *Antioxid Redox Signal*, Vol. 11, No. 7, pp. 1587-1602.
Fornai, F., Longone, P., Cafaro, L., Kastsiuchenka, O., Ferrucci, M., Manca, M.L., Lazzeri, G., Spalloni, A., Bellio, N., Lenzi, P., Modugno, N., Siciliano, G., Isidoro, C., Murri, L.,

Ruggieri, S. & Paparelli, A. (2008). Lithium delays progression of amyotrophic lateral sclerosis. *Proc Natl Acad Sci U S A*, Vol. 105, No. 6, pp. 2052-2057.

Fornai, F., Meininger, V. & Silani, V. (2011). Future therapeutical strategies dictated by pre-clinical evidence in ALS. *Arch Ital Biol*, Vol. 149, No. 1, pp. 169-174.

Garnock-Jones, K.P. (2011). Dextromethorphan/Quinidine: in pseudobulbar affect. *CNS Drugs*, Vol. 25, No. 5, pp. 435-445.

Geser, F., Lee, V.M. & Trojanowski, J.Q. (2010). Amyotrophic lateral sclerosis and frontotemporal lobar degeneration: a spectrum of TDP-43 proteinopathies. *Neuropathology*, Vol. 30, No. 2, pp. 103-112.

Geser, F., Martinez-Lage, M., Robinson, J., Uryu, K., Neumann, M., Brandmeir, N.J., Xie, S.X., Kwong, L.K., Elman, L., McCluskey, L., Clark, C.M., Malunda, J., Miller, B.L., Zimmerman, E.A., Qian, J., Van Deerlin, V., Grossman, M., Lee, V.M. & Trojanowski, J.Q. (2009). Clinical and pathological continuum of multisystem TDP-43 proteinopathies. *Arch Neurol*, Vol. 66, No. 2, pp. 180-189.

Gillies, P.S. & Dunn, C.J. (2000). Pioglitazone. *Drugs*, Vol. 60, No. 2, pp. 333-343; discussion 344-335.

Giordana, M.T., Ferrero, P., Grifoni, S., Pellerino, A., Naldi, A. & Montuschi, A. (2011). Dementia and cognitive impairment in amyotrophic lateral sclerosis: a review. *Neurol Sci*, Vol. 32, No. 1, pp. 9-16.

Gordon, P.H., Cheung, Y.K., Levin, B., Andrews, H., Doorish, C., Macarthur, R.B., Montes, J., Bednarz, K., Florence, J., Rowin, J., Boylan, K., Mozaffar, T., Tandan, R., Mitsumoto, H., Kelvin, E.A., Chapin, J., Bedlack, R., Rivner, M., McCluskey, L.F., Pestronk, A., Graves, M., Sorenson, E.J., Barohn, R.J., Belsh, J.M., Lou, J.S., Levine, T., Saperstein, D., Miller, R.G. & Scelsa, S.N. (2008). A novel, efficient, randomized selection trial comparing combinations of drug therapy for ALS. *Amyotroph Lateral Scler*, Vol. 9, No. 4, pp. 212-222.

Gordon, P.H., Moore, D.H., Miller, R.G., Florence, J.M., Verheijde, J.L., Doorish, C., Hilton, J.F., Spitalny, G.M., MacArthur, R.B., Mitsumoto, H., Neville, H.E., Boylan, K., Mozaffar, T., Belsh, J.M., Ravits, J., Bedlack, R.S., Graves, M.C., McCluskey, L.F., Barohn, R.J. & Tandan, R. (2007). Efficacy of minocycline in patients with amyotrophic lateral sclerosis: a phase III randomised trial. *Lancet Neurol*, Vol. 6, No. 12, pp. 1045-1053.

Gourie-Devi, M., Nalini, A. & Subbakrishna, D.K. (1997). Temporary amelioration of symptoms with intravenous cyclophosphamide in amyotrophic lateral sclerosis. *J Neurol Sci*, Vol. 150, No. 2, pp. 167-172.

Graber, J.J. & Dhib-Jalbut, S. (2009). Protective autoimmunity in the nervous system. *Pharmacol Ther*, Vol. 121, No. 2, pp. 147-159.

Graf, M., Ecker, D., Horowski, R., Kramer, B., Riederer, P., Gerlach, M., Hager, C., Ludolph, A.C., Becker, G., Osterhage, J., Jost, W.H., Schrank, B., Stein, C., Kostopulos, P., Lubik, S., Wekwerth, K., Dengler, R., Troeger, M., Wuerz, A., Hoge, A., Schrader, C., Schimke, N., Krampfl, K., Petri, S., Zierz, S., Eger, K., Neudecker, S., Traufeller, K., Sievert, M., Neundorfer, B. & Hecht, M. (2005). High dose vitamin E therapy in amyotrophic lateral sclerosis as add-on therapy to riluzole: results of a placebo-controlled double-blind study. *J Neural Transm*, Vol. 112, No. 5, pp. 649-660.

Green, A.R. (2002). Why do neuroprotective drugs that are so promising in animals fail in the clinic? An industry perspective. *Clin Exp Pharmacol Physiol*, Vol. 29, No. 11, pp. 1030-1034.

Gribkoff, V.K. & Bozik, M.E. (2008). KNS-760704 [(6R)-4,5,6,7-tetrahydro-N6-propyl-2, 6-benzothiazole-diamine dihydrochloride monohydrate] for the treatment of amyotrophic lateral sclerosis. *CNS Neurosci Ther*, Vol. 14, No. 3, pp. 215-226.

Groeneveld, G.J., Veldink, J.H., van der Tweel, I., Kalmijn, S., Beijer, C., de Visser, M., Wokke, J.H., Franssen, H. & van den Berg, L.H. (2003). A randomized sequential trial of creatine in amyotrophic lateral sclerosis. *Ann Neurol*, Vol. 53, No. 4, pp. 437-445.

Harrington, H., Hallett, M. & Tyler, H.R. (1984). Ganglioside therapy for amyotrophic lateral sclerosis: a double-blind controlled trial. *Neurology*, Vol. 34, No. 8, pp. 1083-1085.

Hawley, R.J., Kratz, R., Goodman, R.R., McCutchen, C.B., Sirdofsky, M. & Hanson, P.A. (1987). Treatment of amyotrophic lateral sclerosis with the TRH analog DN-1417. *Neurology*, Vol. 37, No. 4, pp. 715-717.

Hetta, J. & Jansson, I. (1997). Sleep in patients with amyotrophic lateral sclerosis. *J Neurol*, Vol. 244, No. 4 Suppl 1, pp. S7-9.

Hillel, A.D., Miller, R.M., Yorkston, K., McDonald, E., Norris, F.H. & Konikow, N. (1989). Amyotrophic lateral sclerosis severity scale. *Neuroepidemiology*, Vol. 8, No. 3, pp. 142-150.

Holmoy, T. (2008). T cells in amyotrophic lateral sclerosis. *Eur J Neurol*, Vol. 15, No. 4, pp. 360-366.

Howland, R.H. (1990). Schizophrenia and amyotrophic lateral sclerosis. *Compr Psychiatry*, Vol. 31, No. 4, pp. 327-336.

Huey, E.D., Koppel, J., Armstrong, N., Grafman, J. & Floeter, M.K. (2010). A pilot study of the prevalence of psychiatric disorders in PLS and ALS. *Amyotroph Lateral Scler*, Vol. 11, No. 3, pp. 293-297.

Ilieva, H., Polymenidou, M. & Cleveland, D.W. (2009). Non-cell autonomous toxicity in neurodegenerative disorders: ALS and beyond. *J Cell Biol*, Vol. 187, No. 6, pp. 761-772.

Imoto, K., Saida, K., Iwamura, K., Saida, T. & Nishitani, H. (1984). Amyotrophic lateral sclerosis: a double-blind crossover trial of thyrotropin-releasing hormone. *J Neurol Neurosurg Psychiatry*, Vol. 47, No. 12, pp. 1332-1334.

Izumi, Y. & Kaji, R. (2007). [Clinical trials of ultra-high-dose methylcobalamin in ALS]. *Brain Nerve*, Vol. 59, No. 10, pp. 1141-1147.

Jackson, C.E. & Bryan, W.W. (1998). Amyotrophic lateral sclerosis. *Semin Neurol*, Vol. 18, No. 1, pp. 27-39.

Jonas, S., Wichter, M. & Spitler, L. (1979). Amyotrophic lateral sclerosis: failure of transfer factor therapy. *Ann Neurol*, Vol. 6, No. 1, pp. 84.

Jossan, S.S., Ekblom, J., Gudjonsson, O., Hagbarth, K.E. & Aquilonius, S.M. (1994). Double blind cross over trial with deprenyl in amyotrophic lateral sclerosis. *J Neural Transm Suppl*, Vol. 41, pp. 237-241.

Kaji, R., Kodama, M., Imamura, A., Hashida, T., Kohara, N., Ishizu, M., Inui, K. & Kimura, J. (1998). Effect of ultrahigh-dose methylcobalamin on compound muscle action potentials in amyotrophic lateral sclerosis: a double-blind controlled study. *Muscle Nerve*, Vol. 21, No. 12, pp. 1775-1778.

Kalmar, B. & Greensmith, L. (2009). Activation of the heat shock response in a primary cellular model of motoneuron neurodegeneration-evidence for neuroprotective and neurotoxic effects. *Cell Mol Biol Lett*, Vol. 14, No. 2, pp. 319-335.

Kalra, S., Cashman, N.R., Caramanos, Z., Genge, A. & Arnold, D.L. (2003). Gabapentin therapy for amyotrophic lateral sclerosis: lack of improvement in neuronal integrity shown by MR spectroscopy. *AJNR Am J Neuroradiol*, Vol. 24, No. 3, pp. 476-480.

Kaufmann, P., Thompson, J.L., Levy, G., Buchsbaum, R., Shefner, J., Krivickas, L.S., Katz, J., Rollins, Y., Barohn, R.J., Jackson, C.E., Tiryaki, E., Lomen-Hoerth, C., Armon, C., Tandan, R., Rudnicki, S.A., Rezania, K., Sufit, R., Pestronk, A., Novella, S.P., Heiman-Patterson, T., Kasarskis, E.J., Pioro, E.P., Montes, J., Arbing, R., Vecchio, D., Barsdorf, A., Mitsumoto, H. & Levin, B. (2009). Phase II trial of CoQ10 for ALS finds insufficient evidence to justify phase III. *Ann Neurol*, Vol. 66, No. 2, pp. 235-244.

Kaur, C. & Ling, E.A. (2008). Antioxidants and neuroprotection in the adult and developing central nervous system. *Curr Med Chem*, Vol. 15, No. 29, pp. 3068-3080.

Keene, C.D., Rodrigues, C.M., Eich, T., Chhabra, M.S., Steer, C.J. & Low, W.C. (2002). Tauroursodeoxycholic acid, a bile acid, is neuroprotective in a transgenic animal model of Huntington's disease. *Proc Natl Acad Sci U S A*, Vol. 99, No. 16, pp. 10671-10676.

Kelemen, J., Hedlund, W., Murray-Douglas, P. & Munsat, T.L. (1982). Lecithin is not effective in amyotrophic lateral sclerosis. *Neurology*, Vol. 32, No. 3, pp. 315-316.

Kiaei, M. (2008). Peroxisome Proliferator-Activated Receptor-gamma in Amyotrophic Lateral Sclerosis and Huntington's Disease. *PPAR Res*, Vol. 2008, pp. 418765.

Kiernan, M.C., Vucic, S., Cheah, B.C., Turner, M.R., Eisen, A., Hardiman, O., Burrell, J.R. & Zoing, M.C. (2011). Amyotrophic lateral sclerosis. *Lancet*, Vol. 377, No. 9769, pp. 942-955.

Klimek, A., Stepien, H. & Szulc-Kuberska, J. (1989). [THyroliberin test in patients with amyotrophic lateral sclerosis]. *Pol Tyg Lek*, Vol. 44, No. 43-45, pp. 918-920.

Klimek, A., Szulc-Kuberska, J., Czernielewska-Rutkowska, I. & Gluszcz-Zielinska, A. (1988). [Treatment of amyotrophic lateral sclerosis with TRH]. *Neurol Neurochir Pol*, Vol. 22, No. 3, pp. 206-210.

Kurt, A., Nijboer, F., Matuz, T. & Kubler, A. (2007). Depression and anxiety in individuals with amyotrophic lateral sclerosis: epidemiology and management. *CNS Drugs*, Vol. 21, No. 4, pp. 279-291.

Lacomblez, L., Bensimon, G., Douillet, P., Doppler, V., Salachas, F. & Meininger, V. (2004). Xaliproden in amyotrophic lateral sclerosis: early clinical trials. *Amyotroph Lateral Scler Other Motor Neuron Disord*, Vol. 5, No. 2, pp. 99-106.

Lacomblez, L., Bensimon, G., Leigh, P.N., Guillet, P. & Meininger, V. (1996). Dose-ranging study of riluzole in amyotrophic lateral sclerosis. Amyotrophic Lateral Sclerosis/Riluzole Study Group II. *Lancet*, Vol. 347, No. 9013, pp. 1425-1431.

Lacomblez, L., Bouche, P., Bensimon, G. & Meininger, V. (1989). A double-blind, placebo-controlled trial of high doses of gangliosides in amyotrophic lateral sclerosis. *Neurology*, Vol. 39, No. 12, pp. 1635-1637.

Lai, E.C., Felice, K.J., Festoff, B.W., Gawel, M.J., Gelinas, D.F., Kratz, R., Murphy, M.F., Natter, H.M., Norris, F.H. & Rudnicki, S.A. (1997). Effect of recombinant human insulin-like growth factor-I on progression of ALS. A placebo-controlled study. The North America ALS/IGF-I Study Group. *Neurology*, Vol. 49, No. 6, pp. 1621-1630.

Lange, D. (2008). Pyrimethamine as a therapy for SOD1 associated fALS: early findings. *Amyotrophic Lateral Sclerosis*, No. Suppl. 1, pp. 46.

Lange, D.J., Murphy, P.L., Diamond, B., Appel, V., Lai, E.C., Younger, D.S. & Appel, S.H. (1998). Selegiline is ineffective in a collaborative double-blind, placebo-controlled trial for treatment of amyotrophic lateral sclerosis. *Arch Neurol*, Vol. 55, No. 1, pp. 93-96.

Lanka, V., Wieland, S., Barber, J. & Cudkowicz, M. (2009). Arimoclomol: a potential therapy under development for ALS. *Expert Opin Investig Drugs*, Vol. 18, No. 12, pp. 1907-1918.

Lauria, G., Campanella, A., Filippini, G., Martini, A., Penza, P., Maggi, L., Antozzi, C., Ciano, C., Beretta, P., Caldiroli, D., Ghelma, F., Ferrara, G., Ghezzi, P. & Mantegazza, R. (2009). Erythropoietin in amyotrophic lateral sclerosis: a pilot, randomized, double-blind, placebo-controlled study of safety and tolerability. *Amyotroph Lateral Scler*, Vol. 10, No. 5-6, pp. 410-415.

Lee, H.P., Casadesus, G., Zhu, X., Lee, H.G., Perry, G., Smith, M.A., Gustaw-Rothenberg, K. & Lerner, A. (2009). All-trans retinoic acid as a novel therapeutic strategy for Alzheimer's disease. *Expert Rev Neurother*, Vol. 9, No. 11, pp. 1615-1621.

Levy, G., Kaufmann, P., Buchsbaum, R., Montes, J., Barsdorf, A., Arbing, R., Battista, V., Zhou, X., Mitsumoto, H., Levin, B. & Thompson, J.L. (2006). A two-stage design for a phase II clinical trial of coenzyme Q10 in ALS. *Neurology*, Vol. 66, No. 5, pp. 660-663.

Li, W.W., Yang, R. & Cai, D.F. (2008). [Protective effects of Cistanche total glycosides on dopaminergic neuron in substantia nigra of model mice of Parkinson's disease]. *Zhongguo Zhong Xi Yi Jie He Za Zhi*, Vol. 28, No. 3, pp. 248-251.

Lill, C.M., Abel, O., Bertram, L. & Al-Chalabi, A. (2011). Keeping up with genetic discoveries in amyotrophic lateral sclerosis: The ALSoD and ALSGene databases. *Amyotroph Lateral Scler*, Vol. 12, No. 4, pp. 238-249.

Lillo, P. & Hodges, J.R. (2009). Frontotemporal dementia and motor neurone disease: overlapping clinic-pathological disorders. *J Clin Neurosci*, Vol. 16, No. 9, pp. 1131-1135.

Lillo, P., Mioshi, E., Zoing, M.C., Kiernan, M.C. & Hodges, J.R. (2011). How common are behavioural changes in amyotrophic lateral sclerosis? *Amyotroph Lateral Scler*, Vol. 12, No. 1, pp. 45-51.

Lipton, S.A., Gu, Z. & Nakamura, T. (2007). Inflammatory mediators leading to protein misfolding and uncompetitive/fast off-rate drug therapy for neurodegenerative disorders. *Int Rev Neurobiol*, Vol. 82, pp. 1-27.

Liu, P.Q., Rebar, E.J., Zhang, L., Liu, Q., Jamieson, A.C., Liang, Y., Qi, H., Li, P.X., Chen, B., Mendel, M.C., Zhong, X., Lee, Y.L., Eisenberg, S.P., Spratt, S.K., Case, C.C. & Wolffe, A.P. (2001). Regulation of an endogenous locus using a panel of designed zinc finger proteins targeted to accessible chromatin regions. Activation of vascular endothelial growth factor A. *J Biol Chem*, Vol. 276, No. 14, pp. 11323-11334.

Lou, J.S. (2008). Fatigue in amyotrophic lateral sclerosis. *Phys Med Rehabil Clin N Am*, Vol. 19, No. 3, pp. 533-543, ix.

Louwerse, E.S., Weverling, G.J., Bossuyt, P.M., Meyjes, F.E. & de Jong, J.M. (1995). Randomized, double-blind, controlled trial of acetylcysteine in amyotrophic lateral sclerosis. *Arch Neurol*, Vol. 52, No. 6, pp. 559-564.

Ludolph, A.C., Kassubek, J., Meyer, T. & Group, T.G.A.S. (2010). Phase II study of pioglitazone in ALS. *Abstract Book of the 21st International Symposium on ALS/MND*, pp. 45.

Ludolph, A.C. & Sperfeld, A.D. (2005). Preclinical trials--an update on translational research in ALS. *Neurodegener Dis*, Vol. 2, No. 3-4, pp. 215-219.
Maragakis, N.J. (2009). Rethinking a drug treatment failure on a traditional ALS target. *Exp Neurol*, Vol. 216, No. 2, pp. 254-257.
Martin, L.J. (2010). Olesoxime, a cholesterol-like neuroprotectant for the potential treatment of amyotrophic lateral sclerosis. *IDrugs*, Vol. 13, No. 8, pp. 568-580.
Maurer, M.H., Schabitz, W.R. & Schneider, A. (2008). Old friends in new constellations--the hematopoetic growth factors G-CSF, GM-CSF, and EPO for the treatment of neurological diseases. *Curr Med Chem*, Vol. 15, No. 14, pp. 1407-1411.
Mazzini, L., Balzarini, C., Colombo, R., Mora, G., Pastore, I., De Ambrogio, R. & Caligari, M. (2001). Effects of creatine supplementation on exercise performance and muscular strength in amyotrophic lateral sclerosis: preliminary results. *J Neurol Sci*, Vol. 191, No. 1-2, pp. 139-144.
Mazzini, L., Testa, D., Balzarini, C. & Mora, G. (1994). An open-randomized clinical trial of selegiline in amyotrophic lateral sclerosis. *J Neurol*, Vol. 241, No. 4, pp. 223-227.
McGuire, D., Garrison, L., Armon, C., Barohn, R.J., Bryan, W.W., Miller, R., Parry, G.J., Petajan, J.H. & Ross, M.A. (1997). A brief quality-of-life measure for ALS clinical trials based on a subset of items from the sickness impact profile. The Syntex-Synergen ALS/CNTF Study Group. *J Neurol Sci*, Vol. 152 Suppl 1, No. 1, pp. S18-22.
McLeod, J.E. & Clarke, D.M. (2007). A review of psychosocial aspects of motor neurone disease. *J Neurol Sci*, Vol. 258, No. 1-2, pp. 4-10.
Meininger, V., Asselain, B., Guillet, P., Leigh, P.N., Ludolph, A., Lacomblez, L., Robberecht, W. & Pentoxifylline European Group. (2006). Pentoxifylline in ALS: a double-blind, randomized, multicenter, placebo-controlled trial. *Neurology*, Vol. 66, No. 1, pp. 88-92.
Meininger, V., Bensimon, G., Bradley, W.R., Brooks, B., Douillet, P., Eisen, A.A., Lacomblez, L., Leigh, P.N. & Robberecht, W. (2004). Efficacy and safety of xaliproden in amyotrophic lateral sclerosis: results of two phase III trials. *Amyotroph Lateral Scler Other Motor Neuron Disord*, Vol. 5, No. 2, pp. 107-117.
Meininger, V., Drory, V.E., Leigh, P.N., Ludolph, A., Robberecht, W. & Silani, V. (2009). Glatiramer acetate has no impact on disease progression in ALS at 40 mg/day: a double- blind, randomized, multicentre, placebo-controlled trial. *Amyotroph Lateral Scler*, Vol. 10, No. 5-6, pp. 378-383.
Meissner, F., Molawi, K. & Zychlinsky, A. (2010). Mutant superoxide dismutase 1-induced IL-1beta accelerates ALS pathogenesis. *Proc Natl Acad Sci U S A*, Vol. 107, No. 29, pp. 13046-13050.
Miller, M.C. (2011). Commentary. Did Lou Gehrig have Lou Gehrig's disease? *Harv Ment Health Lett*, Vol. 27, No. 8, pp. 8.
Miller, R., Bradley, W., Cudkowicz, M., Hubble, J., Meininger, V., Mitsumoto, H., Moore, D., Pohlmann, H., Sauer, D., Silani, V., Strong, M., Swash, M. & Vernotica, E. (2007). Phase II/III randomized trial of TCH346 in patients with ALS. *Neurology*, Vol. 69, No. 8, pp. 776-784.
Miller, R.G., Bryan, W.W., Dietz, M.A., Munsat, T.L., Petajan, J.H., Smith, S.A. & Goodpasture, J.C. (1996). Toxicity and tolerability of recombinant human ciliary neurotrophic factor in patients with amyotrophic lateral sclerosis. *Neurology*, Vol. 47, No. 5, pp. 1329-1331.

Miller, R.G., Gelinas, D. & O'Connor, P. (2005). *Amyotrophic lateral sclerosis* Demos Medical Publishing, 1-932603-06-9, New York.

Miller, R.G., Mitchell, J.D., Lyon, M. & Moore, D.H. (2007). Riluzole for amyotrophic lateral sclerosis (ALS)/motor neuron disease (MND). *Cochrane Database Syst Rev*, Vol. 24, No. 1, pp. CD001447.

Miller, R.G., Moore, D., Young, L.A., Armon, C., Barohn, R.J., Bromberg, M.B., Bryan, W.W., Gelinas, D.F., Mendoza, M.C., Neville, H.E., Parry, G.J., Petajan, J.H., Ravits, J.M., Ringel, S.P. & Ross, M.A. (1996). Placebo-controlled trial of gabapentin in patients with amyotrophic lateral sclerosis. WALS Study Group. Western Amyotrophic Lateral Sclerosis Study Group. *Neurology*, Vol. 47, No. 6, pp. 1383-1388.

Miller, R.G., Moore, D.H., 2nd, Gelinas, D.F., Dronsky, V., Mendoza, M., Barohn, R.J., Bryan, W., Ravits, J., Yuen, E., Neville, H., Ringel, S., Bromberg, M., Petajan, J., Amato, A.A., Jackson, C., Johnson, W., Mandler, R., Bosch, P., Smith, B., Graves, M., Ross, M., Sorenson, E.J., Kelkar, P., Parry, G. & Olney, R. (2001). Phase III randomized trial of gabapentin in patients with amyotrophic lateral sclerosis. *Neurology*, Vol. 56, No. 7, pp. 843-848.

Miller, R.G., Munsat, T.L., Swash, M. & Brooks, B.R. (1999). Consensus guidelines for the design and implementation of clinical trials in ALS. World Federation of Neurology committee on Research. *J Neurol Sci*, Vol. 169, No. 1-2, pp. 2-12.

Miller, R.G., Petajan, J.H., Bryan, W.W., Armon, C., Barohn, R.J., Goodpasture, J.C., Hoagland, R.J., Parry, G.J., Ross, M.A. & Stromatt, S.C. (1996). A placebo-controlled trial of recombinant human ciliary neurotrophic (rhCNTF) factor in amyotrophic lateral sclerosis. rhCNTF ALS Study Group. *Ann Neurol*, Vol. 39, No. 2, pp. 256-260.

Miller, R.G., Shepherd, R., Dao, H., Khramstov, A., Mendoza, M., Graves, J. & Smith, S. (1996). Controlled trial of nimodipine in amyotrophic lateral sclerosis. *Neuromuscul Disord*, Vol. 6, No. 2, pp. 101-104.

Miller, R.G., Smith, S.A., Murphy, J.R., Brinkmann, J.R., Graves, J., Mendoza, M., Sands, M.L. & Ringel, S.P. (1996). A clinical trial of verapamil in amyotrophic lateral sclerosis. *Muscle Nerve*, Vol. 19, No. 4, pp. 511-515.

Miller, S.C. & Warnick, J.E. (1989). Protirelin (thyrotropin-releasing hormone) in amyotrophic lateral sclerosis. The role of androgens. . *Arch Neurol*, Vol. 46, No. 3, pp. 330-335.

Mitsumoto, H. (1997). Diagnosis and progression of ALS. *Neurology*, Vol. 48, No. S4, pp. 2S-8S.

Mitsumoto, H. (Eds.). (2009). *Amyotrophic lateral sclerosis. A guide for patients and families.* (3rd), Demos Medical Publishing, New York.

Mitsumoto, H., Przedborski, S. & Gordon, P. (Eds.). (2006). *Amyotrophic Lateral Sclerosis. Current Science and Approaches to Therapy* Taylor & Francis Group, 978-0-8247-2924-0, New York.

Mitsumoto, H., Salgado, E.D., Negroski, D., Hanson, M.R., Salanga, V.D., Wilber, J.F., Wilbourn, A.J., Breuer, A.C. & Leatherman, J. (1986). Amyotrophic lateral sclerosis: effects of acute intravenous and chronic subcutaneous administration of thyrotropin-releasing hormone in controlled trials. *Neurology*, Vol. 36, No. 2, pp. 152-159.

Montanari, M. & Pessina, G. (1955). [Trypan red in therapy of amyotrophic lateral sclerosis and of myelopathic muscular atrophy]. *Rass Int Clin Ter*, Vol. 35, No. 6, pp. 197-206.

Mora, J.S., Munsat, T.L., Kao, K.P., Finison, L.J., Hedlund, W., Bradley, G.A., Scheife, R. & Georgiades, J.A. (1986). Intrathecal administration of natural human interferon alpha in amyotrophic lateral sclerosis. *Neurology*, Vol. 36, No. 8, pp. 1137-1140.

Mück-Seler, D. & Pivac, N. (2000). TCH-346 (Novartis). *IDrugs*, Vol. 3, No. 5, pp. 530-535.

Munsat, T.L., Easterday, C.S., Levy, S., Wolff, S.M. & Hiatt, R. (1981). Amantadine and guanidine are ineffective in ALS. *Neurology*, Vol. 31, No. 8, pp. 1054-1055.

Munsat, T.L., Taft, J., Jackson, I.M., Andres, P.L., Hollander, D., Skerry, L., Ordman, M., Kasdon, D. & Finison, L. (1992). Intrathecal thyrotropin-releasing hormone does not alter the progressive course of ALS: experience with an intrathecal drug delivery system. *Neurology*, Vol. 42, No. 5, pp. 1049-1053.

Nakano, I. (2000). Frontotemporal dementia with motor neuron disease (amyotrophic lateral sclerosis with dementia). *Neuropathology*, Vol. 20, No. 1, pp. 68-75.

Nandedkar, S.D., Barkhaus, P.E. & Stalberg, E.V. (2010). Motor unit number index (MUNIX): principle, method, and findings in healthy subjects and in patients with motor neuron disease. *Muscle Nerve*, Vol. 42, No. 5, pp. 798-807.

Nefussy, B., Artamonov, I., Deutsch, V., Naparstek, E., Nagler, A. & Drory, V.E. (2010). Recombinant human granulocyte-colony stimulating factor administration for treating amyotrophic lateral sclerosis: A pilot study. *Amyotroph Lateral Scler*, Vol. 11, No. 1-2, pp. 187-193.

Neuwirth, C., Nandedkar, S., Stalberg, E., Barkhaus, P.E., Carvalho, M.D., Furtula, J., Dijk, J.P., Baldinger, R., Castro, J., Costa, J., Otto, M., Sandberg, A. & Weber, M. (2011). Motor Unit Number Index (MUNIX): A novel neurophysiological marker for neuromuscular disorders; test-retest reliability in healthy volunteers. *Clin Neurophysiol*, Vol. 2011, pp. 9.

Norris, F.H., Jr., Calanchini, P.R., Fallat, R.J., Panchari, S. & Jewett, B. (1974). The administration of guanidine in amyotrophic lateral sclerosis. *Neurology*, Vol. 24, No. 8, pp. 721-728.

Norris, F.H., Jr., Fallat, R.J. & Calanchini, P.R. (1974). Increased paralysis induced by guanidine in motor neuron disease. *Neurology*, Vol. 24, No. 2, pp. 135-137.

Norris, F.H., Tan, Y., Fallat, R.J. & Elias, L. (1993). Trial of oral physostigmine in amyotrophic lateral sclerosis. *Clin Pharmacol Ther*, Vol. 54, No. 6, pp. 680-682.

Norris, L., Que, G. & Bayat, E. (2010). Psychiatric aspects of amyotrophic lateral sclerosis (ALS). *Curr Psychiatry Rep*, Vol. 12, No. 3, pp. 239-245.

Ochs, G., Penn, R.D., York, M., Giess, R., Beck, M., Tonn, J., Haigh, J., Malta, E., Traub, M., Sendtner, M. & Toyka, K.V. (2000). A phase I/II trial of recombinant methionyl human brain derived neurotrophic factor administered by intrathecal infusion to patients with amyotrophic lateral sclerosis. *Amyotroph Lateral Scler Other Motor Neuron Disord*, Vol. 1, No. 3, pp. 201-206.

Olarte, M.R., Gersten, J.C., Zabriskie, J. & Rowland, L.P. (1979). Transfer factor is ineffective in amyotrophic lateral sclerosis. *Ann Neurol*, Vol. 5, No. 4, pp. 385-388.

Olarte, M.R. & Shafer, S.Q. (1985). Levamisole is ineffective in the treatment of amyotrophic lateral sclerosis. *Neurology*, Vol. 35, No. 7, pp. 1063-1066.

Oliveira, A.S. & Pereira, R.D. (2009). Amyotrophic lateral sclerosis (ALS): three letters that change the people's life. For ever. *Arq Neuropsiquiatr*, Vol. 67, No. 3A, pp. 750-782.

Olney, N. & Rosen, H. (2010). AVP-923, a combination of dextromethorphan hydrobromide and quinidine sulfate for the treatment of pseudobulbar affect and neuropathic pain. *IDrugs*, Vol. 13, No. 4, pp. 254-265.

Olson, W.H., Simons, J.A. & Halaas, G.W. (1978). Therapeutic trial of tilorone in ALS: lack of benefit in a double-blind, placebo-controlled study. *Neurology*, Vol. 28, No. 12, pp. 1293-1295.

Orrell, R.W. (2006). AEOL-10150 (Aeolus). *Curr Opin Investig Drugs*, Vol. 7, No. 1, pp. 70-80.

Orrell, R.W., Lane, R.J. & Ross, M. (2008). A systematic review of antioxidant treatment for amyotrophic lateral sclerosis/motor neuron disease. *Amyotroph Lateral Scler*, Vol. 9, No. 4, pp. 195-211.

Pascuzzi, R.M., Shefner, J., Chappell, A.S., Bjerke, J.S., Tamura, R., Chaudhry, V., Clawson, L., Haas, L. & Rothstein, J.D. (2010). A phase II trial of talampanel in subjects with amyotrophic lateral sclerosis. *Amyotroph Lateral Scler*, Vol. 11, No. 3, pp. 266-271.

Pasinelli, P. & Brown, R.H. (2006). Molecular biology of amyotrophic lateral sclerosis: insights from genetics. *Nat Rev Neurosci*, Vol. 7, No. 9, pp. 710-723.

Patrignani, J., Proano, J. & Morales, M.D. (1992). [Treatment of amyotrophic lateral sclerosis with daily intrathecal TRH. A year's experience. Pilot study II]. *Neurologia*, Vol. 7, No. 1, pp. 4-9.

Pattee, G.L., Post, G.R., Gerber, R.E. & Bennett, J.P., Jr. (2003). Reduction of oxidative stress in amyotrophic lateral sclerosis following pramipexole treatment. *Amyotroph Lateral Scler Other Motor Neuron Disord*, Vol. 4, No. 2, pp. 90-95.

Percy, A.K., Davis, L.E., Johnston, D.M. & Drachman, D.B. (1971). Failure of isoprinosine in amyotropic lateral sclerosis. *N Engl J Med*, Vol. 285, No. 12, pp. 689.

Phukan, J. (2010). Arimoclomol, a coinducer of heat shock proteins for the potential treatment of amyotrophic lateral sclerosis. *IDrugs*, Vol. 13, No. 7, pp. 482-496.

Piepers, S., Veldink, J.H., de Jong, S.W., van der Tweel, I., van der Pol, W.L., Uijtendaal, E.V., Schelhaas, H.J., Scheffer, H., de Visser, M., de Jong, J.M., Wokke, J.H., Groeneveld, G.J. & van den Berg, L.H. (2009). Randomized sequential trial of valproic acid in amyotrophic lateral sclerosis. *Ann Neurol*, Vol. 66, No. 2, pp. 227-234.

Pradat, P.F., Attarian, S., Camdessanche, J.P., Carluer, L., Cintas, P., Corcia, P., Echaniz-Laguna, A., Gonzalez-Bermejo, J., Guy, N., Nicolas, G., Perez, T., Soriani, M.H., Vandenberghe, N. & Verschueren, A. (2010). [Research in amyotrophic lateral sclerosis: what is new in 2009?]. *Rev Neurol (Paris)*, Vol. 166, No. 8-9, pp. 683-698.

Rapport, M.M. (1990). Implications of altered brain ganglioside profiles in amyotrophic lateral sclerosis (ALS). *Acta Neurobiol Exp (Wars)*, Vol. 50, No. 4-5, pp. 505-513.

Rivera, V.M., Grabois, M., Deaton, W., Breitbach, W. & Hines, M. (1980). Modified snake venom in amyotrophic lateral sclerosis. Lack of clinical effectiveness. *Arch Neurol*, Vol. 37, No. 4, pp. 201-203.

Robberecht, W. (2002). Genetics of familial amyotrophic lateral sclerosis and ethical aspects, In: *Motor Neuron Disease*, Kuncl, R.W. (Eds.), pp. 75-93, Saunders, Philadelphia, PA.

Rodrigues, C.M., Spellman, S.R., Sola, S., Grande, A.W., Linehan-Stieers, C., Low, W.C. & Steer, C.J. (2002). Neuroprotection by a bile acid in an acute stroke model in the rat. *J Cereb Blood Flow Metab*, Vol. 22, No. 4, pp. 463-471.

Rosenbloom, A.L. (2009). Mecasermin (recombinant human insulin-like growth factor I). *Adv Ther*, Vol. 26, No. 1, pp. 40-54.

Rosenfeld, J., King, R.M., Jackson, C.E., Bedlack, R.S., Barohn, R.J., Dick, A., Phillips, L.H., Chapin, J., Gelinas, D.F. & Lou, J.S. (2008). Creatine monohydrate in ALS: effects on strength, fatigue, respiratory status and ALSFRS. *Amyotroph Lateral Scler*, Vol. 9, No. 5, pp. 266-272.

Ross, E. (2009). Unapproved drug use: compassionate or cause for concern? *Lancet Neurol*, Vol. 8, No. 2, pp. 136-137.

Ross, M.A., Miller, R.G., Berchert, L., Parry, G., Barohn, R.J., Armon, C., Bryan, W.W., Petajan, J., Stromatt, S., Goodpasture, J. & McGuire, D. (1998). Toward earlier diagnosis of amyotrophic lateral sclerosis: revised criteria. rhCNTF ALS Study Group. *Neurology*, Vol. 50, No. 3, pp. 768-772.

Rowland, L.P. (2001). How amyotrophic lateral sclerosis got its name: the clinical-pathologic genius of Jean-Martin Charcot. *Arch Neurol*, Vol. 58, No. 3, pp. 512-515.

Rowland, L.P. (2009). T.L. Bunina, Asao Hirano, and the post mortem cellular diagnosis of amyotrophic lateral sclerosis. *Amyotroph Lateral Scler*, Vol. 10, No. 2, pp. 74-78.

Ryberg, H., Askmark, H. & Persson, L.I. (2003). A double-blind randomized clinical trial in amyotrophic lateral sclerosis using lamotrigine: effects on CSF glutamate, aspartate, branched-chain amino acid levels and clinical parameters. *Acta Neurol Scand*, Vol. 108, No. 1, pp. 1-8.

Sacca, F., Quarantelli, M., Rinaldi, C., Tucci, T., Piro, R., Perrotta, G., Carotenuto, B., Marsili, A., Palma, V., De Michele, G., Brunetti, A., Brescia Morra, V., Filla, A. & Salvatore, M. (2011). A randomized controlled clinical trial of growth hormone in amyotrophic lateral sclerosis: clinical, neuroimaging, and hormonal results. *J Neurol*, Vol. 2011, pp. [Epub ahead of print].

Sathasivam, S. (2010). Motor neurone disease: clinical features, diagnosis, diagnostic pitfalls and prognostic markers. *Singapore Med J*, Vol. 51, No. 5, pp. 367-372; quiz 373.

Sathasivam, S., Ince, P.G. & Shaw, P.J. (2001). Apoptosis in amyotrophic lateral sclerosis: a review of the evidence. *Neuropathol Appl Neurobiol*, Vol. 27, No. 4, pp. 257-274.

Scelsa, S.N., MacGowan, D.J., Mitsumoto, H., Imperato, T., LeValley, A.J., Liu, M.H., DelBene, M. & Kim, M.Y. (2005). A pilot, double-blind, placebo-controlled trial of indinavir in patients with ALS. *Neurology*, Vol. 64, No. 7, pp. 1298-1300.

Schwob, R.A. & Bonduelle, M. (1952). [Trypan blue and trypan red in the treatment of amyotrophic lateral sclerosis; application to the treatment of multiple sclerosis]. *Sem Hop*, Vol. 28, No. 39, pp. 1637-1642.

Scott, S., Kranz, J.E., Cole, J., Lincecum, J.M., Thompson, K., Kelly, N., Bostrom, A., Theodoss, J., Al-Nakhala, B.M., Vieira, F.G., Ramasubbu, J. & Heywood, J.A. (2008). Design, power, and interpretation of studies in the standard murine model of ALS. *Amyotroph Lateral Scler*, Vol. 9, No. 1, pp. 4-15.

Serratrice, G., Desnuelle, C., Guelton, C., Meyer-Dutour, A., Richard, P., Braguer, D. & Crevat, A. (1985). [Trial of thyrotropin-releasing factor in amyotrophic lateral sclerosis]. *Presse Med*, Vol. 14, No. 8, pp. 487-488.

Shefner, J.M., Cudkowicz, M.E., Schoenfeld, D., Conrad, T., Taft, J., Chilton, M., Urbinelli, L., Qureshi, M., Zhang, H., Pestronk, A., Caress, J., Donofrio, P., Sorenson, E., Bradley, W., Lomen-Hoerth, C., Pioro, E., Rezania, K., Ross, M., Pascuzzi, R., Heiman-Patterson, T., Tandan, R., Mitsumoto, H., Rothstein, J., Smith-Palmer, T., MacDonald, D. & Burke, D. (2004). A clinical trial of creatine in ALS. *Neurology*, Vol. 63, No. 9, pp. 1656-1661.

Shefner, J.M., Watson, M.L., Simionescu, L., Caress, J.B., Burns, T.M., Maragakis, N.J., Benatar, M., David, W.S., Sharma, K.R. & Rutkove, S.B. (2011). Multipoint incremental motor unit number estimation as an outcome measure in ALS. *Neurology*, Vol. 2011, No. [epub ahead of print], pp. 15.

Shi, P., Gal, J., Kwinter, D.M., Liu, X. & Zhu, H. (2010). Mitochondrial dysfunction in amyotrophic lateral sclerosis. *Biochim Biophys Acta*, Vol. 1802, No. 1, pp. 45-51.

Siciliano, G., Carlesi, C., Pasquali, L., Piazza, S., Pietracupa, S., Fornai, F., Ruggieri, S. & Murri, L. (2010). Clinical trials for neuroprotection in ALS. *CNS Neurol Disord Drug Targets*, Vol. 9, No. 3, pp. 305-313.

Silani, V., Meininger, V. & Fornai, F. (2011). Introducing Amyotrophic lateral sclerosis. *Arch Ital Biol*, Vol. 149, No. 1, pp. 1-4.

Silani, V., Messina, S., Poletti, B., Morelli, C., Doretti, A., Ticozzi, N. & Maderna, L. (2011). The diagnosis of Amyotrophic lateral sclerosis in 2010. *Arch Ital Biol*, Vol. 149, No. 1, pp. 5-27.

Silani, V., Perini, M., Fayoumi, Z.M. & Scarlato, G. (1983). Naloxone of no benefit in amyotrophic lateral sclerosis. *Ann Neurol*, Vol. 13, No. 2, pp. 222.

Sleegers, K., Cruts, M. & Van Broeckhoven, C. (2010). Molecular pathways of frontotemporal lobar degeneration. *Annu Rev Neurosci*, Vol. 33, pp. 71-88.

Smith, R.A., Miller, T.M., Yamanaka, K., Monia, B.P., Condon, T.P., Hung, G., Lobsiger, C.S., Ward, C.M., McAlonis-Downes, M., Wei, H., Wancewicz, E.V., Bennett, C.F. & Cleveland, D.W. (2006). Antisense oligonucleotide therapy for neurodegenerative disease. *J Clin Invest*, Vol. 116, No. 8, pp. 2290-2296.

Sorenson, E.J., Windbank, A.J., Mandrekar, J.N., Bamlet, W.R., Appel, S.H., Armon, C., Barkhaus, P.E., Bosch, P., Boylan, K., David, W.S., Feldman, E., Glass, J., Gutmann, L., Katz, J., King, W., Luciano, C.A., McCluskey, L.F., Nash, S., Newman, D.S., Pascuzzi, R.M., Pioro, E., Sams, L.J., Scelsa, S., Simpson, E.P., Subramony, S.H., Tiryaki, E. & Thornton, C.A. (2008). Subcutaneous IGF-1 is not beneficial in 2-year ALS trial. *Neurology*, Vol. 71, No. 22, pp. 1770-1775.

Stober, T., Schimrigk, K., Dietzsch, S. & Thielen, T. (1985). Intrathecal thyrotropin-releasing hormone therapy of amyotrophic lateral sclerosis. *J Neurol*, Vol. 232, No. 1, pp. 13-14.

Stommel, E.W., Cohen, J.A., Fadul, C.E., Cogbill, C.H., Graber, D.J., Kingman, L., Mackenzie, T., Channon Smith, J.Y. & Harris, B.T. (2009). Efficacy of thalidomide for the treatment of amyotrophic lateral sclerosis: a phase II open label clinical trial. *Amyotroph Lateral Scler*, Vol. 10, No. 5-6, pp. 393-404.

Szulc-Kuberska, J., Klimek, A., Stepien, H. & Woszczak, M. (1990). [Clinical trial of the treatment of amyotrophic lateral sclerosis with bromocriptine]. *Neurol Neurochir Pol*, Vol. 24, No. 1-2, pp. 37-41.

Takahashi, R. (2009). Edaravone in ALS. *Exp Neurol*, Vol. 217, No. 2, pp. 235-236.

Tandan, R., Bromberg, M.B., Forshew, D., Fries, T.J., Badger, G.J., Carpenter, J., Krusinski, P.B., Betts, E.F., Arciero, K. & Nau, K. (1996). A controlled trial of amino acid therapy in amyotrophic lateral sclerosis: I. Clinical, functional, and maximum isometric torque data. *Neurology*, Vol. 47, No. 5, pp. 1220-1226.

Thatte, U. & Dahanukar, S. (1997). Apoptosis: clinical relevance and pharmacological manipulation. *Drugs*, Vol. 54, No. 4, pp. 511-532.

The ALS CNTF treatment study (ACTS) phase I-II Study Group. (1996). The Amyotrophic Lateral Sclerosis Functional Rating Scale. Assessment of activities of daily living in patients with amyotrophic lateral sclerosis. . *Arch Neurol*, Vol. 53, No. 2, pp. 141-147.

The BDNF Study Group (Phase III). (1999). A controlled trial of recombinant methionyl human BDNF in ALS. *Neurology*, Vol. 52, No. 7, pp. 1427-1433.

Thielen, T., Stober, T. & Schimrigk, K. (1987). Therapeutic trial of intrathecal thyrotropin-releasing hormone (TRH) and a TRH-analogue in amyotrophic lateral sclerosis (ALS). *Adv Exp Med Biol*, Vol. 209, pp. 305-308.

Ticozzi, N., Tiloca, C., Morelli, C., Colombrita, C., Poletti, B., Doretti, A., Maderna, L., Messina, S., Ratti, A. & Silani, V. (2011). Genetics of familial Amyotrophic lateral sclerosis. *Arch Ital Biol*, Vol. 149, No. 1, pp. 65-82.

Traynor, B.J., Alexander, M., Corr, B., Frost, E. & Hardiman, O. (2003). An outcome study of riluzole in amyotrophic lateral sclerosis--a population-based study in Ireland, 1996-2000. *J Neurol*, Vol. 250, No. 4, pp. 473-479.

Traynor, B.J., Bruijn, L., Conwit, R., Beal, F., O'Neill, G., Fagan, S.C. & Cudkowicz, M.E. (2006). Neuroprotective agents for clinical trials in ALS: a systematic assessment. *Neurology*, Vol. 67, No. 1, pp. 20-27.

Tsujimoto, M., Senda, J., Ishihara, T., Niimi, Y., Kawai, Y., Atsuta, N., Watanabe, H., Tanaka, F., Naganawa, S. & Sobue, G. (2011). Behavioral changes in early ALS correlate with voxel-based morphometry and diffusion tensor imaging. *J Neurol Sci*, Vol. 307, No. 1-2, pp. 34-40.

Turner, M.R., Grosskreutz, J., Kassubek, J., Abrahams, S., Agosta, F., Benatar, M., Filippi, M., Goldstein, L.H., van den Heuvel, M., Kalra, S., Lule, D. & Mohammadi, B. (2011). Towards a neuroimaging biomarker for amyotrophic lateral sclerosis. *Lancet Neurol*, Vol. 10, No. 5, pp. 400-403.

Valentine, J.S., Doucette, P.A. & Zittin Potter, S. (2005). Copper-zinc superoxide dismutase and amyotrophic lateral sclerosis. *Annu Rev Biochem*, Vol. 74, pp. 563-593.

van der Meer, J.W. & Simon, A. (2010). Blocking IL-1beta to slow down progression of ALS? *Proc Natl Acad Sci U S A*, Vol. 107, No. 29, pp. 12741-12742.

Veldink, J.H., Kalmijn, S., Groeneveld, G.J., Wunderink, W., Koster, A., de Vries, J.H., van der Luyt, J., Wokke, J.H. & Van den Berg, L.H. (2007). Intake of polyunsaturated fatty acids and vitamin E reduces the risk of developing amyotrophic lateral sclerosis. *J Neurol Neurosurg Psychiatry*, Vol. 78, No. 4, pp. 367-371.

von Haehling, S., Stepney, R. & Anker, S.D. (2010). Advances in understanding and treating cardiac cachexia: highlights from the 5th Cachexia Conference. *Int J Cardiol*, Vol. 144, No. 3, pp. 347-349.

Wang, H., Larriviere, K.S., Keller, K.E., Ware, K.A., Burns, T.M., Conaway, M.A., Lacomis, D., Pattee, G.L., Phillips, L.H., 2nd, Solenski, N.J., Zivkovic, S.A. & Bennett, J.P., Jr. (2008). R+ pramipexole as a mitochondrially focused neuroprotectant: initial early phase studies in ALS. *Amyotroph Lateral Scler*, Vol. 9, No. 1, pp. 50-58.

Weber, M., Goldman, B. & Truniger, S. (2010). Tetrahydrocannabinol (THC) for cramps in amyotrophic lateral sclerosis: a randomised, double-blind crossover trial. *J Neurol Neurosurg Psychiatry*, Vol. 81, No. 10, pp. 1135-1140.

Welty, D.F., Schielke, G.P. & Rothstein, J.D. (1995). Potential treatment of amyotrophic lateral sclerosis with gabapentin: a hypothesis. *Ann Pharmacother*, Vol. 29, No. 11, pp. 1164-1167.

Werdelin, L., Boysen, G., Jensen, T.S. & Mogensen, P. (1990). Immunosuppressive treatment of patients with amyotrophic lateral sclerosis. *Acta Neurol Scand*, Vol. 82, No. 2, pp. 132-134.

Westarp, M.E., Bartmann, P., Rossler, J., Geiger, E., Westphal, K.P., Schreiber, H., Fuchs, D., Westarp, M.P. & Kornhuber, H.H. (1993). Antiretroviral therapy in sporadic adult amyotrophic lateral sclerosis. *Neuroreport*, Vol. 4, No. 6, pp. 819-822.

Weydt, P. & Moller, T. (2005). Neuroinflammation in the pathogenesis of amyotrophic lateral sclerosis. *Neuroreport*, Vol. 16, No. 6, pp. 527-531.

Wijesekera, L.C. & Leigh, P.N. (2009). Amyotrophic lateral sclerosis. *Orphanet J Rare Dis*, Vol. 4, No. 3, pp. 3.

Williams, M.T., Donnelly, J.P., Holmlund, T. & Battaglia, M. (2008). ALS: Family caregiver needs and quality of life. *Amyotroph Lateral Scler*, Vol. 9, No. 5, pp. 279-286.

Witgert, M., Salamone, A.R., Strutt, A.M., Jawaid, A., Massman, P.J., Bradshaw, M., Mosnik, D., Appel, S.H. & Schulz, P.E. (2009). Frontal-lobe mediated behavioral dysfunction in amyotrophic lateral sclerosis. *Eur J Neurol*, Vol. 17, No. 1, pp. 103-110.

Woolley, S.C. & Jonathan, S.K. (2008). Cognitive and behavioral impairment in amyotrophic lateral sclerosis. *Phys Med Rehabil Clin N Am*, Vol. 19, No. 3, pp. 607-617, xi.

Worrall, B.B., Rowland, L.P., Chin, S.S. & Mastrianni, J.A. (2000). Amyotrophy in prion diseases. *Arch Neurol*, Vol. 57, No. 1, pp. 33-38.

Yamane, K., Osawa, M., Kobayashi, I. & Maruyama, S. (1986). Treatment of amyotrophic lateral sclerosis with thyrotropin-releasing hormone (TRH). *Jpn J Psychiatry Neurol*, Vol. 40, No. 2, pp. 179-187.

Yase, Y., Matsumoto, N., Azuma, K., Nakai, Y. & Shiraki, H. (1972). Amyotrophic lateral sclerosis. Association with schizophrenic symptoms and showing Alzheimer's tangles. *Arch Neurol*, Vol. 27, No. 2, pp. 118-128.

Yoshida, M. (2004). Amyotrophic lateral sclerosis with dementia: the clinicopathological spectrum. *Neuropathology*, Vol. 24, No. 1, pp. 87-102.

Yoshino, H. & Kimura, A. (2006). Investigation of the therapeutic effects of edaravone, a free radical scavenger, on amyotrophic lateral sclerosis (Phase II study). *Amyotroph Lateral Scler*, Vol. 7, No. 4, pp. 241-245.

Zago, S., Poletti, B., Morelli, C., Doretti, A. & Silani, V. (2011). Amyotrophic lateral sclerosis and frontotemporal dementia (ALS-FTD). *Arch Ital Biol*, Vol. 149, No. 1, pp. 39-56.

Zhang, Y., Wang, L., Fu, Y., Song, H., Zhao, H., Deng, M., Zhang, J. & Fan, D. (2009). Preliminary investigation of effect of granulocyte colony stimulating factor on amyotrophic lateral sclerosis. *Amyotroph Lateral Scler*, Vol. 10, No. 5-6, pp. 430-431.

Zinman, L. & Cudkowicz, M. (2011). Emerging targets and treatments in amyotrophic lateral sclerosis. *Lancet Neurol*, Vol. 10, No. 5, pp. 481-490.

Zoccolella, S., Beghi, E., Palagano, G., Fraddosio, A., Guerra, V., Samarelli, V., Lepore, V., Simone, I.L., Lamberti, P., Serlenga, L. & Logroscino, G. (2007). Riluzole and amyotrophic lateral sclerosis survival: a population-based study in southern Italy. *Eur J Neurol*, Vol. 14, No. 3, pp. 262-268.

Zoccolella, S., Santamato, A. & Lamberti, P. (2009). Current and emerging treatments for amyotrophic lateral sclerosis. *Neuropsychiatr Dis Treat*, Vol. 5, pp. 577-595.

2

Dynamic Meta-Analysis as a Therapeutic Prediction Tool for Amyotrophic Lateral Sclerosis

Cassie S. Mitchell and Robert H. Lee
Georgia Institute of Technology and Emory University, Atlanta, Georgia, United States

1. Introduction

In this chapter, we present a new method, dynamic meta-analysis, which allows the examination of the underlying system dynamics of ALS utilizing the wealth of existing published experimental and/or clinical literature. We perform a small-scale feasibility study of the G93A SOD1 mouse model to show that dynamic meta-analysis can also be utilized to predict treatment outcomes in a high-throughput manner.

1.1 Leveraging the wealth of data

In 2010 alone, 980 articles were specifically published on the fatal neurodegenerative disease Amyotrophic Lateral Sclerosis (ALS), and the cumulative total literature base for this single intractable pathology exceeds 10,300 articles, according to a PubMed search. One might think that with this wealth of information we would have ALS well in hand. Yet, there is no available, life-extending treatment despite the extensive and detailed information obtained by thousands of researchers at the cost of billions of dollars. ALS remains one of the most intractable neurological diseases; there is no apparent quick fix, no smoking gun, and no obvious answers—just mountains of intertwined experimental observations recorded across a host of individual publications. Furthermore, ALS has been remarkably resistant to reductionistic attempts to pinpoint the underlying problem. Potential contributing defects, mutations, and regulatory failures have been cited across a broad range of categories, including axonal transport (Bilsland, Sahai et al.), cellular chemistry (Hayward, Rodriguez et al. 2002), energetics (Shi, Gal et al.), excitotoxicity (Roy, Minotti et al. 1998), free radicals (Bogdanov, Ramos et al. 1998), genetic damage (Nagano, Murakami et al. 2002), inflammation (King, Dickson et al. 2009), necro-apoptosis (Vukosavic, Dubois-Dauphin et al. 1999), proteomics (Wood, Beaujeux et al. 2003), as well as systemic origin (Dobrowolny, Aucello et al. 2008). Yet experimental correction or "treatment" of any individually identified potential contributor has failed to translate into clinically significant and reproducible results (Peviani, Caron et al.).

1.2 Identifying and utilizing the system dynamics of ALS for combination therapy

Based on current evidence, ALS may exhibit system-level abnormalities that emerge from the complexities and interactions of their underlying mechanisms (Mitchell 2009; Rothstein

2009). Like an engineering control loop with many elements that ends up with an unstably high feedback gain, ALS may initiate from the combined effects of many small deviations that, in and of themselves, might be considered normal. To address multiple contributors and their interactions, a distributed intervention like combination therapy is necessary. Combination treatment strategies are typically based on the assumed presence of system-level synergistic interactions, which could amplify the desired treatment effects. Thus, before a combination treatment can even be developed, the system dynamics and potential synergistic interactions must first be revealed. That is, we cannot "treat", for example, a high-loop gain abnormality if we are not aware of its existence and have no means to measure it. A further limitation to combination treatment research is the combinatorial explosion of treatment possibilities (often hundreds to thousands) that must be experimentally explored—a daunting task that is neither financially nor temporally feasible. What is needed is a tool or method that can both identify and utilize ALS pathology dynamics to pre-screen treatment combinations in silico, such that treatment combinations predicted to have the highest efficacies could be experimentally assessed first, and thus greatly speed the time from ALS treatment discovery to potential clinical treatment success.

1.3 Dynamic meta-analysis as a means of experimental and clinical prediction

Here we examine the use of a novel and innovative form of meta-analysis, which we call *dynamic meta-analysis*, as a tool that enables the necessary examination of system-level ALS pathology dynamics as well as the prediction of ALS combination treatment outcomes. Traditional meta-analysis, which aggregates the results of multiple, heavily overlapping clinical/epidemiological studies into a larger virtual study from which relationships across a broader array of conditions can be examined and overall statistical power can be increased, has been successfully used to examine individual clinical treatments (Miller, Mitchell et al. 2007; Pastula, Moore et al. 2010).

Much can and has been honed from using traditonal meta-analysis to examine clinical trials. However, clinical trials lack the advantages of in vitro and in vivo experimental models where we can perform protocols and obtain mechanistic insight that is not possible in human studies alone. To examine the dynamics of ALS in order to develop successful ombination therapies, we really need to examine the individual interactions and regulation of multipe cellular- and system-level interactions, which are either too complex, too inaccessible, or inappropriate for human experimentation. The ALS literature, particularly through superoxide dismutase 1 mouse models (G93A, G85R, etc), identified several such interactions and their regulation. What is needed is a method by which we can integrate the individual studies, each of which study different aspects of ALS (axonal transport, excitotoxicity, apoptosis, etc.), into the quilt that is ALS. This indeed does sound like a task for meta-analysis.

However, traditional meta-analysis is not an option for examining experimental literature. The ALS experimental literature base is simultaneously much larger than any single collection of clinical trials, and much less overlapping than clinical protocols. Dynamic meta-analysis overcomes the constraints of traditional meta-analysis by allowing the implicit inclusion of system interactions and explicit inclusion of time, two key ingredients necessary to examine pathology dynamics and subsequent combination treatments. In short, dynamic meta-analysis provides a manageable means to integrate the experimental data published by thousands of researchers into a unified view from which new ALS treatments and treatment combinations can be explored.

While a major strength of dynamic meta-analysis is that it does provide an approach for aggregating and recapitulating experimental studies, its application is by no means limited to experimental studies. The same method can certainly be used to dynamically examine clinical stuides. The advantages of the implicit inclusion of interactions and explict inclusion of time still apply.

1.4 G93A SOD1 mouse model as a test bed for dynamic meta-analysis

In this chapter we perform a small dynamic meta-analysis feasibility study utilizing the G93A SOD1 ALS mouse model literature to illustrate the potential power of dynamic meta-analysis to reveal key system dynamics, identify treatment strategies, and predict combination treatment outcomes in ALS. This model, developed over 15 years ago, is still the primary experimental model used to investigate ALS mechanisms and treatments.

2. The dynamic meta-analysis method

In this section, we provide the foundation, overview, and detailed processes involved in dynamic meta-analysis. The methods are generalized, such that they could be applied to any experimental or clinical dataset. We use the G93A SOD1 model as our detailed example of the construction, implementation, and analysis required for dynamic meta-analysis in this section. However, we reserve the specific dynamic meta-analysis predictions for the G93A SOD1 mouse model for the 3. Results section.

2.1 Traditional meta-analysis as a foundation

Traditional meta-analysis leverages an a priori model of relationships to generate a system-wide phenomenological model of the system. What makes this approach effective is the statistical weight of all the measured data behind the regressed coefficients. However, its limitations are that it does not explicitly permit the inclusion of time or the implicit examination of metric interactions. The a priori model used in traditional meta-analysis is based on the idea that all systems can be locally approximated algebraically as first order (essentially $\Delta Y = B \cdot \Delta X$ where X and Y are metrics within the system and B is a regression constant of proportionality). The a priori model is typically illustrated in the form of the meta-regression equation:

$$Y = B_1 \cdot X_1 + B_2 \cdot X_2 + B_3 \cdot X_3 + B_4 \cdot X_4 \ldots \quad (1)$$

2.2 Mathematical basis of "dynamic" meta-analysis

The central novel premise behind dynamic meta-analysis is that relationships in biological systems are better conceptualized as a first order differential equation ($dY/dt = B \cdot X$). Such an a priori model utilizing rates of change treats system relationships much like chemical reactions. Clearly, for much of what constitutes a biological system a reaction metaphor is not just a good approximation, it is literally true. Thus, the meta-regression equation for dynamic meta-analysis becomes

$$dY_1/dt = B_1 \cdot X_1 + B_2 \cdot X_2 + B_3 \cdot X_3 + B_4 \cdot X_4 \ldots \quad (2)$$

where X's are various effectors within the system, Y is one (of many) affected metrics and B's are the interaction gain coefficients. With this meta-regression equation, the concept of time is introduced explicitly. Therefore, dynamic meta-analysis can incorporate experimental data from differing time-points and predict effects over time. These traits make dynamic meta-analysis unique, even when compared to advanced meta-analysis methods such as network analysis (Trelle, Reichenbach et al. 2011). While network analysis does use comparative relationships, it does not include interactions or show how relationship ratios change over time. Thus, where traditional or even advanced meta-analysis produces a static set of linear relationships, dynamic meta-analysis produces a set of differential equations. This results in an innovative way to examine pathology dynamics as we can look at how metrics change and interact over time rather than being limited to how they correlate at a single point in time. Currently, the only other available technique capable of implictly including interactions and explicity including time is relational modeling (Mitchell, 2009; Mitchell and Lee, 2008). In fact, dynamic meta-analysis is, itself, one form of relational modeling. However, traditional relational models typically do not provide the desired statistical weight of dynamic meta-analysis since only one primary study is included per interaction.

2.3 Overview of the dynamic meta-analysis process

Dynamic meta-analysis is similar to traditional meta-analysis in that it utilizes literature searches, inclusion/exclusion critieria, and data aggregation techniques. A key difference in the dynamic meta-analysis process, however, is the study structure and data extraction. In the following sub-sections of the chapter we provide the details necessary to perform each step of dynamic meta-analysis: determining the study scope, performing literature searches and study inclusion/excusion, developing structure, extracting data, aggregating extracted data, implementing dynamic meta-analysis, and analyzing dynamic meta-analysis results.

2.4 Defining the study scope

Just as in traditional meta-analysis, defining the scope is an important step. There are several things to consider, including the outcome goals of the project, the measures and timepoints to be included, the statistical weight, and the desired timeline of the project. There is no methodological limit on the number of studies, measures, and timepoints that can be included in dynamic meta-analysis. Rather, the researcher must impose those limits. There is a balance between including enough studies to obtain statistically significant results and the amount of man-hours it takes to perform dynamic meta-analysis. The one drawback of meta-analysis is it is by no means a completely automated process. Rather, humans must be involved at each step, to search and more importantly extract the data from included studies.

To assist in balancing workload and the time it takes to get preliminary results from dynamic meta-analysis, we divide dynamic meta-analysis into two parts: a feasibility study and a full study. A full study, as the name implies, encompasses all of the primary articles that meet the inclusion criteria. In contrast, a feasibility study can potentially have the same number and breadth of outcome measures as the full study, but utilizes a lesser number of included primary studies for each metric (i.e. a lower "n"). That is, the statistical weight is decreased. The advantage of performing an initial feasibility study goes beyond simply obtaining preliminary results more quickly. The initial results of the feasibility study also provide insight and direction, which can be used to fine tune the targeting of the full study (e.g. determining if more or less measures are needed or if the scope of the study needs revised, etc.).

2.5 Literature searches, inclusion and exclusion criteria

Literature searches are performed in a semi-automated manner, similar to a systematic review (see Cochrane Review instructions for a full description of this method). Here, we utilize keyword searches in PubMed. Our strategy is not to be over-limiting in our resulting study selection. Rather, we limit the size of our dynamic meta-analysis by decreasing the study scope instead of using highly selective inclusion/exclusion criteria.

For the dynamic meta-analysis presented in this chapter, we perform two different literature searches, Phase I and Phase II. The first literature search (Phase I) is an all-encompassing literature search for primary research studies/articles. Phase I inclusion results in ~1,803 papers, while Phase I exclusion leaves a remainder of 1,144 papers. These 1,144 articles are the studies/data sets for dynamic meta-analysis. The second literature search (Phase II) is for ALS review articles. Phase II inclusion results in ~200 reviews, while Phase II exclusion reduces the number to 52. The review articles are utilized for the purposes of structure and aggregation (to be discussed in the following sub-sections).

Phase I Inclusion Criteria:

- All studies must be from peer-reviewed journals, which are indexed in the United States National Library of Medicine and National Institute of Health PubMed database.
- Amyotrophic Lateral Sclerosis" or "ALS" in title/abstract
- "G93A" or "transgenic mouse" in title/abstract
- Most Recent 15 years
- Primary research artciles

Phase I Exclusion Criteria:

- articles without verifiable controls for each experimental metric utilized
- articles without quantitative, statistically significant results
- studies not measured at two or more time points

Phase II Inclusion Criteria:

- all studies must be from peer-reviewed journals, which are indexed in the United States National Library of Medicine and National Institute of Health PubMed database.
- "Amytrophic Lateral Sclerosis" or "ALS" in title/abstract
- clinical or experimental review articles
- most recent 5 years

Phase II Exclusion Criteria:

- articles focused on human case studies
- articles focused on assessment metrics
- articles focused on ALS variants with dementia
- articles focused on disease management
- articles focused on non-mechanistic based therapies

2.6 Structure: Outcome measures, interactions, and categories

Similar to traditional meta-analysis, dynamic meta-analysis utilizes outcome measures (measures that are calculated or derived from the included studies) as a means of prediction. Unlike traditional meta-analysis, dynamic meta-analysis also includes *interactions* between the outcome measures. However, due to the larger scope of dynamic meta-analysis compared to traditional meta-analysis, it is helpful to combine individual experimental metrics or outcome metrics into aggregates we refer to as *categories*. The outcome measures, interactions, and their respective categories, together, make up the dynamic meta-analysis structure (Figure 1).

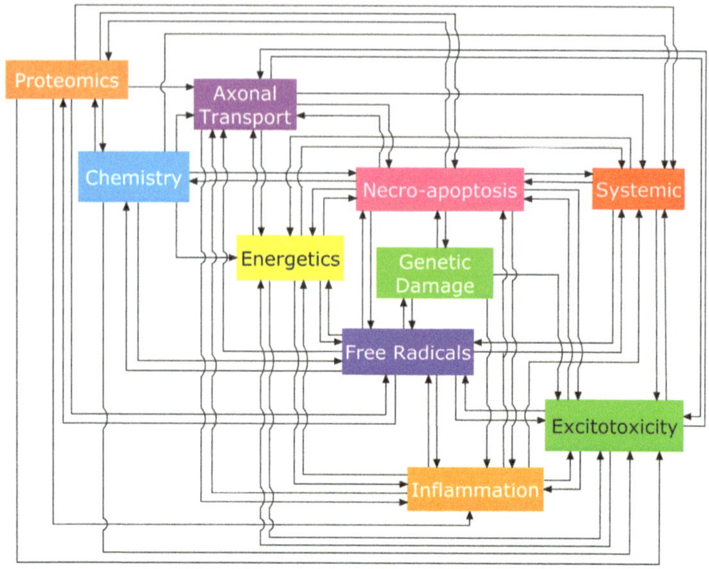

Fig. 1. Dynamic Meta-Analysis Feasibility Study Structure. Boxes represent the ten categories of outcome measures. Lines represent the 72 one-way interactions between categories of outcome measures. Systemics is shown in red as it represents the functional outcome metrics measured the in vivo G93A SOD1 mouse, and is used as the primary outcome for treatment evaluation (see Results). Categories are derived from the Phase II literature reviews. The outcome measures and their interactions are derived from the primary studies obtained from the Phase I literature search.

2.6.1 Category definitions

Aggregation of primary study metrics into categories balances the number and specificity of dynamic meta-analysis outcome measures with statistical weight. Too little aggregation will result in too disparate of a collection of very specific experimental mesasures or outcomes and will reduce the statistical weight of their predictions. In contrast, too much aggregation will result in outcome measures that are too broad; while this will increase their stasticial weight, it will also ultimately reduce the specificity of the dynamic meta-analysis predictions. Thus, the level, type, and implementation of aggregation will depend on the scope of the study, the number or primary studies utilized, as well as the desired statistical weight.

If the quantitative outcome metrics and their measured interactions come from the primary studies of Phase I, where do their categories come from? Categories are derived from the review articles of Phase II. Reviews do a nice job of providing key topics that are being researched by the field. For this feasibility study, reviews were analyzed for common research topics, based on broad categories of related physiological measures. For example, all measures of dynein, kinesin, mitochondrial transport, neurofilament transport, and neurofilament transport, etc, were grouped into the category outcome measure "Axonal Transport". Key terms were then extracted from these topics and used to sort the primary studies, and their respective outcome measures, into the following categories (definitions follow at the end of this sub-section): axonal transport, chemistry, energetics, excitotoxicity, free radicals, genetics, inflammation, necro-apoptosis, proteomics, and systemics. Reviews were also used to preliminarily determine which categories are inter-related (without having to examine each and every primary article). This is extremely helpful for development of the feasibility study. The quantitative specifics of the data aggregation process are discussed in Data Aggregation, while the category definitions are given below.

Excitotoxicity: encompasses measures of electrophysiology; ion, neurotransmitter, and buffer concentrations; activation of ionotropic/metabotropic receptors (Ikonomidou, Qin Qin et al. 1996; Dunlop, Beal McIlvain et al. 2003; Van Damme, Leyssen et al. 2003); altered excitability related to sodium (Kuo, Schonewille et al. 2004; Kuo, Siddique et al. 2005); and transport and pump capacity (Guatteo, Carunchio et al. 2007), causing toxic over-activation.

Axonal transport: encompasses measures of the anterograde and retrograde transport of cargos, such as mitochondria, neurotransmitters, neurofilaments, and endosomes/ lysosomes, as well as the measures of the involved machinery, such as the molecular motors kinesin and dynein. The most recognized impairments and their measures include mutations to cargos (Meyer and Potter 1995; Wong, He et al. 2000) and molecular motor cargo carriers (Hafezparast, Ahmad-Annuar et al. 2003; Teuchert, Fischer et al. 2006; Mitchell and Lee, 2009) that prevent the cargo from be appropriately bound to either dynein or kinesin. Other deficits include correlations to energetics, such as decreased mitochondrial transport or a decrease in overall transport due to a drop in mitochondrial potential (Ackerley, Grierson et al. 2004).

Energetics: encompasses measures of all machinery and processes related to cellular respiration and production of cellular ATP (Echaniz-Laguna, Zoll et al. 2002). Energetic contributors include impairments to the cellular machinery responsible for the production of ATP, especially mitochondria (Kong and Xu 1998; Sumi, Nagano et al. 2006), whose dysfunction also leads to accumulation of free radicals and calcium. Overburdened energetic capabilities because of increased homeostatic and transport demands from excitotoxicity (Dupuis, Oudart et al. 2004) have also been observed.

Genetic damage: encompasses measures of an extremely diverse spectrum of either inherited or sporadic mutations resulting in cellular dysfunction (Tanaka, Niwa et al. 2006). The most widely known genetic mutation, accounting for 2% of all ALS cases, is superoxide dismutase-1 (SOD1), which has over 100 known different mutations (Banci, Bertini et al. 2008) (for list, see www.alsod.org) that result in a gain of one or more toxic properties that are independent of the levels of SOD1 activity (Stathopulos, Rumfeldt et al. 2003).

Proteomics: encompasses measures of protein folding, degradation, and translation, which become impaired, resulting in defective essential proteins, toxic accumulation of aggregates or aggresomes, and inhibition of organelle function (Watanabe, Dykes-Hoberg et al. 2001; Urushitani, Kurisu et al. 2002; Rumfeldt, Lepock et al. 2009).

Chemistry: encompasses measures of aberrant cellular chemistry, enzymatics, or catalysis (Tiwari, Xu et al. 2005; Tokuda, Ono et al. 2008) that results in oxidative damage and metal mishandling that can be seen alone or in conjunction with SOD1 mutations.

Inflammation: encompasses measures of immune-induced inflammation, including astrocyte (Nagai, Re et al. 2007) and microglia (Hall, Andrus et al. 1998) counts, gliosis and the release of nitric oxide and proinflammatory cytokines, which in combination with impaired growth factors/trophic support (Narai, Nagano et al. 2005; Kadoyama, Funakoshi et al. 2007), further inhibit the neural environment.

Free radicals: encompasses measures of oxidation or inflammation-induced nitric oxide, but particularly the accumulation of reactive oxygen species, such as the superoxides and peroxides that are associated with mitochondrial dysfunction or failure. Free radicals initiate reactions that damage DNA (Pehar, Vargas et al. 2007).

Necro-apoptosis: encompasses the measures of cell death, including the signaling cascades, their constituents, and machinery, which promote cell death. The final destination of an ALS affected motoneuron is cell death either through inflammation-induced necrosis or more likely through apoptosis (Mattson and Duan 1999) via the activation of stress response and caspase pathways (Beere 2004; Gifondorwa, Robinson et al. 2007).

Systemic: encompasses invivo measures of function in the G93A mouse model (Derave, Van Den Bosch et al. 2003). It includes measures of muscle weakness, atrophy, fasiculations, denervation and ultimately loss of function that decreases essential stimulatory retrograde signaling, causing further progression of the diseased state.

2.6.2 G93A feasibility study structure

The dynamic meta-analysis structure is best illustrated like an engineering process flow diagram. Here we show in Figure 1 the categories of outcome measures (boxes) and their interactions (lines). Based on the presented study structure, we determined that there are minimally 72 interactions between the 10 categories of outcome measures. Thus, the minimum number of primary studies to be included in the feasibility study is 72, one for each interaction. Note that we define a primary study as an experiment that measures the interaction between two outcome measures. Therefore, a single published primary experimental article can, and often does, contain more than one primary study. However, it is easier to think of each interaction as needing at least one primary article, and thus, approximately 72 primary articles are need for data extraction to complete a minimalistic feasibility study. The differences between the full and feasibility study structure are shown in Figure 2.

Even for a feasibility study, an "n" of one for each interaction may not sound like meta-analysis, but keep in mind that there are multiple interactions contributing to the effect and prediction of each category. For example, in the structure presented in Figure 1, there are 3-10 interactions for each category. Therefore, 3-10 primary studies contribute to the prediction of each category of outcome measures. That range is in line with the number of primary studies per outcome measure that we might expect for a traditional meta-analysis.

2.7 Extracting data

Quantifiable data is extracted from included primary study figures and tables. Figure 3 shows a hypothetical example of the type of data figure one typically seen in the G93A literature. The Y-axis is typically the affected measure (in this case, percent of cargos travelling retrogradely) and the X-axis is typically the controlled measure (glutamate concentration in our hypothetical example). Additionally, the measure is usually quantified in both the wild-type and G93A mice populations.

Upon extraction, data is normalized to make it unitless. That is, we only look at the relative changes between measures. In this example data, the wild-type retrograde transport went down by ~20% with a 40% increase in glutamate concentration, whereas the SOD1 retrograde transport went down by ~25% with a 40% increase in glutamate concentration.

Therefore, the slope or gain (dY/dX) for wild-type is -0.2 for the interaction from glutamate to retrograde transport. Correspondingly, the gain, for SOD1, is -0.25. Because we only calculate relative changes in dynamic meta-analysis, the magnitude of the gain utilized is actually the relative difference between the wild-type and SOD1 gain magnitudes, (|SOD1| - |wild-type|)/|wild-type|, or [(0.25) - (0.20)]/(0.25) = 0.25, and the sign of this final gain value for this example is net negative (-). Applying the gain of the experimental outcome measures to the category measures, the interaction *from* the category outcome measure of excitotoxicity *to* the category outcome measure of axonal transport is -0.25. Finally, we divide the gain by the time point (or in the case of a feasibility study, the *to* category time constant) to obtain the interaction coefficient (B) used in Equation 2.

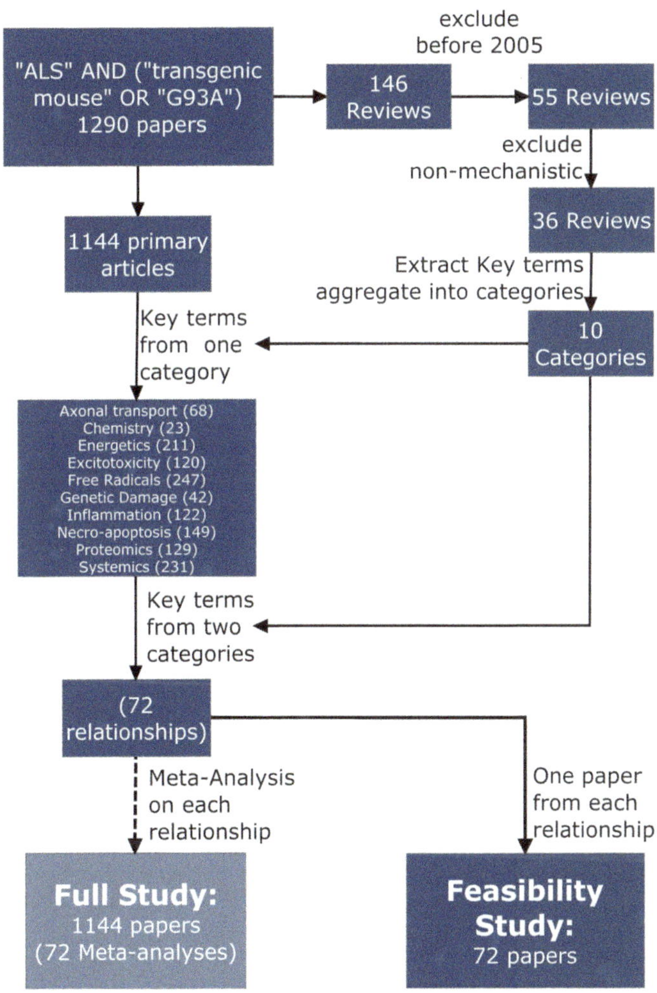

Fig. 2. Scope of dynamic meta-analysis study for the G93A SOD1 mouse model of ALS: feasibility study versus a full study.

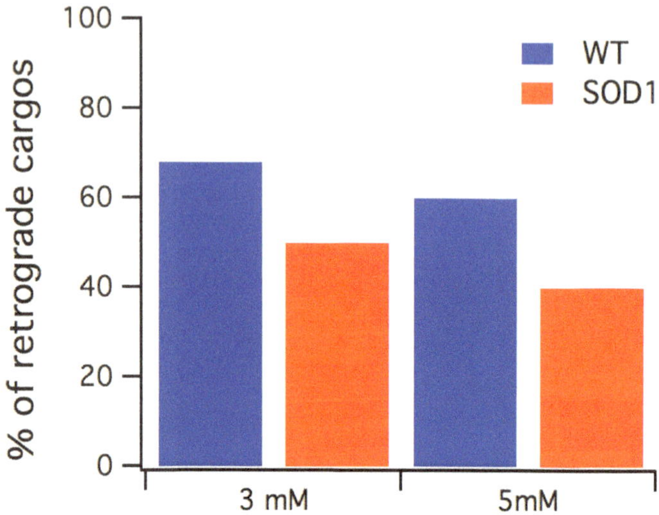

Fig. 3. Example data from a prototypical primary study.

2.8 Quantified data aggregation

For a category-level feasiblity study, such as presented here, it is appropriate to take a non-parametric approach to aggregating the quantitative experimental measures, as the aggregated relationships too disparate to make normalization practical. Consequently, gains were first qualitatively grouped into "small," "medium," or "large". Based on the overall range and resolution of the quantified category interaction magnitudes obtained from the primary studies, numerical gain values for small, medium, and large were set to 0.33, 1, and 3, respectively. However, other values were also explored (e.g. 0.5, 1, and 2; 0.25, 0.5, and 1 etc.) with no qualitative change in result. Table 1 lists the relative magnitude and sign of the category relationships and the primary references from which data was extracted.

Additionally, the corresponding time points for each category utilize a qualitative grouping of small, medium, and large. Based on our mathematical implementaiton of the time points, which is analagous to that used with time constants, we refer to the time points as time constants. Their numerical values and scaling are chosen based on the average onset of associated changes documented for a particular category using the G93A SOD1 mouse model time course. For example, measurable changes are occurring by day 40 in axonal transport, such as the appearance of aggregates and changes in cargo distribution (Kieran, Hafezparast et al. 2005; Teuchert, Fischer et al. 2006); thus, 40 days is used as the time constant for that category. Using the range and resolution of documented changes in G93A over all of the categories, the small, medium, and large time constants are set to 40, 80, and 120 days, respectively (Table 2).

From	To	Size	Sign	Primary Reference(s)
Axonal Transport	Axonal Transport	M	-	(Kieran, 2005; De Vos, 2007; Zhang, Strom 2007)
	Energetics	S	-	(Sakama, 2003; Miller , 2004; De Vos, 2007)
	Excitotoxicity	S	-	(Hiruma, 2003; Stevenson, 2009; Tateno, Kato, 1999)
	Necro-Apoptosis	M	+	(Collard, 1995; Ackerley, 2004)
	Inflammation	S	-	(Brooks,1991; Sasaki, 1996)
Chemistry	Systemic	M	+	(Tiwari, 2005; Ludolph, 2006; Watanabe, 2007; Hozumi, 2008)
	Axonal Transport	S	-	(LaMonte, 2002; Strom, 2008)
	Excitotoxicity	S	+	(Kawahara, 2004; Sasabe, 2007)
	Energetics	S	-	(Wendt, 2002; Lee, Shin, 2008)
	Free Radicals	S	+	(Poon, 2005; Furukawa, 2006)
	Necro-Apoptosis	M	+	(Elam, 2003; Kiaei, 2007; Lee, Shin, 2008)
	Proteomics	M	+	(Lindberg, 2002; Bergemalm, 2006; Rumfeldt, Stathopulos,2006)
Excitotoxicity	Axonal Transport	S	-	(Hiruma, 2003; Tateno, 2008; Stevenson, Yates. 2009)
	Excitotoxicity	M	+	(Rothstein, 1990; Rothstein, 1995; Kuo, 2004; Damiano, Starkov, 2006; Kuwabara, 2007)
	Energetics	L	-	(Beal, 1992; Nicholls, 1998; Jabaudon, 2000; Ellis, 2003)
	Free Radicals	L	+	(Kruman, 1999; Kruman, 1999; Carriedo, 2000; Ellis, 2003)
	Inflammation	L	+	(Hewett, 1994; Cholet, 2002; Barbeito, 2004)
	Necro-Apoptosis	L	+	(Liu, 1999; Sun, 2006; Gibb, 2007; Boutahar, 2008)
	Systemic	S	+	(Bittigau, 1997; Corona, 2007)
Energetics	Axonal Transport	M	+	(Sickles, 1990; Magrane, 2009)
	Excitotoxicity	L	+	(Beal, 1992; Agrawal, 1996; Ellis, 2003; Nicholls, 2003)
	Energetics	M	+	(Mattson, 1999; Mattiazzi, 2002)
	Free Radicals	L	+	(Mattson, 1999; Liu, 2002; Cassina, 2008)
	Inflammation	M	+	(Levine, 1999; Bilsland, 2008)
	Necro-Apoptosis	L	+	(Kruman, 1999; Kaal, 2000; Guegan, 2001; Dupuis, Gonzalez de Aguilar, 2004; Ilzecka, 2007; Knudson, 2008)
	Systemic	M	+	(Verstreken, 2005)
Free Radicals	Axonal Transport	S	-	(Chou, 1996; Chou, 1996; Ferrante, 1997)
	Chemistry	S	+	(Poon, 2005; Furukawa, 2006)
	Excitotoxicity	S	+	(Kruman,1999; Kruman, 1999; Ellis, 2003)
	Energetics	L	-	(Liu, 1996; Liu, 1999; Mattson, 1999; Liu, 2002; Cassina, 2005)
	Free Radicals	M	-	(Liu 1996; Liu. 1999; Cookson, 2002; Cassina, Pehar 2005; Pehar 2007)

From	To	Size	Sign	Primary Reference(s)
	Genetic Damage	M	+	(Aguirre, 2005; Mitsumoto, 2008)
	Inflammation	M	+	(Hensley, 2006; Liu, 2008; Nagai, 2007; Pehar, 2005)
	Necro-Apoptosis	L	+	(Chen, 2009; Estevez, 1999; Pehar, 2005; Pehar, 2007; Wood, 1995)
	Proteomics	S	+	(Dalle-Donne, 2007; Poon, 2005)
	Systemic	S	+	(Dalle-Donne, 2007; Poon, 2005; Kato, 2005; Mahoney, 2006; Mitsumoto, 2008; Sohmiya, 2005)
Genetic Damage	Excitotoxicity	M	+	(Kawahara, 2004; Ignacio, Moore, 2005; Kawahara, 2006)
	Free Radicals	S	+	(Armon, 2005; Wiedau-Pazos, 1996)
	Genetic Damage	M	-	(Armon, 2005; Jiang, 2005; Muller, 2008)
	Inflammation	S	-	(Puttaparthi, 2005; Di Giorgio, 2007; Puttaparthi, 2007)
	Necro-Apoptosis	M	+	(Locatelli, 2007; Lu, 2000)
Inflammation	Axonal Transport	S	-	(Chou, 1996; Kaasik, 2007; King, 2009; Morimoto, 2007)
	Excitotoxicity	M	+	(Hewett, 1994; Cholet, 2002; Pehar, 2004)
	Energetics	S	-	(Cassina, 2008; Cassina, 2005; Takeuchi, 2005; Bilsland, 2008)
	Free Radicals	L	+	(Hensley, 2006; Nagai, 2007; Pehar, 2007)
	Inflammation	M	-	(Gowing, 2008; Puttaparthi, 2005; Schiffer, 1996)
	Necro-Apoptosis	L	+	(Collard, 1995; Ackerley, 2004)
	Systemic	S	+	(Hall, 1998; Cassina, 2005; Cho, 1999)
Necro-Apoptosis	Axonal Transport	S	+	(Ackerley, 2004; Collard, 1995)
	Chemistry	S	-	(Kiaei, 2007; Elam, 2003; Lee, 2009)
	Excitotoxicity	L	+	(Gibb, 2007; Sun, 2002; Liu, 1999)
	Energetics	L	-	(Guegan, 2001; Guegan, 2002)
	Free Radicals	M	+	(Raoul, 2002; Raoul, 2005)
	Genetic Damage	S	+	(Muller, 2007; Raoul, 2006)
	Inflammation	L	+	(Hall, 1998; Cassina, 2005)
	Necro-Apoptosis	L	-	(Gonzalez de Aguilar, 2000; Gonzalez de Aguilar, 1999)
	Proteomics	M	+	(Gal, 2007; Gal, 2009; Yamashita, 2007)
	Systemic	M	+	(Li, 2007; Narai, 2005)
Proteomics	Axonal Transport	M	+	(Eaton, 2005; De Vos, 2007; Sasaki, 2005)
	Chemistry	M	+	(Rumfeldt, 2009; Atkin, 2006)
	Excitotoxicity	S	+	(Rothstein, 2005; Vanoni, 20040
	Free Radicals	S	+	(Aquilano, Rotilio et al. 2003; Clement, 2003)
	Inflammation	M	+	(Stieber, 2000)
	Necro-Apoptosis	M	+	(Urushitani, 2008; Atkin, 2008; Gal, 2007)

From	To	Size	Sign	Primary Reference(s)
	Proteomics	S	-	(Puttaparthi, 2007; Morimoto, 2007; Cheroni, 2009)
	Systemic	M	+	(Turner, 2005; Bucher, 2007)
Systemic	Excitotoxicity	S	+	(Kuner, 2005 ; Pieri, 2008)
	Energetics	S	-	(Wendt, 2002; Zhao, 2006)
	Free Radicals	S	+	(Mahoney, 2006; Pierce, 2008)
	Necro-Apoptosis	S	+	(Martin, 2000; Patel, 2010)
	Systemic	S	-	(Nagano, 2005; Deforges, 2009)

Table 1. Parametric gains for category interactions. Interactions are listed directionally-oriented *from* the category imposing the effected *to* the category being affected. The sign indicates whether the interaction is increasing or decreasing the category, and size (small, medium, large) qualitatively represents the gain magnitude (see Extracted Data Aggregation).

Category	Time Point (days)
Axonal Transport	40
Chemistry	40
Excitotoxicity	80
Energetics	80
Free Radicals	80
Genetic Damage	40
Inflammation	120
Necro-Apoptosis	120
Proteomics	40
Systemic	120

Table 2. Feasibility study time constants utilized for the calculation of the interaction term (B), as shown in Equation 2. Time points are aggregated from primary studies.

2.9 Implementation

Differential equations, in the form shown in Equation 2, are use to construct the dynamic meta-analysis computations. Thus, each category has its own first order differential equation, which includes the effects of each interaction as well as the category time point (or in the case of a feasibility study, a time constant). Each interaction gain coefficient (B) in Equation 2 is simply the change in the affected interaction measure divided by the time point (or in the case of a feasibility study, the category time constant). Because the effect of time is included, the dynamic meta-analysis can predict outcome measures at multiple time points over the entire disease course. Thus, a dynamic meta-analysis can be "simulated" much like a traditional mechanistic model. Because the time-based differential equation computations of dynamic meta-analysis are inherently more complicated than the algebraic regression equations of traditional meta-analysis, the use of a computer simulator assists in its implementation. For this feasibility study, the dynamic meta-analysis was coded, simulated, and analyzed in Matlab (Mathworks, Inc.).

2.10 Post-result analysis and prediction

The basic results of dynamic meta-analysis are quantitative predictions of each outcome measure or category outcome measure changes over time. Additional, higher level results can be obtained by performing sensitivity analyses, which perturb the system and measure the resulting affects. Perturbation can include varying the initial conditions of each category individually or en masse, or varying the interaction gain coefficients (B). Changing initial conditions provides an assessment of the effect size whereas varying specific or category gains provides an assessment of their sensitivity/specificity. For more detail on sensitivity analyses, see (Mitchell, Feng et al. 2007; Mitchell and Lee 2007; Mitchell and Lee 2009).

Traditional meta-analysis analytical tools, such as statistical linear regression and effect size prediction, are still useful to analyze dynamic meta-analysis results. However, the dynamic and multi-variate nature of dynamic meta-analysis also provides possibilities for richer analyses like those typically seen in the analysis of complex or dynamical systems. Given that the two greatest advantages of dynamic analysis are the implicit inclusion of interactions and explicit inclusion of time, analyses that examine how relationships change over time are particularly telling. Analyses such as cross-correlation (or landscapes) of outcome measures or category outcome measures at specific disease time points, such was done in (Mitchell and Lee 2008) and (Mitchell and Lee 2007), provide a overview of what the system is doing without becoming mired in detail.

Finally, the implicit inclusion of interactions allows combination treatments to be examined. All clinical treatments, in some form, exploit a cellular interaction at some level. For example, pharmaceutical modulators typically exploit the interaction between a receptor and its ligand. Thus, every potential interaction within the dynamic meta-analysis structure can be evaluated as a hypothetical treatment possibility. Furthermore, the structure of dynamic meta-analysis allows every single interaction (whether between outcome measures or between categories of outcome measures) to be varied and simulated individually and in combination. Measuring the resultant effect size of an interaction or combination of interactions predicts its potential treatment efficacy. For more methodological detail on simulating combination therapies, see our previous work with combination treatments and spinal cord injury (Mitchell and Lee 2008).

3. Results of a G93A SOD1 feasibility study

We begin by examing the effect size of each category, an analysis that is typically seen with traditional meta-analysis. Table 3 reveals the average, standard deviation, maximum, and minimum effect size of each category based on a sensitivity analysis that perturbed the intial conditions. Note that "N" is the connectivity, or number of interactions (as shown in Figure 1), affecting the category measure. This examination reveals that the average effect of, for example, treating energetics is a relatively unimpressive 19% outcome change for a 100% treatment effect on energetics itself. (Note that a "real" treatment would have effects substantially smaller than 100%, often only 10% or so.). However, this type of analysis misses the potential for interactions completely and to some extent even minimizes the potential significance of targeted treatments by averaging.

Category	Avg	Stdev	Min	Max	N
Axon Transport	-1%	12%	-21%	16%	6
Chemistry	11%	27%	-6%	71%	7
Energetics	-19%	71%	-98%	102%	7
Excitotoxicity	0%	39%	-80%	36%	7
Free Radical	2%	24%	-53%	44%	10
Genetics	3%	6%	-3%	12%	5
Inflammation	14%	21%	-6%	49%	7
Necro-Apoptosis	16%	26%	-35%	59%	10
Proteomics	13%	24%	-17%	56%	8
Systemic	-2%	5%	-10%	2%	5

Table 3. Standard meta-analysis result table illustrating the effect of each category on disease outcome measures (survival and function).

3.1 Dynamics of the G93A SOD1 mouse pathology

Next, we examine the relative changes in the category outcome measures over time in order to get a better feel of the system dynamics. As shown in Figure 4, initially, the system exhibits a period of relative quiescence (days 0-80) in which there appears to be little variation from the baseline operating point. However, closer examination reveals a few fluctuations, which appear as small oscillations from baseline (Figure 5). Over time each oscillation grows in magnitude, with the first notable oscillation starting around day 40. However, the component trajectories do eventually explode at approximately day 150.

These qualitative system features of ALS align well with the characterization of the G-93A SOD-1 experimental paradigm. In fact, the first large oscillation corresponds to the average onset of measurable functional deficits and the final explosion aligns with the average time of death for the G-93A SOD-1 mouse model (Xu, Jung et al. 2004; Kieran, Hafezparast et al. 2005; Gould, Buss et al. 2006; Teuchert, Fischer et al. 2006). It should be noted that the oscillations of this system do not necessarily represent the relapsing and remitting of functional deficits, such as is seen with multiple sclerosis, but rather the oscillations of individual mechanisms and pathways. In fact, such oscillations could be responsible for small fluctuations sometimes seen within and among mechanistic studies, such as those examining axonal transport (De Vos, Chapman et al. 2007) and protein aggregation (Stieber, Gonatas et al. 2000; Gould, Buss et al. 2006). How oscillations correlating with specific losses in muscle function remains to be seen. It is likely that the overall loss of systemic control aligns with what is typically seen as continuously degenerating function or degenerative function with intermixed plateaus.

From a system dynamics point of view, it is likely that the exploding oscillations of ALS are the result of an unstable system. Initially, the regulatory systems, including excitability, ionic and axonal transport, cellular energetics and others, are able to maintain partial control, as evidenced by the smaller oscillations, which are an attempt to regulate. However, as the disease progresses the control mechanisms simply fail to keep up.

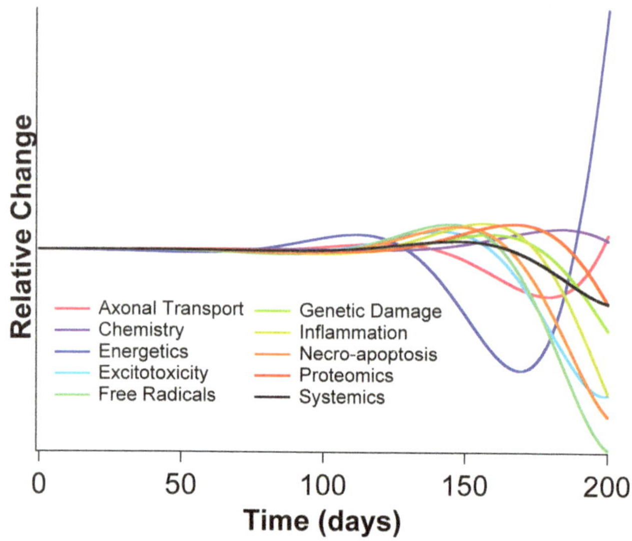

Fig. 4. Unstable, oscillatory dynamics of ALS predicted by dynamic meta-analysis .

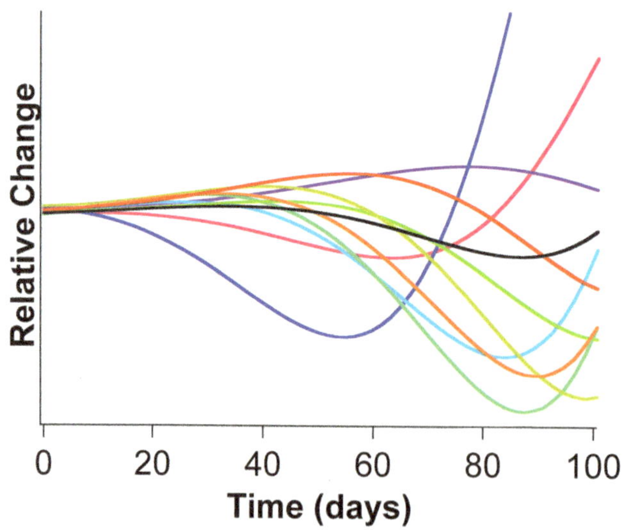

Fig. 5. Expansion of oscillations initiating during the pre-symptomatic quiescent period.

3.2 Combination therapy predictions

We examine how hypothetical therapeutics that exploit single and multi-category interactions can potentially "treat" the system. We utilize the systemic category as our primary outcome measure since it includes known functional metrics. Two different combination treatment types are examined: 1.) combination treatments that stabilize the system (e.g. dampen the oscillations) and 2.) synergistic combination treatments.

Stabilizing Treatments: If pathological progression is driven by, or is the result of, system instability, then one potential therapeutic strategy is to develop treatments that rectify the instability. We tested single treatments that targeted individual category interactions as well as combination treatments that simultaneously targeted up to 3 category interactions. A small percentage of the over 44,000 different combinations treatments investigated rectified the system instability (See example in Figure 6), thereby preventing the "explosion" typically seen between days 150-200 at the average time of death. That is, these treatments have the potential to greatly extend the life span of the typical G-93A mouse.

Of note is that many of the most successful treatment combinations did not include the component that was responsible for the initiating perturbation. Also in some cases, the directions (sign of the relationship) that components best treated the system could be non-intuitive, again likely owing to the highly interactive nature of the ALS system.

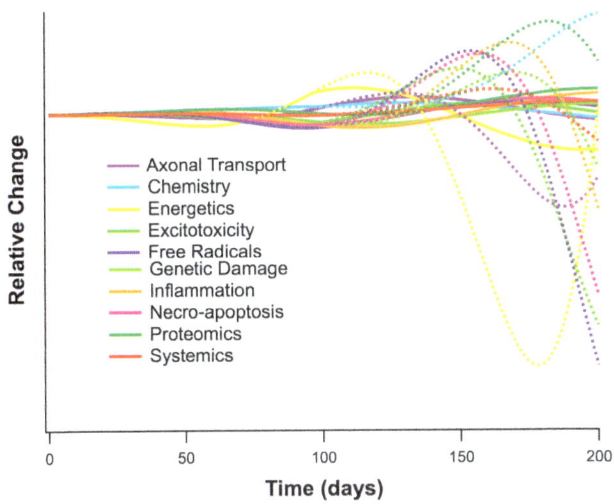

Fig. 6. Dynamics of ALS predicted by dynamic analysis of the G93A SOD1 mouse model. ALS dynamics are unstable, (dashed lines) characterized by growing oscillations that "explode" near the average time of death. Dynamic meta-analysis of potential treatment combinations predicts that a small percentage of 3-way treatment combinations can assist in re-stabilization of the system (solid lines).

Treatment synergism: Whether stabilizing or not, or just purely interaction-based, many of the ALS treatments have a synergistic effect. That is, their combined effects are substantially greater than the sum of their individual effects. For two-way treatments (treatments addressing two category interactions), 16% of the total possible 10,000 combinations are synergistic. (Note that treatment direction was made in the more favorable direction.) For three-way combinations, approximately 22% of the possible 900,000 combinations are synergistic (Figure 7).

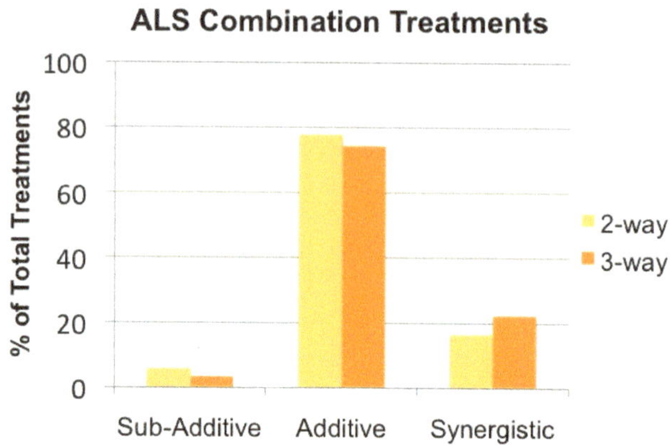

Fig. 7. Percentage of total treatment combinations belonging to each efficacy type.

Tables 4 and 5, show the efficacies of 2-way and 3-way synergistic combination treatments. A linearly additive treatment (combination A&B effect = A effect + B effect) was assigned an efficacy factor of 1.0. Thus, synergistic treatments have efficacy factors >1 and sub-additive treatments have efficacy factors <1. Therefore, categories with higher average and maximum efficacy factors have a tendency to produce greater synergistic effects in combination.

Category	Avg	Stdev	Max	Count
Axonal Transport	1.08	0.16	1.74	59
Chemistry	1.02	0.05	1.39	107
Energetics	1.23	0.32	2.44	229
Excitotoxicity	1.09	0.24	2.33	160
Free Radical	1.06	0.14	1.93	311
Genetics	1.01	0.02	1.21	86
Inflammation	1.03	0.07	1.66	195
Necro-Apoptosis	1.10	0.23	2.35	327
Proteomics	1.04	0.15	2.05	154
Systemic	1.05	0.07	1.23	22

Table 4. Synergistic two-way combination treatment predictions.

Category	Avg	Stdev	Max	Count
Axonal Transport	1.08	0.17	2.82	17395
Chemistry	1.19	0.26	4.85	23101
Energetics	1.09	0.19	2.82	22332
Excitotoxicity	1.05	0.13	2.13	33020
Free Radical	1.04	0.12	2.01	12929
Genetics	1.05	0.12	3.26	22589
Inflammation	1.09	0.19	2.67	35586
Necro-Apoptosis	1.09	0.20	2.60	22603
Proteomics	1.06	0.14	2.05	11322
Systemic	1.00	0.00	1.00	0

Table 5. Synergistic three-way combination treatment predictions.

4. Conclusions

System dynamics revealed. Conventional wisdom in ALS research has been that there is a single, specific root cause. However, dynamic meta-analysis predicts that a system-level instability is the actual problem (see oscillations in Figure 4). Lending credence to the predictions of dynamic meta-analysis is the mounting evidence from recent studies that indicates that multiple mutations or underlying mechanisms can result in the symptoms characterized as ALS (Rothstein 2009).

Novel treatment strategies identified. In this small scale feasibility study of ALS, dynamic meta-analysis predicts that reducing the overall feedback gain will be more effective than identifying and ameliorating a single "source" or point of initiation (Mitchell and Lee 2010). That is, inducing small changes across multiple categories of mechanisms is more effective than inducing a large change in a single category. Additionally, treatments that target the underyling system dyanmics, such as stabilizing oscillations, could be another potentially effective path.

Combination treatment prediction enabled. Another key opportunity afforded by dynamic meta-analysis is an innovative approach to predicting combination treatment effectiveness in a high-throughput manner. The interacting differential equations of dynamic meta-analysis implicitly include all possible treatment interactions. Thus, potential synergistic combinations can be identified before they are explicitly examined experimentally. For example, in spinal cord injury, a sweep of all possible combinations of virtual treatments revealed that none were synergistic (Mitchell and Lee 2008). While disappointing, we were at least able to discover treatments that combined linearly. On the other hand, in our initial evaluation of ALS, a small percentage of treatment combinations show very profound synergism! It appears that in ALS, the broader the treatment the more effective it becomes. (Figure 6 illustrates an example of a 3-way combination that appears to arrest the oscillatory explosion observed in the control case.) Finally, dynamic meta-analysis is not only well suited to identify promising combinations but can be used to prioritize them as well.

5. Acknowledgments

This work was supported by the National Institute of Health (NS069616 and NS062200).

6. References

Ackerley, S., A. J. Grierson, et al. (2004). "p38alpha stress-activated protein kinase phosphorylates neurofilaments and is associated with neurofilament pathology in amyotrophic lateral sclerosis." *Mol Cell Neurosci* 26(2): 354-364.

Banci, L., I. Bertini, et al. (2008). "SOD1 and amyotrophic lateral sclerosis: mutations and oligomerization." *PLoS One* 3(2): e1677.

Beere, H. M. (2004). ""The stress of dying": the role of heat shock proteins in the regulation of apoptosis." *J Cell Sci* 117(Pt 13): 2641-2651.

Bilsland, L. G., E. Sahai, et al. "Deficits in axonal transport precede ALS symptoms in vivo." *Proc Natl Acad Sci U S A.*

Bogdanov, M. B., L. E. Ramos, et al. (1998). "Elevated "hydroxyl radical" generation in vivo in an animal model of amyotrophic lateral sclerosis." *J Neurochem* 71(3): 1321-1324.

De Vos, K. J., A. L. Chapman, et al. (2007). "Familial amyotrophic lateral sclerosis-linked SOD1 mutants perturb fast axonal transport to reduce axonal mitochondria content." *Hum Mol Genet* 16(22): 2720-2728.

Derave, W., L. Van Den Bosch, et al. (2003). "Skeletal muscle properties in a transgenic mouse model for amyotrophic lateral sclerosis: effects of creatine treatment." *Neurobiol Dis* 13(3): 264-272.

Dobrowolny, G., M. Aucello, et al. (2008). "Skeletal muscle is a primary target of SOD1G93A-mediated toxicity." *Cell Metab* 8(5): 425-436.

Dunlop, J., H. Beal McIlvain, et al. (2003). "Impaired spinal cord glutamate transport capacity and reduced sensitivity to riluzole in a transgenic superoxide dismutase mutant rat model of amyotrophic lateral sclerosis." *J Neurosci* 23(5): 1688-1696.

Dupuis, L., H. Oudart, et al. (2004). "Evidence for defective energy homeostasis in amyotrophic lateral sclerosis: benefit of a high-energy diet in a transgenic mouse model." *Proc Natl Acad Sci U S A* 101(30): 11159-11164.

Echaniz-Laguna, A., J. Zoll, et al. (2002). "Mitochondrial respiratory chain function in skeletal muscle of ALS patients." *Ann Neurol* 52(5): 623-627.

Gifondorwa, D. J., M. B. Robinson, et al. (2007). "Exogenous delivery of heat shock protein 70 increases lifespan in a mouse model of amyotrophic lateral sclerosis." *J Neurosci* 27(48): 13173-13180.

Gould, T. W., R. R. Buss, et al. (2006). "Complete dissociation of motor neuron death from motor dysfunction by Bax deletion in a mouse model of ALS." *J Neurosci* 26(34): 8774-8786.

Guatteo, E., I. Carunchio, et al. (2007). "Altered calcium homeostasis in motor neurons following AMPA receptor but not voltage-dependent calcium channels' activation in a genetic model of amyotrophic lateral sclerosis." *Neurobiol Dis* 28(1): 90-100.

Hafezparast, M., A. Ahmad-Annuar, et al. (2003). "Paradigms for the identification of new genes in motor neuron degeneration." *Amyotroph Lateral Scler Other Motor Neuron Disord* 4(4): 249-257.

Hall, E. D., P. K. Andrus, et al. (1998). "Relationship of oxygen radical-induced lipid peroxidative damage to disease onset and progression in a transgenic model of familial ALS." *J Neurosci Res* 53(1): 66-77.

Hayward, L. J., J. A. Rodriguez, et al. (2002). "Decreased metallation and activity in subsets of mutant superoxide dismutases associated with familial amyotrophic lateral sclerosis." *J Biol Chem* 277(18): 15923-15931.

Ikonomidou, C., Y. Qin Qin, et al. (1996). "Motor neuron degeneration induced by excitotoxin agonists has features in common with those seen in the SOD-1 transgenic mouse model of amyotrophic lateral sclerosis." *J Neuropathol Exp Neurol* 55(2): 211-224.

Kadoyama, K., H. Funakoshi, et al. (2007). "Hepatocyte growth factor (HGF) attenuates gliosis and motoneuronal degeneration in the brainstem motor nuclei of a transgenic mouse model of ALS." *Neurosci Res* 59(4): 446-456.

Kieran, D., M. Hafezparast, et al. (2005). "A mutation in dynein rescues axonal transport defects and extends the life span of ALS mice." *J Cell Biol* 169(4): 561-567.

King, A. E., T. C. Dickson, et al. (2009). "Neuron-glia interactions underlie ALS-like axonal cytoskeletal pathology." *Neurobiol Aging*.

Kong, J. and Z. Xu (1998). "Massive mitochondrial degeneration in motor neurons triggers the onset of amyotrophic lateral sclerosis in mice expressing a mutant SOD1." *J Neurosci* 18(9): 3241-3250.

Kuo, J. J., M. Schonewille, et al. (2004). "Hyperexcitability of cultured spinal motoneurons from presymptomatic ALS mice." *J Neurophysiol* 91(1): 571-575.

Kuo, J. J., T. Siddique, et al. (2005). "Increased persistent Na(+) current and its effect on excitability in motoneurones cultured from mutant SOD1 mice." *J Physiol* 563(Pt 3): 843-854.

Mattson, M. P. and W. Duan (1999). "Apoptotic" biochemical cascades in synaptic compartments: roles in adaptive plasticity and neurodegenerative disorders." *J Neurosci Res* 58(1): 152-166.

Meyer, M. A. and N. T. Potter (1995). "Sporadic ALS and chromosome 22: evidence for a possible neurofilament gene defect." *Muscle Nerve* 18(5): 536-539.

Miller, R. G., J. D. Mitchell, et al. (2007). "Riluzole for amyotrophic lateral sclerosis (ALS)/motor neuron disease (MND)." *Cochrane Database Syst Rev*(1): CD001447.

Mitchell, C. S. (2009). Viewpoint aggregation via relational modeling and analysis: A new approach to systems physiology. *Wallace H. Coulter Department of Biomedical Engineering*. Atlanta, GA, Georgia Institute of Technology and Emory University.

Mitchell, C. S., S. S. Feng, et al. (2007). "An analysis of glutamate spillover on the N-methyl-D-aspartate receptors at the cerebellar glomerulus." *J Neural Eng* 4(3): 276-282.

Mitchell, C. S. and R. H. Lee (2007). "Output-based comparison of alternative kinetic schemes for the NMDA receptor within a glutamate spillover model." *J Neural Eng* 4(4): 380-389.

Mitchell, C. S. and R. H. Lee (2008). "Pathology dynamics predict spinal cord injury therapeutic success." *J Neurotrauma* 25(12): 1483-1497.

Mitchell, C. S. and R. H. Lee (2009). "A quantitative examination of the role of cargo-exerted forces in axonal transport." *J Theor Biol* 257(3): 430-437.

Mitchell, C. S. and R. H. Lee (2010). *Dynamic Meta-Analysis of the G93A SOD1 mouse model: Pathology dynamics and combination treatment predictions*. 21st International Symposium on ALS/MND, Orlando, FL.

Nagai, M., D. B. Re, et al. (2007). "Astrocytes expressing ALS-linked mutated SOD1 release factors selectively toxic to motor neurons." *Nat Neurosci* 10(5): 615-622.

Nagano, I., T. Murakami, et al. (2002). "Early decrease of survival factors and DNA repair enzyme in spinal motor neurons of presymptomatic transgenic mice that express a mutant SOD1 gene." *Life Sci* 72(4-5): 541-548.

Narai, H., I. Nagano, et al. (2005). "Prevention of spinal motor neuron death by insulin-like growth factor-1 associating with the signal transduction systems in SODG93A transgenic mice." *J Neurosci Res* 82(4): 452-457.

Pastula, D. M., D. H. Moore, et al. (2010). "Creatine for amyotrophic lateral sclerosis/motor neuron disease." *Cochrane Database Syst Rev*(6): CD005225.

Pehar, M., M. R. Vargas, et al. (2007). "Mitochondrial superoxide production and nuclear factor erythroid 2-related factor 2 activation in p75 neurotrophin receptor-induced motor neuron apoptosis." *J Neurosci* 27(29): 7777-7785.

Peviani, M., I. Caron, et al. "Unraveling the complexity of amyotrophic lateral sclerosis: recent advances from the transgenic mutant SOD1 mice." *CNS Neurol Disord Drug Targets* 9(4): 491-503.

Rothstein, J. D. (2009). "Current hypotheses for the underlying biology of amyotrophic lateral sclerosis." *Ann Neurol* 65 Suppl 1: S3-9.

Roy, J., S. Minotti, et al. (1998). "Glutamate potentiates the toxicity of mutant Cu/Zn-superoxide dismutase in motor neurons by postsynaptic calcium-dependent mechanisms." *J Neurosci* 18(23): 9673-9684.

Rumfeldt, J. A., J. R. Lepock, et al. (2009). "Unfolding and folding kinetics of amyotrophic lateral sclerosis-associated mutant Cu,Zn superoxide dismutases." *J Mol Biol* 385(1): 278-298.

Shi, P., J. Gal, et al. "Mitochondrial dysfunction in amyotrophic lateral sclerosis." *Biochim Biophys Acta* 1802(1): 45-51.

Stathopulos, P. B., J. A. Rumfeldt, et al. (2003). "Cu/Zn superoxide dismutase mutants associated with amyotrophic lateral sclerosis show enhanced formation of aggregates in vitro." *Proc Natl Acad Sci U S A* 100(12): 7021-7026.

Stieber, A., J. O. Gonatas, et al. (2000). "Aggregation of ubiquitin and a mutant ALS-linked SOD1 protein correlate with disease progression and fragmentation of the Golgi apparatus." *J Neurol Sci* 173(1): 53-62.

Sumi, H., S. Nagano, et al. (2006). "Inverse correlation between the formation of mitochondria-derived vacuoles and Lewy-body-like hyaline inclusions in G93A superoxide-dismutase-transgenic mice." *Acta Neuropathol* 112(1): 52-63.

Tanaka, F., J. Niwa, et al. (2006). "Gene expression profiling toward understanding of ALS pathogenesis." *Ann N Y Acad Sci* 1086: 1-10.

Teuchert, M., D. Fischer, et al. (2006). "A dynein mutation attenuates motor neuron degeneration in SOD1(G93A) mice." *Exp Neurol* 198(1): 271-274.

Tiwari, A., Z. Xu, et al. (2005). "Aberrantly increased hydrophobicity shared by mutants of Cu,Zn-superoxide dismutase in familial amyotrophic lateral sclerosis." *J Biol Chem* 280(33): 29771-29779.

Trelle, S., S. Reichenbach, et al. (2011). "Cardiovascular safety of non-steroidal anti-inflammatory drugs: network meta-analysis." *BMJ* 342: c7086.

Tokuda, E., S. Ono, et al. (2008). "Ammonium tetrathiomolybdate delays onset, prolongs survival, and slows progression of disease in a mouse model for amyotrophic lateral sclerosis." *Exp Neurol* 213(1): 122-128.

Urushitani, M., J. Kurisu, et al. (2002). "Proteasomal inhibition by misfolded mutant superoxide dismutase 1 induces selective motor neuron death in familial amyotrophic lateral sclerosis." *J Neurochem* 83(5): 1030-1042.

Van Damme, P., M. Leyssen, et al. (2003). "The AMPA receptor antagonist NBQX prolongs survival in a transgenic mouse model of amyotrophic lateral sclerosis." *Neurosci Lett* 343(2): 81-84.

Vukosavic, S., M. Dubois-Dauphin, et al. (1999). "Bax and Bcl-2 interaction in a transgenic mouse model of familial amyotrophic lateral sclerosis." *J Neurochem* 73(6): 2460-2468.

Watanabe, M., M. Dykes-Hoberg, et al. (2001). "Histological evidence of protein aggregation in mutant SOD1 transgenic mice and in amyotrophic lateral sclerosis neural tissues." *Neurobiol Dis* 8(6): 933-941.

Wong, N. K., B. P. He, et al. (2000). "Characterization of neuronal intermediate filament protein expression in cervical spinal motor neurons in sporadic amyotrophic lateral sclerosis (ALS)." *J Neuropathol Exp Neurol* 59(11): 972-982.

Wood, J. D., T. P. Beaujeux, et al. (2003). "Protein aggregation in motor neurone disorders." *Neuropathol Appl Neurobiol* 29(6): 529-545.

Xu, Z., C. Jung, et al. (2004). "Mitochondrial degeneration in amyotrophic lateral sclerosis." *J Bioenerg Biomembr* 36(4): 395-399.

3

Insights Arising from Gene Expression Profiling in Amyotrophic Lateral Sclerosis

Johnathan Cooper-Knock, Joanna J. Bury, Laura Ferraiuolo, Emily F. Goodall, Pamela J. Shaw and Janine Kirby
Sheffield Institute for Translational Neuroscience, University of Sheffield, Sheffield, United Kingdom

1. Introduction

Gene expression profiling has been used extensively in multiple fields of research to compare disease and control samples, to investigate mechanisms of disease, to identify subtypes within a heterogeneous clinical phenotype and to establish responses to a specific treatment. In addition, it can also be used to determine the function of a gene, to monitor changes over time, or for discovering cell specific expression or responses.

This chapter will initially explain the principles of gene expression profiling, before discussing the sources of samples, along with their advantages and limitations, and will then summarise the research to date regarding the application of gene expression profiling to amyotrophic lateral sclerosis (ALS).

2. What is gene expression profiling?

The primary application of gene expression profiling is to use a glass slide containing oligonucleotides or cDNA sequences, termed a microarray, to quantify the amount of individual RNA transcripts that are present in a particular cell or tissue. RNA is extracted, fluorescently labelled and then hybridized to the microarray. A linear amplification step can also be performed prior to labelling to ensure sufficient RNA is generated from low yields of RNA extracted from small sample sizes. The quantity of labelled RNA binding to each oligonucleotide or cDNA sequence on the microarray determines the intensity of fluorescence at that location and thus allows quantification of the RNA transcripts in the initial sample (Stoughton 2005).

Comparison of the expression of transcripts between sample groups allows identification of transcripts which are differentially expressed between the groups. The large number of genes simultaneously interrogated by a microarray means that the resulting data are amenable to study the expression of inter-related clusters of genes such as those involved in known functional categories or specific pathways. Changes in expression level of a particular gene do not take into account regulation at the level of translation. However, the functional impact of a differentially expressed gene can be subsequently established by assaying the encoded protein expression or function.

The advent of next generation sequencing, and specifically the sequencing of all RNA molecules in a quantitative manner, has recently become an alternative, though expensive method for measuring levels of gene expression. However, this has the potential to add further knowledge and value to the application of gene expression profiling to disease.

3. Uses of gene expression profiling

Quantification of the transcriptome has been a useful mechanism for both discovering and defining mechanisms of pathogenesis in ALS (Cox et al 2010; Ferraiuolo et al 2007; Kirby et al 2005; Kirby et al 2011). In particular lists of differentially expressed genes can be usefully converted to functional 'themes' by an enrichment analysis (Hosack et al 2003). Various categorisations exist, including the gene ontology (GO) and Kyoto encyclopaedia of genes and genomes (KEGG), which classify genes according to molecular function, biological process, cellular component or a known biological pathway.

A frequent application of gene expression profiling has been the development of putative biomarkers via a supervised classification approach (Booij et al 2011; Nagasaka et al 2005; Scherzer et al 2007). The large number of targets quantified simultaneously by gene expression profiling is essential for biomarker discovery, as it allows an unbiased survey of the most informative RNA transcripts. A reliable biomarker(s) for defining pathogenesis and prognosis in ALS has yet to be established, though gene expression profiling is one of the methodologies currently being used to establish an ALS biomarker(s).

4. Sources of material for studying ALS

In ALS, the vulnerable cells are the motor neurones, located in the motor cortex, brainstem and spinal cord. Since motor neurones cannot be sampled during life, model systems, such as neuronal-like cells in culture and animals carrying mutant transgenes, have been used to study the neurodegenerative process. In addition to sampling post-mortem material from patients, peripheral tissue from living patients (and neurologically normal controls) has been used as a source material for applying gene expression profiling to ALS.

4.1 Cellular models of ALS

Neuronal cell lines, both human (e.g. SH-SY5Y) and rodent (e.g. PC12), have been used as a model to investigate mechanisms of neurodegeneration. However, one of the most widely used cellular models for examining the molecular pathophysiology underpinning the neurodegenerative disease process in ALS is the mouse spinal cord/neuroblastoma cell line NSC-34 (Cashman et al 1992). Immortalized NSC-34 cells recapitulate many of the characteristics of motor neurones whilst maintaining their ability to proliferate in culture; thus providing a continual resource of motor neurone-like cells (Cashman et al 1992; Durham et al 1993). In particular, they have proved a robust model of mutant copper zinc superoxide dismutase-1 (*SOD1*) associated familial ALS (FALS), as they can be transfected with vectors carrying normal or mutant forms of the human *SOD1* gene (Durham et al 1997; Menzies et al 2002a; Menzies et al 2002b). Cellular models of TDP-43-related ALS, caused by mutation of the TAR DNA binding protein gene (*TARDBP*) are being generated (Duan et al 2010; Igaz et al 2009), though sustained over-expression of the wild-type and mutant proteins is proving problematic due to the toxicity of both the wild-type and mutant over-expressed proteins and the tight auto-regulation of TDP-43 (Budini & Buratti 2011).

Gene expression profiling of cell lines transfected with ALS associated genes provides a genetically homogenous cell population uncontaminated by non-neuronal astrocytes and other types of glial cells, which are present in the central nervous system (CNS). Furthermore, environmental conditions can easily be manipulated and tightly controlled *in vitro* so as to reduce the impact of external confounding factors on gene expression. The limitations of this type of model system include the fact that NSC-34 cell lines (or other neuronal cell lines) are continually dividing cells, rather than post-mitotic cells and they are unable to mirror the effects of cellular interactions that occur between the different cell populations *in situ* (Kirby et al 2011).

Primary neuronal and astrocytic cells can be isolated from embryonic mice and short-term cultures generated for microarray analysis. These cells more closely mirror those present in the CNS, though the primary neuronal cultures, as they are post-mitotic cells, have a limited lifespan of 7-10 days. In contrast, cultured primary astrocytes are able to proliferate in culture. Whilst co-cultures or separated co-cultures allow a degree of interaction between the two cell types, these types of mixed cultures have not yet been used for microarray analysis in ALS.

4.2 Animal models of ALS

Transgenic mice expressing mutant forms of ALS-related genes provide a source of RNA for microarray analysis. For investigating the mechanisms of *SOD1*-related neurodegeneration, mice over-expressing the human p.G93A or mouse p.G86R mutant forms of the SOD1 protein ($SOD1^{G93A}$ or $SOD1^{G86R}$) have been used as they develop an age dependent neuromuscular condition; the motor function symptoms and histopathological features have been extensively characterised and resemble those observed in both *SOD1*-related ALS and classical ALS patients (Gurney et al 1994; Ripps et al 1995). In contrast, over-expression of wild-type human SOD1 ($SOD1^{WT}$) does not produce an overt motor phenotype, supporting a toxic gain of function by the mutant SOD1 protein as the mechanism by which the mutant proteins cause cell death. In contrast, mouse models over-expressing either wild-type or mutant TDP-43 show a neurodegenerative phenotype (Igaz et al 2011; Stallings et al 2010).

One of the major advantages of using animal models for microarray analysis is the ability to examine animals at different ages in order to investigate the progression of disease, an approach that is unattainable in human post-mortem tissue. Valuable insights regarding onset of disease can be established in pre-symptomatic and early symptomatic disease stages since these represent time points at which the identification of key novel targets for therapeutic intervention could be best placed to rescue vulnerable neuronal cell populations before the development of irreversible neuronal injury (Ferraiuolo et al 2007). In addition, sampling of specific cell types from the CNS allow gene expression changes to be identified which include the effects of interactions with neighbouring cells.

Backcrossing of the $SOD1^{WT}$ and $SOD1^{G93A}$ mice with C57Bl6 mice has led to the formation of $SOD1^{WT}$ and $SOD1^{G93A}$ mice on a homogeneous background (Ferraiuolo et al 2007). The use of these mice for microarray analysis and the use of non-transgenic littermates as controls have proven effective in reducing inter-individual genetic variability to ensure the generation of consistent and reliable gene expression data.

4.3 Human post-mortem material

Human post-mortem brain and spinal cord specimens derived from clinically and pathologically confirmed cases of ALS can be used in comparisons with age, gender and ethnically matched neurologically normal controls and are a pivotal source of RNA for gene expression profiling in ALS. Brain and spinal cord represent the tissues that are most susceptible to the underlying neurodegenerative disease process. However, there are a number of limitations that should be taken into account when using this tissue. First and foremost, the transcriptional changes that are detected are reflecting the terminal stage of disease, with the majority of vulnerable neuronal cells having already undergone cell death (Sharp et al 2006). Therefore, it can be difficult to distinguish whether the changes detected are due to the survival response in the remaining cells, initiation of a cell death pathway (if the cells are beginning to die), or whether the changes are present in response to a pathogenic trigger (Lederer et al 2007). Secondly, samples, and particularly control material, are difficult to obtain and often in short supply. This restricts the sample sizes that can be used, which has a negative impact upon the statistical power of such studies. Considerable heterogeneity exists between individuals in disease and control groups and gene expression changes may also be influenced by post-mortem interval, variability in brain pH, degree of neuroinflammation and sample type including white versus grey matter or cortical motor neurones versus spinal motor neurones. Furthermore, *ex vivo* RNA degradation, particularly during sample preparation, should also be taken into consideration (Maes et al 2007).

RNA extraction protocols are faster and more straightforward for whole tissue homogenates. However, the inclusion of a heterogeneous mixture of cell populations may in effect blur the distinctive profile emanating from the neuronal cells that are most affected in ALS (Kirby et al 2011). In comparing the gene expression profiles generated from diseased tissue to that of healthy controls there is also the added issue of a shift in the proportion of different cell populations within the sample as neurodegeneration is characterised by the loss of motor neurones and the active proliferation of non-neuronal microglia and macrophages (Dangond et al 2004). Laser capture microdissection (LCM) may be a more expensive and laborious technique but is beneficial in studying a neuronal enriched cell population (Jiang et al 2005). It also is noteworthy that in comparison to primary cultures these cells have had the benefit of being embedded within their natural environment where physiologically relevant cross talk has taken place with neighbouring cells and tissues (Ferraiuolo et al 2007).

4.4 Human peripheral tissue samples

Peripheral tissue such as whole venous blood, cultured skin fibroblasts and muscle biopsy material offer an attractive and readily accessible resource for microarray analysis in ALS. Samples can be collected longitudinally, particularly as the collection of blood is relatively non-invasive and sampling techniques can be standardized across research centres (Highley et al 2011; Saris et al 2009; Shtilbans et al 2011; Tsuang et al 2005).

Blood is classified as a fluid connective tissue composed of plasma (55%), erythrocytes (43%), leukocytes (0.5%) and platelets (1.5%) which continuously permeates and interacts with every other tissue and organ of the mammalian body. It is in a permanent state of renewal and is known to play a pivotal role in physiological homeostasis, cellular immunity and inflammation (Mohr & Liew 2007). Since 80% of the genes routinely expressed within the CNS have also been detectable in circulating blood cells it is anticipated that there are quantifiable changes in the levels of these gene transcripts which have the potential to act as a sentinel of disease (Liew et al 2006). Evidence suggests that the shear abundance of endogenous alpha and beta globin messenger RNA (mRNA), which constitutes up to 70% of erythrocytic mRNA transcripts, masks the expression of less abundant genes of potential biological significance as a result of their high signal intensity on the microarray (Wright et al 2008). Thus, strategies have been developed and evaluated to remove these transcripts present in the RNA samples from whole blood (Liu et al 2006). Alternatively, fractionation of peripheral blood mononuclear cells (PBMCs) can also be used though the additional processing steps involved in isolating the PBMCs can introduce spurious artifactual alterations in gene expression that are not attributable to the disease (Whitney et al 2003).

Fibroblasts are not known to have any direct involvement in ALS, though they provide a model with the genetic background of the individual and have the added value of being a source for the generation of induced pluripotent stem cells (iPS) or for the direct manipulation into motor neuronal cells (Dimos et al 2008; Son et al 2011). In addition, fibroblasts have been shown to reflect changes in patients with neurodegenerative disease (Aguirre et al 1998; Hoepken et al 2008; Mortiboys et al 2008) and their gene expression profiles distinguish pre-symptomatic individuals from those of controls (Nagasaka et al 2005). In contrast to fibroblasts, skeletal muscle is severely affected by the disease. Whilst muscle biopsies are the most invasive sample to collect, they are a useful source for gene expression profiling, as they provide a window into the mechanisms involved in the neuromuscular degeneration that occur in ALS during life (Dadon-Nachum et al 2011; Dupuis & Loeffler 2009).

5. Results from use of cellular models of ALS

Gene expression profiling of the widely used NSC34 cellular model of *SOD1*-related FALS identified a marked degree of transcriptional repression in the presence of the $SOD1^{G93A}$ mutation (Kirby et al 2005). These repressed genes included a group of antioxidant response (ARE) genes or "programmed cell life" genes that are regulated by the Nrf2 transcription factor (Figure 1). Reduced expression of *Nrf2* and selected downstream targets was seen at both the RNA and protein levels in the cellular model and *NRF2* dysregulation was also demonstrated in isolated motor neurones from *SOD1*-related ALS cases. Subsequent work by Sarlette and colleagues has shown that *NRF2* transcription and translation is also decreased in SALS cases (Sarlette et al 2008). Most recently, it has been demonstrated that activation of *Nrf2* in NSC34 *SOD1*-related ALS cell models, primary motor neurone and astrocyte co-cultures and in the $SOD1^{G93A}$ mouse model all improve neuronal survival (Neymotin et al 2011; Vargas et al 2008a).

Primary astrocyte cultures prepared from mutant SOD1 rodent models have been shown to increase motor neuronal death in co-cultures (Nagai et al 2007; Vargas et al 2006). To investigate this effect, gene expression profiling was performed on RNA isolated from astrocyte cultures generated from $SOD1^{G93A}$ rats (and litter mate controls). Perhaps surprisingly, there were limited differences in the transcriptional profiles of transgenic and non-transgenic astrocytes (Vargas et al 2008b). However, of the two genes most dysregulated, regulator of differentiation (*Rod1*) and decorin (*Dcn*), both showed consistent changes in asymptomatic and early symptomatic rats, implicating components of RNA processing and the extracellular matrix as contributors early in the disease process (Figure 1).

Primary neuronal cultures originating from $SOD1^{G93A}$ mice and subjected to oxidative stress (H_2O_2) or excitotoxicity (NMDA), demonstrated a greater level of cell death, compared to non-transgenic cultures (Boutahar et al 2011). Microarray analysis detected cytoskeletal remodelling and vesicular transport related genes as increased in response to oxidative stress, whilst genes involved in the ubiquitin-proteasome system and cytokines were increased following excitotoxicity (Figure 1). Several of these pathways have already been implicated as playing a pathogenic role in ALS and add further support to the idea that the proposed disease mechanisms are mutually compatible.

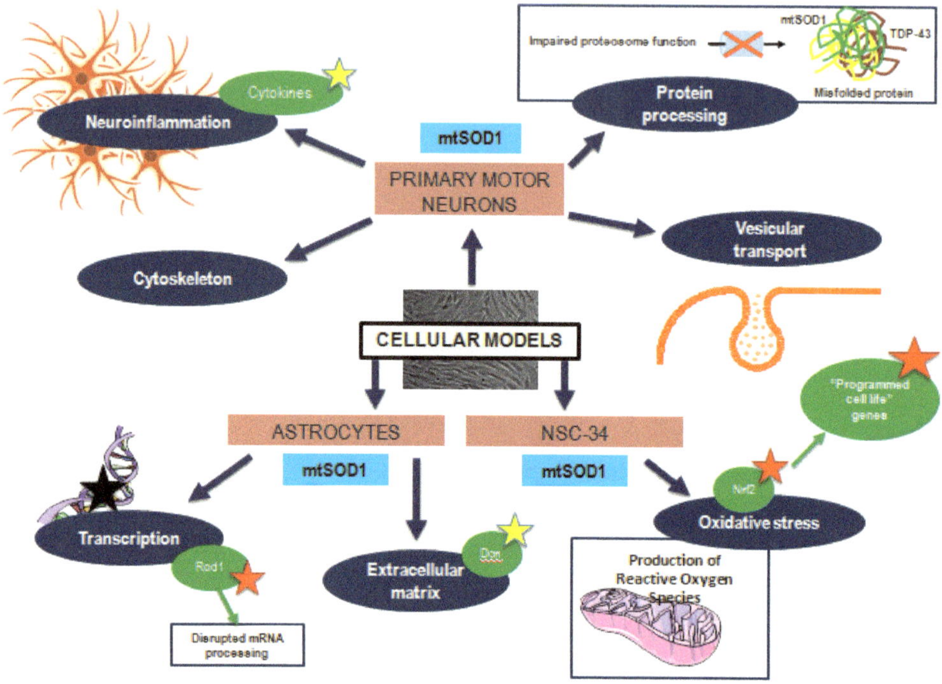

Fig. 1. Summary of prominent pathways arising from GEP of Cellular Models. Important changes in the transcriptome have been highlighted by green labels; yellow stars indicate up-regulation, red stars indicate down-regulation. Blue squares outline functional consequences of changes in the transcriptome. Further details are discussed in the text.

6. Results from use of animal models of ALS

6.1 Gene expression profiling of mixed cell type CNS samples

Microarray analysis of whole spinal cord homogenates from ALS mouse models have been performed by several research groups in order to obtain a global view of changes in the CNS prior to and during disease. Results from SOD1^{G93A} mice have shown that inflammation, apoptosis and adaptive responses to metal ion dysregulation are the main pathways activated in both pre-symptomatic mice and during the disease process (Olsen et al 2001; Yoshihara et al 2002) (Figure 2). Analysis of the SOD1^{L126delTT} transgenic mouse, which results in a truncated SOD1 protein, also showed pre-symptomatic changes related to the reactive gliosis which is occurring in the spinal cord (Fukada et al 2007).

Recently, transgenic mice carrying mutant TDP-43 have also contributed to better understanding the different mechanisms involved in ALS. Transgenic mice induced to express human TDP-43 without the nuclear localization signal (hTDP43-delNLS) developed signs of motor spasticity, neurone loss in forebrain regions and corticospinal tract degeneration (Igaz et al 2011). Microarray analysis of hTDP43-delNLS expression in the cortex of mutant mice, following 2 weeks induction of the mutant protein, detected dramatic changes in gene expression, with the most enriched pathway being chromatin assembly (Figure 2). Interestingly, after only 2 weeks of hTDP43-delNLS induction, markers of inflammation and neuronal loss were unchanged.

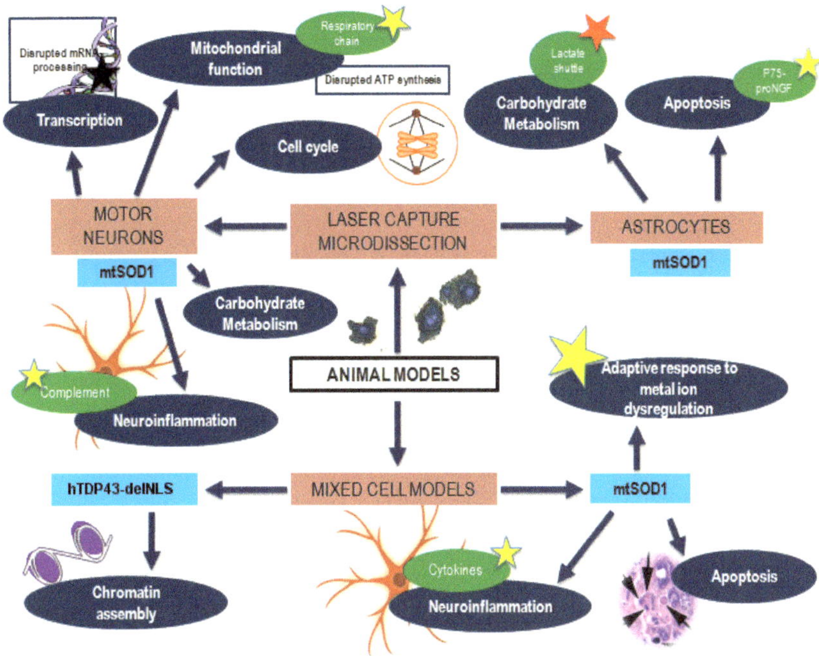

Fig. 2. Summary of prominent pathways arising from GEP of Animal Models. Important changes in the transcriptome have been highlighted by green labels; yellow stars indicate up-regulation, red stars indicate down-regulation. Blue squares outline functional consequences of changes in the transcriptome. Further details are discussed in the text.

Although these studies have greatly contributed to present knowledge on the transcriptional changes occurring in ALS, the analysis of a mixed cell population within the CNS has several disadvantages. This kind of approach does not identify which cell population is responsible for the transcriptional changes observed and only detects those transcripts most highly differentially expressed, with subtle but potential pivotal gene expression changes masked as well as changes in genes differentially expressed in one cell type, but not in others.

6.2 Gene expression profiling of laser capture microdissection isolated cell types

In order to overcome the limitations of using mixed cell population samples, dissection of single cells from complex tissues using LCM has been applied to identify the contribution of different cell types to the degenerative process occurring in ALS.

Several studies have determined the changes in gene expression occurring in motor neurones isolated from the spinal cord of mutant SOD1^{G93A} mice at different stages during the disease; from the pre-symptomatic stage to paralysis (Ferraiuolo et al 2007; Perrin et al 2005). The first report described transcriptional analysis of motor neurones isolated from SOD1^{G93A} mice bred on a mixed background and no differentially expressed genes were detected in the pre-symptomatic mice (Perrin et al 2005). However, in contrast to the whole tissue homogenates, motor neurones did not show activation of apoptotic genes, suggesting that cell death signals derive from other cell types in the spinal cord (Figure 2).

In the second publication, microarray analysis was carried out on SOD1^{G93A} mice bred on a homogeneous background; this enabled important changes in the motor neurones at the pre-symptomatic stage of disease, mainly involved in carbohydrate metabolism and transcription, to be detected (Ferraiuolo et al 2007). The upregulation of transcripts encoding proteins involved in the energy production pathway, i.e. tricarboxylic acid cycle and respiratory chain, suggested that motor neurones were trying to compensate for their increased energy needs in response to ongoing stress. At the late stage of disease, increased expression of transcripts involved in reactivation of the cell cycle (as an alternative pathway of cell death), and complement activation (a mechanism through which motor neurones can attract cells from the immune system), and down-regulation of transcription-related genes were identified (Figure 2).

To complement the gene expression profiling of motor neurones, astrocytes isolated from SOD1^{G93A} mice at the pre-symptomatic stage of disease were isolated and used for microarray analysis (Ferraiuolo et al 2011a). This enabled the cross-talk between the motor neurones and astrocytes at this very early time point to be interrogated. Interestingly, astrocytes displayed a marked impairment of carbohydrate metabolism (Figure 2). Comparing the expression profiles of the two cell types from the same SOD1^{G93A} mice highlighted that the metabolic impairment observed in motor neurones could derive from the lack of provision of substrates, i.e. lactate, from the astrocytes, and led to the conclusion that the lactate shuttle (the mechanism through which motor neurones and astrocytes combine metabolism and signalling through lactate and glutamate), is impaired. In addition, the activation of an important neuronal cell death pathway involving p75 and its ligand pro nerve growth factor (proNGF) was established. Gene expression profiling of SOD1^{G93A} astrocytes demonstrated that these cells expressed high levels of *Ngf*, while the motor neurones over-expressed the p75 receptor. *In vitro* data confirmed the dysregulation of both pathways and preliminary data from human ALS biosamples supported these findings from the murine model.

6.3 Gene expression profiling of peripheral tissue from mouse models

Microarray technology has also been applied to peripheral tissues from the SOD1^{G86R} mouse model (Gonzalez de Aguilar et al 2008). Profiling of the skeletal muscles revealed that the major expression changes happen at onset of disease, when muscles are activating pathways involved in detoxification and regeneration, but also cell death and tissue degradation. These findings revealed that while motor neurones are degenerating, muscles are undergoing major remodelling trying to compensate for muscle damage with new myogenesis. Whilst over-expression of transcripts such as cyclin-dependent kinase inhibitor-1A (*Cdkn1a*) and growth arrest-and DNA damage-inducible gene-45 (*Gadd45*) could be mediating apoptosis of myofibres resulting in muscle atrophy, increased expression B cell translocation gene-1 (*Btg1*), growth differentiation factor-5 (*Gdf5*) and myogenic factor-6 (*Myf6*) are potent activators of new fibre formation.

7. Results from use of human post-mortem material

7.1 Gene expression profiling of mixed cell type CNS samples

Multiple studies have utilised gene expression profiling of post mortem mixed cell samples from ALS patients and controls; these have either focused on using samples from the motor cortex (Lederer et al 2007; Wang et al 2006) or from the spinal cord (Dangond et al 2004; Malaspina et al 2001; Offen et al 2009). The majority used sporadic ALS (SALS) cases, though Dangond et al also sampled two FALS cases, one of which carried an *SOD1* mutation (Dangond et al 2004). Despite the different tissues profiled and the different platforms utilised, the studies showed some consistent results: All of the studies recorded altered gene expression related to inflammation and Malaspina and colleagues detected an increase in glial fibrillary acidic protein (*GFAP*), indicating active astrogliosis (Figure 3). In addition, a number of the studies discovered differential expression related to cytoskeleton function, protein processing and the antioxidant response, in agreement with other lines of research in ALS (Ferraiuolo et al 2011b).

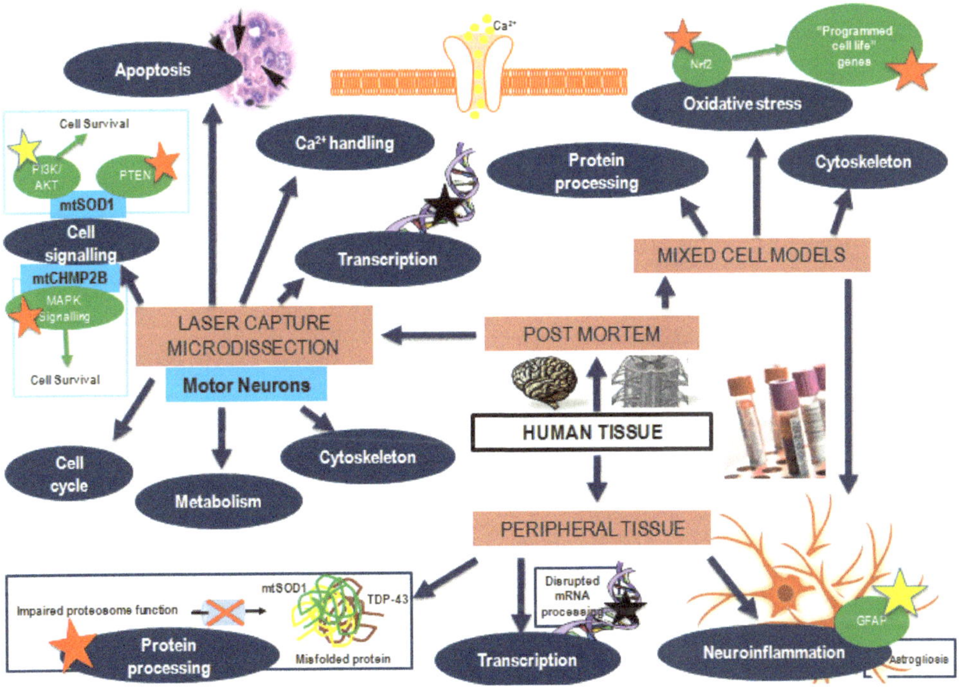

Fig. 3. Summary of prominent pathways arising from GEP of Human Tissue. Important changes in the transcriptome have been highlighted by green labels; yellow stars indicate up-regulation, red stars indicate down-regulation. Blue squares outline functional consequences of changes in the transcriptome. Further details can be found in the text.

7.2 Gene expression profiling of laser capture microdissection isolated cell types

As with the mouse models, in order to determine those genes differentially expressed in the vulnerable cell type, LCM has been used in post-mortem material to isolate the motor neurones from the spinal cord.

Motor neurones isolated from SALS cases and neurologically normal controls were shown to have distinct gene expression profiles compared to those generated from ventral horn homogenates, particularly with respect to those genes down-regulated in motor neurones (Jiang et al 2005). The motor neurones showed differential expression of genes associated with the cytoskeleton and evidence of decreased transcription, whilst cell death-associated genes and those involved in cell signalling were increased (Figure 3). In addition, cell cycle related genes were also reported as dysregulated, supporting the theory that inappropriate activation of the cell cycle in these post-mitotic cells leads to cell death. A follow-up study demonstrated that expression of several of these genes also correlated with pathological markers, such as phosphorylated neurofilament and ubiquitinated protein accumulations as well as motor neurone loss (Jiang et al 2007).

Gene expression profiling of isolated motor neurones has also been performed on ALS cases which carry genetic mutations in the *SOD1* and chromatin modifying protein 2B (*CHMP2B*) genes (Cox et al 2010; Kirby et al 2011). Motor neurones from *SOD1*-related cases of ALS showed increases in genes in the protein kinase B/phosphatidylinositol-3 kinase (AKT/PI3K) cell survival pathway, with concomitant decreases in negative regulators such as phophastase and tensin homologue (*PTEN*) (Kirby et al 2011) (Figure 3). Further work demonstrated that inhibition of PTEN led to increased activation of the AKT/PI3K pathway and increased neuronal survival in cell models including primary motor neurone cultures. Thus, activation of the AKT/PI3K pathway was proposed as a candidate for future therapeutic strategies.

The transcriptional profiles from motor neurones isolated from the *CHMP2B*-related ALS cases were distinct from those in *SOD1*-related cases (Cox et al 2010). These motor neurones showed dysregulation of genes involved in the classical and p38 MAPK signalling pathways, gene changes predicted to reflect reduced autophagy and repression of translation (Figure 3). The functional implication of *CHMP2B* mutations on cellular mechanisms was demonstrated by the presence of large cytoplasmic vacuoles and impairment of autophagy in a cellular model transfected with mutant *CHMP2B*, consistent with the microarray findings (Cox et al 2010). Interestingly, differential expression of genes encoding proteins responsible for calcium handling and cell cycle genes, as well as those genes involved in transcription, signalling and metabolism, was detected in both genetic subtypes.

8. Results from use of human peripheral tissue

Gene expression profiling has been conducted on blood and fibroblasts from ALS patients (Highley et al 2011; Saris et al 2009; Zhang et al 2011). Microarray analysis of SALS and control blood samples was followed by hierarchical clustering of all genes found to be significantly expressed in all samples after normalisation (Saris et al 2009). The method identified five clusters; two of which were able to differentiate between ALS and control samples. These clusters were replicated in a further two cohorts of patients and controls, demonstrating that such an analysis, which takes into account the interdependence of gene expression, is a means of reducing the false negative rate when subsequently detecting differential gene expression. This work also provided evidence that peripheral blood is a valuable medium for studying ALS. In addition, there was a correlation with the CNS tissue studies, as the blood in ALS patients showed a decrease in genes associated with protein processing and RNA post-transcriptional modification, as well as increases in genes associated with inflammation.

A more recent study performed gene expression profiling on peripheral blood mononuclear cells from patients with SALS (Zhang et al 2011). These cells showed an up-regulation of genes associated with immune activation in response to lipopolysaccharide (LPS), which correlated with an elevation of plasma LPS. Unfortunately, no correlation between expression of these genes and disease progression was provided.

Transcriptional profiles of fibroblasts from patients with SALS, FALS and controls have been shown to be informative in distinguishing the different genetic variants from each other, as well as from SALS patients, by their gene expression profiles and specifically the level of alternative splicing (Highley et al 2011). The FALS samples were derived from patients with mutations in *SOD1* and *TARDBP*. Using microarrays which interrogate every exon of every gene, it was demonstrated that there was a significant amount of aberrant splicing in the samples with a *TARDBP* mutation which was replicated to a lesser degree in the SALS samples and virtually absent in the samples with a *SOD1* mutation (Figure 3). In support of this, other work has identified aberrant splicing in cell and animal models with depletion of TDP-43 (Polymenidou et al 2011; Tollervey et al 2011).

9. The future of gene expression profiling in ALS

9.1 RNA sequencing (RNA-seq)

The advent of next generation sequencing has evolved to enable quantitative parallel sequencing of RNA transcripts from isolated cells and tissues. There are a number of advantages of next generation RNA sequencing over the microarray platform which in general extend from the fact that there is no reliance on the pre-designed probes which are present on the microarrays. In contrast, the methodology aims to sequence every base of every transcript of RNA. This leads to a better detection rate of known transcripts and splicing events and the detection of RNA transcripts (both coding and non-coding) which have not previously been described and therefore have no specific probe (Sultan et al 2008). As there is no reliance on probes, the problem of cross hybridisation is avoided. In addition, because each base in each transcript is sequenced, as well as providing information about expression level and alternative splicing, the sequencing also provides information about sequence variability within the RNA (Wang et al 2009). The biggest challenge to RNA sequencing, however, is the analysis of the large amounts of data produced which is substantially more than the read out of even the most comprehensive microarray. Not least among these challenges is the problem of mapping the RNA sequences to the genome, as in contrast to DNA sequencing, the absence of introns can lead to substantial difficulties (Sutherland et al 2011).

9.2 Role of microRNAs in ALS

This chapter has focused on the mRNA that is translated into protein. However, although 90% of eukaryotic genomic DNA is transcribed, only 1-2% actually encodes protein. The vast majority of transcribed material is comprised of non-coding RNA (ncRNA) and there is increasing evidence to support functional roles for at least a subset of these transcripts (Kaikkonen et al 2011). There are broadly two types of ncRNA, infrastructural (including transfer RNA and small nuclear RNA) and regulatory RNA (including microRNA, Piwi-interacting RNA and small interfering RNA). The function of ncRNAs remains largely unknown. However, research into microRNA (miRNA) has led the field in recent years. miRNAs are a class of small, ncRNA molecules predicted to post-transcriptionally regulate at least one third of human genes (Lewis et al 2005). Each miRNA can potentially target hundreds of genes and play key regulatory roles in a diverse range of pathways including development, differentiation and pathological processes such as neurodegeneration (Enciu et al 2011). The study of miRNA in ALS is at a very early stage. However, given the proposed role for TDP-43 in miRNA biogenesis and the recent discovery of a beneficial effect of miRNA-206 in the mutant SOD1 mouse model, this will be an interesting area of investigation for the future (Buratti et al 2010; Williams et al 2009)

9.3 Biomarkers in ALS

There is no diagnostic test for ALS, so diagnosis currently relies upon clinical assessment involving the exclusion of "ALS-mimic" syndromes (such as multifocal motor neuropathy and cervical radiculomyelopathy), causing an average delay of one year from symptom onset to a confirmed diagnosis (Silani et al 2011; Zoccolella et al 2006). In such a rapidly progressive disease this delay is a significant obstacle to potential neuroprotective therapies. ALS is clinically heterogeneous, with multiple subtypes associated with different survival times and symptoms making prognosis challenging. This heterogeneity is also a confounding factor for clinical trials as patient phenotype will impact upon survival data and may influence responses to therapeutic intervention, with some subtypes more responsive to therapy than others (Turner et al 2009). Robust biomarkers would therefore be valuable for the initial diagnosis of disease, the classification of various subtypes, monitoring responses to therapeutic agents and tracking disease progression (Turner et al 2009). Gene expression profiling offers a useful tool for biomarker discovery allowing patient and control biofluids, such as blood and CSF, to be compared on a genome wide scale. These tools have already been employed to improve classification and diagnosis of multiple diseases including neurodegenerative conditions such as Huntington's disease and Parkinson's disease (Borovecki et al 2005; Scherzer et al 2007).

10. Conclusion

In conclusion, microarray analysis has been pivotal in understanding the transcriptional alterations occurring in response to genetic mutations associated with ALS and the sporadic disease (SALS). The cellular model has generated a therapeutic target and transcriptional activation of *Nrf2* is currently being assessed *in-vivo*. Use of spinal cord and peripheral tissues from transgenic mouse models has provided a mechanism to look at the progression of the disease and specifically to identify early changes in the motor neurones and astrocytes. These dysregulated pathways provide future therapeutic targets. In addition, gene expression profiling has allowed crucial insights into the mechanisms affecting different areas of the motor system, with the combination of LCM and microarray technology able to discriminate changes in specific cell types and understand how these affect each other and contribute to disease progression. Finally, the use of human material has begun to allow the distinctions between genetic and sporadic disease to be differentiated as well as providing further candidates for therapeutic approaches. In the future, gene expression profiling of larger, consistently collected patient samples has the potential to generate robust and reliable prognostic and diagnostic biomarkers, which will ultimately be applicable for use in the clinic.

11. Acknowledgments

PJS and JK are funded by the European Community's Health Seventh Framework Programme (FP7/2007-2013) under grant agreement 259867 and by the Motor Neurone Disease Association (MNDA). EFG is also funded by the MNDA.

12. References

Aguirre T, Van Den Bosch L, Goetschalckx K, Tilkin P, Mathijs G, et al. 1998. Increased sensitivity of fibroblasts from amyotrophic lateral sclerosis patients to oxidative stress. *Ann Neurol* 43:452-7

Booij BB, Lindahl T, Wetterberg P, Skaane NV, Saebo S, et al. 2011. A gene expression pattern in blood for the early detection of Alzheimer's disease. *J Alzheimers Dis* 23:109-19

Borovecki F, Lovrecic L, Zhou J, Jeong H, Then F, et al. 2005. Genome-wide expression profiling of human blood reveals biomarkers for Huntington's disease. *Proc Natl Acad Sci U S A* 102:11023-8

Boutahar N, Wierinckx A, Camdessanche JP, Antoine JC, Reynaud E, et al. 2011. Differential effect of oxidative or excitotoxic stress on the transcriptional profile of amyotrophic lateral sclerosis-linked mutant SOD1 cultured neurons. *J Neurosci Res* 89:1439-50

Budini M, Buratti E. 2011. TDP-43 Autoregulation: Implications for Disease. *J Mol Neurosci*

Buratti E, De Conti L, Stuani C, Romano M, Baralle M, Baralle F. 2010. Nuclear factor TDP-43 can affect selected microRNA levels. *FEBS J* 277:2268-81

Cashman NR, Durham HD, Blusztajn JK, Oda K, Tabira T, et al. 1992. Neuroblastoma x spinal cord (NSC) hybrid cell lines resemble developing motor neurons. *Dev Dyn* 194:209-21

Cox LE, Ferraiuolo L, Goodall EF, Heath PR, Higginbottom A, et al. 2010. Mutations in CHMP2B in lower motor neuron predominant amyotrophic lateral sclerosis (ALS). *PLoS ONE* 5:e9872

Dadon-Nachum M, Melamed E, Offen D. 2011. The "dying-back" phenomenon of motor neurons in ALS. *J Mol Neurosci* 43:470-7

Dangond F, Hwang D, Camelo S, Pasinelli P, Frosch MP, et al. 2004. Molecular signature of late-stage human ALS revealed by expression profiling of postmortem spinal cord gray matter. *Physiol Genomics* 16:229-39

Dimos JT, Rodolfa KT, Niakan KK, Weisenthal LM, Mitsumoto H, et al. 2008. Induced pluripotent stem cells generated from patients with ALS can be differentiated into motor neurons. *Science* 321:1218-21

Duan W, Li X, Shi J, Guo Y, Li Z, Li C. 2010. Mutant TAR DNA-binding protein-43 induces oxidative injury in motor neuron-like cell. *Neuroscience* 169:1621-9

Dupuis L, Loeffler JP. 2009. Neuromuscular junction destruction during amyotrophic lateral sclerosis: insights from transgenic models. *Curr Opin Pharmacol* 9:341-6

Durham HD, Dahrouge S, Cashman NR. 1993. Evaluation of the spinal cord neuron X neuroblastoma hybrid cell line NSC-34 as a model for neurotoxicity testing. *Neurotoxicology* 14:387-95

Durham HD, Roy J, Dong L, Figlewicz DA. 1997. Aggregation of mutant Cu/Zn superoxide dismutase proteins in a culture model of ALS. *J Neuropathol Exp Neurol* 56:523-30

Enciu AM, Popescu BO, Gheorghisan-Galateanu A. 2011. MicroRNAs in brain development and degeneration. *Mol Biol Rep* 10.1007/s11033-011-0973-1:(Epub ahead of print)

Ferraiuolo L, Heath PR, Holden H, Kasher P, Kirby J, Shaw PJ. 2007. Microarray analysis of the cellular pathways involved in the adaptation to and progression of motor neuron injury in the SOD1 G93A mouse model of familial ALS. *J Neurosci* 27:9201-19

Ferraiuolo L, Higginbottom A, Heath P, Barber S, Greenald D, et al. 2011a. Dysregulation of astrocyte-motor neuron cross-talk in mutant SOD1 related amyotrophic lateral sclerosis. *Brain* (In Press)

Ferraiuolo L, Kirby J, Grierson AJ, Sendtner M, Shaw PJ. 2011b. Molecular and cellular pathways of motor neuron injury in amyotrophic lateral sclerosis. *Nat Rev Neurology* (In Press)

Fukada Y, Yasui K, Kitayama M, Doi K, Nakano T, et al. 2007. Gene expression analysis of the murine model of amyotrophic lateral sclerosis: studies of the Leu126delTT mutation in SOD1. *Brain Res* 1160:1-10

Gonzalez de Aguilar JL, Niederhauser-Wiederkehr C, Halter B, De Tapia M, Di Scala F, et al. 2008. Gene profiling of skeletal muscle in an amyotrophic lateral sclerosis mouse model. *Physiol Genomics* 32:207-18

Gurney ME, Pu H, Chiu AY, Dal Canto MC, Polchow CY, et al. 1994. Motor neuron degeneration in mice that express a human Cu,Zn superoxide dismutase mutation. *Science* 264:1772-5

Highley JR, Hewamadduma C, Jansweijer JA, Kirby J, Heath PR, et al. 2011. Amyotrophic lateral sclerosis-causing TARDBP (TDP-43) mutations cause widespread dysregulation of mRNA splicing in cell lines from human patients. *PLoS ONE* (Under Review)

Hoepken HH, Gispert S, Azizov M, Klinkenberg M, Ricciardi F, et al. 2008. Parkinson patient fibroblasts show increased alpha-synuclein expression. *Exp Neurol* 212:307-13

Hosack DA, Dennis G, Jr., Sherman BT, Lane HC, Lempicki RA. 2003. Identifying biological themes within lists of genes with EASE. *Genome Biol* 4:R70

Igaz LM, Kwong LK, Chen-Plotkin A, Winton MJ, Unger TL, et al. 2009. Expression of TDP-43 C-terminal Fragments in Vitro Recapitulates Pathological Features of TDP-43 Proteinopathies. *J Biol Chem* 284:8516-24

Igaz LM, Kwong LK, Lee EB, Chen-Plotkin A, Swanson E, et al. 2011. Dysregulation of the ALS-associated gene TDP-43 leads to neuronal death and degeneration in mice. *J Clin Invest* 121:726-38

Jiang YM, Yamamoto M, Kobayashi Y, Yoshihara T, Liang Y, et al. 2005. Gene expression profile of spinal motor neurons in sporadic amyotrophic lateral sclerosis. *Ann Neurol* 57:236-51

Jiang YM, Yamamoto M, Tanaka F, Ishigaki S, Katsuno M, et al. 2007. Gene expressions specifically detected in motor neurons (dynactin 1, early growth response 3, acetyl-CoA transporter, death receptor 5, and cyclin C) differentially correlate to pathologic markers in sporadic amyotrophic lateral sclerosis. *J Neuropathol Exp Neurol* 66:617-27

Kaikkonen MU, Lam MT, Glass CK. 2011. Non-coding RNAs as regulators of gene expression and epigenetics. *Cardiovasc Res* 90:430-40

Kirby J, Halligan E, Baptista MJ, Allen S, Heath PR, et al. 2005. Mutant SOD1 alters the motor neuronal transcriptome: implications for familial ALS. *Brain* 128:1686-706

Kirby J, Ning K, Ferraiuolo L, Heath PR, Ismail A, et al. 2011. Phosphatase and tensin homologue/protein kinase B pathway linked to motor neuron survival in human superoxide dismutase 1-related amyotrophic lateral sclerosis. *Brain* 134:506-17

Lederer CW, Torrisi A, Pantelidou M, Santama N, Cavallaro S. 2007. Pathways and genes differentially expressed in the motor cortex of patients with sporadic amyotrophic lateral sclerosis. *BMC Genomics* 8:26

Lewis BP, Burge CB, Bartel DP. 2005. Conserved seed pairing, often flanked by adenosines, indicates that thousands of human genes are microRNA targets. *Cell* 120:15-20

Liew CC, Ma J, Tang HC, Zheng R, Dempsey AA. 2006. The peripheral blood transcriptome dynamically reflects system wide biology: a potential diagnostic tool. *The Journal of Laboratory and Clinical Medicine* 147:126-32

Liu J, Walter E, Stenger D, Thach D. 2006. Effects of globin mRNA reduction methods on gene expression profiles from whole blood. *J Mol Diagn* 8:551-8

Maes OC, Xu S, Yu B, Chertkow HM, Wang E, Schipper HM. 2007. Transcriptional profiling of Alzheimer blood mononuclear cells by microarray. *Neurobiology of Aging* 28:1795-809

Malaspina A, Kaushik N, de Belleroche J. 2001. Differential expression of 14 genes in amyotrophic lateral sclerosis spinal cord detected using gridded cDNA arrays. *J Neurochem* 77:132-45

Menzies FM, Cookson MR, Taylor RW, Turnbull DM, Chrzanowska-Lightowlers ZM, et al. 2002a. Mitochondrial dysfunction in a cell culture model of familial amyotrophic lateral sclerosis. *Brain* 125:1522-33

Menzies FM, Grierson AJ, Cookson MR, Heath PR, Tomkins J, et al. 2002b. Selective loss of neurofilament expression in Cu/Zn superoxide dismutase (SOD1) linked amyotrophic lateral sclerosis. *J Neurochem* 82:1118-28

Mohr S, Liew CC. 2007. The peripheral-blood transcriptome: new insights into disease and risk assessment. *Trends Mol Med* 13:422-32

Mortiboys H, Thomas KJ, Koopman WJ, Klaffke S, Abou-Sleiman P, et al. 2008. Mitochondrial function and morphology are impaired in parkin-mutant fibroblasts. *Ann Neurol* 64:555-65

Nagai M, Re DB, Nagata T, Chalazonitis A, Jessell TM, et al. 2007. Astrocytes expressing ALS-linked mutated SOD1 release factors selectively toxic to motor neurons. *Nat Neurosci* 10:615-22

Nagasaka Y, Dillner K, Ebise H, Teramoto R, Nakagawa H, et al. 2005. A unique gene expression signature discriminates familial Alzheimer's disease mutation carriers from their wild-type siblings. *Proc Natl Acad Sci U S A* 102:14854-9

Neymotin A, Calingasan NY, Wille E, Naseri N, Petri S, et al. 2011. Neuroprotective effect of Nrf2/ARE activators, CDDO ethylamide and CDDO trifluoroethylamide, in a mouse model of amyotrophic lateral sclerosis. *Free Radic Biol Med* 51:88-96

Offen D, Barhum Y, Melamed E, Embacher N, Schindler C, Ransmayr G. 2009. Spinal cord mRNA profile in patients with ALS: comparison with transgenic mice expressing the human SOD-1 mutant. *J Mol Neurosci* 38:85-93

Olsen MK, Roberds SL, Ellerbrock BR, Fleck TJ, McKinley DK, Gurney ME. 2001. Disease mechanisms revealed by transcription profiling in SOD1-G93A transgenic mouse spinal cord. *Ann Neurol* 50:730-40

Perrin FE, Boisset G, Docquier M, Schaad O, Descombes P, Kato AC. 2005. No widespread induction of cell death genes occurs in pure motoneurons in an amyotrophic lateral sclerosis mouse model. *Hum Mol Genet* 14:3309-20

Polymenidou M, Lagier-Tourenne C, Hutt KR, Huelga SC, Moran J, et al. 2011. Long pre-mRNA depletion and RNA missplicing contribute to neuronal vulnerability from loss of TDP-43. *Nat Neurosci* 14:459-68

Ripps ME, Huntley GW, Hof PR, Morrison JH, Gordon JW. 1995. Transgenic mice expressing an altered murine superoxide dismutase gene provide an animal model of amyotrophic lateral sclerosis. *Proc Natl Acad Sci U S A* 92:689-93

Saris CG, Horvath S, van Vught PW, van Es MA, Blauw HM, et al. 2009. Weighted gene co-expression network analysis of the peripheral blood from Amyotrophic Lateral Sclerosis patients. *BMC Genomics* 10:405

Sarlette A, Krampfl K, Grothe C, Neuhoff N, Dengler R, Petri S. 2008. Nuclear erythroid 2-related factor 2-antioxidative response element signaling pathway in motor cortex and spinal cord in amyotrophic lateral sclerosis. *J Neuropathol Exp Neurol* 67:1055-62

Scherzer CR, Eklund AC, Morse LJ, Liao Z, Locascio JJ, et al. 2007. Molecular markers of early Parkinson's disease based on gene expression in blood. *Proc Natl Acad Sci U S A* 104:955-60

Sharp FR, Lit L, Xu H, Apperson M, Walker W, et al. 2006. Genomics of brain and blood: progress and pitfalls. *Epilepsia* 47:1603-7

Shtilbans A, Choi SG, Fowkes ME, Khitrov G, Shahbazi M, et al. 2011. Differential gene expression in patients with amyotrophic lateral sclerosis. *Amyotroph Lateral Scler* 12:250-6

Silani V, Messina S, Poletti B, Morelli C, Doretti A, et al. 2011. The diagnosis of Amyotrophic lateral sclerosis in 2010. *Arch Ital Biol* 149:5-27

Son EY, Ichida JK, Wainger BJ, Toma JS, Rafuse VF, et al. 2011. Conversion of Mouse and Human Fibroblasts into Functional Spinal Motor Neurons. *Cell Stem Cell* DOI: 10.1016/j.stem.2011.07.014:(Epub ahead of print)

Stallings NR, Puttaparthi K, Luther CM, Burns DK, Elliott JL. 2010. Progressive motor weakness in transgenic mice expressing human TDP-43. *Neurobiol Dis* 40:404-14

Stoughton RB. 2005. Applications of DNA microarrays in biology. *Annu Rev Biochem* 74:53-82

Sultan M, Schulz MH, Richard H, Magen A, Klingenhoff A, et al. 2008. A global view of gene activity and alternative splicing by deep sequencing of the human transcriptome. *Science* 321:956-60

Sutherland GT, Janitz M, Kril JJ. 2011. Understanding the pathogenesis of Alzheimer's disease: will RNA-Seq realize the promise of transcriptomics? *J Neurochem* 116:937-46

Tollervey JR, Curk T, Rogelj B, Briese M, Cereda M, et al. 2011. Characterizing the RNA targets and position-dependent splicing regulation by TDP-43. *Nat Neurosci* 14:452-8

Tsuang MT, Nossova N, Yager T, Tsuang MM, Guo SC, et al. 2005. Assessing the validity of blood-based gene expression profiles for the classification of schizophrenia and bipolar disorder: a preliminary report. *Am J Med Genet B Neuropsychiatr Genet* 133B:1-5

Turner MR, Kiernan MC, Leigh PN, Talbot K. 2009. Biomarkers in amyotrophic lateral sclerosis. *Lancet Neurol* 8:94-109

Vargas MR, Johnson DA, Sirkis DW, Messing A, Johnson JA. 2008a. Nrf2 activation in astrocytes protects against neurodegeneration in mouse models of familial amyotrophic lateral sclerosis. *J Neurosci* 28:13574-81

Vargas MR, Pehar M, Cassina P, Beckman JS, Barbeito L. 2006. Increased glutathione biosynthesis by Nrf2 activation in astrocytes prevents p75NTR-dependent motor neuron apoptosis. *J Neurochem* 97:687-96

Vargas MR, Pehar M, Diaz-Amarilla PJ, Beckman JS, Barbeito L. 2008b. Transcriptional profile of primary astrocytes expressing ALS-linked mutant SOD1. *J Neurosci Res* 86:3515-25

Wang XS, Simmons Z, Liu W, Boyer PJ, Connor JR. 2006. Differential expression of genes in amyotrophic lateral sclerosis revealed by profiling the post mortem cortex. *Amyotroph Lateral Scler* 7:201-10

Wang Z, Gerstein M, Snyder M. 2009. RNA-Seq: a revolutionary tool for transcriptomics. *Nat Rev Genet* 10:57-63

Whitney AR, Diehn M, Popper SJ, Alizadeh AA, Boldrick JC, et al. 2003. Individuality and variation in gene expression patterns in human blood. *Proc Natl Acad Sci U S A* 100:1896-901

Williams AH, Valdez G, Moresi V, Qi X, McAnally J, et al. 2009. MicroRNA-206 delays ALS progression and promotes regeneration of neuromuscular synapses in mice. *Science* 326:1549-54

Wright C, Bergstrom D, Dai H, Marton M, Morris M, et al. 2008. Characterization of globin RNA interference in gene expression profiling of whole-blood samples. *Clinical chemistry* 54:396-405

Yoshihara T, Ishigaki S, Yamamoto M, Liang Y, Niwa J, et al. 2002. Differential expression of inflammation- and apoptosis-related genes in spinal cords of a mutant SOD1 transgenic mouse model of familial amyotrophic lateral sclerosis. *J Neurochem* 80:158-67

Zhang R, Hadlock KG, Do H, Yu S, Honrada R, et al. 2011. Gene expression profiling in peripheral blood mononuclear cells from patients with sporadic amyotrophic lateral sclerosis (sALS). *J Neuroimmunol* 230:114-23

Zoccolella S, Beghi E, Palagano G, Fraddosio A, Samarelli V, et al. 2006. Predictors of delay in the diagnosis and clinical trial entry of amyotrophic lateral sclerosis patients: a population-based study. *J Neurol Sci* 250:45-9

4

In Vivo and *In Vitro* Models to Study Amyotrophic Lateral Sclerosis

François Berthod and François Gros-Louis
Centre LOEX de l'Université Laval,
Centre de recherche FRSQ du Centre hospitalier affilié universitaire de Québec,
Département de Chirurgie, Faculté de Médecine, Université Laval, Québec,
Canada

1. Introduction

Amyotrophic Lateral Sclerosis (ALS) is the most common adult-onset neurodegenerative disorder characterized by the death of large motor neurons in the cerebral cortex and spinal cord (Tandan and Bradley, 1985). Dysfunction and death of these cell populations lead to progressive muscle weakness, atrophy, fasciculations, spasticity and ultimately, paralysis and death usually within 3 to 5 years after disease onset (Mulder, 1982). The estimated worldwide incidence for this disease is around 2 per 100,000 in the general population and the life-long risk to develop ALS is approximately 1:2000. The disease occurs in sporadic (90%) and familial forms (10%) (Gros-Louis, et al., 2006). With the exception of few FALS cases in which other neurodegenerative disorders can simultaneously occur, FALS and SALS are clinically indistinguishable. To date, mutations in the Cu/Zn superoxide dismutase 1 (*SOD1*) gene have remained the major known genetic causes associated with ALS. However, the mechanism whereby mutant SOD1 causes specific degeneration of motor neurons remains unclear. Nonetheless, many neuronal death pathways have been revealed through studies with transgenic mice expressing SOD1 mutants. Other vertebrate, invertebrate and *in vitro* models of ALS have also been described. Here, we will review various animal and cellular models that have been used to study the toxicity of ALS-linked gene mutations and also to investigate pathological hallmarks of the disease.

1.1 Familial ALS

Though most cases of ALS are sporadic, 10% of cases have affected relatives, some with clear Mendelian inheritance and high penetrance (Gros-Louis, et al., 2006). The landmark discovery in 1993 of missense mutations in the *SOD1* gene in subsets of familial cases directed most ALS research to elucidate the mechanism of SOD1-mediadted disease (Rosen, et al., 1993). More recently, mutations in two other genes, *TARDBP* and *FUS/TLS* have been found in ALS patients (Kabashi, et al., 2008; Sreedharan, et al., 2008; Vance, et al., 2009). Rare mutations in other genes such as *ANG, ALS2, DCTN1, MAPT, SETX* and *VAPB* have also been described (for reviews see (Gros-Louis, et al., 2006)). Various other genetic mutations in the *ELP3* ((Simpson, et al., 2009), *FIG4* (Chow, et al., 2009), *DAO* (Mitchell, et al., 2010), *OPTN* (Maruyama, et al., 2010) and *CHGB* (Gros-Louis, et al., 2009a) genes have also been associated with the disease through several candidate gene-based association studies. Given the high degree of genetic and clinical heterogeneity seen in ALS patients, along with population-specific genetic risk factors for ALS, independent replication of these genetic association studies would be crucial in order to better understand the different mechanisms involved in these disease. As there are several excellent reviews in the literature describing these genes and their relevance to ALS, we will mainly describe the most recent and exciting advances involving *SOD1*, *TARDBP* and *FUS* in this area.

To date, family-based linkage studies and positional cloning have led to the identification of fifteen ALS-associated genes in which mutations have been identified in familial ALS cases (Table 1). Different research groups or consortiums have replicated these results in several populations. To date, a number of genes have been discovered as causative for the classical adult onset form of familial ALS with typical symptoms, namely *SOD1*, *TARDBP*, *FUS/TLS*, and *C9ORF72* (DeJesus-Hernandez, et al., 2011; Kabashi, et al., 2008; Kwiatkowski, et al., 2009; Renton, et al., 2011; Rosen, et al., 1993; Sreedharan, et al., 2008). These genes cumulatively account for about 25% of familial cases, indicating that other causative genes remain to be identified. The difficulties to identify gene responsible for FALS arise in part because large families with sufficient statistical power for linkage analysis are hard to come by, due to the late-onset and age-dependant penetrance of the disease, and the relative short survival time of affected ALS patients. Furthermore, the high degree of genetic heterogeneity, i.e. many rare variants in many different genes individually having a modest effect on the total number of ALS cases, is also certainly a limiting factor for the identification of causative ALS-predisposing genes. Four other genes, namely *DAO*, *OPTN*, *ATAX2* and *VCP* have also been included in this category, but the evidence for their role in predisposing to classical ALS needs to be confirmed in replication studies, and more families linked to these genes also need to be described (Elden, et al., 2010; Johnson, et al., 2010; Maruyama, et al., 2010; Mitchell, et al., 2010).

FALS-associated known genes (gene symbol)	Inheritance	Onset	Mutation types	References
Superoxyde dismutase 1 (SOD1)	AD	Adult	Missense and truncation mutation	Rosen et al., 1993
TAR DNA-binding protein (TARDBP)	AD	Adult	Missense and nonsense mutations	Kabashi et al., 2008; Sreedharan et al., 2008
Fused in sarcoma/translated in liposarcoma (FUS/TL	AD and AR	Adult	Missense mutations, indels	Kwiatkowski et al., 2009; Vance et al., 2009
Chromosome 9 opend reading frame 72 (C9ORF72)	AD	Adult	Hexanucleotide GGGGCC expansion repea	enton et al., 2011, DeJesus-Hernandez et al., 201
Ataxin 2 (ATAX2)	AD	Adult	Trinucleotide CAG expansion repeat	Elden et al., 2010
Ubiquitin-like protein ubiquilin2 (UBQLN2)	X-linked	Adult	Missense mutations	Deng et al., 2011
Optineurin (OPTN)	AD	Adult	Missense and nonsense mutations	Maruyama et al., 2010
D-amino acid oxidase (DAO)	AD	Adult	One R199W missense mutation	Mitchell et al., 2010
Amyotrophic lateral sclerosis 2 (ALS2)	AR	Juvenile	Missense and nonsense mutations	Hadano et al., 2002, Yang et al., 2002
Valosin-containing protein (VCP)	AD	Adult	Missense mutations	Johnson et al., 2010
Vesicle-associated membrane protein B (VAPB)	AD	Adult	Missense mutations	Nishimura et al., 2004
Microtubule-associated protein tau (MAPT)	AD	Adult	Missense and 5'-splice-site mutations	Hutton et al., 1998
Dynactin 1 (DCTN1)	AD	Adult	Missense mutations	Puls et al., 2003
Angiogenin	AD	Adult	Missense mutations	Chen et al., 2004
Senataxin (SETX)	AD	Juvenile	Missense mutations	Greeway et al., 2006

Table 1. Identified genes predisposing for familial ALS and/or ALS-FTLD
FALS: Familial ALS, ALS-FTLD: ALS with frontotemporal lobar degeneration,
AD: autosomal dominant, AR: autosomal recessive, Indels: insertions, deletions

The identification of other genes responsible for the disease and the understanding of the molecular pathways involved will bring some new insights into the mechanisms of disease pathogenesis, and may also elucidate the underlying mechanism(s) for specific motor neuron degeneration observed in ALS.

1.2 Sporadic ALS

For most cases of ALS, the causes are unknown. A genetic component is also thought to contribute to the pathogenesis of sporadic ALS, which accounts for the majority of ALS cases. However, identification of gene mutations associated with SALS has met with limited success so far. Several groups have reported on gene variants and association studies found in individuals with sporadic ALS, each accounting for a small number of the total cases reflecting a complex pattern of inheritance with very low penetrance, a high degree of heterogeneity and/or the existence of environmental factors predisposing to ALS. Because familial and sporadic forms of the disease are clinically and pathologically similar, understanding the familial form will shed light on possible epidemiological and pathophysiological mechanisms in SALS.

Many divergent data generated by different research groups who have studied different populations around the world have been published. The use of an adequate size population with appropriate control individuals is needed in order to reach enough statistical power and to observe any significant results. Homogeneity regarding ethnical origin, age, age of onset, disease duration, site of the first symptoms and gender among the studied populations is essential to design a good and robust genetic study. The requirement for larger sample sizes and possibly more sensitive and efficient analytic tools allowing for reliable detection across studied populations are now becoming more and more available as non cost-effective genotyping strategies are being developed.

The identifications of different genes and genetic risk factors associated with ALS over the past years have highlighted common molecular pathways mainly involving intracellular cell trafficking and RNA metabolism. To what extent these pathways are implicated in ALS remain to be determined and studied further. However, it is interesting to note that genes such as *ALS2, VAPB, MAPT, DCTN1, EAAT2, NEFH, PRPH, FIG4, CNTF, CHGB* and *OPTN* in which mutations have been found in a subset of FALS and/or SALS patients, are all related to intracellular trafficking either via axonal transport, vesicle docking and transport, or microtubule and neurofilament stabilization. Furthermore, this common theme is also seen in other motor neuron diseases and neurodegenerative disorders such as hereditary spastic paraplegia, Parkinson's disease, spinal muscular atrophy and Charcot-Marie-tooth disease. It is also noteworthy that RNA metabolism via alternative splicing abnormalities or RNA binding is also a common theme observed amongst the different ALS related genes such as *ALS2, MAPT, EAAT2, PRPH, GluR2, CNTF, SETX, SMN1, SMN2, TARDBP and FUS/TLS.* The high degree of genetic heterogeneity observed in ALS suggests that an individual phenotype could result from the sum of several contributing gene defects and/or epigenetic influences, which individually do not cause disease, and may explain the difficulties in identifying genes associated with SALS. The identification of other genes associated with motor neuron disease, as well as the determination of genetic and/or environmental factors that predispose to SALS is crucial in the development of novel therapies for ALS. The generation of cellular or animal models to study SALS, in which the disease can be closely replicated, would also be the utmost importance to reach a full understanding of the molecular mechanisms and environmental factors associated with SALS.

1.3 ALS with cognitive impairments

In recent years, key developments have revealed a novel neurodegenerative disease spectrum with clinical symptoms overlapping between ALS and frontotemporal lobar degeneration (FTLD) (Strong and Yang, 2011). Cognitive and behavioral impairment is well described in ALS with a significant proportion of patients meeting strict diagnostic criteria for FTLD. Neuroimaging and pathological studies have shown clear involvement of non-motor areas of the brain. More recently, distinct subtypes of frontotemporal lobar dysfunction have been identified in ALS and further work to distinguish these phenotypes and their correlate neuropathology is under way. Attention has been devoted lately to a gene coding for a DNA/RNA binding protein, which have been implicated in the pathogenesis of ALS with cognitive impairments. Indeed, dominant mutations in the *TARDBP* gene, encoding for TDP-43, were reported by several groups as a primary cause of ALS in about 3% familial cases and 1.5% sporadic cases (Chio, et al., 2011; Corrado, et al., 2009; Daoud, et al., 2009; Gitcho, et al., 2008; Kabashi, et al., 2008; Millecamps, et al., 2010; Sreedharan, et al., 2008; Van Deerlin, et al., 2008). The discovery of gene mutations linked to human ALS has provided plethora opportunities to develop model systems for investigating mechanisms of TDP-43 associated disease.

Motor neuron degeneration can also occasionally occurs in patients with Parkinson's disease and frontotemporal dementia (FTD). This disease is also called Disinhibition-dementia-parkinsonism-amyotrophy complex (DDPAC) or FTDP17 (Lynch, et al., 1994). The pathologic features distinguish this disease from the ALS-parkinsonism-dementia complex of Guam seen in the peninsula of Japan and from ALS-FTD linked to chromosome 9. Mutations in the *microtubule-associated protein tau* gene (*MAPT*) have been shown to be associated with FTD and Parkinsonism (Hutton, et al., 1998). Tau is a member of the microtubule-associated protein family, which have the principal function stabilizing microtubules and promoting their assembly by binding to tubulin. As a number of reviews (Gros-Louis, et al., 2006; Julien and Kriz, 2006) have already described the relationship between MAPT and ALS, the following sections will not discuss in details about this gene and FTDP17 models that have been generated.

2. In vivo models to study ALS

The exact mechanisms by which all the above-described gene products are involved in ALS pathogenesis are the subject of many ongoing researches. Current thinking about ALS pathogenesis revolves around the interplay between pre-existing genetic susceptibility and environmental factors that may trigger disease. The search for putative environmental factors has remained elusive however; transgenic animal studies have yielded the greatest wealth of information to date. Through these studies, multiple cellular pathways have been identified including, protein misfolding, RNA processing, oxidative stress, excitotoxicity, axonal transport, mitochondrial dysfunction and abnormal secretion of proteins. Nevertheless, how accurately these animal models replicate all ALS clinical symptoms of the human illness remains an unanswered and troublesome question. This section will include the complete description of all published invertebrate and vertebrate models of ALS. Other considerations such as advantages, disadvantages, cost and availability of each model will also be discussed. Each model organism has its own advantages and disadvantages. Choosing an appropriate model depends on the question being asked. Many laboratories find it useful to perform parallel experiments in two or more model systems to understand different aspects of a biochemical process.

2.1 Invertebrate models

Invertebrate model organisms include systems such as the simple yeast (fungi), fly, and nematode. The study of these experimental systems began with genetics and development, moved into molecular and cellular biology prior to most recently propelled into functional genomics and proteomics. These model organisms have highly manipulable genomes allowing for rapid generation of transgenic lines to provide insight on gene functions and protein network interactions. In 2002, Sydner Brenner, Robert Horvitz and John Sulston received the Nobel Prize in Physiology and Medicine for their establishment of the nematode *Caenorhadditis elegans* as a novel model organism to explore the molecular bases of organ development and cell death. Their discoveries identified key genes involved in cell division, differentiation and apoptosis. They determined that these genes were in fact highly conserved both structurally and functionally with higher organisms, including humans. Their studies provided the framework in which simpler organisms can be used to define key pathways and processes of relevance with the important benefit that the results are often directly applicable to understand human diseases.

The key points into generating models for human disease using smaller invertebrate organisms should encompass high degree of conservation with mammals in order for the model to be useful for the identification of the molecular components implicated in disease pathogenesis. A fully sequenced genome of the studied organism should ideally be also easily accessible for genome comparison with higher vertebrates and mammals in order to facilitate evolutionary genomics studies and to quickly generate transgenic animals through DNA transformation. The model organism should also provide significant experimental advantages over their mammalian counterparts, including a short generation time, small size, ease and reasonable cost of maintenance. It should be also amenable to both forward (phenotype to gene) and reverse (gene to phenotype) genetic approaches, which are essential molecular tools to dissect out and understand gene function. Classic forward genetic characteristics allow for the identification of novel molecules or pathways involved in a particular cellular process. This can be one of the most powerful attributes of invertebrate models. Forward-genetic screens using chemical mutagens are one of the most universal ways to generate mutants to elucidate gene function. On the other side, reverse genetics allows the quick identification of pathways on which a particular gene acts. Genetic knockdown mutants, using RNA interference (RNAi) technology in which a gene product is dramatically reduced by introducing double-stranded RNA (dsRNA) into the organism, can also provide invaluable information on the role a gene plays in a biological process.

The obvious disadvantage of using invertebrate model organisms such as fly or worm models is that there are evolutionarily far from mammals and that many physiological functions are not conserved, e.g. the immune system. Furthermore, their organs are extremely undeveloped and simple compared to other animals. The limited cellular diversity also represents a major disadvantage.

2.1.1 Caenorhabditis elegans

Yet, for the vast majority of neurodegenerative disorders including ALS, the mechanisms underlying neuronal dysfunction and death remain poorly understood despite the identification of relevant disease genes. Given the fact that molecular conservation in neuronal signaling pathways across vertebrate and invertebrate is relatively high and since the *Caenorhabditis elegans* nervous system contains almost all of the known signaling and neurotransmitter systems found in mammals (Bargmann, 1998), many researchers have turned to this model organism to identify the mechanisms underlying neurodegenerative disease pathology.

Research in *C. elegans* has been instrumental, especially over the last decade, for the elucidation of molecular pathways implicated in many human diseases. This is highly related to the fact that the *C. elegans* genome was the first multicellular organism to be completely sequenced in 1998 (Anonymous, 1998). The worm genome contains approximately 20,000 genes, compared with 25,000 in the human genome highlighting that *C. elegans* is a powerful model system for genetic analysis and for exploring the molecular mechanisms of neuron development, function, and disease. Furthermore, at least 42% of human disease related genes have a *C. elegans* ortholog, suggesting that most biochemical pathways are conserved across evolution (Culetto and Sattelle, 2000).

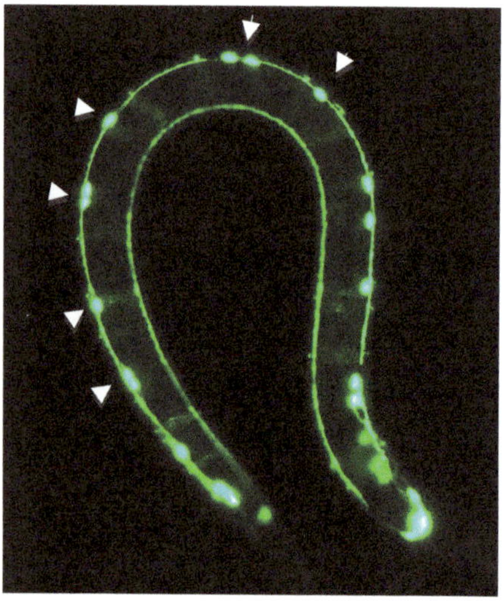

Fig. 1. Transgenic UNC-47:GFP *C. elegans*
In *C. elegans*, 26 neurons of 5 different classes express the neurotransmitter Gamma-Aminobutyric Acid (GABA) (McIntire, et al., 1993). Nineteen of these GABAergic neurons, known as the type D neurons, are required for normal locomotion by providing dorsoventral cross-inhibition to body wall muscles (McIntire, et al., 1993; White, et al., 1986). Therefore, this transgenic worm would be a good model to depict pathological changes associated with locomotor dysfunction. Arrowheads point to type D neurons (only some of the D neurons are indicated). *Courtesy of Dr Alex J. Parker from the Centre of Excellence in Neuromics, University of Montreal, Quebec, Canada.*

C. elegans is a free-living nematode of about 1 millimeter in length with a short generation cycle (3 days) and lifespan (around 3 weeks), large brood size (approximately 300 progeny from a single hermaphrodite), and a transparent anatomically simple body that allows for the visualization of all cell types at all stages of development (Brenner, 1974). This last feature allows researchers to easily detect and quantify neuronal cell death and protein inclusions using optical techniques. The complete *C. elegans* embryonic cell-lineage is also known, making it possible to follow organogenesis from the earliest stages of embryos formation to the terminal steps of differentiation and morphogenesis (Sulston, et al., 1983). Additionally, *C. elegans* have a simple nervous system of 302 neurons out of 959 cells in the adult hermaphrodite, in which each neuron has a unique position (Sulston, 1983). Twenty of these neurons are located inside the pharynx, which has its own nervous system. The remaining 282 neurons are located in various ganglia in the head and tail and also along the ventral cord, the main longitudinal axon tract (Fig. 1). The majority of the neurons develop during embryogenesis. However, 80 of them, mainly motor neurons, develop post-embryonically. The structure of the nervous system is highly reproducible from animal to animal and has been described in detail by electron microscopic reconstruction (White, et al., 1986) This technique allowed White and colleague to obtain high-resolution images to identify all the synapses formed in *C. elegans* (about 5000 chemical synapses, 2000 neuromuscular junctions and some 500 gap junctions) and to map all the connections in order to work out the entire neuronal circuit of this model organism.

In addition, gene knockdown by RNA interference can be relatively easily achieved in most cell types *in vivo* or *in vitro* by injecting the double stranded RNA for a specific gene of interest, by simply soaking the animals in dsRNA, or by feeding the animals with bacteria expressing the desired dsRNA (Fire, et al., 1998; Maeda, et al., 2001). Primary neuronal and muscular cell cultures obtained by dissecting this animal have also been optimized to allow for stable growth of embryonic cells (Christensen, et al., 2002).

For all these reasons, *C. elegans* has emerged as an attractive and powerful *in vivo* model system for studying pathological mechanisms in several major neurodegenerative disorders, including ALS, providing clear leads towards the identification of potential targets for the development of new therapeutic interventions against human diseases.

2.1.1.1 C. Elegans SOD1 models

A number of *C. elegans* models have been developed that recapitulate many aspects of ALS pathogenesis. These transgenic models mainly expressed either the SOD1 or the TDP-43 protein under the control of various gene promoters. The first *C. elegans* ALS model was first generated in 2001 (Oeda, et al., 2001). This transgenic *C. elagans* model has been generated by introducing human wild type and various human FALS *SOD1*-linked mutations (A4V, G37R and G93A) under the control of hsp16-2 heat shock and myo-3 muscle-specific promoters. The heat inducible hsp16-2 promoter allows expression of mutant SOD1 in almost all tissues, including neurons, while the myo-3 muscle-specific promoter allows high level of protein expression in all of the muscle tissues except for the pharynx. Unfortunately, no morphological abnormalities and no discernable changes in survival or behavior were observed. However, the authors reported some interesting findings. The mutant SOD1 expressing nematodes showed a reduced resistance to paraquat-induced oxidative stress. Furthermore, oxidative stress significantly reduced the degradation rate of mutant SOD1 protein, and finally aberrant accumulation of mutant human SOD1 proteins was also observed when expressed in muscle cells. Interestingly, this later pathological phenotype is in line with the pathology observed in human post-mortem ALS tissues.

In a subsequent study, pan-neuronal expression of the G85R ALS-linked mutant form of human SOD1, using the *C. elegans* syntobrevin gene promoter (*snb-1*), coupled to a yellow fluorescent protein (YFP) produces strong locomotor defects and paralysis in this transgenic snb-1/G85RSOD1-YFP *C. elegans* model (Wang, et al., 2009a). Interestingly, the observed phenotype correlated with intra-neuronal SOD1 aggregation. Another SOD1 mutant *C. elegans* model in which aggregation, toxicity, and cellular interactions can be directly compared between different SOD1 mutants was also reported. This mutant SOD1-YFP model, expressing various SOD1 mutants (G85R, G93A, 127X) in *C. elegans* muscle cells by the use of the muscle specific *unc-54* gene promoter resulted in mild cellular dysfunction (Gidalevitz, et al., 2009). However, when mutant SOD1 was introduced into genetic backgrounds harboring destabilizing temperature-sensitive mutations, the toxicity was enhanced significantly and a variety of toxic phenotypes were observed. Based on theses results, the authors concluded that the specific toxic phenotypes may not be simply due to aggregation toxicity of the causative mutant proteins, but may be modulated by the genetic interactions with cellular pathways harboring mildly destabilizing polymorphisms in the genetic background.

2.1.1.2 C. Elegans TDP-43 models

In order to study TDP-43 function and neurotoxicity, transgenic *C. elegans* model was generated allowing pan-neuronal expression of the wild-type TDP-43 human protein (Ash, et al., 2010). This was done using the *snb-1* gene promoter driving the expression of human TDP-43 cDNA in all neurons. The transgenic snb-1/hTDP-43 worms displayed a distinctive uncoordinated phenotype characterized by non-sinusoidal, slow movement and inappropriate responses to stimulus. Transgenic worms first display this phenotype during larval stages, and the phenotype remains constant throughout the adulthood. The authors have also found that this uncoordinated phenotype correlated with abnormal motor neuron synapses. The mechanism by which nuclear TDP-43 activity leads to abnormal synapses is still unknown, but the authors hypothesized that excessive TDP-43 activity may alters some component of RNA metabolism (e.g. alternative splicing), subsequently leading to altered production of specific proteins required for proper synaptic function. In another study, also describing a *C. elegans* model of TDP-43 proteinopathy, Liachko and colleagues similarly found that overexpression of normal human TDP-43 in all *C. elegans* neurons causes motor defects (Liachko, et al., 2010). However, they also found that overexpression of various human ALS-associated TDP-43 mutants (G290A, A315T, or M337V) cause a more severe motor dysfunction phenotype. Interestingly, the authors also demonstrated that the observed motor phenotype worsen over time and that the described mutant TDP-43 *C. elegans* model recapitulates some characteristic features seen in ALS and FTLD-U patients including progressive paralysis, reduced lifespan, and degeneration of motor neurons accompanied by hyperphosphorylation, truncation, and ubiquitination of the TDP-43 protein that accumulates in detergent insoluble protein deposits.

All the above described *C. elegans* models provide a good *in vivo* system to further dissect cellular and molecular mechanisms underlying disease. Further investigations using these models may reveal insights into SOD1 and TDP-43 functions, potentially reveal neurotoxic mechanisms relevant to ALS and other neurodegenerative diseases, and ultimately lead to the development of novel therapeutic targets.

2.1.2 Drosophila melanogaster

The fruit fly *Drosophila melanogaster* is a powerful genetic tool to study neurodegenerative diseases. *Drosophila* is a complex organism, with a functioning brain and nervous system, capable of many behaviors like learning, motility, and visual acuity. This model organism is one of the oldest multi cellular eukaryotic genetic models and has been used for almost a century to examine a variety of basic biological principles, including genetic inheritance, behavioral and developmental processes, and the first experimental description of the gene as a functional unit. Its importance for human health was recognized by the award of the Nobel Prize in Physiology and Medicine to Ed Lewis, Christiane Nusslein-Volhard and Eric Wieschaus in 1995 for their discoveries concerning the genetic control of early embryonic development using *D. melanogaster* as a model.

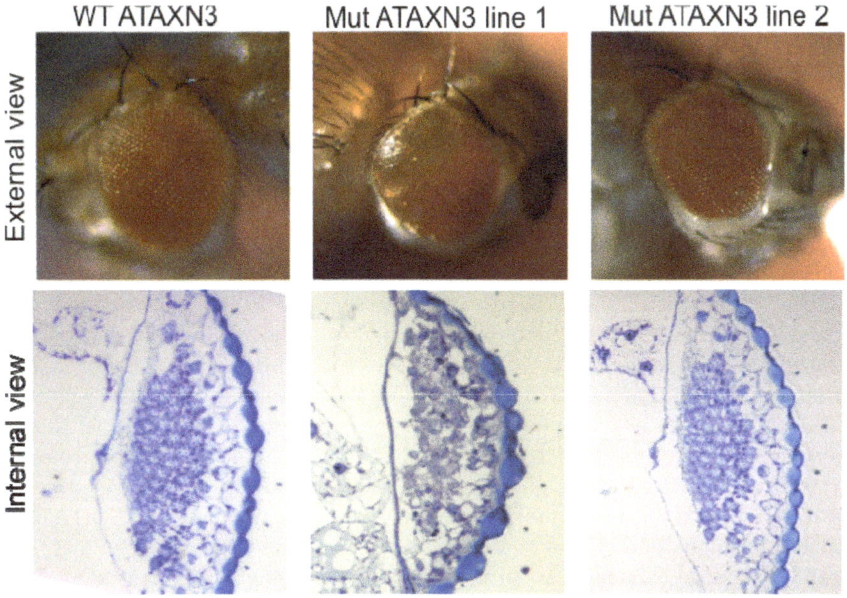

Fig. 2. Expression of human *Ataxin3* gene in the compound eye of transgenic flies using the GAL4/UAS system.
Transgenic *drosophila* expressing human full-length WT or mutated Ataxin 3 (ATXN3) gene in the compound eye. Only mutant ATAXN3 flies showed an external and internal degeneration, which is characterized by cell death and irregular ommatidia and photoreceptor distribution. *Courtesy of Dr Guy A. Rouleau from the Centre of Excellence in Neuromics, University of Montreal, Quebec, Canada.*

Drosophila is cheap, of small size (approximately 2.5mm) and easy to maintain in the laboratory. One of the most attractive aspects of *Drosophila* for use as a model organism is its short reproductive cycle and large number of genetically identical progeny. Adult females can lay, following a circadian pattern, over 400 eggs within 10 days and their short 2-week generation time allows for quick analysis of mutant animals. The fly has only four pairs of chromosomes, including three autosomal chromosomes and one set of sexual X/Y chromosomes which can be directly visualized in the giant polytene chromosome of the larval salivary gland. The *Drosophila* genome has been completely sequenced (Adams, et al., 2000). Its entire genome is encoded by roughly 13,600 genes as compared to 25,000 human genes. Another interesting feature of the fly is that it is relatively easy to drive time- and tissue-specific expression of any gene of interest using the yeast transcription activator protein Gal4 in combination with the Upstream Activation Sequence (UAS) to which Gal4 specifically binds to activate gene transcription (Brand and Perrimon, 1993). To study neurodegenerative diseases, the compound eye is predominantly used because it allows the

generation of a neurodegenerative phenotype (rough eye phenotype) that can be easily appreciated under a standard light microscope (Fig. 2). In turn, the Gal4/UAS system can be also used to screen for genetic modifier (enhancer or suppressor) genes.
Based on these observations, it is obvious that *Drosophila melanogaster* can offer unique opportunities in the study of human neurodegeneration. Nonetheless, the major disadvantage of using *D. melanogaster* as a model is that forward genetic screen using RNA interference technology is more tedious than in the *C.elegans* model. For instance, at the moment, knockdown of genes by RNAi cannot be carried out by simply feeding flies with double-stranded RNA (as in the worm model); it has to be injected into the embryo. Although very laborious, this problem could be overcome by generating transgenic constructs expressing dsRNA for each transcript.

2.1.2.1 Drosophila SOD1 models

Initial ALS studies in *Drosophila* showed either reduced longevity and fertility, increased susceptibility to oxidative stress, motor deficits and/or necrotic cell death in the fly eye of *Sod* null flies (Phillips, et al., 1989). Surprisingly, subsequent studies in transgenic fly model, overexpressing human WT SOD1 only in motor neurons, showed an extension of lifespan, without affecting locomotion or motor neuron survival (Parkes, et al., 1998). In contrast, another study showed that selective expression of WT or human SOD1 (hSOD1) disease-linked (A4V, G85R) mutants in motor neurons induced progressive motor dysfunctions, coupled with electrophysiological defects and abnormal accumulation of the protein and a stress response in surrounding glial cells (Watson, et al., 2008). These effects were accompanied by synaptic transmission deficits, focal accumulation of hSOD1 in motor neurons, and up-regulation of heat shock protein in glia. This work suggests that SOD can cause cell-autonomous damage to motor neurons, and highlights that motor neuron selective expression of hSOD1 can induces change in glial cells. These results are in line with findings that disease is not strictly autonomous to motor neurons and that toxicity can propagate from one cell to another (Boillee, et al., 2006; Clement, et al., 2003). Expression of a human *SOD1* transgene in *Drosophila* motor neurons was achieved by using the yeast GAL4/UAS system. Interestingly, Mocket and colleagues showed that human WT SOD1 expression, placed in a *Drosophila* Cu-Zn Sod null background, at very low levels was sufficient to rescue the life-span reduction, increased oxidative stress, and impaired physiological function associated with the *Drosophila* Sod null model described above (Mockett, et al., 2003). However, the introduction of FALS-linked SOD1 alleles (A4V, G37R, G41D, G93C, and I113T) only partly reversed these effects. These results, in conjunction with earlier findings from FALS SOD1 expression restricted to motor neurons, suggest that the introduction of FALS mutant SOD1 alleles in *Drosophila* does not result in a dominant gain-of-function, as it is observed in human patients.

2.1.2.2 Drosophila TDP-43 models

A number of models for TDP-43 toxicity in flies have also been generated, revealing that the protein shows toxicity *in vivo*. Mainly, these independent studies have examined phenotypes associated with manipulation of both endogenous *Drosophila* TDP-43 ortholog (dTDP) and transgenic expression of human TDP-43. The major findings of these complementary studies were largely consistent with one other. Flies lacking dTDP appeared externally normal but presented deficient locomotive behaviors, reduced life span, anatomical defects at the neuromuscular junctions and decreased dendritic branching

(Feiguin, et al., 2009; Lin, et al., 2011; Lu, et al., 2009). These phenotypes were rescued by expression of the human TDP-43 protein in a restricted group of neurons including motor neurons (Feiguin, et al., 2009). These findings support the notion that loss of normal TDP-43 function may contribute to the pathogenesis of ALS and FTLD. On the other hand, ubiquitous or tissue-specific overexpression of either dTDP or human TDP-43 also recapitulated key hallmark features of ALS pathology including premature lethality, neuronal loss, neuromuscular junctions architecture defects and locomotor deficits (Elden, et al., 2010; Estes, et al., 2011; Hanson, et al., 2010; Li, et al., 2010; Lu, et al., 2009; Miguel, et al., 2011; Ritson, et al., 2010; Voigt, et al., 2010). Furthermore, TDP-43 expression appears to be independent of ALS/FTLD-linked mutations (Elden, et al., 2010; Estes, et al., 2011; Ritson, et al., 2010; Voigt, et al., 2010). These results also support the view of a toxic dominant gain-of-function mechanism(s) associated with TDP-43 proteinopathies.

To further explore the role of TDP-43 pathogenesis and identify pathogenic mechanisms, several independent research groups have used different genetic approaches to identify modifier genes that could suppress or enhance TDP-43 toxicity (Elden, et al., 2010; Hanson, et al., 2010; Ritson, et al., 2010). Interestingly, upregulation of Pab1-binding protein 1 (Pbp1), an ortholog of the human *ATXN2* gene, in a transgenic model of TDP-43 enhanced TDP-43 toxicity and led to a more severe TDP-43 associated phenotypes (Elden, et al., 2010). Similarly, overexpression of ubiquilin 1, a previously identified TDP- 43 interacting partner (Kim, et al., 2009), reduced steady-state TDP-43 expression but enhanced the severity of TDP-43 phenotypes (Hanson, et al., 2010). Another study also showed that the TDP-43 associated phenotypes observed in a transgenic *Drosophila* TDP-43 model was modulated by coexpression of valosin-containing protein (VCP), a member of the ATPases associated with multiple cellular activities (AAA+) family of proteins regulating a wide array of cellular processes (Ritson, et al., 2010). Further investigations on these interesting findings may enable the development of novel therapeutics targets that can regulate TDP-43 expression in patients and hopefully delay or cure TDP-43-linked patients.

2.1.2.3 Drosophila FUS models

The pathogenic mechanisms underlying FUS proteinopathy remain largely unknown, although it is clear that *FUS* mutations affects motor neurons and other neuronal populations such as cortical neurons. In order to study FUS related function *in vivo*, a FUS/TLS Drosophila model was generated in which targeted expression of mutant human FUS/TLS (R518K, R521C and R521H) caused severe neurodegeneration in Drosophila eyes, whereas expression of WT human FUS/TLS resulted in very mild eye degeneration (Lanson, et al., 2011). Locomotor dysfunction and premature lethality was also observed in the mutant FUS/TLS transgenic flies. In addition, overexpression of mutant FUS/TLS caused an accumulation of ubiquitinated proteins, a pathological hallmark feature of ALS. Similarly, a pathogenic role of human ALS-associated FUS/TLS mutations (R524S and P525L) using Drosiphila has been described (Chen, et al., 2011). In this model overexpression of either Wt or ALS-mutant in different neuronal subpopulations, including photoreceptors, mushroom bodies and motor neurons led to an age-dependent progressive neuronal degeneration, including axonal loss, morphological changes and functional impairment in motor neurons. The human FUS/TLS drosophila ortholog (*caz*) has been also disrupted in order to study FUS function. The *caz* deficient fly exhibited reduced life span and locomotor deficits as compared with controls. Interestingly, these phenotypes were fully rescued by WT human FUS, but not ALS-associated mutant FUS proteins suggesting that ALS-associated FUS/TLS mutations are toxics (Walker, et al., 2011). Through cross-rescue analysis, it has been demonstrated that FUS acted together with and downstream of TDP-43 in a common genetic pathway in neurons. Furthermore, the authors found that these proteins associated with each other in an RNA-dependent complex. These results establish that FUS and TDP-43 function together *in vivo* and suggest that molecular pathways requiring the combined activities of both of these proteins may be disrupted in ALS and FTD.

2.2 Vertebrate models

Projecting the human genome sequence into our understanding of human health and disease has been a new challenge faced in the post-genomic era. As described above, unicellular and invertebrate model systems can be of great value in defining the molecular components of pathways or processes that depend on the function of several interacting proteins. However, vertebrate models offer the best opportunity for defining landmarks of disease progression and for understanding the functional consequences of gene mutations. The great advantage of using vertebrates to model human diseases is clearly the possibility they offer for evaluation of new treatments. Indeed, testing new drugs on mice or other vertebrate models is often mandatory and asked by the Food and Drug Administration, for safety reasons, prior to approve new drug treatments. This step is also fundamental for paving the way towards human clinical trials, with both larger and smaller vertebrate model organisms.

Other advantages of using vertebrate models include: the ability to make efficient targeted gene knockouts by homologous recombination, they are evolutionary closer to human, the developmental overview is similar for all mammals, the availability of material at all stages of development, their brains are more similar to human, they respond to injury and can be conditioned (great advantages to study learning, neuronal connectivity and plasticity) and they provide a valuable source of primary cells for culture. The later feature will be discussed in more details in the next section of this book chapter.

On the contrary, the high maintenance cost, a relatively slow life cycle development, lower number of progeny, genetically identical offspring more difficult to obtain and the difficulty to manipulate embryos (intrauterine development) represent the major disadvantages of using vertebrate as disease model organisms.

2.2.1 Mice

Over the past century, the laboratory mouse (*Mus musculus*) has become the premier mammalian model organism for experimental studies and genetic research. Scientists from a wide range of biomedical fields have used the mouse because of its close genetic and physiological similarities to humans, as well as the ease with which its genome can be manipulated and analyzed, ease of handling and it's relatively high reproductive rate. Although yeasts, worms and flies are excellent models for studying many developmental processes, mice are far better models for studying diverse physiological systems such as the immune system, the endocrine system, the nervous system, the cardiovascular system, the skeletal system and other complex physiological systems that mammals share. Like humans and many other mammals, mice naturally develop diseases that affect these systems, including cancer, atherosclerosis, hypertension, diabetes, osteoporosis and glaucoma. In addition, manipulating the mouse genome and environment can induce certain diseases that afflict humans but normally do not strike mice, such as cystic fibrosis, obesity, blindness, anxiety, aggressive behavior, alcoholism, drug addiction and neurodegenerative disorders such as Alzheimer's disease, Parkinson's disease, Huntington's disease and ALS. Immunodeficient mice can also be used as hosts to facilitate cancer and AIDS research.

Researchers have used a collection of innovative genetic technologies to produce custom-made mouse models for a broad array of specific diseases, as well as to study the function of targeted genes. One of the most important technological advances has been the ability to produce transgenic mice, in which a new gene (cloned from human or other various species, wild-type or mutated) is inserted into the mouse's germline. Indeed, the 2007 Nobel Prize in Physiology and Medicine was awarded to Drs Mario R. Capecchi, Martin J. Evans and Oliver Smithies for their discoveries of principles for introducing specific gene modifications in mice by the use of embryonic stem cells. Even more potent approaches, it is now possible to knockout or to artificially drive the expression of an inserted gene in specific tissue or at various time during development or adulthood using the Cre/Loxp system (Sauer, 1998). There are many mouse models commercially available for genetic research including thousands of unique inbred strains and genetically engineered mutants.

Researches using the laboratory mouse led to major advances in our ability to treat a number of serious diseases and conditions. Genetically, mice are more closely related to humans than invertebrates in the sense that most human genes have functional mouse counterparts and the mouse genome is organized in a very similar manner to the human genome. The mouse and human genomes are approximately the same size. They most likely contain the same number of genes and show extensive synteny and conserved gene order. Importantly, mice have also genes that are often not represented in other models, such as *C. elegans* and *Drosophila*. All these advantages make the laboratory mouse the model organism of choice to study human diseases. Although mice are widely used in research, questions remain however about their reliability as a model for human diseases. In occurrence, how to explain that many drugs worked well during preclinical trials in mice, but turned out to be ineffective when used in clinical trials on humans? Here, we will review the mouse studies that contributed toward understanding the pathogenic pathways of motor neuron disease and the testing of therapeutic approaches.

2.2.1.1 Mice SOD1 models

The use of mouse models has been of particular importance in studying the pathogenesis of Amyotrophic Lateral Sclerosis. The initial description of *SOD1* gene mutations in familial ALS patients, in 1993, first led to the hypothesis that the disease resulted from compromised enzymatic activity due to the loss of the enzyme function (Rosen, et al., 1993). However, this loss of function hypothesis was rapidly refuted, as *Sod1* KO mice in which the murine *Sod1* gene was disrupted, do not develop disease (Reaume, et al., 1996). To date, over 150 different *SOD1* missense mutations have been reported. In contrast, transgenic mice ubiquitously overexpressing various *SOD1* gene mutations with different biochemical properties, even in the presence of endogenous mouse *Sod1* gene, develop a neurodegenerative disease that is quite similar to the human illness. Of particular interest, transgenic mice overexpressing WT human SOD1 or specifically expressing mutant SOD1 only in neurons or only in glial cells do not develop disease (Bruijn, et al., 1998; Gong, et al., 2000; Pramatarova, et al., 2001). A toxic gain-of-function rather than a loss-of-function of mutant *SOD1* gene is therefore believe to be involved in ALS-linked SOD1 patients. All published mouse models have used the endogenous murine *Sod1* promoter resulting in high levels of expression of the mutant transgene in all tissues. Although these models implicate mutant SOD1 in the development of motor neuron degeneration, many questions regarding the mechanism of pathogenesis remain unanswered. One of the central mysteries in ALS research is why an ubiquitously expressed gene such as *SOD1* causes selective devastation to motor neurons in the absence of pathology in other tissues. One possible explanation is that expression of the mutant protein in motor neurons may not be sufficient to lead to the development of a neurodegenerative disease in mice, suggesting that mutant *SOD1* expression in other cells may be necessary for the development of the disease. Although there are indications that neurodegeneration in ALS may not strictly result from a cell-autonomous process, the selective motor neuron vulnerability observed in the disease pathogenesis remains enigmatic.

The favored hypothesis at this time of SOD1-mediated disease is that toxicity of SOD1 mutants is related to the misfolding and aggregation of SOD1 species (Gros-Louis, et al., 2009b). However, it is not clear which conformational SOD1 species and oligomers cause ALS and the exact mechanism of toxicity of the misfolded SOD1 species remains unknown. Deleterious effects could result from the interaction of misfolded SOD1 species with essential cellular components such as Bcl-2 (Pasinelli, et al., 2004), from their recruitment to outer membrane of mitochondria or from overwhelming the capacity of the protein folding chaperones and/or of ubiquitin proteasome pathway to degrade important cellular regulatory factors (Turner, et al., 2005; Urushitani, et al., 2008; Urushitani, et al., 2002). The misfolded SOD1 protein may also form aggregates that might sequester important cellular components causing cytotoxicity. Recent studies demonstrated that a fraction of SOD1 could be translocated via the ER-Golgi network and that chromogranins, which are abundant proteins in motor neurons, interneurons and activated astrocytes, may act as chaperone-like proteins to promote secretion of misfolded SOD1 mutants (Urushitani, et al., 2008; Urushitani, et al., 2006). Moreover, it has been reported that extracellular mutant SOD1 can induce microgliosis and motor neuron death (Urushitani, et al., 2006). Such ALS pathogenic mechanism based on toxicity of secreted SOD1 mutant is in line with findings that disease is not strictly autonomous to motor neurons and that toxicity can propagate from one cell to another. Interestingly, it has been proposed that endoplasmic reticulum (ER) stress response might exert a critical role in the disease pathogenesis. The ER is the site of synthesis and folding of secretory and membrane bound proteins. The capacity of the ER to process proteins is limited and the accumulation of misfolded proteins may activate different ER stress pathways. The challenges in the future are to find out which somatic insults are causing the initial protein change, and to discover ways of preventing the misfolded proteins from spreading through the nervous system.

The overexpression of either G37R, G85R, G86R, D90A, G93A, H46R/H48Q or H46R/H48Q/H63G/H120G, L126Z and G127X mutant SOD1 protein in mice leads to motor neuron degeneration (Borchelt, et al., 1994; Bruijn, et al., 1997; Gurney, et al., 1994; Jonsson, et al., 2004; Jonsson, et al., 2006; Ripps, et al., 1995; Tu, et al., 1996; Wang, et al., 2003; Wang, et al., 2002; Wong, et al., 1995). In all of these mouse models, massive death of motor neurons in the ventral horn of the spinal cord and loss of myelinated axons in ventral motor roots ultimately leads to paralysis and muscle atrophy. Histopathological findings observed in these transgenic animals include progressive accumulation of detergent-resistant aggregates containing SOD1 and ubiquitin, aberrant neurofilament accumulations in degenerating motor neurons. In addition to neuronal degeneration, similar to that observed in ALS patients, Golgi fragmentation and neuroinflammation noted by the presence of reactive astroglia and microglia in diseased tissue are also observed. However, the severity of the phenotype (in term of age of onset, disease progression and disease duration) varies from one model to another and may be dependant on mouse genetic background (Heiman-Patterson, et al., 2005) and gene dosage. In deed, the life span of these ALS mice is inversely proportional to gene dosage, i.e. the number of transgene insertion within the mouse genome, leading to different steady state level of mutant SOD1 protein in the central nervous system. Such variation in the steady state protein levels must reflect different stabilities and degradation of the various human SOD1 mutants.

The G93A-SOD1 mouse line is currently the most widely used experimental model in ALS research and drug testing. Unfortunately, several pharmacological approaches tested so far have produced only modest beneficial effects. Riluzole, a glutamate antagonist, extended the life span of G93A-SOD1 mice by 10 to 15 days without affecting disease onset (Gurney, et al., 1996). Today, riluzole is the only drug currently approved for ALS treatment. This treatment only produces modest beneficial effect in some ALS patients. Interestingly, is has been shown that treatment with the ER stress-protective agent salubrinal attenuated disease manifestations and delayed progression in a G93A-SOD1 mouse model (Saxena, et al., 2006). This result suggests a role of ER stress in ALS. Furthermore, it has been also shown that immunization therapy, using specific anti-misfolded SOD1 monoclonal antibodies, succeeded in reducing the level of mutant SOD1 by 23% in the spinal cord of immunized animals, in delaying disease onset and in prolonging the lifespan of G93A-SOD1 mice in proportion to the duration of treatment (Gros-Louis, et al., 2010). These results suggest that accumulation of misfolded SOD1 species is toxic, and reducing the burden of these toxic species leads to beneficial effect. Interestingly, it has been recently reported that WT SOD1 can acquire properties of ALS-linked mutant SOD1 species possibly implying a shared pathophysiological pathway between SALS and FALS (Bosco, et al., 2010b; Ezzi, et al., 2007). Another study also demonstrated that WT SOD1 may acquire toxic properties upon oxidative damage and that WT SOD1 expression dramatically exacerbated disease in transgenic mice expressing mutant SOD1 forms such as A4V, G85R, L126Z, and G93A SOD1 mutants (Wang, et al., 2009b). It is noteworthy that overexpression of WT SOD1 conferred ALS disease to unaffected A4V SOD1 mice. Based on these results, the possibility that WT SOD1 may be a contributor of pathogenesis in sporadic ALS must be considered.

2.2.1.2 Mice TDP-43 models

As previously mentioned, several research groups have reported that dominant mutations in the *TARDBP* gene, which encodes for TDP-43, cause ALS (Kabashi, et al., 2008; Sreedharan, et al., 2008; Van Deerlin, et al., 2008). Following these initials studies, a number of TDP-43 ALS mouse model has been described. Embryonic lethality is observed in homozygous mouse knockouts for TDP-43 (Kraemer, et al., 2010; Sephton, et al., 2010; Wu, et al., 2010). The TDP-43 deficient embryos die at embryonic day 7.5 thereby demonstrating the essential function of TDP-43 protein in development. Mice heterozygous for TDP-43 disruption only exhibit subtle muscle weakness with no evidence of motor neuron pathology.

Many of the transgenic mouse lines overexpressing WT or mutant TDP-43 reported to date have showed some ALS features including early paralysis leading to premature death (Stallings, et al., 2010; Wegorzewska, et al., 2009; Wils, et al., 2010). These pan-neuronal TDP-43 transgenic mouse models expressing high-level of either WT or mutant (A315T and

M337V) TDP-43 transgene in neurons both showed aggressive paralysis accompanied by increased ubiquitination in specific neuronal populations (Stallings, et al., 2010; Wegorzewska, et al., 2009; Wils, et al., 2010; Xu, et al., 2010). However, many concerns have been raised regarding the biological validity of these models, as they do not completely mimics disease. Since TDP-43 is a moderately and ubiquitously expressed protein, restricted non-physiological neuronal expression of TDP-43 is one of them, along with the use of the TDP-43 cDNA as transgene and the lack of cytoplasmic ubiquitinated TDP-43 inclusions. In order to better mimic the ubiquitous and moderate levels of TDP-43 expression seen in humans, another transgenic mouse models have been generated allowing the expression of genomic TDP-43 fragments (Swarup, et al., 2011). This TDP-43 mouse model exhibited age-related phenotypic defects as seen in the human condition including both cognitive and motor deficits. Other pathological features as seen in human patients were also observed including, cytoplasmic TDP-43-positive ubiquitinated inclusions, intermediate filament abnormalities, axonopathy and neuroinflammation. These phenotypes were more severe in the transgenic TDP-43 mutant (G348C and A315T) models than the transgenic TDP-43 WT model.

2.2.1.3 Mice intermediate filament models

Several transgenic mouse lines and knockout mice implicating different neurofilament subunits have been extensively studied over the past years (for complete review, see: (Julien and Kriz, 2006; Lariviere and Julien, 2004)). Even though genetic mutations in intermediate filament (IF) genes are not major causes of ALS, it is of potential relevance to ALS that transgenic mice with altered stoichiometry of neuronal intermediate filament develop pathological features of the disease (Beaulieu, et al., 2000; Beaulieu and Julien, 2003; Cote, et al., 1993; Millecamps, et al., 2006). Of particular interest was the finding that overexpression of WT peripherin, a type III intermediate filament, in *NEFL* null background mice caused age-dependant selective motor neurons degeneration (Beaulieu, et al., 1999). This mouse model is also characterized by the formation of perikaryal and axonal intermediate filament inclusions resembling spheroids in motor neurons of human ALS. The precise mechanism by which accumulation of intermediate neurofilament leads to neurodegenerative disorders is not fully understood. Neurofilament and peripherin proteins are two types of intermediate filaments detected in the majority of axonal inclusion bodies, called spheroids, in motor neurons of ALS patients (Corbo and Hays, 1992). Multiple factors can potentially cause the accumulation of intermediate filament proteins including deregulation of intermediate filament protein synthesis, proteolysis, defective axonal transport, abnormal phosphorylation, and other protein modifications.

2.2.1.4 Mice ALS2 models

Truncating mutations were discovered in coding exons of a the *ALS2* gene encoding for Alsin, from patients with an autosomal recessive form of juvenile ALS, primary lateral sclerosis (PLS) and infantile-onset ascending hereditary spastic paralysis (IAHSP) (Devon, et al., 2003; Eymard-Pierre, et al., 2002; Eymard-Pierre, et al., 2006; Gros-Louis, et al., 2003; Hadano, et al., 2001; Kress, et al., 2005; Yang, et al., 2001). The pattern of inheritance and the nature of the mutations identified in this gene suggest that motor neuron degeneration seen in patients results from a loss of protein function. Six different groups have reported the generation of an alsin knockout mouse (Cai, et al., 2005; Deng, et al., 2007; Devon, et al., 2003; Gros-Louis, et al., 2008; Hadano, et al., 2006; Yamanaka, et al., 2006). Despite an age-

dependent loss of motor coordination revealed by rotarod and grip strength performances of the Als2 KO mice, no major motor deficits consistent with ALS or other motor neuron diseases were present in these models. All Als2-deficient mice appear to be grossly normal, viable and fertile with lifespan expectancy similar to WT littermates. However, some differences are noteworthy and may explain the heterogeneity of the phenotype, ranging from ALS to less severe PLS or IAHSP. The diversity of the apparent phenotypes among different Als2 KO mouse models may be due in part by different gene targeting strategies used to generate each mice models, ES cell lines used leading to differences in the genetic background, housing conditions or approaches taken to evaluate the mice.
Interestingly, thorough molecular analysis of one of these *Als2* KO mouse model revealed the presence of a number of novel *Als2* isoforms expressed in the central nervous system of these animals (Gros-Louis, et al., 2008). These results suggest that other alternatively spliced *Als2* isoforms may exist and that some of these novel *Als2* mRNA species still can be transcribed in *Als2* null animals and may compensate for the loss of the full-length protein.

2.2.1.5 Mice models associated with other motor neuron diseases

Different other transgenic mice models overexpressing different human proteins either ubiquitously or specifically in neurons have been generated (for review see (Gros-Louis, et al., 2006; Julien and Kriz, 2006). These mice acquire age-dependent central nervous system pathology similar to other related motor neuron diseases such as FTDP17, progressive supranuclear palsy, spinal muscular atrophy or hereditary spastic paraplegia. Interesting pathological features, which are also associated with ALS, can be seen in these different mouse models including axonal degeneration in brain and spinal cord, progressive motor disturbance, behavioral impairment, and the presence of cellular aggregates and intermediate filament inclusions.

2.2.2 Rat

As a model of human disease, the laboratory rat (*Rattus norvegicus*) offers some advantages over the mouse and other organisms. The main advantage is in fact that rats are physiologically more similar to humans compare to mice. The size of the animal also confers a valuable advantage and enhances its use as a disease model. The later advantage is especially true when performing surgical procedures, microdialysis, intravenous cannulation and for pharmacodynamic drug studies as its size enables serial blood sampling. Thereby, the rat would be a better model than the mouse to study cardiovascular disease, hypertension, diabetes, arthritis, and many autoimmune, behavioral, and addiction disorders. The rat is also a good model in neurobehavioral and stereotaxic neurological studies. The size of the rat brain offers unique possibilities for the application of microsurgical techniques, intrathecal administration of drugs, stem cell transplantation, serial sampling of the cerebrospinal fluid (CSF), *in vivo* nerve recordings, and neuroimaging procedures.
However, even though its size is considered as an advantage over mice, the higher cost of maintenance (bigger cages, food, less animals can be housed per cages) and limited housing capacity in animal facilities directly related to its size also confers the principal limitation of using rats as a model.

2.2.2.1 Rat SOD1 models

Transgenic rat models of ALS have also been generated. In these models overexpression of G93A or H46R mutant SOD1 led to an ALS-like phenotype (Howland, et al., 2002; Nagai, et al., 2001). These transgenic rat models reproduce the major phenotypic features of human ALS, such as selective motor neuron loss, ubiquitination, hyaline inclusions, vacuolation, and neuroinflammation. However, several differences between the rat and mouse ALS models can be denoted including a more rapid progression of disease and the transient appearance of vacuoles in the transgenic SOD1 rats. As the CSF volume of a rat is 10- to 20-fold greater than that of a mouse (Nagai, et al., 2001), transgenic *SOD1* rats may facilitate to study the CSF proteome and to detect SOD1 activity or drug concentrations, even in an age-dependent manner. Therefore, ALS rat models may be useful to demonstrate therapeutic efficacy, blood-brain barrier filtration and to assess the toxicity of novel therapeutic compounds in drug development.

2.2.2.2 Rat TDP-43 models

In order to generate a TDP-43 rodent model that is more suitable for pharmacological studies, rat models ubiquitously overexpressing either WT TDP-43 or the M337V-associated *TARDBP* mutation were generated (Zhou, et al., 2010). In contrast to what it is observed in TDP-43 transgenic mouse models, overexpression of mutant TDP-43 only, but not the WT protein, caused widespread neurodegeneration. Despite the fact that this transgenic mutant TDP-43 rat model exhibited progressive degeneration of motor neurons, neurodegeneration was not only restricted to motor neurons. However, TDP-43 mutation affected motor neurons earlier and more severely than other neurons in the CNS at end stage of the disease. In some aspects, this rat model recapitulated TDP-43 pathological features both seen in the different mouse models and in ALS patients indicating that this model could be used in future pharmalogical studies in order to identify novel therapeutic avenues to treat TDP-43 related disorders.

2.2.3 Zebrafish

In the last decade, a new vertebrate model has emerged in the study of human diseases. The principal attraction of using zebrafish (*Danio renio*) as model organisms is that its genome can be much more easily manipulated and studied in terms of genetics and development than other vertebrate model organisms. As being a vertebrate with common organs and tissues with conserved organization such as brain and spinal cord, the attractiveness of zebrafish to model human diseases lies therefore in its biology and genetics. Although there are obvious differences in the physiology of fish and humans the zebrafish offers several advantages that make it an important complement to mouse models of disease. These advantages include the embryo and larvae optical clarity (which allows easy visualization of developmental processes), the external fertilization (which facilitates gene expression manipulation), high fecundity (adult female can lay hundreds of eggs per day), and rapid development (swimming behavior appears less than 48 hours post-fertilization). As in invertebrate models, it is also relatively easy to perform forward and reverse genetic screens for gene identification and to understand specific gene function.

Forward-genetic screens in zebrafish, using random mutagenesis, can be used to identify novel genes involved in embryogenesis, organogenesis or different specific biological processes. To generate mutants, male fish are exposed to the mutagen ethyl-nitroso-urea (ENU), which typically induces point mutations within zebrafish genome (Driever, et al., 1996; Haffter, et al., 1996; Henion, et al., 1996; Solnica-Krezel, et al., 1996). Random mutagenesis has also been successfully carried out in zebrafish using retroviral methods (Amsterdam, et al., 1999). Treated males are then crossed to wildtype females to produce the

F1 heterozygous progeny and so on so forth in order to generate homozygous progeny and to facilitate the identification of gene mutation by positional cloning. Forward-genetic screens in zebrafish are greatly facilitated by the transparency of embryos and larvae, simplifying phenotypic screening and allowing large scale screening without sophisticated expansive equipments. These features provide an advantage over other vertebrate models in which aspects of organogenesis and disease pathology cannot be examined without surgical interventions. Large-scale forward-genetic screens have allowed the identification of numerous mutations in zebrafish genes (Amsterdam and Hopkins, 2006). Comparative genomic can be then used in order to identify the corresponding orthologous gene in humans and, in some instances, the mutant phenotypes have been sufficiently similar to the human pathology to allow the identification of gene mutations by a candidate gene approach.

On the other hand, reverse genetics refers to the study of the phenotypic consequences following manipulation of gene expression. An essential tool for investigating gene function during development is the ability to perform gene knockdown, overexpression, and misexpression studies. The external egg fertilization in zebrafish enables microinjection of RNA, DNA, proteins, antisense oligonucleotides and other small molecules into the developing embryo thereby providing researchers a quick and robust assay for exploring gene function *in vivo*. Antisense morpholino oligonucleotides (AMO) are now widely used to modify gene expression by blocking translation of a targeted protein or by modifying pre-mRNA splicing (Nasevicius and Ekker, 2000)). The ability to examine the course of a pathological process *in vivo* and in real time using AMO reverse genetic is a particular strength of zebrafish models. In particular, AMO are powerful reverse genetic tools for the biological validation of genetic variants identified in human and for defining the pathological nature of a particular gene mutation (Amsterdam and Hopkins, 2006). Finally, high-throughput screening for small-molecule chemical able to modify disease pathogenesis, firmly establishing a role for zebrafish in the field of pharmaceutical drug discovery.

2.2.3.1 Zebrafish SOD1 models

In order to generate a SOD1 zebrafish model of ALS, transient overexpression of human SOD1 mutants (A4V, G37R and G93A) was achieved using mRNA microinjection into 2 to 4 cell stage blastulae (Lemmens, et al., 2007). Overexpression of mutant human SOD1 in zebrafish embryos induced a dose-dependant motor axonopathy in all studied mutations. Likewise in ALS patients, ubiquitous expression of the mutant protein produced motor neuron specific neuropathology, suggesting that this model may be useful to elucidate the mechanisms underlying specific vulnerability of motor neurons in *SOD1*-linked ALS. Interestingly, the observed motor neuron phenotype in this transient SOD1mutant zebrafish embryo expresser suggests that ALS may be a developmental disease.

With the goal of achieving constitutive mutant SOD1 expression in zebrafish, Ramesh and colleagues generated transgenic zebrafish models overexpressing either WT or mutant SOD1 (Ramesh, et al., 2010). Zebrafish overexpressing mutant SOD1 exhibited many hallmark phenotypes of ALS including neuromuscular junction defects, spinal motor neuron loss, muscle degeneration, decreased endurance to swim, partial paralysis and premature death. Interestingly, all of these pathological features are consistent with those seen in SOD1 transgenic mice and rats, supporting the idea that overexpression of SOD1 in vertebrate models results in the development of common pathologies. As zebrafish are highly amenable to chimeric analysis, this zebrafish model will offer a tool to hopefully address in future studies the cell autonomous hypothesis seen in SOD1-linked ALS.

2.2.3.2 Zebrafish TDP-43 models

In order to test the toxicity associated with various *TARDBP* mutations (A315T, G348C and A382T), transient overexpression of WT and mutant TDP-43 was achieved by *TARDBP* mRNA microinjection (Kabashi, et al., 2010). Mutant TDP-43 overexpression resulted in motor neuron defects, including shorter axons, abnormal axonal branching and swimming deficits in the absence of sensory deficits. These phenotypes were also observed in WT *TARDBP* overexpressing zebrafish, but were less severe. These results confirmed that the studied *TARDBP* mutations are toxic and suggested that TDP-43 linked mutations preferentially target motor neurons for degeneration. Interestingly, knocking down the zebrafish *Tardbp* gene (z*Tardbp*), using a specific AMO designed to block z*Tardbp* translation, led to a similar phenotype, which was rescued by co-expressing WT but not mutant human TDP-43 (Kabashi, et al., 2010). Together these two reverse genetic approaches showed that *TARDBP* mutations cause motor neuron defects and toxicity, suggesting that mutant TDP-43 contributes to disease pathogenesis by both a toxic gain-of-function and a loss-of-function molecular mechanisms.

2.2.3.3 Zebrafish FUS models

To test the FUS/TLS-linked mutations toxicity, transient expression of mRNAs encoding green fluorescent protein (GFP)-FUS (WT, H517Q, R521G, R495X or G515X) fused proteins was achieved by injecting these mRNA into zebrafish eggs at the 1 to 2 cells stage of development (Bosco, et al., 2010a). Interestingly, the expression of human FUS WT and the H517Q and R521G mutants each exhibited a predominantly nuclear pattern in the spinal cord, whereas the R495X and G515X truncation mutants accumulated in the cytoplasm. Noteworthy, abnormal accumulation of protein in the cytoplasm has been frequently observed in post-mortem tissues collected from ALS patients. This phenotype was exacerbated after heat shock treatment. These results suggest that the studied FUS-linked mutations induce toxicity and that multiple factors may influence the subcellular localization of GFP-FUS *in vivo*, including various cellular stresses. Similarly, upon transient overexpression of a FUS-linked ALS mutation (R521H) in zebrafish embryos, motor deficits characterized by abnormal touch-evoke escape response was observed in 57% of the mRNA injected zebrafish larvae as compared to 23% in controls (Kabashi, et al., 2011). These results, from both studies, indicate that ALS-linked FUS/TLS mutants can cause motor neuron deficits by a toxic gain-of-function. On the other hand, loss-of-function cannot be totally excluded as knockdown of the zebrafish *Fus* (z*Fus*) gene, using antisense morpholino oligo, also yielded a motor phenotype characterized by a deficient touch-evoked escape response, reduced motor neuron outgrowth and axonal branching (Kabashi, et al., 2011). Interestingly, these phenotypes could be rescued upon co-expression of WT human FUS but not ALS-linked *FUS/TLS* mutations.

2.2.3.4 Zebrafish ALS2 models

To investigate *ALS2* gene function and to elucidate if the identified mouse Als2 splicing isoforms may compensate for the loss of the full length protein in Als2 KO mice described earlier, a knock-down of the zebrafish Als2 ortholog (z*Als2*) in zebrafish was performed using an AMO directed against the start codon of the z*Als2* gene (Gros-Louis, et al., 2008).

Consistent with this hypothesis, Gros-Louis and colleagues found that the zAls2 knocked down zebrafish led to both severe developmental abnormalities and an obvious behavioral phenotype, including swimming impairment and motor neuron disruption. This model is still the only ALS2 animal model mimicking the severe motor neuron degeneration observed in ALS2 patients. Interestingly, some of these Als2 splice variants rescued the zebrafish phenotype suggesting that these identified spliced variants, observed in Als2 null mice and in ALS2 patients, prevented the Als2 KO mice from developing severe neurodegenerative disease. These findings may also explain the variable phenotype observed in ALS2-linked patients.

2.2.4 Dog

The domestic dog (*Canis familiaris*), with over 450 naturally-occurring hereditary diseases, is a valuable model organism for the study of human genetic diseases and complex traits. In humans, common diseases show complex modes of inheritance, and as a result, genetic analysis and gene mapping could be tedious. Rodent systems are more tractable genetically, but studies using transgenic mouse models represent an induction of a particular mutation rather than naturally arising alleles, and results are often of limited direct relevance to human disease because of profound differences in physiology. In contrast, the physiology, disease presentation and clinical response of dogs to drugs often mimic human diseases closely. The dog genome is similar in size to the human genome; containing an estimated 2.8 billion DNA base pairs (Lindblad-Toh, et al., 2005). Canine models have played an important role in advancing biomedical knowledge and techniques. Due to a long history of selective breeding, many breeds of dogs are naturally prone to genetic diseases including cancer, autoimmune and neurological disorders afflicting humans. These dog models, in which naturally occurring mutations in different genes was described, may help the study of genetic diseases difficult to study in humans. The structure of the canine population offers specific advantages for genetic mapping studies. The dog enjoys a genetic diversity unrivaled by any other mammalian species. A thousand centuries of directed breeding by humans has been responsible for that diversity leading to an unequaled variety of morphologies and behaviors, and also into a number of inherited diseases. The top 10 diseases in dogs include cancer, epilepsy, allergy, retinal disease, cataracts, and heart disease. Several of these diseases constitute also a major health concerns to humans.

The disadvantages of using dog as a model are its size, cost of maintenance and housing limitations in order to provide adequate area for the dogs to run. Furthermore, there use in research has been more controversial and of public concerns than other animal models because of an obvious emotional tie toward dogs.

2.2.4.1 Dog SOD1 model

A genome-wide association analysis reveals a *SOD1* mutation in canine degenerative myelopathy (Awano, et al., 2009). This disease has been recognized for more than 35 years as a spontaneously occurring, adult-onset spinal cord disorder of dogs (Averill, 1973). The resequencing of the canine *Sod1* gene revealed a recessive E40K missense mutation. Pathological studies of spinal cords from affected dogs showed myelin and axonal loss, SOD1-positive neuronal cytoplasmic inclusions similar to those seen in patients. The disease is also fatal in dogs and, typically, presents with progressive upper motor neuron spasticity and general proprioceptive ataxia in the pelvic limbs leading to paraplegia. Dogs develop disease generally around 8 years of age or older and disease duration will not exceed, if euthanasia is delayed, 3 years. These findings suggest that this disease afflicting dogs is closely related to ALS and identify canine degenerative myelopathy to be the first recognized spontaneously occurring animal model for ALS. The canine ALS model may be particularly valuable for evaluating therapeutic interventions as the environmental conditions and the SOD1 level of expression mimic better the human ALS situation.

2.2.5 Pig

Pigs, although not easily kept for laboratory research, are readily available for biomedical research through the large-scale industrial production of pigs produced for human consumption. Recent research has facilitated the biological experimentation with pigs, and helped develop the pig into a novel model organism for biomedical research.

The domesticated pig (*Sus scrofa*) shares several similarities with human, in particular the size of organs and various aspects of anatomy and physiology. The development of somatic cloning technology and the merger with techniques of targeted genetic modification and conditional gene expression will enhance the possibilities for creating useful models for human diseases in pigs. The pig has also evolved as the major target species for producing xenografts in order to provide appropriate human organs. The sequencing of the domestic pig genome has not yet been fully completed. However, initial draft revealed that the size and composition of the porcine genome is comparable to that of humans; comprising about 2.7 billion base pairs (Hart, et al., 2007). Furthermore, both gene content and sequence are highly conserved between pig and human. Detailed information on the porcine genome together with emerging transgenic technologies, such as siRNA or conditional knockouts will enhance our possibilities to create useful pig models. Other advantages of using domestic pigs to model human diseases include high fertility, great abundance, rapid growth, anatomy and physiology not too different from human and the possibility to introduce genetic modifications in its genome. The pig has been an essential and very successful model in biomedical research and is particularly suited to close the gap between basic research in current models and clinical application. The future will certainly see several promising porcine models for human diseases.

The high resemblance between the central nervous systems of humans and pigs makes the pig an ideal model organism for studying human neurodegenerative diseases. For neurodegenerative disorders such as ALS, Parkinson's disease and Alzheimer's disease, the pig may represent a model superior to other models presently available. Large animals, including pigs and non-human primates in neuroscience enable the use of conventional clinical brain imaging and the direct testing of surgical procedures. The evaluation of novel therapeutic avenues in an animal model with higher brain complexity will allow a more direct translation to human diseases.

3. In vitro models to study ALS

In vitro models are extremely helpful to study human diseases because they allow to analyze different cell types independently from each other and to perform dynamic studies on isolated cells. Moreover, diseased cells can be combined with healthy ones to better understand which cell type is the most critical in the different stages of the disease.

Some of these *in vitro* models were developed using the ALS animal models previously discussed. However, neural cells are impossible to obtain from patients and their extraction from post-mortem tissues is limited due to the difficulty to isolate living cells from adult brain or spinal cord, especially motor neurons.

Thus, such postmortem tissue biopsies are mostly used to perform histological and immunohistochemical, genetic as well as proteomic studies. More recently, they were also used to extract neural precursor cells that were further differentiated into motor neurons and glial cells to develop innovative models of the disease.

3.1 Organotypic cultures of spinal cord slices

The best way to preserve all the cellular content and the complex electrophysiological and biochemical organization of cells in the spinal cord is to maintain a whole tissue slice in an organotypic culture. In addition, organotypic slice cultures can be obtained from both embryos and postnatal animals, conferring a major advantage when using transgenic mice from which the disease genotype has to be ascertained after birth (Kosuge, et al., 2009; Mazzone and Nistri, 2011). After dissection of the lumbar spinal cord and removal of the meninges, 200 to 400μm-thick transversal sections are sectioned and transferred into membrane inserts fitting six-well or 12-well culture plates (Caldero, et al., 2010). These organotypic cultures can be used for more than 2 months (Delfs, et al., 1989). Various types of molecules can be added in the culture medium, such as kainate or lithium, to modulate neurotoxicity (Caldero, et al., 2010; Mazzone and Nistri, 2011).

These tissue sections can then be used to perform various analysis like recording the neuron rhythmic activity by placing the tissue on a multielectrode array (Tscherter, et al., 2001; Young, et al., 2007), or studying real-time glutamate release using a biosensor and redox reaction current using a multichannel potentiostat (Mazzone and Nistri, 2011), in addition to the conventional immunohistochemical staining and electrophysiological recordings (Caldero, et al., 2010; Young, et al., 2007). Neonatal brainstem slices can be used to analyze excitotoxicity on hypoglossal motor neurons that control the respiratory drive. These neurons are particularly useful for electrophysiological studies because they exhibit a range of rhythmic patterns that will be altered during early onset of ALS (Cifra, et al., 2011a; Cifra, et al., 2011b).

Organotypic culture is a convenient culture system that closely reproduces the *in vivo* situation and allows dynamic studies with various drugs and useful analysis systems. However, it does not always fully recapitulate what is happening *in vivo* (Tovar, et al., 2009). In addition, it does not easily allow the study of different mixed cell combinations by removing or by adding specific cell types to the tissue slices. These organotypic spinal cord slice cultures are difficult to obtain from postmortem patients due to limited availability and it is obviously impossible to study disease progression using human spinal cord biopsies as opposed to biopsies obtained from animal models.

3.2 Spinal cord cell cultures

The isolation of individual cells is extremely useful to study various intracellular mechanisms from proliferation to mRNA expression, mitochondrial function, protein aggregation, intermediate filament assembly or axonal transport. However, neurons cannot proliferate and are difficult to maintain in culture. In addition, adult nervous tissues are difficult to access and the viability of the cells extracted from them is very low. Actually, most of the cells that can be maintained in culture after extraction are neural precursor cells (Haidet-Phillips, et al., 2011).

To overcome this limitation, embryos are preferred for nervous tissue harvesting. Indeed, at the E12-13 embryonic developmental stage, the spinal cord of mice embryos is easy to access and remove, and motor neurons, astrocytes and microglia can be extracted, purified and maintain in culture with high viability yields (Gingras, et al., 2007b; Sanelli, et al., 2007; Schnaar and Schaffner, 1981). These cells can be dissociated from the spinal cord and cultured together to facilitate motor neuron survival (Tradewell, et al., 2011; Tradewell and Durham, 2010). Motor neurons will be easy to identify because of their large cell body (>20μm in diameter) and dendritic trees, and can be stained for expression of the transcription factor Hb9 and choline acetyltransferase, specific molecular markers of motor neuron (Fig 3) (Gingras, et al., 2007b; Tradewell, et al., 2011).

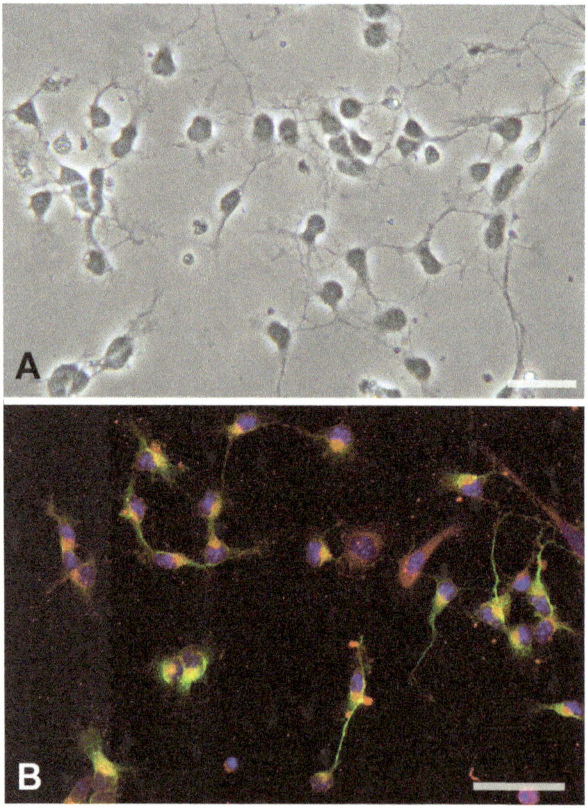

Fig. 3. E12 mouse embryo-purified motor neurons.
A: phase contrast microscopy of purified motor neurons 24h after seeding. B: Motor neurons were labeled in red with Hb9 and in green with MAP2. Bar represent 30 μm in A and 50μm in B. *Courtesy of Dr. Marie Gingras.*

Cultures of purified motor neurons without the trophic support of glial cells are difficult to maintain for more than 2 weeks (Bar, 2000; Lunn, et al., 2009). In order to perform studies on a chronic disease like ALS, especially while looking for long-term cell survival effects, dissociated spinal cord cell cultures constitute a better choice as they can be maintain in culture for up to 7 weeks (Tradewell, et al., 2011). Purified motor neurons can also be cultured on an astrocyte feeder layer for several weeks on which they display characteristics (neurite pattern) closer to adult motor neurons (Bar, 2000). To reproduce an ALS phenotype, motor neurons can be induced to express multiple copies of the gene of interest, for example, mutated human G93A SOD1, by microinjection of the vectors into the cells identified by their specific morphology (Tradewell, et al., 2011; Tradewell and Durham, 2010). Motor neurons can also be purified and cultured separately, to allow their adenoviral transduction with G93A SOD1 (Lunn, et al., 2009), and then, to enhance their survival, they can be plated on a glial cell feeder layer treated with arabinofuranosyl cytidine (AraC), to prevent cell proliferation (De Paola, et al., 2008). These *in vitro* cultures are particularly useful to study cellular morphometry (axon length), gene expression using RT-PCR (ideally with only one purified cell type), apoptosis, signaling pathways, calcium imaging, mitochondrial membrane potential, glutamate uptake, excitotoxicity, etc.

The major drawbacks of spinal cord cell cultures are the need to perform cell extraction from embryos for each new experiment. In addition, cells cultured on plastic dishes cannot recapitulate the *in vivo* environment and some results obtained *in vitro* may not be reproducible *in vivo* at least in part because the complex interactions developed in the nervous system are lost. Furthermore, another disadvantage to use primary cells from embryos is that some features of the adult phenotype may not be expressed at this early stage (Park, et al., 2004).

3.3 NCS-34 motor neuron cell line

To greatly facilitate *in vitro* studies, motor neuron-enriched embryonic mouse spinal cord cells were fused with mouse neuroblastoma to generate the hybrid cell line NCS-34 (Cashman, et al., 1992; Durham, et al., 1993; Hunter, et al., 1991). This cell line contains small proliferative and undifferentiated cells and larger multinucleate cells. These cells express properties of motor neurons such as choline acetyltransferase, acethylcholine synthesis and neurofilament expression. They respond to agents affecting voltage-gated ion channels, cytoskeletal organization and axonal transport similarly with primary motor neurons, but failed to reproduce synaptic connections (Durham, et al., 1993). This cell line is widely used in several studies related to ALS (Foran, et al., 2011; Tabata, et al., 2008; Vijayalakshmi, et al., 2009; Yang, et al., 2010). For example, NCS-34 cells were treated with the cerebrospinal fluid (CSF) collected from sporadic ALS patients. It induced intracellular aggregates formation, ubiquitin immunoreactivity, neurofilament phosphorylation and choline acetyl transferase expression through induction of endoplasmic reticular stress. This effect was attenuated by addition of VEGF prior to exposition to CSF (Kulshreshtha, et al., 2011; Vijayalakshmi, et al., 2011; Vijayalakshmi, et al., 2009). NCS-34 cells can also be used to screen antioxidant molecules capable of rescuing them from expression of mutated SOD1 (Barber, et al., 2009).

3.4 Xenopus oocyte model for electrophysiological recordings

The *Xenopus Laevi* is an African frog from which the oocyte (egg) is a commonly used model for electrophysiological recording because of its large size (about 1mm in diameter) which facilitates its handling. The oocyte has been used for decades to study various ion channels, transporters and receptors. This cell can be transduced with a molecules of interest for co-expression studies including the human glutamate transporter GLT1 (EAAT2) or NMDA receptors (Boehmer, et al., 2006; Texido, et al., 2011; Trotti, et al., 2001). This model has been used in some studies related to ALS, such as the analysis of the properties of the GLT1 transporter activities under controlled voltage clamp in presence or not of mutant SOD1 (Trotti, et al., 1999).

3.5 Neural precursor cells (NPCs) and induced pluripotent stem cells (iPS)

One important advantage of *in vitro* cell cultures could gain over animal models would be to collect neural precursor cells directly from patients. These cells can be differentiated into all neural cell types, including motor neurons. As previously discussed, most of animal and cell culture models developed to study ALS so far were derived from known FALS-associated mutations in the *SOD1*, *TARDBP* or *FUS/TLS* genes. While these models are particularly useful to study FALS, they are not ideal for the study of SALS. Therefore, trying to understand the cause of the disease through the study of motor neurons and glial cells obtained from SALS patients would be challenging but potentially highly promising. However, motor neurons, and even glial cells are extremely difficult to isolate from brain and spinal cord samples obtained from post-mortem ALS patients.

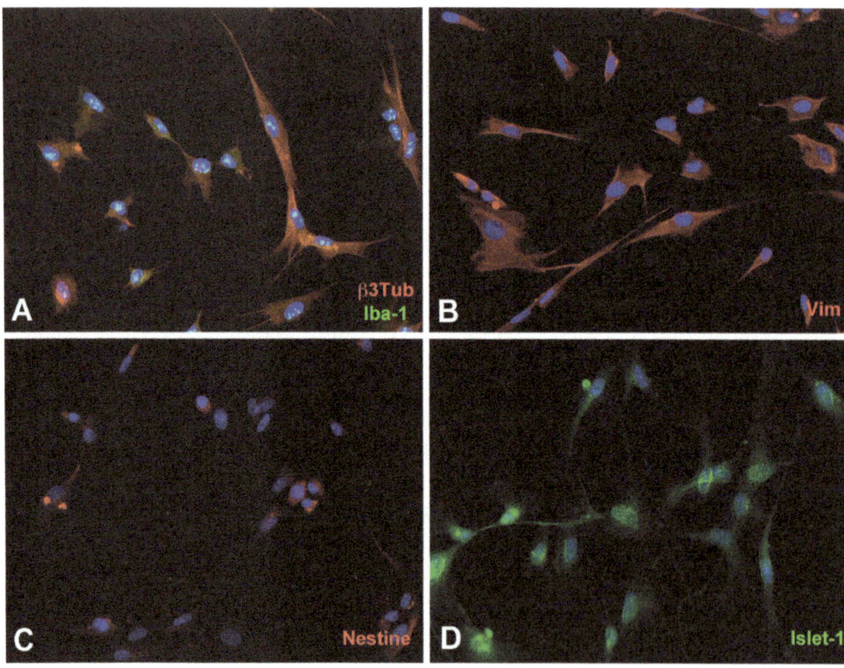

Fig. 4. Characterization of neural precursor cells (NPCs) extracted from postmortem ALS patient's spinal cord.
Cells express Iba1 (a marker of microglia) and β3-tubulin (early marker of neuronal differentiation) (A), Vimentin (transiently expressed in neuronal precursors) (B), Nestin (transiently expressed in neuronal precursors) (C) and Islet-1 (an early marker for motor neuron differentiation) (C) that highlight their NPC status when co-expressed together in the same cells. *Courtesy of Dr. Marie-Josée Beaulieu.*

One very promising alternative is to take advantage of the neural precursor cells that can be extracted from adult tissues. Indeed, in a first step, the potential of mouse embryonic stem cells (ESCs) to differentiate into motor neurons has been well established (Wichterle, et al., 2002) and applied to the development of *in vitro* ALS models using ALS-linked G93A *SOD1* gene mutation and WT SOD1 mouse embryos as source of stem cells (Di Giorgio, et al.,

2007). It was shown that G93A-SOD1 ESCs differentiated into motor neurons had a lower survival over 2 to 4 weeks in culture than their WT counterparts and showed ALS pathology hallmarks such as SOD1 protein aggregates and increase in activated caspase-3 expression after 21 days of culture (Di Giorgio, et al., 2007). Motor neurons have also been successfully differentiated from human ESCs (Hester, et al., 2011; Hu and Zhang, 2009). However, to obtain a source of multipotent stem cells from adult ALS patients, other approaches needed to be developed. These cells can be obtained from easily accessible tissues such as skin (Gingras, et al., 2007a; Toma, et al., 2001), but their limited proliferation capacity *in vitro* needs a relatively large amount of starting materials that up to now preclude their extraction from patients. Another possibility is to obtain postmortem biopsies of brain and spinal cord from ALS patients. It has been shown that if living glial cells and neurons are difficult to isolate from these tissues, neural precursor cells (NPCs) with a good proliferation rate are oppositely easy to purify and culture *in vitro*. These cells can then be differentiated in the cell type of interest. Neurons, astrocytes and oligodendrocytes were differentiated from NPCs purified from familial and sporadic ALS patient postmortem spinal cord samples (Fig 4) to study the toxic properties of patients-derived astrocytes on motor neurons (Haidet-Phillips, et al., 2011). Both FALS and SALS-derived astrocytes were shown to be toxic to motor neurons, and the knock-down of SOD1 in SALS-derived astrocytes was demonstrated to attenuate this toxicity (Haidet-Phillips, et al., 2011). But postmortem tissues are difficult to obtain.

A much more versatile technique to generate multipotent stem cells from adults is to generate induced pluripotent stem cells (iPS cells) starting from somatic cells. This technique only requires a small punch biopsy of a few millimeters in diameter collected from the patient's skin, which will heal spontaneously without scarring. From this biopsy, dermal fibroblasts will be extracted and expanded to generate iPS cells. Generation of IPs cells is possible via overexpression of a defined set of transcription factors (*c-Myc*, *Oct3/4*, *Klf4* and *SOX2*) (Takahashi, et al., 2007a; Takahashi, et al., 2007b). The genetic transduction of these oncogenes is usually achieved by using retroviral or lentiviral vectors. However, the use of integrating viral vectors represent a major obstacle to the therapeutic translation of iPS cells as this technology can produce insertional mutagenic lesions that are potentially tumorigenic. Other methods to reprogram cells are now being intensively tested, such as the use of secreted recombinant reprogramming factors present in the culture media. These iPS cells are morphologically and phenotypically similar to embryonic stem (ES) cells and thus offer exciting possibilities in stem cell research and regenerative medicine. This method has been successfully applied to ALS patients and allowed to study iPS-derived motor neurons *in vitro* (Dimos, et al., 2008; Mitne-Neto, et al., 2011). Since this technology is still recent, it is not clear whether motor neurons and glial cells derived from ALS patients-iPS cells will efficiently recapitulate the disease *in vitro*. However, these cells seem to behave like ESCs and even if they only partly mimic the ALS phenotype in culture, they certainly will be extremely interesting to use, especially for a better understanding of sporadic ALS.

3.6 Three-dimensional in vitro models

Now that iPS or NPCs ALS patient-derived motor neurons and glial cells will be available to develop better ALS *in vitro* models, their design could also be improved. The culture of neural cells in two dimensions on plastic does not mimic properly the *in vivo* situation. Building three-dimensional environment around ALS patient-derived neural cells could be a major improvement in the development of *in vitro* models of the disease. The culture of NPCs in methylcellulose scaffold enriched with laminin has been shown to reduce apoptosis and enhance survival, differentiation into neurons, astrocytes or oligodendrocytes and neurite extension (Cullen, et al., 2007; Stabenfeldt, et al., 2010). Motor neurons axonal migration can also be analyzed when these cells are cultured on the top of a three-dimensional reconstructed connective tissue made of a collagen sponge populated with fibroblasts. The addition of neurotrophic factors underneath the construct promotes neurite growth from the top to the bottom of the tissue. The main advantage of this model is to enable myelin sheath formation by Schwann cells around axons in the connective tissue and the possibility to add various glial cells (astrocytes, microglia) in the motor neuron layer (Fig 5) (Gingras, et al., 2008). In addition, it is possible to easily combine cells from different origin, like WT motor neurons with ALS glial cells, and vice-versa in order to further explore the non-cell autonomous effect observed in SOD1-linked ALS pathology. Such combinations could also be very informative in the study of sporadic ALS. Alternatively, a 3 dimensional reconstructed muscle model has been developed to study *in vitro* the effect of muscle stretching on mRNA expression of muscle cells. This model was prepared using primary muscle cultures from human control subjects and ALS patients. The cells were embedded in a collagen gel tethered to a Culture Force Monitor to analyze gel contraction (Cheema, et al., 2003; Evans, et al., 2010).

Finally, the combination of ALS patient NPC-derived neural cells in tissue-engineered reconstructed spinal cord models is a promising strategy to develop the next generation of *in vitro* models of ALS.

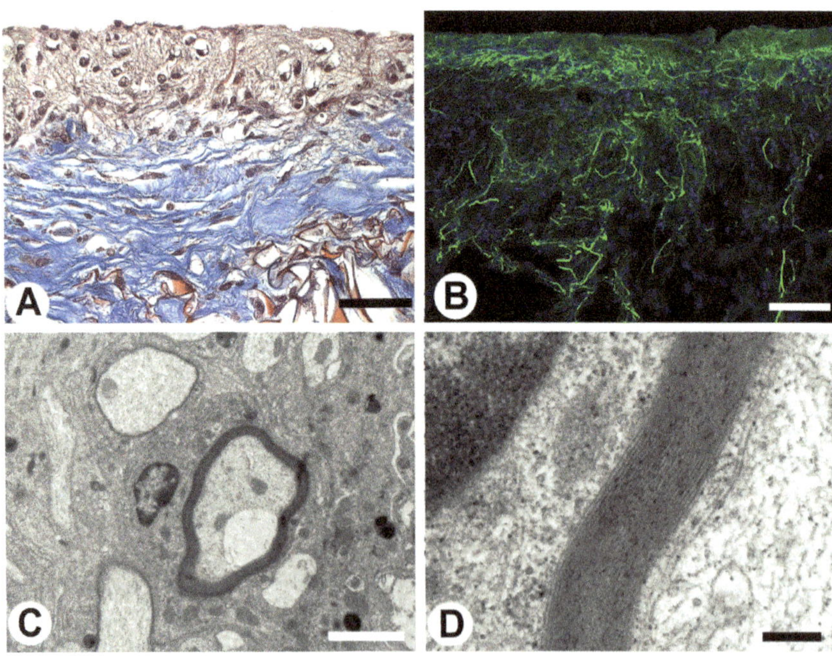

Fig. 5. Three-dimensional model of motor neuron axonal migration and myelin sheath formation.

In A, after the culture of fibroblasts and Schwann cells for 21 days in a collagen sponge (blue area), mouse motor neurons were seeded on top of the sponge (purple area) and cultured for an additional 14 days and observed by histology staining with Masson's trichrom. In B, axonal migration (stained in green with an antibody against Neurofilament-M) originating from the top layer was shown migrating through the connective tissue. In C, a transmission electron microscopic picture showed that some neurites were wrapped with thick myelin sheaths, observed at higher magnification in D. Bar in A, 60µm; bar in B, 100µm; bar in C, 2µm; bar in F, 0,2µm *(Modified from Gingras, et al., 2008).*

4. Conclusion

A very large body of knowledge has been built over the years with the development of various *in vivo* models to better understand ALS. Particularly, the generation of a large number of different transgenic mice has been extremely useful to study familial ALS, but has met with limited success so far to study SALS or to identify drugs alleviating the disease symptoms. This could be explained by the existence of redundant compensatory mechanisms present in higher vertebrates. The use of invertebrates together with higher animal models will hopefully allow the identification of novel pathogenic pathways and novel therapeutic avenues in order to cure this devastating disease.

In parallel, the development of *in vitro* models will give valuable information about the intracellular modulations induced by the disease. In addition, the promise of building sophisticated *in vitro* models using patient's cells will also be crucial to better understand the disease. However, the results obtained from *in vitro* models may not always be relevant because they are oversimplified compared to the *in vivo* situation. Therefore, the best strategy to reduce the limitations inherent to all these different models, and to benefit from their specific advantages is to combine both *in vivo* and *in vitro* models in order to better model the disease. Future work, focusing on different neuronal in vitro system and animal models, will certainly increases our knowledge in the biology of ALS and hopefully leads to more translational researches in order to find a cure or to slow down the course of this yet untreatable disease.

5. Acknowledgment

We would like to thank Dr. Alex J. Parker and Dr Guy A. Rouleau, from the Centre of Excellence in Neuromics, University of Montreal, Quebec, Canada, for having provided respectively the figure 1 and 2 of this book chapter. We also thank Marie Gingras and Marie-Josée Beaudet for their assistance in generating figure 3 to 5. Dr François Gros-Louis is supported by the Fond de la recherche en santé du Québec (FRSQ) and by the Fondation des hôpitaux Enfant-Jésus–St-Sacrement. Dr François Berthod is supported by the Muscular Dystrophy Association USA (www.mda.org). The authors declare no conflict of interest.

6. References

Adams, M. D., Celniker, S. E., Holt, R. A., Evans, C. A., Gocayne, J. D., Amanatides, P. G., Scherer, S. E., Li, P. W., Hoskins, R. A., Galle, R. F., George, R. A., Lewis, S. E., Richards, S., Ashburner, M., Henderson, S. N., Sutton, G. G., Wortman, J. R., Yandell, M. D., Zhang, Q., Chen, L. X., Brandon, R. C., Rogers, Y. H., Blazej, R. G., Champe,

M., Pfeiffer, B. D., Wan, K. H., Doyle, C., Baxter, E. G., Helt, G., Nelson, C. R., Gabor, G. L., Abril, J. F., Agbayani, A., An, H. J., Andrews-Pfannkoch, C., Baldwin, D., Ballew, R. M., Basu, A., Baxendale, J., Bayraktaroglu, L., Beasley, E. M., Beeson, K. Y., Benos, P. V., Berman, B. P., Bhandari, D., Bolshakov, S., Borkova, D., Botchan, M. R., Bouck, J., Brokstein, P., Brottier, P., Burtis, K. C., Busam, D. A., Butler, H., Cadieu, E., Center, A., Chandra, I., Cherry, J. M., Cawley, S., Dahlke, C., Davenport, L. B., Davies, P., de Pablos, B., Delcher, A., Deng, Z., Mays, A. D., Dew, I., Dietz, S. M., Dodson, K., Doup, L. E., Downes, M., Dugan-Rocha, S., Dunkov, B. C., Dunn, P., Durbin, K. J., Evangelista, C. C., Ferraz, C., Ferriera, S., Fleischmann, W., Fosler, C., Gabrielian, A. E., Garg, N. S., Gelbart, W. M., Glasser, K., Glodek, A., Gong, F., Gorrell, J. H., Gu, Z., Guan, P., Harris, M., Harris, N. L., Harvey, D., Heiman, T. J., Hernandez, J. R., Houck, J., Hostin, D., Houston, K. A., Howland, T. J., Wei, M. H., Ibegwam, C., Jalali, M., Kalush, F., Karpen, G. H., Ke, Z., Kennison, J. A., Ketchum, K. A., Kimmel, B. E., Kodira, C. D., Kraft, C., Kravitz, S., Kulp, D., Lai, Z., Lasko, P., Lei, Y., Levitsky, A. A., Li, J., Li, Z., Liang, Y., Lin, X., Liu, X., Mattei, B., McIntosh, T. C., McLeod, M. P., McPherson, D., Merkulov, G., Milshina, N. V., Mobarry, C., Morris, J., Moshrefi, A., Mount, S. M., Moy, M., Murphy, B., Murphy, L., Muzny, D. M., Nelson, D. L., Nelson, D. R., Nelson, K. A., Nixon, K., Nusskern, D. R., Pacleb, J. M., Palazzolo, M., Pittman, G. S., Pan, S., Pollard, J., Puri, V., Reese, M. G., Reinert, K., Remington, K., Saunders, R. D., Scheeler, F., Shen, H., Shue, B. C., Siden-Kiamos, I., Simpson, M., Skupski, M. P., Smith, T., Spier, E., Spradling, A. C., Stapleton, M., Strong, R., Sun, E., Svirskas, R., Tector, C., Turner, R., Venter, E., Wang, A. H., Wang, X., Wang, Z. Y., Wassarman, D. A., Weinstock, G. M., Weissenbach, J., Williams, S. M., WoodageT, Worley, K. C., Wu, D., Yang, S., Yao, Q. A., Ye, J., Yeh, R. F., Zaveri, J. S., Zhan, M., Zhang, G., Zhao, Q., Zheng, L., Zheng, X. H., Zhong, F. N., Zhong, W., Zhou, X., Zhu, S., Zhu, X., Smith, H. O., Gibbs, R. A., Myers, E. W., Rubin, G. M. and Venter, J. C. (2000). The genome sequence of Drosophila melanogaster. *Science*, 287, 2185-95.

Amsterdam, A., Burgess, S., Golling, G., Chen, W., Sun, Z., Townsend, K., Farrington, S., Haldi, M. and Hopkins, N. (1999). A large-scale insertional mutagenesis screen in zebrafish. *Genes Dev*, 13, 2713-24.

Amsterdam, A. and Hopkins, N. (2006). Mutagenesis strategies in zebrafish for identifying genes involved in development and disease. *Trends Genet*, 22, 473-8.

Anonymous (1998). Genome sequence of the nematode C. elegans: a platform for investigating biology. *Science*, 282, 2012-8.

Ash, P. E., Zhang, Y. J., Roberts, C. M., Saldi, T., Hutter, H., Buratti, E., Petrucelli, L. and Link, C. D. (2010). Neurotoxic effects of TDP-43 overexpression in C. elegans. *Hum Mol Genet*, 19, 3206-18.

Averill, D. R., Jr. (1973). Degenerative myelopathy in the aging German Shepherd dog: clinical and pathologic findings. *J Am Vet Med Assoc*, 162, 1045-51.

Awano, T., Johnson, G. S., Wade, C. M., Katz, M. L., Johnson, G. C., Taylor, J. F., Perloski, M., Biagi, T., Baranowska, I., Long, S., March, P. A., Olby, N. J., Shelton, G. D., Khan, S., O'Brien, D. P., Lindblad-Toh, K. and Coates, J. R. (2009). Genome-wide association analysis reveals a SOD1 mutation in canine degenerative myelopathy that resembles amyotrophic lateral sclerosis. *Proc Natl Acad Sci U S A*, 106, 2794-9.

Bar, P. R. (2000). Motor neuron disease in vitro: the use of cultured motor neurons to study amyotrophic lateral sclerosis. *Eur J Pharmacol*, 405, 285-95.

Barber, S. C., Higginbottom, A., Mead, R. J., Barber, S. and Shaw, P. J. (2009). An in vitro screening cascade to identify neuroprotective antioxidants in ALS. *Free Radic Biol Med*, 46, 1127-38.

Bargmann, C. I. (1998). Neurobiology of the Caenorhabditis elegans genome. *Science*, 282, 2028-33.

Beaulieu, J. M., Jacomy, H. and Julien, J. P. (2000). Formation of intermediate filament protein aggregates with disparate effects in two transgenic mouse models lacking the neurofilament light subunit. *J Neurosci*, 20, 5321-8.

Beaulieu, J. M. and Julien, J. P. (2003). Peripherin-mediated death of motor neurons rescued by overexpression of neurofilament NF-H proteins. *J Neurochem*, 85, 248-56.

Beaulieu, J. M., Nguyen, M. D. and Julien, J. P. (1999). Late onset of motor neurons in mice overexpressing wild-type peripherin. *J Cell Biol*, 147, 531-44.

Boehmer, C., Palmada, M., Rajamanickam, J., Schniepp, R., Amara, S. and Lang, F. (2006). Post-translational regulation of EAAT2 function by co-expressed ubiquitin ligase Nedd4-2 is impacted by SGK kinases. *J Neurochem*, 97, 911-21.

Boillee, S., Yamanaka, K., Lobsiger, C. S., Copeland, N. G., Jenkins, N. A., Kassiotis, G., Kollias, G. and Cleveland, D. W. (2006). Onset and progression in inherited ALS determined by motor neurons and microglia. *Science*, 312, 1389-92.

Borchelt, D. R., Lee, M. K., Slunt, H. S., Guarnieri, M., Xu, Z. S., Wong, P. C., Brown, R. H., Jr., Price, D. L., Sisodia, S. S. and Cleveland, D. W. (1994). Superoxide dismutase 1 with mutations linked to familial amyotrophic lateral sclerosis possesses significant activity. *Proc Natl Acad Sci U S A*, 91, 8292-6.

Bosco, D. A., Lemay, N., Ko, H. K., Zhou, H., Burke, C., Kwiatkowski, T. J., Jr., Sapp, P., McKenna-Yasek, D., Brown, R. H., Jr. and Hayward, L. J. (2010a). Mutant FUS proteins that cause amyotrophic lateral sclerosis incorporate into stress granules. *Hum Mol Genet*, 19, 4160-75.

Bosco, D. A., Morfini, G., Karabacak, N. M., Song, Y., Gros-Louis, F., Pasinelli, P., Goolsby, H., Fontaine, B. A., Lemay, N., McKenna-Yasek, D., Frosch, M. P., Agar, J. N., Julien, J. P., Brady, S. T. and Brown, R. H., Jr. (2010b). Wild-type and mutant SOD1 share an aberrant conformation and a common pathogenic pathway in ALS. *Nat Neurosci*, 13, 1396-403.

Brand, A. H. and Perrimon, N. (1993). Targeted gene expression as a means of altering cell fates and generating dominant phenotypes. *Development*, 118, 401-15.

Brenner, S. (1974). The genetics of Caenorhabditis elegans. *Genetics*, 77, 71-94.

Bruijn, L. I., Becher, M. W., Lee, M. K., Anderson, K. L., Jenkins, N. A., Copeland, N. G., Sisodia, S. S., Rothstein, J. D., Borchelt, D. R., Price, D. L. and Cleveland, D. W. (1997). ALS-linked SOD1 mutant G85R mediates damage to astrocytes and promotes rapidly progressive disease with SOD1-containing inclusions. *Neuron*, 18, 327-38.

Bruijn, L. I., Houseweart, M. K., Kato, S., Anderson, K. L., Anderson, S. D., Ohama, E., Reaume, A. G., Scott, R. W. and Cleveland, D. W. (1998). Aggregation and motor neuron toxicity of an ALS-linked SOD1 mutant independent from wild-type SOD1. *Science*, 281, 1851-4.

Cai, H., Lin, X., Xie, C., Laird, F. M., Lai, C., Wen, H., Chiang, H. C., Shim, H., Farah, M. H., Hoke, A., Price, D. L. and Wong, P. C. (2005). Loss of ALS2 function is insufficient to trigger motor neuron degeneration in knock-out mice but predisposes neurons to oxidative stress. *J Neurosci*, 25, 7567-74.

Caldero, J., Brunet, N., Tarabal, O., Piedrafita, L., Hereu, M., Ayala, V. and Esquerda, J. E. (2010). Lithium prevents excitotoxic cell death of motoneurons in organotypic slice cultures of spinal cord. *Neuroscience*, 165, 1353-69.

Cashman, N. R., Durham, H. D., Blusztajn, J. K., Oda, K., Tabira, T., Shaw, I. T., Dahrouge, S. and Antel, J. P. (1992). Neuroblastoma x spinal cord (NSC) hybrid cell lines resemble developing motor neurons. *Dev Dyn*, 194, 209-21.

Cheema, U., Yang, S. Y., Mudera, V., Goldspink, G. G. and Brown, R. A. (2003). 3-D in vitro model of early skeletal muscle development. *Cell Motil Cytoskeleton*, 54, 226-36.

Chen, Y., Yang, M., Deng, J., Chen, X., Ye, Y., Zhu, L., Liu, J., Ye, H., Shen, Y., Li, Y., Rao, E. J., Fushimi, K., Zhou, X., Bigio, E. H., Mesulam, M., Xu, Q. and Wu, J. Y. (2011). Expression of human FUS protein in Drosophila leads to progressive neurodegeneration. *Protein Cell*, 2, 477-86.

Chio, A., Borghero, G., Pugliatti, M., Ticca, A., Calvo, A., Moglia, C., Mutani, R., Brunetti, M., Ossola, I., Marrosu, M. G., Murru, M. R., Floris, G., Cannas, A., Parish, L. D., Cossu, P., Abramzon, Y., Johnson, J. O., Nalls, M. A., Arepalli, S., Chong, S., Hernandez, D. G., Traynor, B. J. and Restagno, G. (2011). Large proportion of amyotrophic lateral sclerosis cases in Sardinia due to a single founder mutation of the TARDBP gene. *Arch Neurol*, 68, 594-8.

Chow, C. Y., Landers, J. E., Bergren, S. K., Sapp, P. C., Grant, A. E., Jones, J. M., Everett, L., Lenk, G. M., McKenna-Yasek, D. M., Weisman, L. S., Figlewicz, D., Brown, R. H. and Meisler, M. H. (2009). Deleterious variants of FIG4, a phosphoinositide phosphatase, in patients with ALS. *Am J Hum Genet*, 84, 85-8.

Christensen, M., Estevez, A., Yin, X., Fox, R., Morrison, R., McDonnell, M., Gleason, C., Miller, D. M., 3rd and Strange, K. (2002). A primary culture system for functional analysis of C. elegans neurons and muscle cells. *Neuron*, 33, 503-14.

Cifra, A., Nani, F. and Nistri, A. (2011a). Respiratory motoneurons and pathological conditions: Lessons from hypoglossal motoneurons challenged by excitotoxic or oxidative stress. *Respir Physiol Neurobiol*, doi:10.1016/j.resp.2011.03.017.

Cifra, A., Nani, F. and Nistri, A. (2011b). Riluzole is a potent drug to protect neonatal rat hypoglossal motoneurons in vitro from excitotoxicity due to glutamate uptake block. *Eur J Neurosci*, 33, 899-913.

Clement, A. M., Nguyen, M. D., Roberts, E. A., Garcia, M. L., Boillee, S., Rule, M., McMahon, A. P., Doucette, W., Siwek, D., Ferrante, R. J., Brown, R. H., Jr., Julien, J. P., Goldstein, L. S. and Cleveland, D. W. (2003). Wild-type nonneuronal cells extend survival of SOD1 mutant motor neurons in ALS mice. *Science*, 302, 113-7.

Corbo, M. and Hays, A. P. (1992). Peripherin and neurofilament protein coexist in spinal spheroids of motor neuron disease. *J Neuropathol Exp Neurol*, 51, 531-7.

Corrado, L., Ratti, A., Gellera, C., Buratti, E., Castellotti, B., Carlomagno, Y., Ticozzi, N., Mazzini, L., Testa, L., Taroni, F., Baralle, F. E., Silani, V. and D'Alfonso, S. (2009). High frequency of TARDBP gene mutations in Italian patients with amyotrophic lateral sclerosis. *Hum Mutat*, 30, 688-94.

Cote, F., Collard, J. F. and Julien, J. P. (1993). Progressive neuronopathy in transgenic mice expressing the human neurofilament heavy gene: a mouse model of amyotrophic lateral sclerosis. *Cell*, 73, 35-46.

Culetto, E. and Sattelle, D. B. (2000). A role for Caenorhabditis elegans in understanding the function and interactions of human disease genes. *Hum Mol Genet*, 9, 869-77.

Cullen, D. K., Stabenfeldt, S. E., Simon, C. M., Tate, C. C. and LaPlaca, M. C. (2007). In vitro neural injury model for optimization of tissue-engineered constructs. *J Neurosci Res*, 85, 3642-51.

Daoud, H., Valdmanis, P. N., Kabashi, E., Dion, P., Dupre, N., Camu, W., Meininger, V. and Rouleau, G. A. (2009). Contribution of TARDBP mutations to sporadic amyotrophic lateral sclerosis. *J Med Genet*, 46, 112-4.

De Paola, M., Diana, V., Bigini, P. and Mennini, T. (2008). Morphological features and responses to AMPA receptor-mediated excitotoxicity of mouse motor neurons: comparison in purified, mixed anterior horn or motor neuron/glia cocultures. *J Neurosci Methods*, 170, 85-95.

DeJesus-Hernandez, M., Mackenzie, I. R., Boeve, B. F., Boxer, A. L., Baker, M., Rutherford, N. J., Nicholson, A. M., Finch, N. A., Flynn, H., Adamson, J., Kouri, N., Wojtas, A., Sengdy, P., Hsiung, G. R., Karydas, A., Seeley, W. W., Josephs, K. A., Coppola, G., Geschwind, D. H., Wszolek, Z. K., Feldman, H., Knopman, D. S., Petersen, R. C., Miller, B. L., Dickson, D. W., Boylan, K. B., Graff-Radford, N. R. and Rademakers, R. (2011). Expanded GGGGCC Hexanucleotide Repeat in Noncoding Region of C9ORF72 Causes Chromosome 9p-Linked FTD and ALS. *Neuron*.

Delfs, J., Friend, J., Ishimoto, S. and Saroff, D. (1989). Ventral and dorsal horn acetylcholinesterase neurons are maintained in organotypic cultures of postnatal rat spinal cord explants. *Brain Res*, 488, 31-42.

Deng, H. X., Zhai, H., Fu, R., Shi, Y., Gorrie, G. H., Yang, Y., Liu, E., Dal Canto, M. C., Mugnaini, E. and Siddique, T. (2007). Distal axonopathy in an alsin-deficient mouse model. *Hum Mol Genet*, 16, 2911-20.

Devon, R. S., Helm, J. R., Rouleau, G. A., Leitner, Y., Lerman-Sagie, T., Lev, D. and Hayden, M. R. (2003). The first nonsense mutation in alsin results in a homogeneous phenotype of infantile-onset ascending spastic paralysis with bulbar involvement in two siblings. *Clin Genet*, 64, 210-5.

Di Giorgio, F. P., Carrasco, M. A., Siao, M. C., Maniatis, T. and Eggan, K. (2007). Non-cell autonomous effect of glia on motor neurons in an embryonic stem cell-based ALS model. *Nat Neurosci*, 10, 608-14.

Dimos, J. T., Rodolfa, K. T., Niakan, K. K., Weisenthal, L. M., Mitsumoto, H., Chung, W., Croft, G. F., Saphier, G., Leibel, R., Goland, R., Wichterle, H., Henderson, C. E. and Eggan, K. (2008). Induced pluripotent stem cells generated from patients with ALS can be differentiated into motor neurons. *Science*, 321, 1218-21.

Driever, W., Solnica-Krezel, L., Schier, A. F., Neuhauss, S. C., Malicki, J., Stemple, D. L., Stainier, D. Y., Zwartkruis, F., Abdelilah, S., Rangini, Z., Belak, J. and Boggs, C. (1996). A genetic screen for mutations affecting embryogenesis in zebrafish. *Development*, 123, 37-46.

Durham, H. D., Dahrouge, S. and Cashman, N. R. (1993). Evaluation of the spinal cord neuron X neuroblastoma hybrid cell line NSC-34 as a model for neurotoxicity testing. *Neurotoxicology*, 14, 387-95.

Elden, A. C., Kim, H. J., Hart, M. P., Chen-Plotkin, A. S., Johnson, B. S., Fang, X., Armakola, M., Geser, F., Greene, R., Lu, M. M., Padmanabhan, A., Clay-Falcone, D., McCluskey, L., Elman, L., Juhr, D., Gruber, P. J., Rub, U., Auburger, G., Trojanowski, J. Q., Lee, V. M., Van Deerlin, V. M., Bonini, N. M. and Gitler, A. D. (2010). Ataxin-2 intermediate-length polyglutamine expansions are associated with increased risk for ALS. *Nature*, 466, 1069-75.

Estes, P. S., Boehringer, A., Zwick, R., Tang, J. E., Grigsby, B. and Zarnescu, D. C. (2011). Wild-type and A315T mutant TDP-43 exert differential neurotoxicity in a Drosophila model of ALS. *Hum Mol Genet*, 20, 2308-21.

Evans, R. M., Harridge, S. D., Velloso, C. P., Yang, S. Y., Goldspink, G. and Orrell, R. W. (2010). Investigation of MGF mRNA expression in patients with amyotrophic lateral sclerosis using parallel in vivo and in vitro approaches. *Amyotroph Lateral Scler*, 11, 172-7.

Eymard-Pierre, E., Lesca, G., Dollet, S., Santorelli, F. M., di Capua, M., Bertini, E. and Boespflug-Tanguy, O. (2002). Infantile-onset ascending hereditary spastic paralysis is associated with mutations in the alsin gene. *Am J Hum Genet*, 71, 518-27.

Eymard-Pierre, E., Yamanaka, K., Haeussler, M., Kress, W., Gauthier-Barichard, F., Combes, P., Cleveland, D. W. and Boespflug-Tanguy, O. (2006). Novel missense mutation in ALS2 gene results in infantile ascending hereditary spastic paralysis. *Ann Neurol*, 59, 976-80.

Ezzi, S. A., Urushitani, M. and Julien, J. P. (2007). Wild-type superoxide dismutase acquires binding and toxic properties of ALS-linked mutant forms through oxidation. *J Neurochem*, 102, 170-8.

Feiguin, F., Godena, V. K., Romano, G., D'Ambrogio, A., Klima, R. and Baralle, F. E. (2009). Depletion of TDP-43 affects Drosophila motoneurons terminal synapsis and locomotive behavior. *FEBS Lett*, 583, 1586-92.

Fire, A., Xu, S., Montgomery, M. K., Kostas, S. A., Driver, S. E. and Mello, C. C. (1998). Potent and specific genetic interference by double-stranded RNA in Caenorhabditis elegans. *Nature*, 391, 806-11.

Foran, E., Bogush, A., Goffredo, M., Roncaglia, P., Gustincich, S., Pasinelli, P. and Trotti, D. (2011). Motor neuron impairment mediated by a sumoylated fragment of the glial glutamate transporter EAAT2. *Glia*.

Gidalevitz, T., Krupinski, T., Garcia, S. and Morimoto, R. I. (2009). Destabilizing protein polymorphisms in the genetic background direct phenotypic expression of mutant SOD1 toxicity. *PLoS Genet*, 5, e1000399.

Gingras, M., Beaulieu, M. M., Gagnon, V., Durham, H. D. and Berthod, F. (2008). In vitro study of axonal migration and myelination of motor neurons in a three-dimensional tissue-engineered model. *Glia*, 56, 354-64.

Gingras, M., Champigny, M. F. and Berthod, F. (2007a). Differentiation of human adult skin-derived neuronal precursors into mature neurons. *J Cell Physiol*, 210, 498-506.

Gingras, M., Gagnon, V., Minotti, S., Durham, H. D. and Berthod, F. (2007b). Optimized protocols for isolation of primary motor neurons, astrocytes and microglia from embryonic mouse spinal cord. *J Neurosci Methods*, 163, 111-8.

Gitcho, M. A., Baloh, R. H., Chakraverty, S., Mayo, K., Norton, J. B., Levitch, D., Hatanpaa, K. J., White, C. L., 3rd, Bigio, E. H., Caselli, R., Baker, M., Al-Lozi, M. T., Morris, J. C., Pestronk, A., Rademakers, R., Goate, A. M. and Cairns, N. J. (2008). TDP-43 A315T mutation in familial motor neuron disease. *Ann Neurol*, 63, 535-8.

Gong, Y. H., Parsadanian, A. S., Andreeva, A., Snider, W. D. and Elliott, J. L. (2000). Restricted expression of G86R Cu/Zn superoxide dismutase in astrocytes results in astrocytosis but does not cause motoneuron degeneration. *J Neurosci*, 20, 660-5.

Gros-Louis, F., Andersen, P. M., Dupre, N., Urushitani, M., Dion, P., Souchon, F., D'Amour, M., Camu, W., Meininger, V., Bouchard, J. P., Rouleau, G. A. and Julien, J. P. (2009a). Chromogranin B P413L variant as risk factor and modifier of disease onset for amyotrophic lateral sclerosis. *Proc Natl Acad Sci U S A*.

Gros-Louis, F., Gaspar, C. and Rouleau, G. A. (2006). Genetics of familial and sporadic amyotrophic lateral sclerosis. *Biochim Biophys Acta*, 1762, 956-72.

Gros-Louis, F., Gowing, G. and Julien, J. P. (2009b). Development of immunotherapeutic approaches to amyotrophic lateral sclerosis. *Future Neurol*, 4, 435-47.

Gros-Louis, F., Kriz, J., Kabashi, E., McDearmid, J., Millecamps, S., Urushitani, M., Lin, L., Dion, P., Zhu, Q., Drapeau, P., Julien, J. P. and Rouleau, G. A. (2008). Als2 mRNA splicing variants detected in KO mice rescue severe motor dysfunction phenotype in Als2 knock-down zebrafish. *Hum Mol Genet*, 17, 2691-702.

Gros-Louis, F., Meijer, I. A., Hand, C. K., Dube, M. P., MacGregor, D. L., Seni, M. H., Devon, R. S., Hayden, M. R., Andermann, F., Andermann, E. and Rouleau, G. A. (2003). An ALS2 gene mutation causes hereditary spastic paraplegia in a Pakistani kindred. *Ann Neurol*, 53, 144-5.

Gros-Louis, F., Soucy, G., Lariviere, R. and Julien, J. P. (2010). Intracerebroventricular infusion of monoclonal antibody or its derived Fab fragment against misfolded forms of SOD1 mutant delays mortality in a mouse model of ALS. *J Neurochem*, 113, 1188-99.

Gurney, M. E., Cutting, F. B., Zhai, P., Doble, A., Taylor, C. P., Andrus, P. K. and Hall, E. D. (1996). Benefit of vitamin E, riluzole, and gabapentin in a transgenic model of familial amyotrophic lateral sclerosis. *Ann Neurol*, 39, 147-57.

Gurney, M. E., Pu, H., Chiu, A. Y., Dal Canto, M. C., Polchow, C. Y., Alexander, D. D., Caliendo, J., Hentati, A., Kwon, Y. W., Deng, H. X. and et al. (1994). Motor neuron degeneration in mice that express a human Cu,Zn superoxide dismutase mutation. *Science*, 264, 1772-5.

Hadano, S., Benn, S. C., Kakuta, S., Otomo, A., Sudo, K., Kunita, R., Suzuki-Utsunomiya, K., Mizumura, H., Shefner, J. M., Cox, G. A., Iwakura, Y., Brown, R. H., Jr. and Ikeda, J. E. (2006). Mice deficient in the Rab5 guanine nucleotide exchange factor ALS2/alsin exhibit age-dependent neurological deficits and altered endosome trafficking. *Hum Mol Genet*, 15, 233-50.

Hadano, S., Hand, C. K., Osuga, H., Yanagisawa, Y., Otomo, A., Devon, R. S., Miyamoto, N., Showguchi-Miyata, J., Okada, Y., Singaraja, R., Figlewicz, D. A., Kwiatkowski, T., Hosler, B. A., Sagie, T., Skaug, J., Nasir, J., Brown, R. H., Jr., Scherer, S. W., Rouleau, G. A., Hayden, M. R. and Ikeda, J. E. (2001). A gene encoding a putative GTPase regulator is mutated in familial amyotrophic lateral sclerosis 2. *Nat Genet*, 29, 166-73.

Haffter, P., Granato, M., Brand, M., Mullins, M. C., Hammerschmidt, M., Kane, D. A., Odenthal, J., van Eeden, F. J., Jiang, Y. J., Heisenberg, C. P., Kelsh, R. N., Furutani-Seiki, M., Vogelsang, E., Beuchle, D., Schach, U., Fabian, C. and Nusslein-Volhard, C. (1996). The identification of genes with unique and essential functions in the development of the zebrafish, Danio rerio. *Development*, 123, 1-36.

Haidet-Phillips, A. M., Hester, M. E., Miranda, C. J., Meyer, K., Braun, L., Frakes, A., Song, S., Likhite, S., Murtha, M. J., Foust, K. D., Rao, M., Eagle, A., Kammesheidt, A., Christensen, A., Mendell, J. R., Burghes, A. H. and Kaspar, B. K. (2011). Astrocytes from familial and sporadic ALS patients are toxic to motor neurons. *Nat Biotechnol*.

Hanson, K. A., Kim, S. H., Wassarman, D. A. and Tibbetts, R. S. (2010). Ubiquilin modifies TDP-43 toxicity in a Drosophila model of amyotrophic lateral sclerosis (ALS). *J Biol Chem*, 285, 11068-72.

Hart, E. A., Caccamo, M., Harrow, J. L., Humphray, S. J., Gilbert, J. G., Trevanion, S., Hubbard, T., Rogers, J. and Rothschild, M. F. (2007). Lessons learned from the initial sequencing of the pig genome: comparative analysis of an 8 Mb region of pig chromosome 17. *Genome Biol*, 8, R168.

Heiman-Patterson, T. D., Deitch, J. S., Blankenhorn, E. P., Erwin, K. L., Perreault, M. J., Alexander, B. K., Byers, N., Toman, I. and Alexander, G. M. (2005). Background and gender effects on survival in the TgN(SOD1-G93A)1Gur mouse model of ALS. *J Neurol Sci*, 236, 1-7.

Henion, P. D., Raible, D. W., Beattie, C. E., Stoesser, K. L., Weston, J. A. and Eisen, J. S. (1996). Screen for mutations affecting development of Zebrafish neural crest. *Dev Genet*, 18, 11-7.

Hester, M. E., Murtha, M. J., Song, S., Rao, M., Miranda, C. J., Meyer, K., Tian, J., Boulting, G., Schaffer, D. V., Zhu, M. X., Pfaff, S. L., Gage, F. H. and Kaspar, B. K. (2011). Rapid and Efficient Generation of Functional Motor Neurons From Human Pluripotent Stem Cells Using Gene Delivered Transcription Factor Codes. *Mol Ther*.

Howland, D. S., Liu, J., She, Y., Goad, B., Maragakis, N. J., Kim, B., Erickson, J., Kulik, J., DeVito, L., Psaltis, G., DeGennaro, L. J., Cleveland, D. W. and Rothstein, J. D. (2002). Focal loss of the glutamate transporter EAAT2 in a transgenic rat model of SOD1 mutant-mediated amyotrophic lateral sclerosis (ALS). *Proc Natl Acad Sci U S A*, 99, 1604-9.

Hu, B. Y. and Zhang, S. C. (2009). Differentiation of spinal motor neurons from pluripotent human stem cells. *Nat Protoc*, 4, 1295-304.

Hunter, D. D., Cashman, N., Morris-Valero, R., Bulock, J. W., Adams, S. P. and Sanes, J. R. (1991). An LRE (leucine-arginine-glutamate)-dependent mechanism for adhesion of neurons to S-laminin. *J Neurosci*, 11, 3960-71.

Hutton, M., Lendon, C. L., Rizzu, P., Baker, M., Froelich, S., Houlden, H., Pickering-Brown, S., Chakraverty, S., Isaacs, A., Grover, A., Hackett, J., Adamson, J., Lincoln, S., Dickson, D., Davies, P., Petersen, R. C., Stevens, M., de Graaff, E., Wauters, E., van Baren, J., Hillebrand, M., Joosse, M., Kwon, J. M., Nowotny, P., Che, L. K., Norton, J., Morris, J. C., Reed, L. A., Trojanowski, J., Basun, H., Lannfelt, L., Neystat, M., Fahn, S., Dark, F., Tannenberg, T., Dodd, P. R., Hayward, N., Kwok, J. B., Schofield, P. R., Andreadis, A., Snowden, J., Craufurd, D., Neary, D., Owen, F., Oostra, B. A., Hardy, J., Goate, A., van Swieten, J., Mann, D., Lynch, T. and Heutink, P. (1998). Association of missense and 5'-splice-site mutations in tau with the inherited dementia FTDP-17. *Nature*, 393, 702-5.

Johnson, J. O., Mandrioli, J., Benatar, M., Abramzon, Y., Van Deerlin, V. M., Trojanowski, J. Q., Gibbs, J. R., Brunetti, M., Gronka, S., Wuu, J., Ding, J., McCluskey, L., Martinez-Lage, M., Falcone, D., Hernandez, D. G., Arepalli, S., Chong, S., Schymick, J. C., Rothstein, J., Landi, F., Wang, Y. D., Calvo, A., Mora, G., Sabatelli, M., Monsurro, M. R., Battistini, S., Salvi, F., Spataro, R., Sola, P., Borghero, G., Galassi, G., Scholz, S. W., Taylor, J. P., Restagno, G., Chio, A. and Traynor, B. J. (2010). Exome sequencing reveals VCP mutations as a cause of familial ALS. *Neuron*, 68, 857-64.

Jonsson, P. A., Ernhill, K., Andersen, P. M., Bergemalm, D., Brannstrom, T., Gredal, O., Nilsson, P. and Marklund, S. L. (2004). Minute quantities of misfolded mutant superoxide dismutase-1 cause amyotrophic lateral sclerosis. *Brain*, 127, 73-88.

Jonsson, P. A., Graffmo, K. S., Andersen, P. M., Brannstrom, T., Lindberg, M., Oliveberg, M. and Marklund, S. L. (2006). Disulphide-reduced superoxide dismutase-1 in CNS of transgenic amyotrophic lateral sclerosis models. *Brain*, 129, 451-64.

Julien, J. P. and Kriz, J. (2006). Transgenic mouse models of amyotrophic lateral sclerosis. *Biochim Biophys Acta*, 1762, 1013-24.

Kabashi, E., Bercier, V., Lissouba, A., Liao, M., Brustein, E., Rouleau, G. A. and Drapeau, P. (2011). FUS and TARDBP but Not SOD1 Interact in Genetic Models of Amyotrophic Lateral Sclerosis. *PLoS Genet*, 7, e1002214.

Kabashi, E., Lin, L., Tradewell, M. L., Dion, P. A., Bercier, V., Bourgouin, P., Rochefort, D., Bel Hadj, S., Durham, H. D., Vande Velde, C., Rouleau, G. A. and Drapeau, P. (2010). Gain and loss of function of ALS-related mutations of TARDBP (TDP-43) cause motor deficits in vivo. *Hum Mol Genet*, 19, 671-83.

Kabashi, E., Valdmanis, P. N., Dion, P., Spiegelman, D., McConkey, B. J., Vande Velde, C., Bouchard, J. P., Lacomblez, L., Pochigaeva, K., Salachas, F., Pradat, P. F., Camu, W., Meininger, V., Dupre, N. and Rouleau, G. A. (2008). TARDBP mutations in individuals with sporadic and familial amyotrophic lateral sclerosis. *Nat Genet*, 40, 572-4.

Kim, S. H., Shi, Y., Hanson, K. A., Williams, L. M., Sakasai, R., Bowler, M. J. and Tibbetts, R. S. (2009). Potentiation of amyotrophic lateral sclerosis (ALS)-associated TDP-43 aggregation by the proteasome-targeting factor, ubiquilin 1. *J Biol Chem*, 284, 8083-92.

Kosuge, Y., Sekikawa-Nishida, K., Negi, H., Ishige, K. and Ito, Y. (2009). Characterization of chronic glutamate-mediated motor neuron toxicity in organotypic spinal cord culture prepared from ALS model mice. *Neurosci Lett*, 454, 165-9.

Kraemer, B. C., Schuck, T., Wheeler, J. M., Robinson, L. C., Trojanowski, J. Q., Lee, V. M. and Schellenberg, G. D. (2010). Loss of murine TDP-43 disrupts motor function and plays an essential role in embryogenesis. *Acta Neuropathol*, 119, 409-19.

Kress, J. A., Kuhnlein, P., Winter, P., Ludolph, A. C., Kassubek, J., Muller, U. and Sperfeld, A. D. (2005). Novel mutation in the ALS2 gene in juvenile amyotrophic lateral sclerosis. *Ann Neurol*, 58, 800-3.

Kulshreshtha, D., Vijayalakshmi, K., Alladi, P. A., Sathyaprabha, T. N., Nalini, A. and Raju, T. R. (2011). Vascular endothelial growth factor attenuates neurodegenerative changes in the NSC-34 motor neuron cell line induced by cerebrospinal fluid of sporadic amyotrophic lateral sclerosis patients. *Neurodegener Dis*, 8, 322-30.

Kwiatkowski, T. J., Jr., Bosco, D. A., Leclerc, A. L., Tamrazian, E., Vanderburg, C. R., Russ, C., Davis, A., Gilchrist, J., Kasarskis, E. J., Munsat, T., Valdmanis, P., Rouleau, G. A., Hosler, B. A., Cortelli, P., de Jong, P. J., Yoshinaga, Y., Haines, J. L., Pericak-Vance, M. A., Yan, J., Ticozzi, N., Siddique, T., McKenna-Yasek, D., Sapp, P. C., Horvitz, H. R., Landers, J. E. and Brown, R. H., Jr. (2009). Mutations in the FUS/TLS gene on chromosome 16 cause familial amyotrophic lateral sclerosis. *Science*, 323, 1205-8.

Lanson, N. A., Jr., Maltare, A., King, H., Smith, R., Kim, J. H., Taylor, J. P., Lloyd, T. E. and Pandey, U. B. (2011). A Drosophila model of FUS-related neurodegeneration reveals genetic interaction between FUS and TDP-43. *Hum Mol Genet*, 20, 2510-23.

Lariviere, R. C. and Julien, J. P. (2004). Functions of intermediate filaments in neuronal development and disease. *J Neurobiol*, 58, 131-48.

Lemmens, R., Van Hoecke, A., Hersmus, N., Geelen, V., D'Hollander, I., Thijs, V., Van Den Bosch, L., Carmeliet, P. and Robberecht, W. (2007). Overexpression of mutant superoxide dismutase 1 causes a motor axonopathy in the zebrafish. *Hum Mol Genet*, 16, 2359-65.

Li, Y., Ray, P., Rao, E. J., Shi, C., Guo, W., Chen, X., Woodruff, E. A., 3rd, Fushimi, K. and Wu, J. Y. (2010). A Drosophila model for TDP-43 proteinopathy. *Proc Natl Acad Sci U S A*, 107, 3169-74.

Liachko, N. F., Guthrie, C. R. and Kraemer, B. C. (2010). Phosphorylation promotes neurotoxicity in a Caenorhabditis elegans model of TDP-43 proteinopathy. *J Neurosci*, 30, 16208-19.

Lin, M. J., Cheng, C. W. and Shen, C. K. (2011). Neuronal function and dysfunction of Drosophila dTDP. *PLoS One*, 6, e20371.

Lindblad-Toh, K., Wade, C. M., Mikkelsen, T. S., Karlsson, E. K., Jaffe, D. B., Kamal, M., Clamp, M., Chang, J. L., Kulbokas, E. J., 3rd, Zody, M. C., Mauceli, E., Xie, X., Breen, M., Wayne, R. K., Ostrander, E. A., Ponting, C. P., Galibert, F., Smith, D. R., DeJong, P. J., Kirkness, E., Alvarez, P., Biagi, T., Brockman, W., Butler, J., Chin, C. W., Cook, A., Cuff, J., Daly, M. J., DeCaprio, D., Gnerre, S., Grabherr, M., Kellis, M., Kleber, M., Bardeleben, C., Goodstadt, L., Heger, A., Hitte, C., Kim, L., Koepfli, K. P., Parker, H. G., Pollinger, J. P., Searle, S. M., Sutter, N. B., Thomas, R., Webber, C., Baldwin, J., Abebe, A., Abouelleil, A., Aftuck, L., Ait-Zahra, M., Aldredge, T., Allen, N., An, P., Anderson, S., Antoine, C., Arachchi, H., Aslam, A., Ayotte, L., Bachantsang, P., Barry, A., Bayul, T., Benamara, M., Berlin, A., Bessette, D., Blitshteyn, B., Bloom, T., Blye, J., Boguslavskiy, L., Bonnet, C., Boukhgalter, B., Brown, A., Cahill, P., Calixte, N., Camarata, J., Cheshatsang, Y., Chu, J., Citroen, M., Collymore, A., Cooke, P., Dawoe, T., Daza, R., Decktor, K., DeGray, S., Dhargay, N., Dooley, K., Dorje, P., Dorjee, K., Dorris, L., Duffey, N., Dupes, A., Egbiremolen, O., Elong, R., Falk, J., Farina, A., Faro, S., Ferguson, D., Ferreira, P., Fisher, S., FitzGerald, M., Foley, K., Foley, C., Franke, A., Friedrich, D., Gage, D., Garber, M., Gearin, G., Giannoukos, G., Goode, T., Goyette, A., Graham, J., Grandbois, E., Gyaltsen, K., Hafez, N., Hagopian, D., Hagos, B., Hall, J., Healy, C., Hegarty, R., Honan, T., Horn, A., Houde, N., Hughes, L., Hunnicutt, L., Husby, M., Jester, B., Jones, C., Kamat, A., Kanga, B., Kells, C., Khazanovich, D., Kieu, A. C., Kisner, P., Kumar, M., Lance, K., Landers, T., Lara, M., Lee, W., Leger, J. P., Lennon, N., Leuper, L., LeVine, S., Liu, J., Liu, X., Lokyitsang, Y., Lokyitsang, T., Lui, A., Macdonald, J., Major, J., Marabella, R., Maru, K., Matthews, C., McDonough, S., Mehta, T., Meldrim, J., Melnikov, A., Meneus, L., Mihalev, A., Mihova, T., Miller, K., Mittelman, R., Mlenga, V., Mulrain, L., Munson, G., Navidi, A., Naylor, J., Nguyen, T., Nguyen, N., Nguyen, C., Nicol, R., Norbu, N., Norbu, C., Novod, N., Nyima, T., Olandt, P., O'Neill, B., O'Neill, K., Osman, S., Oyono, L., Patti, C., Perrin, D., Phunkhang, P., Pierre, F., Priest, M., Rachupka, A., Raghuraman, S., Rameau, R., Ray, V., Raymond, C., Rege, F., Rise, C., Rogers, J., Rogov, P., Sahalie, J., Settipalli, S., Sharpe, T., Shea, T., Sheehan, M., Sherpa, N., Shi, J., Shih, D., Sloan, J., Smith, C., Sparrow, T., Stalker, J., Stange-Thomann, N., Stavropoulos, S., Stone, C., Stone, S., Sykes, S., Tchuinga, P., Tenzing, P., Tesfaye, S., Thoulutsang, D., Thoulutsang, Y., Topham, K., Topping, I., Tsamla, T., Vassiliev, H., Venkataraman, V., Vo, A., Wangchuk, T., Wangdi, T., Weiand, M., Wilkinson, J., Wilson, A., Yadav, S., Yang, S., Yang, X., Young, G., Yu, Q., Zainoun, J., Zembek, L., Zimmer, A. and Lander, E. S. (2005). Genome sequence, comparative analysis and haplotype structure of the domestic dog. *Nature*, 438, 803-19.

Lu, Y., Ferris, J. and Gao, F. B. (2009). Frontotemporal dementia and amyotrophic lateral sclerosis-associated disease protein TDP-43 promotes dendritic branching. *Mol Brain*, 2, 30.

Lunn, J. S., Sakowski, S. A., Kim, B., Rosenberg, A. A. and Feldman, E. L. (2009). Vascular endothelial growth factor prevents G93A-SOD1-induced motor neuron degeneration. *Dev Neurobiol*, 69, 871-84.

Lynch, T., Sano, M., Marder, K. S., Bell, K. L., Foster, N. L., Defendini, R. F., Sima, A. A., Keohane, C., Nygaard, T. G., Fahn, S. and et al. (1994). Clinical characteristics of a family with chromosome 17-linked disinhibition-dementia-parkinsonism-amyotrophy complex. *Neurology*, 44, 1878-84.

Maeda, I., Kohara, Y., Yamamoto, M. and Sugimoto, A. (2001). Large-scale analysis of gene function in Caenorhabditis elegans by high-throughput RNAi. *Curr Biol*, 11, 171-6.

Maruyama, H., Morino, H., Ito, H., Izumi, Y., Kato, H., Watanabe, Y., Kinoshita, Y., Kamada, M., Nodera, H., Suzuki, H., Komure, O., Matsuura, S., Kobatake, K., Morimoto, N., Abe, K., Suzuki, N., Aoki, M., Kawata, A., Hirai, T., Kato, T., Ogasawara, K., Hirano, A., Takumi, T., Kusaka, H., Hagiwara, K., Kaji, R. and Kawakami, H. (2010). Mutations of optineurin in amyotrophic lateral sclerosis. *Nature*, 465, 223-6.

Mazzone, G. L. and Nistri, A. (2011). Electrochemical detection of endogenous glutamate release from rat spinal cord organotypic slices as a real-time method to monitor excitotoxicity. *J Neurosci Methods*, 197, 128-32.

McIntire, S. L., Jorgensen, E. and Horvitz, H. R. (1993). Genes required for GABA function in Caenorhabditis elegans. *Nature*, 364, 334-7.

Miguel, L., Frebourg, T., Campion, D. and Lecourtois, M. (2011). Both cytoplasmic and nuclear accumulations of the protein are neurotoxic in Drosophila models of TDP-43 proteinopathies. *Neurobiol Dis*, 41, 398-406.

Millecamps, S., Robertson, J., Lariviere, R., Mallet, J. and Julien, J. P. (2006). Defective axonal transport of neurofilament proteins in neurons overexpressing peripherin. *J Neurochem*, 98, 926-38.

Millecamps, S., Salachas, F., Cazeneuve, C., Gordon, P., Bricka, B., Camuzat, A., Guillot-Noel, L., Russaouen, O., Bruneteau, G., Pradat, P. F., Le Forestier, N., Vandenberghe, N., Danel-Brunaud, V., Guy, N., Thauvin-Robinet, C., Lacomblez, L., Couratier, P., Hannequin, D., Seilhean, D., Le Ber, I., Corcia, P., Camu, W., Brice, A., Rouleau, G., LeGuern, E. and Meininger, V. (2010). SOD1, ANG, VAPB, TARDBP, and FUS mutations in familial amyotrophic lateral sclerosis: genotype-phenotype correlations. *J Med Genet*, 47, 554-60.

Mitchell, J., Paul, P., Chen, H. J., Morris, A., Payling, M., Falchi, M., Habgood, J., Panoutsou, S., Winkler, S., Tisato, V., Hajitou, A., Smith, B., Vance, C., Shaw, C., Mazarakis, N. D. and de Belleroche, J. (2010). Familial amyotrophic lateral sclerosis is associated with a mutation in D-amino acid oxidase. *Proc Natl Acad Sci U S A*, 107, 7556-61.

Mitne-Neto, M., Machado-Costa, M., Marchetto, M. C., Bengtson, M. H., Joazeiro, C. A., Tsuda, H., Bellen, H. J., Silva, H. C., Oliveira, A. S., Lazar, M., Muotri, A. R. and Zatz, M. (2011). Downregulation of VAPB expression in motor neurons derived from induced pluripotent stem cells of ALS8 patients. *Hum Mol Genet.*

Mockett, R. J., Radyuk, S. N., Benes, J. J., Orr, W. C. and Sohal, R. S. (2003). Phenotypic effects of familial amyotrophic lateral sclerosis mutant Sod alleles in transgenic Drosophila. *Proc Natl Acad Sci U S A*, 100, 301-6.

Mulder, D. W. (1982). Clinical limits of amyotrophic lateral sclerosis. *Adv Neurol*, 36, 15-22.

Nagai, M., Aoki, M., Miyoshi, I., Kato, M., Pasinelli, P., Kasai, N., Brown, R. H., Jr. and Itoyama, Y. (2001). Rats expressing human cytosolic copper-zinc superoxide dismutase transgenes with amyotrophic lateral sclerosis: associated mutations develop motor neuron disease. *J Neurosci*, 21, 9246-54.

Nasevicius, A. and Ekker, S. C. (2000). Effective targeted gene 'knockdown' in zebrafish. *Nat Genet*, 26, 216-20.

Oeda, T., Shimohama, S., Kitagawa, N., Kohno, R., Imura, T., Shibasaki, H. and Ishii, N. (2001). Oxidative stress causes abnormal accumulation of familial amyotrophic lateral sclerosis-related mutant SOD1 in transgenic Caenorhabditis elegans. *Hum Mol Genet*, 10, 2013-23.

Park, K. S., Kim, H. J., Choi, W. J., Kim, M. and Lee, K. W. (2004). Detection method of the adjacent motor neuronal death in an in vitro co-culture model of familial ALS-associated Cu/Zn superoxide dismutase. *Biotechnol Lett*, 26, 1201-5.

Parkes, T. L., Elia, A. J., Dickinson, D., Hilliker, A. J., Phillips, J. P. and Boulianne, G. L. (1998). Extension of Drosophila lifespan by overexpression of human SOD1 in motorneurons. *Nat Genet*, 19, 171-4.

Pasinelli, P., Belford, M. E., Lennon, N., Bacskai, B. J., Hyman, B. T., Trotti, D. and Brown, R. H., Jr. (2004). Amyotrophic lateral sclerosis-associated SOD1 mutant proteins bind and aggregate with Bcl-2 in spinal cord mitochondria. *Neuron*, 43, 19-30.

Phillips, J. P., Campbell, S. D., Michaud, D., Charbonneau, M. and Hilliker, A. J. (1989). Null mutation of copper/zinc superoxide dismutase in Drosophila confers hypersensitivity to paraquat and reduced longevity. *Proc Natl Acad Sci U S A*, 86, 2761-5.

Pramatarova, A., Laganiere, J., Roussel, J., Brisebois, K. and Rouleau, G. A. (2001). Neuron-specific expression of mutant superoxide dismutase 1 in transgenic mice does not lead to motor impairment. *J Neurosci*, 21, 3369-74.

Ramesh, T., Lyon, A. N., Pineda, R. H., Wang, C., Janssen, P. M., Canan, B. D., Burghes, A. H. and Beattie, C. E. (2010). A genetic model of amyotrophic lateral sclerosis in zebrafish displays phenotypic hallmarks of motoneuron disease. *Dis Model Mech*, 3, 652-62.

Reaume, A. G., Elliott, J. L., Hoffman, E. K., Kowall, N. W., Ferrante, R. J., Siwek, D. F., Wilcox, H. M., Flood, D. G., Beal, M. F., Brown, R. H., Jr., Scott, R. W. and Snider, W. D. (1996). Motor neurons in Cu/Zn superoxide dismutase-deficient mice develop normally but exhibit enhanced cell death after axonal injury. *Nat Genet*, 13, 43-7.

Renton, A. E., Majounie, E., Waite, A., Simon-Sanchez, J., Rollinson, S., Gibbs, J. R., Schymick, J. C., Laaksovirta, H., van Swieten, J. C., Myllykangas, L., Kalimo, H., Paetau, A., Abramzon, Y., Remes, A. M., Kaganovich, A., Scholz, S. W., Duckworth, J., Ding, J., Harmer, D. W., Hernandez, D. G., Johnson, J. O., Mok, K., Ryten, M., Trabzuni, D., Guerreiro, R. J., Orrell, R. W., Neal, J., Murray, A., Pearson, J., Jansen, I. E., Sondervan, D., Seelaar, H., Blake, D., Young, K., Halliwell, N., Callister, J. B., Toulson, G., Richardson, A., Gerhard, A., Snowden, J., Mann, D., Neary, D., Nalls, M. A., Peuralinna, T., Jansson, L., Isoviita, V., Kaivorinne, A., Holtta-Vuori, M., Ikonen, E., Sulkava, R., Benatar, M., Wuu, J., Chio, A., Restagno, G., Borghero, G., Sabatelli, M., Consortium, T. I., Heckerman, D., Rogaeva, E., Zinman, L., Rothstein, J. D., Sendtner, M., Drepper, C., Eichler, E. E., Alkan, C., Abdullaev, Z., Pack, S. D., Dutra, A., Pak, E., Hardy, J., Singleton, A., Williams, N. M., Heutink, P., Pickering-Brown, S., Morris, H. R., P.J., T. and Traynor, B. J. (2011). A Hexanucleotide Repeat Expansion in C9ORF72 Is the Cause of Chromosome 9p21-Linked ALS-FTD. *Neuron*.

Ripps, M. E., Huntley, G. W., Hof, P. R., Morrison, J. H. and Gordon, J. W. (1995). Transgenic mice expressing an altered murine superoxide dismutase gene provide an animal model of amyotrophic lateral sclerosis. *Proc Natl Acad Sci U S A*, 92, 689-93.

Ritson, G. P., Custer, S. K., Freibaum, B. D., Guinto, J. B., Geffel, D., Moore, J., Tang, W., Winton, M. J., Neumann, M., Trojanowski, J. Q., Lee, V. M., Forman, M. S. and Taylor, J. P. (2010). TDP-43 mediates degeneration in a novel Drosophila model of disease caused by mutations in VCP/p97. *J Neurosci*, 30, 7729-39.

Rosen, D. R., Siddique, T., Patterson, D., Figlewicz, D. A., Sapp, P., Hentati, A., Donaldson, D., Goto, J., O'Regan, J. P., Deng, H. X. and et al. (1993). Mutations in Cu/Zn superoxide dismutase gene are associated with familial amyotrophic lateral sclerosis. *Nature*, 362, 59-62.

Sanelli, T., Ge, W., Leystra-Lantz, C. and Strong, M. J. (2007). Calcium mediated excitotoxicity in neurofilament aggregate-bearing neurons in vitro is NMDA receptor dependant. *J Neurol Sci*, 256, 39-51.

Sauer, B. (1998). Inducible gene targeting in mice using the Cre/lox system. *Methods*, 14, 381-92.

Saxena, S., Cabuy, E. and Caroni, P. (2006). A role for motoneuron subtype-selective ER stress in disease manifestations of FALS mice. *Nat Neurosci*, 12, 627-36.

Schnaar, R. I. and Schaffner, A. E. (1981). Separation of cell types from embryonic chicken and rat spinal cord: characterization of motoneuron-enriched fractions. *J Neurosci*, 1, 204-17.

Sephton, C. F., Good, S. K., Atkin, S., Dewey, C. M., Mayer, P., 3rd, Herz, J. and Yu, G. (2010). TDP-43 is a developmentally regulated protein essential for early embryonic development. *J Biol Chem*, 285, 6826-34.

Simpson, C. L., Lemmens, R., Miskiewicz, K., Broom, W. J., Hansen, V. K., van Vught, P. W., Landers, J. E., Sapp, P., Van Den Bosch, L., Knight, J., Neale, B. M., Turner, M. R., Veldink, J. H., Ophoff, R. A., Tripathi, V. B., Beleza, A., Shah, M. N., Proitsi, P., Van Hoecke, A., Carmeliet, P., Horvitz, H. R., Leigh, P. N., Shaw, C. E., van den Berg, L. H., Sham, P. C., Powell, J. F., Verstreken, P., Brown, R. H., Jr., Robberecht, W. and Al-Chalabi, A. (2009). Variants of the elongator protein 3 (ELP3) gene are associated with motor neuron degeneration. *Hum Mol Genet*, 18, 472-81.

Solnica-Krezel, L., Stemple, D. L., Mountcastle-Shah, E., Rangini, Z., Neuhauss, S. C., Malicki, J., Schier, A. F., Stainier, D. Y., Zwartkruis, F., Abdelilah, S. and Driever, W. (1996). Mutations affecting cell fates and cellular rearrangements during gastrulation in zebrafish. *Development*, 123, 67-80.

Sreedharan, J., Blair, I. P., Tripathi, V. B., Hu, X., Vance, C., Rogelj, B., Ackerley, S., Durnall, J. C., Williams, K. L., Buratti, E., Baralle, F., de Belleroche, J., Mitchell, J. D., Leigh, P. N., Al-Chalabi, A., Miller, C. C., Nicholson, G. and Shaw, C. E. (2008). TDP-43 mutations in familial and sporadic amyotrophic lateral sclerosis. *Science*, 319, 1668-72.

Stabenfeldt, S. E., Munglani, G., Garcia, A. J. and LaPlaca, M. C. (2010). Biomimetic microenvironment modulates neural stem cell survival, migration, and differentiation. *Tissue Eng Part A*, 16, 3747-58.

Stallings, N. R., Puttaparthi, K., Luther, C. M., Burns, D. K. and Elliott, J. L. (2010). Progressive motor weakness in transgenic mice expressing human TDP-43. *Neurobiol Dis*, 40, 404-14.

Strong, M. J. and Yang, W. (2011). The Frontotemporal Syndromes of ALS. Clinicopathological Correlates. *J Mol Neurosci*.

Sulston, J. E. (1983). Neuronal cell lineages in the nematode Caenorhabditis elegans. *Cold Spring Harb Symp Quant Biol*, 48 Pt 2, 443-52.

Sulston, J. E., Schierenberg, E., White, J. G. and Thomson, J. N. (1983). The embryonic cell lineage of the nematode Caenorhabditis elegans. *Dev Biol*, 100, 64-119.

Swarup, V., Phaneuf, D., Bareil, C., Robertson, J., Rouleau, G. A., Kriz, J. and Julien, J. P. (2011). Pathological hallmarks of amyotrophic lateral sclerosis/frontotemporal lobar degeneration in transgenic mice produced with TDP-43 genomic fragments. *Brain*, 134, 2610-26.

Tabata, R. C., Wilson, J. M., Ly, P., Zwiegers, P., Kwok, D., Van Kampen, J. M., Cashman, N. and Shaw, C. A. (2008). Chronic exposure to dietary sterol glucosides is neurotoxic to motor neurons and induces an ALS-PDC phenotype. *Neuromolecular Med*, 10, 24-39.

Takahashi, K., Okita, K., Nakagawa, M. and Yamanaka, S. (2007a). Induction of pluripotent stem cells from fibroblast cultures. *Nat Protoc*, 2, 3081-9.

Takahashi, K., Tanabe, K., Ohnuki, M., Narita, M., Ichisaka, T., Tomoda, K. and Yamanaka, S. (2007b). Induction of pluripotent stem cells from adult human fibroblasts by defined factors. *Cell*, 131, 861-72.

Tandan, R. and Bradley, W. G. (1985). Amyotrophic lateral sclerosis: Part 1. Clinical features, pathology, and ethical issues in management. *Ann Neurol*, 18, 271-80.

Texido, L., Hernandez, S., Martin-Satue, M., Povedano, M., Casanovas, A., Esquerda, J., Marsal, J. and Solsona, C. (2011). Sera from amyotrophic lateral sclerosis patients induce the non-canonical activation of NMDA receptors "in vitro". *Neurochem Int*, doi:10.1016/j.neuint.2011.07.006.

Toma, J. G., Akhavan, M., Fernandes, K. J., Barnabe-Heider, F., Sadikot, A., Kaplan, D. R. and Miller, F. D. (2001). Isolation of multipotent adult stem cells from the dermis of mammalian skin. *Nat Cell Biol*, 3, 778-84.

Tovar, Y. R. L. B., Santa-Cruz, L. D. and Tapia, R. (2009). Experimental models for the study of neurodegeneration in amyotrophic lateral sclerosis. *Mol Neurodegener*, 4, 31.

Tradewell, M. L., Cooper, L. A., Minotti, S. and Durham, H. D. (2011). Calcium dysregulation, mitochondrial pathology and protein aggregation in a culture model of amyotrophic lateral sclerosis: mechanistic relationship and differential sensitivity to intervention. *Neurobiol Dis*, 42, 265-75.

Tradewell, M. L. and Durham, H. D. (2010). Calpastatin reduces toxicity of SOD1G93A in a culture model of amyotrophic lateral sclerosis. *Neuroreport*, 21, 976-9.

Trotti, D., Aoki, M., Pasinelli, P., Berger, U. V., Danbolt, N. C., Brown, R. H., Jr. and Hediger, M. A. (2001). Amyotrophic lateral sclerosis-linked glutamate transporter mutant has impaired glutamate clearance capacity. *J Biol Chem*, 276, 576-82.

Trotti, D., Rolfs, A., Danbolt, N. C., Brown, R. H., Jr. and Hediger, M. A. (1999). SOD1 mutants linked to amyotrophic lateral sclerosis selectively inactivate a glial glutamate transporter. *Nat Neurosci*, 2, 427-33.

Tscherter, A., Heuschkel, M. O., Renaud, P. and Streit, J. (2001). Spatiotemporal characterization of rhythmic activity in rat spinal cord slice cultures. *Eur J Neurosci*, 14, 179-90.

Tu, P. H., Raju, P., Robinson, K. A., Gurney, M. E., Trojanowski, J. Q. and Lee, V. M. (1996). Transgenic mice carrying a human mutant superoxide dismutase transgene develop neuronal cytoskeletal pathology resembling human amyotrophic lateral sclerosis lesions. *Proc Natl Acad Sci U S A*, 93, 3155-60.

Turner, B. J., Atkin, J. D., Farg, M. A., Zang, D. W., Rembach, A., Lopes, E. C., Patch, J. D., Hill, A. F. and Cheema, S. S. (2005). Impaired extracellular secretion of mutant superoxide dismutase 1 associates with neurotoxicity in familial amyotrophic lateral sclerosis. *J Neurosci*, 25, 108-17.

Urushitani, M., Ezzi, S. A., Matsuo, A., Tooyama, I. and Julien, J. P. (2008). The endoplasmic reticulum-Golgi pathway is a target for translocation and aggregation of mutant superoxide dismutase linked to ALS. *Faseb J*, 22, 2476-87.

Urushitani, M., Kurisu, J., Tsukita, K. and Takahashi, R. (2002). Proteasomal inhibition by misfolded mutant superoxide dismutase 1 induces selective motor neuron death in familial amyotrophic lateral sclerosis. *J Neurochem*, 83, 1030-42.

Urushitani, M., Sik, A., Sakurai, T., Nukina, N., Takahashi, R. and Julien, J. P. (2006). Chromogranin-mediated secretion of mutant superoxide dismutase proteins linked to amyotrophic lateral sclerosis. *Nat Neurosci*, 9, 108-18.

Van Deerlin, V. M., Leverenz, J. B., Bekris, L. M., Bird, T. D., Yuan, W., Elman, L. B., Clay, D., Wood, E. M., Chen-Plotkin, A. S., Martinez-Lage, M., Steinbart, E., McCluskey, L., Grossman, M., Neumann, M., Wu, I. L., Yang, W. S., Kalb, R., Galasko, D. R., Montine, T. J., Trojanowski, J. Q., Lee, V. M., Schellenberg, G. D. and Yu, C. E. (2008). TARDBP mutations in amyotrophic lateral sclerosis with TDP-43 neuropathology: a genetic and histopathological analysis. *Lancet Neurol*, 7, 409-16.

Vance, C., Rogelj, B., Hortobagyi, T., De Vos, K. J., Nishimura, A. L., Sreedharan, J., Hu, X., Smith, B., Ruddy, D., Wright, P., Ganesalingam, J., Williams, K. L., Tripathi, V., Al-Saraj, S., Al-Chalabi, A., Leigh, P. N., Blair, I. P., Nicholson, G., de Belleroche, J., Gallo, J. M., Miller, C. C. and Shaw, C. E. (2009). Mutations in FUS, an RNA processing protein, cause familial amyotrophic lateral sclerosis type 6. *Science*, 323, 1208-11.

Vijayalakshmi, K., Alladi, P. A., Ghosh, S., Prasanna, V. K., Sagar, B. C., Nalini, A., Sathyaprabha, T. N. and Raju, T. R. (2011). Evidence of endoplasmic reticular stress in the spinal motor neurons exposed to CSF from sporadic amyotrophic lateral sclerosis patients. *Neurobiol Dis*, 41, 695-705.

Vijayalakshmi, K., Alladi, P. A., Sathyaprabha, T. N., Subramaniam, J. R., Nalini, A. and Raju, T. R. (2009). Cerebrospinal fluid from sporadic amyotrophic lateral sclerosis patients induces degeneration of a cultured motor neuron cell line. *Brain Res*, 1263, 122-33.

Voigt, A., Herholz, D., Fiesel, F. C., Kaur, K., Muller, D., Karsten, P., Weber, S. S., Kahle, P. J., Marquardt, T. and Schulz, J. B. (2010). TDP-43-mediated neuron loss in vivo requires RNA-binding activity. *PLoS One*, 5, e12247.

Walker, L. M., Huber, M., Doores, K. J., Falkowska, E., Pejchal, R., Julien, J. P., Wang, S. K., Ramos, A., Chan-Hui, P. Y., Moyle, M., Mitcham, J. L., Hammond, P. W., Olsen, O. A., Phung, P., Fling, S., Wong, C. H., Phogat, S., Wrin, T., Simek, M. D., Principal Investigators, P. G., Koff, W. C., Wilson, I. A., Burton, D. R. and Poignard, P. (2011). Broad neutralization coverage of HIV by multiple highly potent antibodies. *Nature*, 477, 466-70.

Wang, J., Farr, G. W., Hall, D. H., Li, F., Furtak, K., Dreier, L. and Horwich, A. L. (2009a). An ALS-linked mutant SOD1 produces a locomotor defect associated with aggregation and synaptic dysfunction when expressed in neurons of Caenorhabditis elegans. *PLoS Genet*, 5, e1000350.

Wang, J., Slunt, H., Gonzales, V., Fromholt, D., Coonfield, M., Copeland, N. G., Jenkins, N. A. and Borchelt, D. R. (2003). Copper-binding-site-null SOD1 causes ALS in transgenic mice: aggregates of non-native SOD1 delineate a common feature. *Hum Mol Genet*, 12, 2753-64.

Wang, L., Deng, H. X., Grisotti, G., Zhai, H., Siddique, T. and Roos, R. P. (2009b). Wild-type SOD1 overexpression accelerates disease onset of a G85R SOD1 mouse. *Hum Mol Genet*, 18, 1642-51.

Wang, L. J., Lu, Y. Y., Muramatsu, S., Ikeguchi, K., Fujimoto, K., Okada, T., Mizukami, H., Matsushita, T., Hanazono, Y., Kume, A., Nagatsu, T., Ozawa, K. and Nakano, I. (2002). Neuroprotective effects of glial cell line-derived neurotrophic factor mediated by an adeno-associated virus vector in a transgenic animal model of amyotrophic lateral sclerosis. *J Neurosci*, 22, 6920-8.

Watson, M. R., Lagow, R. D., Xu, K., Zhang, B. and Bonini, N. M. (2008). A drosophila model for amyotrophic lateral sclerosis reveals motor neuron damage by human SOD1. *J Biol Chem*, 283, 24972-81.

Wegorzewska, I., Bell, S., Cairns, N. J., Miller, T. M. and Baloh, R. H. (2009). TDP-43 mutant transgenic mice develop features of ALS and frontotemporal lobar degeneration. *Proc Natl Acad Sci U S A*, 106, 18809-14.

White, J., Southgate, E., Thomson, J. and Brenner, S. (1986). The structure of the nervous system of the nematode Caenorhabditis elegans. *Philos Trans R Soc Lond Biol*, 314, 1-340.

Wichterle, H., Lieberam, I., Porter, J. A. and Jessell, T. M. (2002). Directed differentiation of embryonic stem cells into motor neurons. *Cell*, 110, 385-97.

Wils, H., Kleinberger, G., Janssens, J., Pereson, S., Joris, G., Cuijt, I., Smits, V., Ceuterick-de Groote, C., Van Broeckhoven, C. and Kumar-Singh, S. (2010). TDP-43 transgenic mice develop spastic paralysis and neuronal inclusions characteristic of ALS and frontotemporal lobar degeneration. *Proc Natl Acad Sci U S A*, 107, 3858-63.

Wong, P. C., Pardo, C. A., Borchelt, D. R., Lee, M. K., Copeland, N. G., Jenkins, N. A., Sisodia, S. S., Cleveland, D. W. and Price, D. L. (1995). An adverse property of a familial ALS-linked SOD1 mutation causes motor neuron disease characterized by vacuolar degeneration of mitochondria. *Neuron*, 14, 1105-16.

Wu, L. S., Cheng, W. C., Hou, S. C., Yan, Y. T., Jiang, S. T. and Shen, C. K. (2010). TDP-43, a neuro-pathosignature factor, is essential for early mouse embryogenesis. *Genesis*, 48, 56-62.

Xu, Y. F., Gendron, T. F., Zhang, Y. J., Lin, W. L., D'Alton, S., Sheng, H., Casey, M. C., Tong, J., Knight, J., Yu, X., Rademakers, R., Boylan, K., Hutton, M., McGowan, E., Dickson, D. W., Lewis, J. and Petrucelli, L. (2010). Wild-type human TDP-43 expression causes TDP-43 phosphorylation, mitochondrial aggregation, motor deficits, and early mortality in transgenic mice. *J Neurosci*, 30, 10851-9.

Yamanaka, K., Miller, T. M., McAlonis-Downes, M., Chun, S. J. and Cleveland, D. W. (2006). Progressive spinal axonal degeneration and slowness in ALS2-deficient mice. *Ann Neurol*, 60, 95-104.

Yang, C., Tan, W., Whittle, C., Qiu, L., Cao, L., Akbarian, S. and Xu, Z. (2010). The C-terminal TDP-43 fragments have a high aggregation propensity and harm neurons by a dominant-negative mechanism. *PLoS One*, 5, e15878.

Yang, Y., Hentati, A., Deng, H. X., Dabbagh, O., Sasaki, T., Hirano, M., Hung, W. Y., Ouahchi, K., Yan, J., Azim, A. C., Cole, N., Gascon, G., Yagmour, A., Ben-Hamida, M., Pericak-Vance, M., Hentati, F. and Siddique, T. (2001). The gene encoding alsin, a protein with three guanine-nucleotide exchange factor domains, is mutated in a form of recessive amyotrophic lateral sclerosis. *Nat Genet*, 29, 160-5.

Young, K. C., McGehee, D. S. and Brorson, J. R. (2007). Glutamate receptor expression and chronic glutamate toxicity in rat motor cortex. *Neurobiol Dis*, 26, 78-85.

Zhou, H., Huang, C., Chen, H., Wang, D., Landel, C. P., Xia, P. Y., Bowser, R., Liu, Y. J. and Xia, X. G. (2010). Transgenic rat model of neurodegeneration caused by mutation in the TDP gene. *PLoS Genet*, 6, e1000887.

5

Electrophysiological Abnormalities in SOD1 Transgenic Models in Amyotrophic Lateral Sclerosis: The Commonalities and Differences

Sherif M. Elbasiouny[1], Katharina A. Quinlan[1], Tahra L. Eissa[4] and Charles J. Heckman[1,2,3]
[1]*Departments of Physiology, Northwestern University*
[2]*Physical Medicine and Rehabilitation, Northwestern University*
[3]*Physical Therapy and Human Movement Sciences, Northwestern University*
[4]*Department of Biological and Environmental Engineering, Cornell University*
USA

1. Introduction

Since its first description in 1874 by Charcot, the hallmark feature of ALS is the progressive degeneration of upper and lower motoneurons (Charcot, 1874). In the spinal cord, motoneuron degeneration starts long before symptom onset and advances in a size-related fashion, in which large-size alpha-motoneurons degenerate first followed by small-size alpha-motoneurons (Pun et al., 2006; Hegedus et al., 2007; Hegedus et al., 2008). There are conflicting reports regarding the survival of the smallest-sized spinal motoneurons, the gamma-motoneurons (Swash and Fox, 1974; Sobue et al., 1981). Despite its original description, the neuronal degeneration in ALS is not limited to motoneurons. Recent reports have shown evidence for degeneration of neurons in the brain (Karim et al., 1998; Lloyd et al., 2000; Maekawa et al., 2004) and interneurons in the spinal cord (Konno et al., 1986; Williams et al., 1990; Takahashi et al., 1993; Stephens et al., 2006).

Before their degeneration, spinal motoneurons experience progressive changes in their properties. These changes result from the pathological actions of the disease and the compensatory mechanisms of the nervous system to mitigate the neuronal malfunction. In this chapter, we describe the changes in the anatomical and electrical properties of spinal motoneurons in various genetic mouse models of ALS and critically analyze literature for the common and different pathological features across these models. We also present data from computer simulations showing the consequences of the alterations in properties of mutant motoneurons on cell excitability and dendritic processing of synaptic inputs. The presented computational analysis allowed for the identification of motoneuron alterations undetectable using standard electrophysiological methods. This information is essential for understanding motoneuron pathophysiology in ALS.

2. The changes in motoneuron anatomical properties

One of the earliest abnormalities in transgenic mouse models of ALS is the change in anatomy of spinal motoneurons. In the G85R model, it has been shown that mutant motoneurons exhibit an increase in the overall cell size and branching pattern of dendrites (Amendola et al., 2007; Amendola and Durand, 2008). These changes appear in transgenic mice at 10 days after birth (P10), long before disease onset and life end-stage (225 and 240 days, respectively) (Bruijn et al., 1997). More specifically, in mutant motoneurons the total dendritic surface area and total dendritic length are increased by 58% and 65% relative to wild-type (WT) cells, respectively. For dendritic branching, the number of dendritic branches, terminal branches, branching nodes, and maximum branching order are increased by 93%, 89%, 97%, 37%, respectively (Fig. 1). On the other hand, the soma size (diameter and surface area) and primary dendrites properties (number, diameter, and cross-sectional area) are similar in WT and mutant motoneurons. Interestingly, the increase in number of branches occurs primarily in short branches (dendritic branches with path length < 100μm) and most of the anatomical changes take place over the middle dendrites (200μm - 500μm from the soma). Surprisingly, the longest dendritic length from the soma was not increased in mutant motoneurons, indicating that dendritic overbranching occurs mainly within the cell circumjacent. In other words, the cell does not swell into larger space in the cord but develops more branching within its dendritic spatial field.

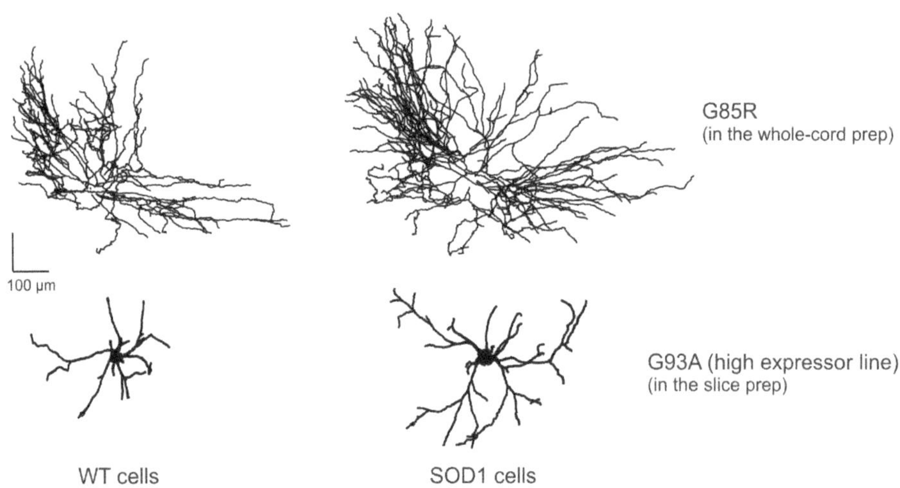

Fig. 1. Anatomical alterations in mutant motoneurons of the G85R (reconstructed from the whole-cord prep[1]) and G93A (high expressor line) (reconstructed from the slice prep.) transgenic models relative to WT cells. [1]: data from Amendola and Durand (2008).

Similar early abnormalities in the anatomical properties of motoneurons have been found in other transgenic mouse models of ALS. In the G93A (low expressor line), which expresses 8 copies of the human SOD1 gene, mutant motoneurons at P9 exhibit increased cell size, dendritic overbranching, and dendritic complexity (Filipchuk et al., 2010). The total dendritic length and number of branching nodes and terminal dendrites in mutant motoneurons were significantly increased relative to WT. Similar to the G85R transgenic model, these anatomical changes in the G93A (low expressor line) model occur early in the disease (at P9) way before symptom development (between 195 and 240 days) and end stage (between 240 and 270 days). Preliminary data from our laboratory obtained in the slice preparation show that neonatal mutant motoneurons (P7) of the G93A (high expressor line), which expresses 25 copies of the human SOD1 gene, experience analogous alterations in their morphology and dendritic branching (Fig. 1), in which the soma surface area, numbers of dendritic branches and terminal dendrites increase significantly relative to WT.

Post-mortem morphological analysis of large neurons in the ventral horn of spinal cord indicated an increase in the initial segment diameter, by 36%, in ALS patients (Sasaki and Maruyama, 1992). Conversely, the soma area of these neurons was smaller by 16% relative to control (Sasaki and Maruyama, 1992).

The similar findings on the anatomical alterations of neonatal motoneurons in various transgenic models of ALS indicate that the increase in cell size and dendritic overbranching are characteristic abnormalities in motoneuron pathophysiology in ALS. However, it is unclear whether the alteration in motoneuron anatomy is a disease mechanism or an adaptive response (see section 7 for discussion). Furthermore, it is important to understand the functional ramifications of the motoneuron anatomical alterations on the cell excitability and electrical properties and to what extent the anatomical alterations contribute to motoneuron degeneration in ALS (see section 6).

3. The changes in motoneuron electrical properties

3.1 The change in input resistance

Changes in a number of motoneuron electrical properties were reported in the transgenic mouse models of ALS. However, one challenge in the field of ALS is the large variability in data of mutant motoneuron electrical properties, which makes recording from a large number of cells is important to allow statistical tests to detect significant differences in electrophysiological properties between WT and mutant motoneuron samples. Table 1 summarizes the changes in electrical properties of mutant motoneurons observed in the various ALS transgenic mouse models. The summary shows that the changes in electrical properties involve the motoneuron passive properties (e.g., cell input resistance), the size and shape of the action potential spike and afterhyperpolarization, the amplitude of voltage-sensitive ionic currents, and the motoneuron excitability and firing activity. However, some of these changes were inconsistent (i.e., not observed consistently) across the ALS transgenic models, whereas others were contradictory (i.e., opposite changes were observed). For instance, the decrease in input resistance of mutant motoneurons relative to WT is an inconsistent finding in ALS transgenic models (see table 1, column 7). This observation was seen in some studies (Bories et al., 2007; ElBasiouny et al., 2010; Quinlan et al., 2011), whereas other studies did not find a statistically significant difference between the input resistance of WT and mutant motoneurons (Pieri et al., 2003; Kuo et al., 2004; Kuo et al., 2005; van Zundert et al., 2008; Pambo-Pambo et al., 2009; Pieri et al., 2009; Filipchuk et al., 2010; Meehan et al., 2010). The changes in action potential size and width in mutant motoneurons, on the other hand, is a conflicting finding in which some studies reported an increase in spike height (van Zundert et al., 2008) and duration (Fuchs et al., 2008, 2009; Pambo-Pambo et al., 2009) relative to WT, whereas others reported reduction in spike height (Kuo et al., 2004; Pambo-Pambo et al., 2009; Filipchuk et al., 2010) and duration (Pieri et al., 2003; Quinlan et al., 2011).

Publication	Model	Preparation	Age	Neuron Type	$[Ca^{2+}]_o$	R_{in} in mutant neurons	V_{rest} and AP properties in mutant neurons	AHP in mutant neurons	PIC properties in mutant neurons	F-I gain & firing properties in mutant neurons
(Pieri et al., 2003)	G93A (high)	Embryonic Culture	E15: 7-12 days	SMNs	2mM	No diff	↓AP duration ↑AP repol rate	No diff	n/a	↑firing freq
(Kuo et al., 2004)	G93A (high)	Organotypic slice culture	P7: 3 weeks	SMNs	2.4mM	No diff	No diff	No diff	n/a	↑F-I gain ↑max firing
	G93A (high)	Embryonic culture	E13: 12-14 days	SMNs	2.8mM	No diff	↓AP height	No diff	n/a	↑F-I gain
(Kuo et al., 2005)	G93A (high)	Embryonic Culture	E13: 10-30 days	SMNs	2.8mM	No diff	Depolarized Vrest in high conductance MNs	No diff	↑NaPIC (measured in VC)	↓rheobase ↑F-I gain ↑spontaneous firing in high conductance MNs
(Bories et al., 2007)	G85R	Whole-cord	P6-10	SMNs	4mM	↓by 30%	No diff	No diff	n/a	↓ F-I gain ↑rheobase
(van Zundert et al., 2008)	G93A (high)	Brainstem slice	P4-10	HGMNs & OINs	2mM	No diff	↑AP height	No diff	↑NaPIC (measured in VC)	↑firing freq
(Fuchs et al., 2008) (Fuchs et al., 2009)	G93A (high)	Brainstem slice	P80-120	HGMNs & OMNs	2mM	No diff	HGMNs (P120): ↑AP duration ↓AP repol rate	At P120: ↓$fAHP_{amp}$ ↑$mAHP_{amp}$	No diff	No diff
(Pambo-Pambo et al., 2009)	G93A (low)	Lumbar slice	P6-10	SMNs	2mM	No diff	↓AP height ↑AP half-width ↓AP rise & decay slopes Depolarized Vrest	No diff	No diff (measured in VC) ↓total PIC (estimated from ΔI data)	↑F-I gain (pulses)

Publication	Model	Preparation	Age	Neuron Type	$[Ca^{2+}]_o$	R_{in} in mutant neurons	V_{rest} and AP properties in mutant neurons	AHP in mutant neurons	PIC properties in mutant neurons	F-I gain & firing properties in mutant neurons
(Pambo-Pambo et al., 2009)	G85R	Lumbar slice	P6-10	SMNs	2mM	No diff	No diff	No diff	No diff (measured in VC) ↓total PIC (estimated from ΔI data)	↓F-I gain (ramp)
(Pieri et al., 2009)	G93A (high)	Cell culture	E15: 11-12 days	CNs	2mM	No diff	↓AP threshold	n/a	↑NaPIC (measured in VC)	↑firing freq ↓rheobase
(Meehan et al., 2010)	G127X	In-vivo lumbar cord	P240	SMNs	n/a	No diff	n/a	No diff	↑PIC (estimated from firing profiles)	No diff ↓Spike freq adaptation
(ElBasiouny et al., 2010)	G85R	Whole-cord	P8-10	SMNs	2mM	↓by 30%	No diff	No diff	n/a	No diff
(Filipchuk et al., 2010)	G93A (low)	Whole-cord	P8-9	SMNs	2mM	No diff	↓ AP height ↓AP rise and decay slopes	No diff	n/a	No diff
(Quinlan et al., 2011)	G93A (high)	Lumbar slice	P0-12	SMNs	2.5mM	↓by 19%	↓AP duration ↑AP rise and decay slopes	↓AHP time constant	↑Na & Ca PICs (measured in VC)	No diff

Table 1. Summary of the alterations in mutant motoneuron properties. SMNs: spinal motoneurons, CNs: cortical neurons, HGMNs: hypoglossal motoneurons, OMNs: ocular motoneurons, OINs: ocular interneurons. $[Ca2+]_o$: extracellular calcium concentration, R_{in}: input resistance, V_{rest}: resting membrane potential, AP: action potential, AHP: afterhyperpolarization, PIC: persistent inward current, F-I: frequency-current relationship. VC: voltage-clamp, ΔI: the difference in injected current at motoneuron recruitment and de-recruitment on a triangular current command, No diff: no difference.

3.1.1 Effect of tissue preparation

The discrepancy in the changes of electrical properties of mutant motoneurons probably results partially from the differences in transgenic model types (e.g., G85R, G93A high or low expressor lines) and is compounded by the variability in experimental conditions such as animal age (e.g., neonatal, pre- or post-symptomatic adult motoneurons) and tissue preparation (e.g., cell culture, slice, whole-cord, or in-vivo), in addition to the recording conditions (e.g., extracellular Ca^{2+} concentrations) and measurement methods (current- or voltage-clamp). However, critical analysis of the changes in electrical properties of mutant motoneurons shows that common pathological features could be identified across the various ALS transgenic models, whereas other features could be related to experimental conditions. For instance, the decrease in input resistance was detected mainly in studies conducted on the whole-cord preparation (in which the brainstem and spinal cord are intact), but was not observed in studies on motoneurons in cell culture or slice preparations (Table 1). Because input resistance is an indirect measure of cell size, it becomes reduced in mutant motoneurons to reflect the enlargement in motoneuron anatomy discussed in the previous section. In the whole-cord preparation, the motoneuron dendrites are completely intact and their effect on input resistance is more easily detected. In the slice preparation, conversely, the motoneuron dendrites are truncated at the surface of the slice. The lack of the middle and distal portions of dendrites could mask the anatomical differences between WT and mutant motoneurons and would explain the disappearance of input resistance differences between WT and mutant motoneurons in the slice preparation. Table 2 shows a comparison of the input resistance values of neonatal motoneurons in the various transgenic models of ALS. In the G85R and G93A (low expressor line) models, the input resistance values in the whole-cord preparation (ElBasiouny et al., 2010; Filipchuk et al., 2010) were on average half of those in the slice preparation (Pambo-Pambo et al., 2009), indicating that nearly half of the dendrites were severed in the slice preparation. Strikingly, the decrease in input resistance of mutant motoneurons of the G93A (high expressor line) model was still detected in the slice preparation in Quinlan et al. (2011). This could indicate that the motoneuron anatomical alterations in the G93A (high expressor line) model are so extensive that they were still substantial in the slice preparation and/or the motoneuron membrane biophysical properties change considerably in the G93A (high expressor line) model and contribute significantly to the decrease in input resistance (see section 4). For cell culture, given that the trigger signal for the alteration in motoneuron anatomy is poorly understood and could result from the alteration in motoneuron excitability and synaptic inputs (Duch et al., 2008), mutant motoneurons in the cell culture preparation might not experience anatomical alterations due to their isolation (in the cell culture) from the pathological neural circuit (in the transgenic mouse spinal cord), leading to absence of differences in input resistance between WT and mutant motoneurons.

3.1.2 Effect of extracellular Ca^{2+} concentration

The measurement of input resistance values, and other electrical properties, in mutant motoneurons also depends on the extracellular concentration of Ca^{2+} ions in the recording solution. For instance, the input resistance value of neonatal motoneurons of the G85R model measured in 4mM of extracellular Ca^{2+} concentration (Bories et al., 2007) was double of that measured in 2mM of extracellular Ca^{2+} concentration (ElBasiouny et al., 2010) (see table 2). Although 2mM is typical, the variability in extracellular Ca^{2+} concentration (ranging between 2mM and 4mM, see table 1) among the various ALS studies could contribute to the discrepancies in electrical properties of mutant motoneurons. This effect is produced because the level of extracellular Ca^{2+} concentration modulates the magnitude of the motoneuronal Ca^{2+}-gated (e.g., Cav 1.2, 1.3, and 2.2 channels) and Ca^{2+}-activated (e.g., SK and Ih channels) ionic currents, which regulate the motoneuron firing activity and affect the action potential and afterhyperpolarization properties.

Model	Publication	Preparation	$[Ca^{2+}]_o$	R_{in} WT/SOD1	Anatomical alterations
G93A (high)	Quinlan et al. (2011)	Slice	2mM	38.5/31.3 MΩ (↓ by 19%)*	Yes[1]
G85R	Bories et al. (2007)	Whole-cord	4mM	33.3/23.8 MΩ (↓ by 29%)*	Yes[2]
	ElBasiouny et al. (2010)	Whole-cord	2mM	16.2/11.4 MΩ (↓ by 30%)*	
	Pambo-Pambo et al. (2009)	Slice	2mM	34.5/33.1 MΩ ns	
G93A (low)	Pambo-Pambo et al. (2009)	Slice	2mM	34.5/37.2 MΩ ns	Yes[3]
	Filipchuk et al. (2010)	Whole-cord	2mM	18.5/16.1 MΩ ns	

Table 2. Comparison of the change in input resistance in mutant motoneurons (P6-P10) in the various ALS transgenic models. [1]: unpublished data, [2]: Amendola and Durand (2008), [3]: Filipchuk et al. (2010), *: statistically-significant ($p<0.05$), ns: not statistically-significant.

In sum, the reduction in input resistance of mutant motoneurons is a common, early pathological feature in the G93A (high expressor line) and G85R transgenic models, but not in the G93A (low expressor line). Also, this abnormality might sometimes not be evident depending on the tissue preparation used in the experiment.

3.2 The changes in action potential and afterhyperpolarization

A change in the action potential properties was frequently seen in mutant motoneurons relative to WT; however, these changes were conflicting across the transgenic models (Table 1, Fig. 2). In the G93A (high expressor line) model, neonatal spinal motoneurons frequently showed faster action potential rate of rise and decay and shorter action potential duration (Pieri et al., 2003; Quinlan et al., 2011), indicating an increase in transient and persistent Na^+ currents, which act to increase the excitability of mutant motoneurons. Signs of increased excitability were differently displayed in other studies as an increase in spike height (van Zundert et al., 2008), depolarization in resting membrane potential (Kuo et al., 2005), or reduction in action potential threshold (Pieri et al., 2009). Conversely, an increase in action potential duration and deceleration in rate of repolarization were observed in post-symptomatic adult hypoglossal motoneurons (Fuchs et al., 2009).

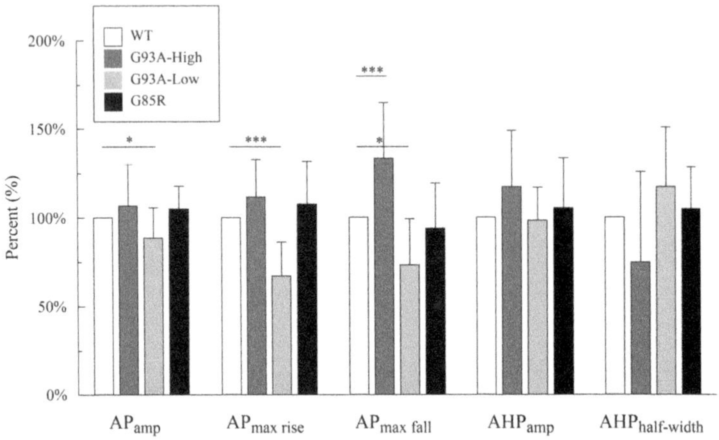

Fig. 2. The changes in action potential height (AP_{amp}), maximum rise ($AP_{max\ rise}$) and fall ($AP_{max\ fall}$) rates, and AHP amplitude (AHP_{amp}) and half-width ($AHP_{half\text{-}width}$) in mutant motoneurons of the G93A (high expressor line) [2nd bars][1], G93A (high expressor line) [3rd bars][2], and the G85R [last bars][2] transgenic models, relative to WT [1st bars]. All reported data from slice preparation. [1]: Quinlan et al. (2011), [2]: Pambo-Pambo et al. (2009).

In the G93A (low expressor line) model, neonatal spinal motoneurons exhibited a reduction in action potential height, increase in half-width, and deceleration in the rates of rise and decay (Pambo-Pambo et al., 2009; Filipchuk et al., 2010). In the G85R model, no changes were observed in the properties of the action potential regardless of the tissue preparation (whole-cord or slice) and extracellular Ca^{2+} concentration (2mM or 4mM) (Bories et al., 2007; Pambo-Pambo et al., 2009; ElBasiouny et al., 2010). Therefore, it appears that the alteration in action potential properties is not a common pathological characteristic, but depends on the ALS transgenic model type.
The after-spike afterhyperpolarization was not consistently altered in mutant motoneurons across the various transgenic models (Table 1, Fig. 2).

3.3 The change in persistent inward currents

Persistent inward currents are intrinsic Na^+ and Ca^{2+} currents that depolarize the membrane potential when activated. Contrary to transient ionic currents, these currents do not inactivate with prolonged membrane depolarization (Schwindt and Crill, 1977). A change in the motoneuron persistent inward current was frequently observed in mutant motoneurons (Table 1, Fig. 3); however, conflicting data were reported on the nature of this change (i.e., increase or decrease). In the G93A (high expressor line) model, an increase in the Na^+ persistent inward current of neonatal mutant motoneurons was consistently reported regardless of tissue preparation (cell culture and slice) or extracellular Ca^{2+} concentration (Table 1). In the G93A (low expressor line) and G85R models, persistent inward current measured in voltage-clamp protocols indicated no change in their amplitude between WT and mutant motoneurons, whereas persistent inward current estimated from the delta I (ΔI) technique indicated a reduction in their amplitude in mutant motoneurons relative to WT (Pambo-Pambo et al., 2009). The former is a more truthful result because voltage-clamp protocols allow direct measurement of the persistent inward current, whereas the ΔI technique (which is obtained from the difference in injected current at motoneuron recruitment and de-recruitment on a triangular current command) provides an indirect estimate of the persistent inward current amplitude (Bennett et al., 2001) and is sensitive to the inactivation of transient Na^+ channels (Miles et al., 2005) and activation of residual outward currents present in the motoneuron membrane (Hamm et al., 2010). However, it should be noted that the number of cells in which the voltage-clamp measurements were obtained was small. In the infrequently studied G127X transgenic model, an increase in the persistent inward current amplitude was estimated from the motoneuron firing profile (Meehan et al., 2010). However, this result is unconfirmed given that firing profile in mutant motoneurons would be also influenced by any differences in inward or outward currents and electrical properties of mutant motoneurons. Accordingly, the change in amplitude of persistent inward currents is not a common abnormality in the various ALS transgenic models. However, it appears that persistent inward currents are increased only in the G93A (high expressor line) transgenic model.

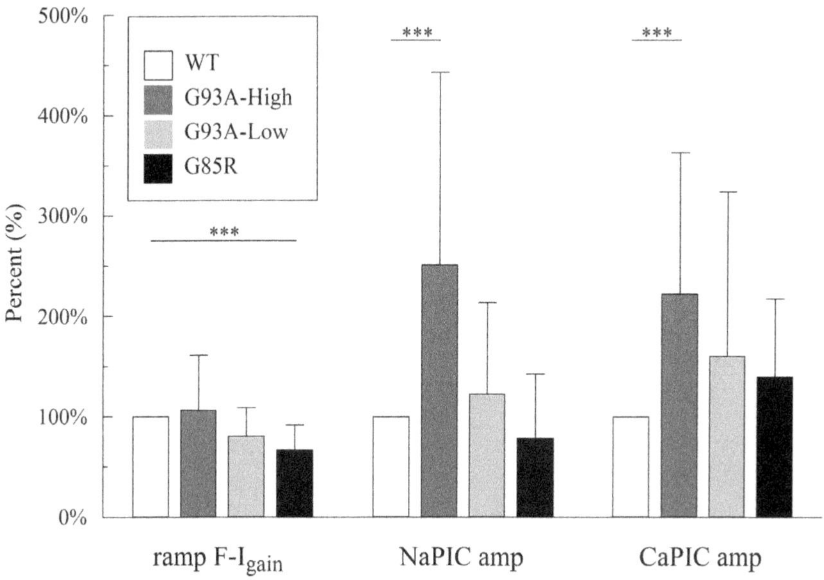

Fig. 3. The changes in ramp frequency-current relationship gain (ramp $F\text{-}I_{gain}$), sodium (NaPIC) and calcium (CaPIC) persistent inward currents in mutant motoneurons of the G93A (high expressor line) [2nd bars][1], G93A (high expressor line) [3rd bars][2], and the G85R [last bars][2] transgenic models, relative to WT [1st bars]. All reported data from slice preparation. [1]: Quinlan et al. (2011), [2]: Pambo-Pambo et al. (2009).

3.4 The change in motoneuron gain and firing activity

A change in the motoneuron gain (i.e., F-I relationship slope) or firing activity was commonly seen in mutant motoneurons, but conflicting observations were also reported. In the G93A (high expressor line) transgenic model, the firing activity and gain of mutant spinal motoneurons were consistently increased in cell culture (Pieri et al., 2003; Kuo et al.,

2004; Kuo et al., 2005; Zona et al., 2006; Pieri et al., 2009), but not in the slice (Quinlan et al., 2011) (Table 1). In the G85R transgenic model, the gain of mutant motoneurons was consistently reduced relative to WT (Bories et al., 2007; Pambo-Pambo et al., 2009). In the G93A (low expressor line) transgenic model, the gain of mutant motoneurons was increased in the slice preparation (Pambo-Pambo et al., 2009), but did not change in the whole-cord preparation (Filipchuk et al., 2010). The disagreement in reports on the change in motoneuron gain in the various transgenic models could be partially due to the variation in tissue preparation and extracellular Ca^{2+} concentration. Motoneuron dendrites have active conductances, which influence the motoneuron gain. Therefore, the portion of the motoneuron dendrites available during recording in the slice preparation would indirectly affect the measurement of the motoneuron gain in WT and mutant motoneurons. Also, the effect of extracellular Ca^{2+} concentration on the amplitude of Ca^{2+}-activated and Ca^{2+}-gated currents would influence the motoneuron gain measurement based on the degree of existence of these channels in WT and mutant motoneurons. Taken collectively, the change in gain and firing activity of mutant motoneurons is inconsistent within and across the various ALS transgenic models.

3.5 Motoneuron excitability in the various ALS transgenic models

Despite the discrepancy in data on the excitability of mutant motoneurons in the various ALS transgenic models, some insights could be attained from the trend in electrical properties change (Table 3). In the G93A (high expressor line) model, most changes in electrical properties push toward increased excitability of mutant motoneurons. For instance, the increases in action potential height and rise and decay rates and the reduction in action potential width are signs of elevated transient and persistent Na^+ currents that enhance the motoneuron excitability of mutant motoneurons. Also, the increase in persistent inward current amplitude further acts to enhance the motoneuron excitability. Collectively, these mechanisms push toward increased excitability of mutant motoneurons (i.e., excitability enhancement mechanisms). On the other hand, the increase in motoneuron size and reduction in input resistance are mechanisms that counteract increased excitability (i.e., excitability suppressive mechanisms) because the motoneuron becomes harder to recruit. It is unclear whether the excitability enhancement or suppressive mechanisms are disease or compensatory processes; however, the net effect of these mechanisms is increased excitability (i.e., hyperexcitability) of mutant motoneurons in the G93A (high expressor line) model (Table 3). This supposition is supported by the numerous reports on increased gain, although from cultured motoneurons, of mutant motoneurons in this transgenic model.

In the G93A (low expressor line) model, all changes in electrical properties indicate a reduction in the excitability of mutant motoneurons (i.e., hypoexcitability) (Table 3). These changes involve increase in motoneuron size, reduction in input resistance, smaller and broader action potential spikes, and slower rise rate (Table 3). The last two observations are indicative of a decrease in transient and persistent Na^+ currents in mutant motoneurons relative to WT. In contrast to these data, the gain of mutant motoneurons measured using long pulses was higher than that of WT motoneurons; however, the gain measured using current ramp was not different from WT motoneurons (Pambo-Pambo et al., 2009). Taken collectively, more evidence is available on reduced excitability of mutant motoneurons in the G93A (low expressor line).

Model	MN size	R_{in}	AP/AHP	PIC	Gain	Excitability
G93A (high)	↑↑	↓↓	Higher & briefer spikes Faster rise & decay rates	↑↑	↑↑/--	Hyperexcitability
G93A (low)	↑↑	--	Smaller & broader spikes Slower rise & decay rates	--	↑↑/--	More evidence on hypoexcitability
G85R	↑↑	↓↓	--	--	↓↓	Hypoexcitability

Table 3. Summary of changes in motoneuron properties in the various ALS transgenic models. MN: motoneuron, Rin: input resistance, AP/AHP: action potential and afterhyperpolarization, ↑↑: increase, ↓↓: decrease, --: no change.

In the G85R transgenic model, not many changes were reported in the electrical properties of mutant motoneurons; however, these changes were consistent with reduced excitability and are supported by the decrease in gain of mutant motoneurons (Table 3). In conclusion, motoneuron pathophysiology is different in the various transgenic mouse models of ALS and their excitability varies from hypo- to hyperexcitability. This disparity could be related to the number of copies of the human SOD1 gene or the severity of the disease (transgenic models with high copy number of SOD1 genes have more aggressive ALS than transgenic models with low copy number of SOD1 genes). Transgenic models with a low number of SOD1 copies (e.g., G85R and G93A-low expressor line) showed a tendency for reduced excitability of mutant motoneurons, whereas transgenic models with a high number of SOD1 copies (e.g., G93A-high expressor line) showed a tendency for increased excitability of mutant motoneurons. These differences should be considered when studying the motoneuron pathophysiology in these ALS transgenic models.

4. Effect of anatomical alterations on motoneuron electrical properties

The enlarged anatomy of mutant motoneurons has consequences for their electrical properties and firing behaviour. Computer simulations have been used to assess the effect of enlargement in motoneuron anatomy and its contribution to the changes in electrical properties (ElBasiouny et al., 2010). Realistic computer models were developed from the reconstructed morphologies of WT and mutant motoneurons of the G85R model and were optimized to replicate the electrophysiological recordings obtained from individual cells. For the 30% reduction in input resistance of mutant motoneurons relative to WT, computer simulations showed that one third of this reduction (i.e., input resistance decrease by 10%) is due to the enlargement of motoneuron anatomy, whereas two thirds of this reduction (i.e., input resistance decrease by additional 20%) is due to a decrease in the specific membrane resistance of the motoneuron membrane. The specific membrane resistance represents the number of leak channels available in a patch of cell membrane and its decrease means that there are more ion channels inserted into the membrane (i.e., the cell has higher conductance). Comparison of WT and mutant motoneuron models indicated a 25% decrease in the somatic and dendritic specific membrane resistance of the mutant models. Therefore, the simulation results indicate that the enlargement in motoneuron anatomy does not fully account for the reduction in input resistance as previously suggested by Bories et al. (2007). This is because the additional dendritic branches causing the increased surface area are electrotonically distant from the soma, the site of input resistance measurement. This electrotonic separation reduces the influence of the additional dendritic area at the soma. Thus, a 60% increase in total surface area of mutant motoneurons causes only a 10% decrease in cell input resistance (not 40% as would be predicted from the reciprocal of surface area increase of an electrotonically compact sphere). Secondly, the simulation results indicate that the reduction in input resistance of mutant motoneurons is a function of two factors: the enlargement in motoneuron anatomy and the decrease in specific membrane resistance; the weights of these factors determine the magnitude of input resistance reduction. This could explain why the enlargement of motoneuron anatomy was not always associated with reduction in input resistance as in the case of the G93A (low expressor line) model (see Table 2), suggesting an insignificant change in the membrane specific membrane resistance in this transgenic model. In contrast, the significant reduction in input resistance of mutant motoneurons of the G93A (high expressor line) model despite the truncation in motoneuron dendrites in the slice preparation in Quinlan et al. (2011) might indicate a substantial change in the specific membrane resistance in that transgenic model.

The effects of enlargement in mutant motoneuron anatomy are not only limited to cell input resistance, but also extend to cell firing properties. For instance, the enlargement in mutant motoneuron anatomy would be expected to cause reductions in the motoneuron F-I gain and initial and maximum firing rates and increases in rheobase current and total cell capacitance. Given that no change was seen in some of these properties of mutant motoneurons indicate that compensatory mechanisms have masked those effects (e.g., upregulation in motoneuron transient and persistent inward currents). Estimating the contribution of anatomy enlargement to the changes in mutant motoneurons firing activity and identifying potential ionic mechanisms for masking these changes using computer simulations would be an important step in revealing hidden alterations in motoneuron properties and improving our understanding of ALS pathogenesis.

5. The changes in synaptic inputs to motoneurons

In ALS patients and transgenic models, synaptic inputs converging onto motoneurons experience changes during disease progression. These changes involve loss of specific types of synaptic inputs, rearrangement of the synaptic contacts, and alteration in the size of synaptic boutons. For instance, it has been shown that cholinergic synapses on lumbar motoneurons are lost in ALS patients (Nagao et al., 1998). This loss starts before motoneuron degeneration. Given that cholinergic synapses provide inhibitory input to motoneurons (Nagy et al., 1993), their loss could alter the balance toward more excitatory inputs, leading to motoneurons overactivation. This prediction has been confirmed in G93A (high expressor line) transgenic mice in which the ratio of inhibitory to excitatory synapses was reduced due to the loss of inhibitory boutons (loss was mediated by nitric oxide) and increase in excitatory boutons (Sunico et al., 2011). Furthermore, residual inhibitory boutons exhibit shorter active zone length and smaller synaptic vesicle density (Sunico et al., 2011). Along the same line, there was a progressive increase in the excitability of interneurons, through NMDA receptors, that starts in the presymptomatic stage of ALS (Jiang et al., 2009).

Computer simulations of mutant motoneuron models predicted a reduction in the efficacy of dendritic processing of synaptic inputs early in ALS (ElBasiouny et al., 2010). The amplitude of somatic excitatory postsynaptic potentials (EPSPs) was reduced in mutant motoneurons by 15%, relative to WT. This reduction was comparable to experimental measurements of EPSP amplitudes in the G85R transgenic model (Bories et al., 2007). The computer simulations showed that the reduction in EPSP amplitude resulted from the alteration in various motoneuron properties such as: the increase in motoneuron morphology, the decrease in specific membrane resistance, and the increase in dendritic active conductance activation. The changes in these properties counteract each other and produce the net reduction in EPSP amplitude. These changes were consistent in synaptic inputs with different dynamics (i.e., slow and fast inputs) (ElBasiouny et al., 2010).

6. The functional ramifications of the alteration in motoneuron properties

The combined changes in motoneuron properties (anatomical, electrical, biophysical) and synaptic inputs converging on them in ALS alter the input-output function of mutant motoneurons and affect their recruitment. For instance, the reduction in input resistance of mutant motoneurons makes them harder to recruit. Similarly, the enlargement in motoneuron anatomy and development of dendritic overbranching increase the attenuation of excitatory and inhibitory post synaptic potentials as they flow to the soma along the dendrites and reduce their efficacy. Computer simulations of reconstructed morphologies of WT and mutant motoneurons indicated a reduction in the efficacy of slow and fast synaptic inputs (by ≈20%) in mutant motoneurons (ElBasiouny et al., 2010). Half of this efficacy reduction was due to the dendritic overbranching, whereas the second half was due to the decrease in specific membrane resistance, leading to increased signal loss through leak conductances. The simulations demonstrated that reduction in synaptic efficacy was still present despite the upregulation in the dendritic active conductances mediating persistent inward current. These combined reductions in cell input resistance and synaptic input efficacy push toward reduced excitability of the cell. It is unclear whether these changes represent disease or protective mechanisms (see next section for discussion).

7. Anatomical alterations versus excitability changes: Disease versus neuroprotective mechanisms?

The individual changes seen in properties of mutant motoneurons could be a disease mechanism, which produces a physiological malfunction, or a neuroprotective (i.e., compensatory) mechanism of the nervous system, which mitigates the physiological malfunction caused by the disease. These mechanisms develop sequentially and act antagonistically. Given that ALS pathogenesis is still poorly understood (i.e., disease mechanisms are not identified yet), it is unfeasible to categorize the changes in mutant motoneurons to disease or compensatory mechanisms with assertion; however, some hypotheses could be formulated from available data regarding the nature of these changes. For instance, the relationship between the alterations in anatomy and excitability of mutant motoneurons is paradoxical. In the G93A (high expressor line) model, the enlargement in motoneuron anatomy and concomitant increase in persistent inward current have opposite actions on the excitability of motoneurons. Two hypotheses are described to infer the nature of these mechanisms. The first hypothesis is based on the effect of endurance training on healthy and transgenic mice. In healthy mice, endurance running exercise reduced the excitability of healthy motoneurons and increased their size, as suggested from their input resistance and cell capacitance measurements (Beaumont and Gardiner, 2002, 2003). In G93A mice, endurance running exercise reduced motor performance and shortened the life span of transgenic mice (Mahoney et al., 2004). Assuming that detrimental effects on transgenic mice would result from approaches that promote disease mechanisms, it is therefore plausible to suggest that anatomy enlargement of motoneurons is potentially an ALS disease mechanism. Consequently, the increase in motoneuron persistent inward current is potentially a compensatory mechanism to enhance the motoneuron excitability and offset the effect of enlarged anatomy. In this scenario, the additional dendrites would not possess active conductances and would reduce the motoneuron excitability by reducing the cell input resistance. However, this hypothesis is challenged by the beneficial effect of riluzole (the only FDA-approved drug available for ALS patients), which reduces motoneuron excitability and extends the life span of ALS patients (Bensimon et al., 1994; Miller et al., 1996) and transgenic mice (Gurney et al., 1998), suggesting increased excitability as the disease mechanism.

The second hypothesis is based on the relationship between the intrinsic motoneuron excitability and dendrite anatomy. When potassium channels were genetically manipulated to increase or decrease the motoneuron excitability, the overall motoneuron size was increased in both conditions with increased dendritic branch formation in the former case or dendritic branch elongation in the latter (Duch et al., 2008). Given that the anatomical alterations seen in mutant motoneurons resemble some features of those produced in response to increased excitability, this suggests that anatomy enlargement of mutant motoneurons is potentially a compensatory mechanism, whereas the increase in motoneuron excitability is potentially the disease mechanism. In this scenario, the pathologically-formed dendrites could contribute to the disease-state by having dendritic active conductances, which would dramatically increase the magnitude of persistent inward currents and enhance the motoneuronal excitability. The reduction in input resistance of mutant motoneurons would result from the increase in cell size. This hypothesis is supported by the beneficial effect of riluzole on mutant motoneurons survival by suppressing their excitability as explained above. Because motoneuron hyperexcitability is not a common feature of ALS transgenic models (hyperexcitability appears in models with high copy number of SOD1 gene, Table 3), riluzole's effect could be more pronounced in the more aggressive models of ALS that exhibit hyperexcitability, but less effective in the mild models of ALS (with less copy number of SOD1 gene) that exhibit hypoexcitability. This prediction might explain the discrepancy in studies on riluzole's efficacy in the various ALS transgenic models (for review see Bellingham, 2011). More data are needed to divulge the nature of these mechanisms.

In the G85R and G93A (low expressor line) models, alterations in anatomy and excitability of mutant motoneurons are observed, with no change in persistent inward current amplitude (Table 3). This disparity in the relationship between persistent inward current amplitude and motoneuron excitability in the various ALS transgenic models could be due to the difference in pace of disease progression in these models. In other words, disease and compensatory mechanisms advance at faster rates in aggressive ALS models (with high copy number of SOD1 genes) than in mild ALS models (with low copy number of SOD1 genes). This supposition is supported by the earlier disease onset and shorter life span in the G93A (high expressor line) than in the G85R and G93A (low expressor line) models (Turner and Talbot, 2008). Longitudinal studies in in-vivo mouse preparations in which the changes in motoneuron excitability, persistent inward currents, and anatomical properties in the various ALS transgenic models could be monitored at short time intervals during disease progression are needed to examine the development of these mechanisms.

8. Conclusion

Numerous alterations in the anatomical and electrical properties of mutant spinal motoneurons take place in the first two postnatal weeks, long before disease onset. Many of these alterations are inconsistent and sometimes contradictory; however, critical analysis of these alterations allowed for the identification of common pathological features within and across the various transgenic models of ALS. The enlargement in anatomy and reduction in input resistance of mutant motoneurons are characteristic features in the various transgenic models of ALS, whereas the alterations in motoneuron excitability and ionic currents (both transient and persistent) differ across transgenic models. To date, it is unfeasible to identify which of these alterations is an action of the disease (i.e., disease mechanism) or a reaction of the nervous system (i.e., compensatory mechanism) and more experiments are needed to elucidate the nature of these alterations. Computer simulations of realistic models of WT and mutant motoneurons allowed for the identification of hidden alteration in the biophysical properties of mutant motoneurons and demonstrated that synaptic efficacy is reduced in mutant motoneurons. It would be important to have extensive computational analysis of motoneuron properties in the various ALS transgenic models at various points in time during disease progression to identify and monitor the immeasurable changes in membrane properties of mutant motoneurons. This information would be expected to improve significantly our understanding of motoneuron pathophysiology in ALS.

9. Acknowledgment

This work was supported by grants to C.J.H. from the National Institutes of Health-National Institute of Neurological Disorders and Stroke (NS034382 and NS051462). S.M.E. was supported by the Tim E. Noel fellowship from the ALS Society of Canada and the Canadian Institutes of Health Research (CIHR). K.A.Q. was supported by the NRSA F32 fellowship (NS063535). T.L.E. was supported by the Joseph A. Blazek Foundation.

10. References

Amendola J, Durand J (2008) Morphological differences between wild-type and transgenic superoxide dismutase 1 lumbar motoneurons in postnatal mice. J Comp Neurol 511:329-341.

Amendola J, Gueritaud J, D'Incamps B, Bories C, Liabeuf S, Allene C, Pambo-Pambo A, Durand J (2007) Postnatal electrical and morphological abnormalities in lumbar motoneurons from transgenic mouse models of amyotrophic lateral sclerosis. Arch Ital Biol 145:311-323.

Beaumont E, Gardiner PF (2002) Effects of daily spontaneous running on the electrophysiological properties of hindlimb motoneurones in rats. J Physiol (Lond) 540:129-138.

Beaumont E, Gardiner PF (2003) Endurance training alters the biophysical properties of hindlimb motoneurons in rats. Muscle Nerve 27:228-236.

Bellingham MC (2011) A review of the neural mechanisms of action and clinical efficiency of riluzole in treating amyotrophic lateral sclerosis: what have we learned in the last decade? CNS Neurosci Ther 17:4-31.

Bennett DJ, Li Y, Siu M (2001) Plateau Potentials in Sacrocaudal Motoneurons of Chronic Spinal Rats, Recorded In Vitro. J Neurophysiol 86:1955-1971.

Bensimon G, Lacomblez L, Meininger V (1994) A controlled trial of riluzole in amyotrophic lateral sclerosis. ALS/Riluzole Study Group. N Engl J Med 330:585-591.

Bories C, Amendola J, Lamotte d'Incamps B, Durand J (2007) Early electrophysiological abnormalities in lumbar motoneurons in a transgenic mouse model of amyotrophic lateral sclerosis. Eur J Neurosci 25:451-459.

Bruijn LI, Becher MW, Lee MK, Anderson KL, Jenkins NA, Copeland NG, Sisodia SS, Rothstein JD, Borchelt DR, Price DL, Cleveland DW (1997) ALS-Linked SOD1 Mutant G85R Mediates Damage to Astrocytes and Promotes Rapidly Progressive Disease with SOD1-Containing Inclusions. Neuron 18:327-338.

Charcot J (1874) De la sclerose laterale amyotrophique. Prog Med 2:325-455.

Duch C, Vonhoff F, Ryglewski S (2008) Dendrite Elongation and Dendritic Branching Are Affected Separately by Different Forms of Intrinsic Motoneuron Excitability. J Neurophysiol 100:2525-2536.

ElBasiouny SM, Amendola J, Durand J, Heckman CJ (2010) Evidence from computer simulations for alterations in the membrane biophysical properties and dendritic processing of synaptic inputs in mutant superoxide dismutase-1 motoneurons. J Neurosci 30:5544-5558.

Filipchuk A, Pambo-Pambo A, Liabeuf S, Brocard C, Kulagina I, Korogod S, Gueritaud J, Durand J (2010) Evidence of early somato-dendritic alterations in lumbar motoneurons of sod1 juvenile mice. Amyotrophic Lat Scler 11:39-40.

Fuchs A, Schuetz B, Liss B, Roeper J (2008) Selective and disease-onset related action potential broadening in vulnerable brainstem motoneurons in the SOD1G93A ALS mouse model. Program No 44510 2008 Neuroscience Meeting Planner Washington, DC: Society for Neuroscience, 2008 Online

Fuchs A, Schuetz B, Liss B, Roeper J (2009) Persistent sodium currents are not altered at disease endstage in vulnerable brainstem motoneurons of the transgenic SOD1G93A ALS mouse model. Program No 6312 2009 Neuroscience Meeting Planner Chicago, IL: Society for Neuroscience, 2009 Online

Gurney ME, Fleck TJ, Himes CS, Hall ED (1998) Riluzole preserves motor function in a transgenic model of familial amyotrophic lateral sclerosis. Neurology 50:62-66.

Hamm TM, Turkin VV, Bandekar NK, O'Neill D, Jung R (2010) Persistent Currents and Discharge Patterns in Rat Hindlimb Motoneurons. J Neurophysiol 104:1566-1577.

Hegedus J, Putman CT, Gordon T (2007) Time course of preferential motor unit loss in the SOD1G93A mouse model of amyotrophic lateral sclerosis. Neurobiol Dis 28:154-164.

Hegedus J, Putman CT, Tyreman N, Gordon T (2008) Preferential motor unit loss in the SOD1G93A transgenic mouse model of amyotrophic lateral sclerosis. J Physiol:jphysiol.2007.149286.

Jiang M, Schuster JE, Fu R, Siddique T, Heckman CJ (2009) Progressive Changes in Synaptic Inputs to Motoneurons in Adult Sacral Spinal Cord of a Mouse Model of Amyotrophic Lateral Sclerosis. J Neuroscience 29:15031-15038.

Karim N, Kibble M, Everall I, Leigh N, Al-Sarraj S (1998) Extra motor neuronal loss in motor neuron disease. Neuropathol Appl Neurobiol 24:161-162.

Konno H, Yamamoto T, Iwasaki Y, Iizuka H (1986) Shy-Drager syndrome and amyotrophic lateral sclerosis. Cytoarchitectonic and morphometric studies of sacral autonomic neurons. J Neurol Sci 73:193-204.

Kuo JJ, Siddique T, Fu R, Heckman CJ (2005) Increased persistent Na+ current and its effect on excitability in motoneurones cultured from mutant SOD1 mice. J Physiol (Lond) 563:843-854.

Kuo JJ, Schonewille M, Siddique T, Schults ANA, Fu R, Bar PR, Anelli R, Heckman CJ, Kroese ABA (2004) Hyperexcitability of Cultured Spinal Motoneurons From Presymptomatic ALS Mice. J Neurophysiol 91:571-575.

Lloyd CM, Richardson MP, Brooks DJ, Al-Chalabi A, Leigh PN (2000) Extramotor involvement in ALS: PET studies with the GABA(A) ligand [(11)C]flumazenil. Brain 123 (Pt 11):2289-2296.

Maekawa S, Al-Sarraj S, Kibble M, Landau S, Parnavelas J, Cotter D, Everall I, Leigh PN (2004) Cortical selective vulnerability in motor neuron disease: a morphometric study. Brain 127:1237-1251.

Mahoney DJ, Rodriguez C, Devries M, Yasuda N, Tarnopolsky MA (2004) Effects of high-intensity endurance exercise training in the G93A mouse model of amyotrophic lateral sclerosis. Muscle Nerve 29:656-662.

Meehan CF, Moldovan M, Marklund SL, Graffmo KS, Nielsen JB, Hultborn H (2010) Intrinsic properties of lumbar motor neurones in the adult G127insTGGG superoxide dismutase-1 mutant mouse in vivo: evidence for increased persistent inward currents. Acta Physiol (Oxf) 200:361-376.

Miles GB, Dai Y, Brownstone RM (2005) Mechanisms underlying the early phase of spike frequency adaptation in mouse spinal motoneurones. J Physiol (Lond) 566:519-532.

Miller RG, Bouchard JP, Duquette P, Eisen A, Gelinas D, Harati Y, Munsat TL, Powe L, Rothstein J, Salzman P, Sufit RL (1996) Clinical trials of riluzole in patients with ALS. ALS/Riluzole Study Group-II. Neurology 47:S86-90; discussion S90-82.

Nagao M, Misawa H, Kato S, Hirai S (1998) Loss of cholinergic synapses on the spinal motor neurons of amyotrophic lateral sclerosis. J Neuropathol Exp Neurol 57:329-333.

Nagy JI, Yamamoto T, Jordan LM (1993) Evidence for the cholinergic nature of C-terminals associated with subsurface cisterns in alpha-motoneurons of rat. Synapse 15:17-32.

Pambo-Pambo AB, Durand J, Gueritaud JP (2009) Early excitability changes in lumbar motoneurons of transgenic SOD1G85R and SOD1G93A-Low mice. J Neurophysiol 102:3627-3642.

Pieri M, Carunchio I, Curcio L, Mercuri NB, Zona C (2009) Increased persistent sodium current determines cortical hyperexcitability in a genetic model of amyotrophic lateral sclerosis. Exp Neurol 215:368-379.

Pieri M, Albo F, Gaetti C, Spalloni A, Bengtson CP, Longone P, Cavalcanti S, Zona C (2003) Altered excitability of motor neurons in a transgenic mouse model of familial amyotrophic lateral sclerosis. Neurosci Lett 351:153-156.

Pun S, Santos AF, Saxena S, Xu L, Caroni P (2006) Selective vulnerability and pruning of phasic motoneuron axons in motoneuron disease alleviated by CNTF. 9:408-419.

Quinlan KA, Schuster JE, Fu R, Siddique T, Heckman CJ (2011) Altered postnatal maturation of electrical properties in spinal motoneurons in an ALS mouse model. J Physiol 589:2245-2260.

Sasaki S, Maruyama S (1992) Increase in diameter of the axonal initial segment is an early change in amyotrophic lateral sclerosis. J Neurol Sci 110:114-120.

Schwindt PC, Crill WE (1977) A persistent negative resistance in cat lumbar motoneurons. Brain Res 120:173-178.

Sobue G, Matsuoka Y, Mukai E, Takayanagi T, Sobue I, Hashizume Y (1981) Spinal and cranial motor nerve roots in amyotrophic lateral sclerosis and X-linked recessive bulbospinal muscular atrophy: morphometric and teased-fiber study. Acta Neuropathol 55:227-235.

Stephens B, Guiloff RJ, Navarrete R, Newman P, Nikhar N, Lewis P (2006) Widespread loss of neuronal populations in the spinal ventral horn in sporadic motor neuron disease. A morphometric study. J Neurol Sci 244:41-58.

Sunico CR, Dominguez G, Garcia-Verdugo JM, Osta R, Montero F, Moreno-Lopez B (2011) Reduction in the motoneuron inhibitory/excitatory synaptic ratio in an early-symptomatic mouse model of amyotrophic lateral sclerosis. Brain Pathol 21:1-15.

Swash M, Fox KP (1974) The pathology of the human muscle spindle: effect of denervation. J Neurol Sci 22:1-24.

Takahashi H, Oyanagi K, Ikuta F (1993) The intermediolateral nucleus in sporadic amyotrophic lateral sclerosis. Acta Neuropathol 86:190-192.

Turner BJ, Talbot K (2008) Transgenics, toxicity and therapeutics in rodent models of mutant SOD1-mediated familial ALS. Prog Neurobiol 85:94-134.

van Zundert B, Peuscher MH, Hynynen M, Chen A, Neve RL, Brown RH, Jr., Constantine-Paton M, Bellingham MC (2008) Neonatal Neuronal Circuitry Shows Hyperexcitable Disturbance in a Mouse Model of the Adult-Onset Neurodegenerative Disease Amyotrophic Lateral Sclerosis. J Neurosci 28:10864-10874.

Williams C, Kozlowski MA, Hinton DR, Miller CA (1990) Degeneration of spinocerebellar neurons in amyotrophic lateral sclerosis. Ann Neurol 27:215-225.

Zona C, Pieri M, Carunchio I (2006) Voltage-Dependent Sodium Channels in Spinal Cord Motor Neurons Display Rapid Recovery From Fast Inactivation in a Mouse Model of Amyotrophic Lateral Sclerosis. J Neurophysiol 96:3314-3322.

6

Molecular and Electrical Abnormalities in the Mouse Model of Amyotrophic Lateral Sclerosis

Katharina A. Quinlan[1], Sherif M. Elbasiouny[1] and C.J. Heckman[1,2,3]
[1]*Department of Physiology, Northwestern University Feinberg School of Medicine*
[2]*Department of Physical Medicine and Rehabilitation, Northwestern University Feinberg School of Medicine*
[3]*Department of Physical Therapy and Human Movement Sciences, Northwestern University Feinberg School of Medicine*
United States of America

1. Introduction

Amyotrophic lateral sclerosis (ALS) is a devastating, fast progressing and fatal disease for which there is little treatment. It is marked by loss of spinal and cortical motoneuron function. Many parameters are altered in the time leading up to this loss, including electrical properties, endoplasmic reticulum (ER) stress, glial functioning, glutamate signaling, protein degradation, mitochondrial functioning, axonal transport, and immune response. This chapter concentrates on the interplay between altered electrophysiological properties and molecular events. Emphasis is placed on the changes that precede overt symptom onset and results are mainly drawn from studies using the rodent models of ALS.

2. ALS animal models

Most cases of ALS are spontaneous (sALS), while the heritable form, familial ALS (fALS), represents about 5% of total ALS cases (Byrne et al., 2011). Of fALS patients, 20% have a mutation in the gene that encodes for the superoxide dismutase 1 (SOD1) copper/zinc enzyme (Rosen et al., 1993), 5% have a mutation in the TARDBP gene which encodes DNA-binding protein 43 (TDP-43), another 5% have a mutation in the FUS gene which encodes for the fused in sarcoma FUS/TLS protein (Mackenzie et al., 2010), some possess a mutation in the gene encoding vesicle-associated membrane protein (VAPB) (Nishimura et al., 2004), and a new study shows that some of those remaining have a mutation in the gene coding for the ubiquitin-like protein ubiquilin-2 (Deng et al., 2011). Transgenic mice expressing one of the various mutations of human SOD1, hereafter referred to as SOD1 mice; (Gurney et al., 1994, Bruijn et al., 1997, Zhang et al., 1997) are very common animal models of ALS; numerous other models of fALS are reviewed by Van Den Bosch (2011). It is not known how the SOD1 mutation leads to the degeneration of motoneurons, though it is probably not due to loss of its normal function converting superoxide into hydrogen peroxide. The mutant, misfolded protein likely possesses a toxic gain-of-function, as some mouse lines retain nearly normal levels of SOD1 enzymatic activity and still develop the disease, while SOD1 knockout mice, which do not possess any SOD1 enzymatic activity, do not develop the disease (Gurney et al., 1994, Reaume et al., 1996, Wong et al., 1995). Whatever the mechanism(s) leading to neurodegeneration, it is not immediate. The SOD1 enzyme is present throughout the nervous system (Pardo et al., 1995) starting embryonically, but does not lead to onset of overt symptoms until well into adulthood, even in mice that express high levels of the protein (Gurney et al., 1994). And within the nervous system, only certain neurons show susceptibility to the disease. This chapter will explore the earliest signs of malfunction in the neurons that are most vulnerable to the disease.

3. Timeline of deficits

In ALS, it is difficult to assess which of all the processes that have been found to be altered are causal to neurodegeneration and which are homeostatic, adaptive mechanisms that are actually allowing the maintenance function. Despite this, it is useful to map out the timing of the various altered properties collected from the mouse models, as presented in Figure 1. Depending on the particular SOD1 mouse model studied, the magnitude and timing of alterations observed does vary (reviewed in Elbasiouny et al, previous chapter). However, for this chapter, the deficits in these mice will be considered in their entirety and not separated based on the particular model from which the results were obtained.

Long before the onset of overt symptoms, within the first week after birth, electrical properties are altered. These properties include an increase in excitability (as measured by both the Na^{+}- and Ca^{2+}- mediated persistent inward current; PIC) and an increased neuronal size (including increased dendritic branching and increased specific input conductance). Significantly larger PICs first appear in cultured embryonic spinal and cortical motoneurons (Kuo et al., 2005, Pieri et al., 2009), persist at an age of about one week in spinal and hypoglossal motoneurons (van Zundert et al., 2008, Quinlan et al., 2011) and are likely still present in the spinal and cortical motoneurons of adults (Carunchio et al., 2010, Meehan et al., 2010). Interestingly, although the PIC is upregulated very early, what might otherwise be the beginning of motoneuron hyperexcitability is instead moderated by changes in size and specific input conductance (Amendola and Durand, 2008, Elbasiouny et al., 2010, Quinlan et al., 2011). In adulthood, but still well before the onset of symptoms, there are signs of defective protein degradation, endoplasmic reticulum (ER) stress, impaired axon transport, and deficiencies in mitochondrial function. Signs of aberrant protein clearance include increased expression of genes related to ubiquitination, UPR, and ER stress (Saxena et al., 2009). As these changes might suggest, there is a buildup of insoluble SOD1 proteins at this time (Johnston et al., 2000, Turner et al., 2003a), followed shortly by fragmentation of the Golgi (Mourelatos et al., 1996). The next signs of impairment appear in the mitochondria and in the cellular transport system (Zhang et al., 1997, Warita et al., 1999, Williamson and Cleveland, 1999, Mattiazzi et al., 2002, Kieran et al., 2005, Damiano et al., 2006, De Vos et al., 2007, Bilsland et al., 2008, Jaiswal et al., 2009, Nguyen et al., 2009, Bilsland et al., 2010, Li et al., 2010). The immune response is initiated next (Alexianu et al., 2001, Chiu et al., 2008, Gowing et al., 2008, Chiu et al., 2009). After this, denervation of the motor units and loss of maximal force begins (Kennel et al., 1996, Frey et al., 2000, Fischer et al., 2004, Hegedus et al., 2007, Hegedus et al., 2008), but the impairment of normal function in the mouse is subtle and onset of overt symptoms is several weeks off, even in the most severe models. Just before the impending functional loss, several of the last changes before overt onset of symptoms involve the glia: activation of astrocytes, expression of different splice variants of EAAT2, decreased expression of the GluR2 subunit, and decreased number of glial K^+ channels (Bruijn et al., 1997, Bendotti et al., 2001, Sasaki et al., 2001, Munch et al., 2002, Warita et al., 2002, Fischer et al., 2004, Ignacio et al., 2005, Kaiser et al., 2006).

It is tempting to assume that the order of appearance of the altered parameters represents a chain reaction of events, but this is not necessarily the case. There is considerable interplay between these components within the neurons, such that one pathway cannot be altered without affecting any other aspect of cellular or synaptic function. These interactions will be considered next.

4. Calcium: No buffer for increased currents

Entry of Ca^{2+} occurs through voltage-gated Ca^{2+} channels and through ligand-gated channels activated by glutamate, particularly the NMDA-type glutamate receptors and those AMPA-type glutamate receptors which lack the Ca^{2+}-impermeable GluR2 subunit. Most voltage-gated Ca^{2+} channels open only when the cell depolarizes; however, the L-type $Ca_v1.3$ channels, which contribute to the PIC, open near the resting membrane potential (-40mV) and allow some Ca^{2+} influx even when the neuron is at rest (Xu and Lipscombe, 2001). There is very little expression of $Ca_v1.3$ channels in spinal motoneurons at birth, but $Ca_v1.3$ channels are increasingly present as the motoneurons mature, reaching adult levels by postnatal day 18 (P18) in mice, (Jiang et al., 1999, Quinlan et al., 2011). The PIC sets the level of excitability in neurons: PICs allow neurons to repetitively fire action potentials, and with large PICs, neurons can sustain firing long after the depolarizing stimulus is removed (Heckman et al., 2008). In addition, motoneurons from SOD1G93A-high-expressor mice show a significantly larger PIC during postnatal development, including significantly larger amplitudes of both Ca^{2+} and Na^+ currents (Quinlan et al., 2011). Larger PICs can increase the overall excitability of a neuron (though other factors, like size, can mitigate this), and the influx of Ca^{2+} could have many other consequences in cell-signaling. An increased PIC is found in cultured, embryonic, SOD1G93A-high motoneurons (both spinal and cortical), though at this point the PIC is completely Na^+-based (Kuo et al., 2005, Pieri et al., 2009). Postnatally, both spinal and brainstem SOD1 motoneurons show an increased PIC (van Zundert et al., 2008, Quinlan et al., 2011), and indirect evidence suggests larger PICs persist into adulthood in SOD1 cortical and spinal motoneurons (Carunchio et al., 2010, Meehan et al., 2010). In addition to the maturation of the PIC, there is an increase in AMPA-type glutamate receptors on motoneurons (Vinay et al., 2000). These receptors normally would not contribute to Ca^{2+} influx since, due to a single amino acid in the pore-forming GluR2 subunit they are impermeable to Ca^{2+}. However, in presymptomatic SOD1 motoneurons, there are fewer Ca^{2+}-impermeable GluR2 subunits; and more Ca^{2+}-permeable GluR3 subunits (Tortarolo et al., 2006). In sALS patients, AMPA receptors also are more Ca^{2+}-permeable, but through a different mechanism. Spinal motoneurons of symptomatic sALS patients, but not SOD1 rats, showed inefficient editing of the mRNA, resulting in mutant, GluR2Q subunits that are Ca^{2+}-permeable (Kawahara et al., 2004, Kwak and Kawahara, 2005, Kawahara et al., 2006). As motoneurons mature they must cope with an ever-increasing burden of Ca^{2+} influx through voltage-gated Ca^{2+} channels (as the Ca^{2+} PIC increases with age) and SOD1 motoneurons have a heavier burden due to potentiation of the Ca^{2+}PIC and altered AMPA receptors which are more Ca^{2+}-permeable.

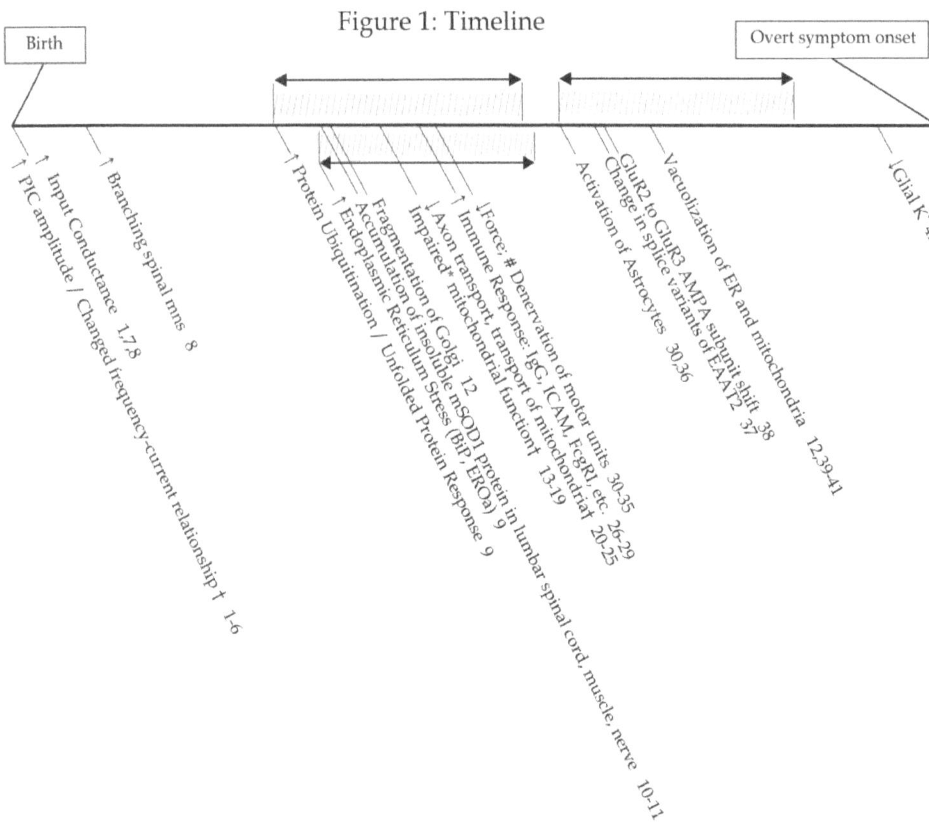

[1](Quinlan et al., 2011),[2](Kuo et al., 2005), [3](van Zundert et al., 2008), [4](Meehan et al., 2010), [5](Carunchio et al., 2010), [6](Pieri et al., 2009), [7](Bories et al., 2007), [8](Amendola and Durand, 2008), [9](Saxena et al., 2009), [10](Johnston et al., 2000), [11](Turner et al., 2003b), [12](Mourelatos et al., 1996), [13](Li et al., 2010), [14](Jaiswal and Keller, 2009),[15](Mattiazzi et al., 2002), [16](Nguyen et al., 2009), [17](Jaiswal et al., 2009), [18](Bilsland et al., 2008), [19](Damiano et al., 2006), [20](Bilsland et al., 2010), [21](De Vos et al., 2007), [22](Williamson and Cleveland, 1999), [23](Zhang et al., 1997), [24](Kieran et al., 2005), [25](Warita et al., 1999), [26](Alexianu et al., 2001), [27](Gowing et al., 2008), [28](Chiu et al., 2008), [29](Chiu et al., 2009), [30](Fischer et al., 2004), [31](Frey et al., 2000), [32](Pun et al., 2006), [33](Hegedus et al., 2007), [34](Hegedus et al., 2008), [35](Kennel et al., 1996), [36](Bruijn et al., 1997), [37](Munch et al., 2002), [38](Tortarolo et al., 2006), [39](Bendotti et al., 2001), [40](Dal Canto and Gurney, 1995), [41](Dal Canto and Gurney, 1994), [42](Kaiser et al., 2006).

Fig. 1. Timeline of deficits in mutant SOD1 mice. Earliest reported deficits in the above properties are used. Different SOD1 mutants were normalized to dates of overt symptom onset. When differences in timing between mouse lines were large (as it was for protein ubiquitination, stress of the ER, and activation of astrocytes), the range is indicated in the timeline with (///). † Also found in embryonic cultured motoneurons. * Different aspects of mitochondrial function were impaired at different time points. The first alteration in function is decreased Ca^{2+} storage capacity[19]. Another property, mitochondrial membrane potential, is not altered until just before symptom onset[17], while the function or regulation of the electron transport chain is impaired slightly before membrane potential[16].

While Ca^{2+} currents are increased in SOD1 motoneurons, large spinal and hypoglossal motoneurons do not have Ca^{2+}-binding proteins calbindin and parvalbumin and thus cannot quickly neutralize large influxes of Ca^{2+}. Instead, they depend heavily on mitochondrial uptake of Ca^{2+} (Ren and Ruda, 1994, Lips and Keller, 1998, Palecek et al., 1999, Bergmann and Keller, 2004). Small ocular motoneurons which have calbindin, parvalbumin and high Ca^{2+}-buffering capacities are unaffected by ALS (Vanselow and Keller, 2000, von Lewinski and Keller, 2005). Ca^{2+}-binding ratio, Ks, depends on Ca^{2+}-binding proteins, the intracellular $[Ca^{2+}]_i$, and the size and geometry of the cell (Neher, 1995). Although Ca^{2+} buffering at the soma of neonatal SOD1 and WT motoneurons was similar (von Lewinski et al., 2008), buffering has not been measured in adult motoneurons or in the processes, where Ca^{2+} channels are located (Sukiasyan et al., 2009). Ca^{2+} buffering could also change postnatally in motoneurons, as in rat Purkinje cells in which the Ca^{2+}-binding ratio more than doubles between P6 and P15 (Fierro and Llano, 1996). The increasing Ca^{2+} entry with postnatal maturation combined with the lack of Ca^{2+}-buffering proteins seems likely to contribute to motoneuronal vulnerability in adulthood.

5. Impaired transport, more places to go

The lack of Ca^{2+}-buffering proteins in vulnerable motoneurons make the mitochondria even more critical to their function. Mitochondria are normally highly mobile both in axons and dendrites (MacAskill et al., 2010). Mitochondrial movement can be halted by increased concentrations of ADP, so they tend to remain in compartments which are highly metabolically-active (Mironov, 2007). Mitochondrial movements are also regulated through Ca^{2+} signaling and synaptic activity (Rintoul et al., 2003, Yi et al., 2004, Macaskill et al., 2009). When glutamate binds NMDA- or certain AMPA-type receptor-channels, it allows the influx of Na^{+} and Ca^{2+} into the cell. The Ca^{2+}-sensitive domain of Miro, the mitochondrial trafficking protein, then interacts with Ca^{2+} and the transport factors TRAK and KIF5, and pauses in its movement at active synapses (Rintoul et al., 2003, MacAskill et al., 2009). Postsynaptic NMDA receptors are also associated with PSD95 and with nitric oxide synthase (NOS) which, through nitric oxide (NO), also pauses mitochondrial movement (Rintoul et al., 2006). Once at a synapse, the mitochondria are probably tethered by neurofilaments, a process that depends both on the state of phosphorylation of the neurofilaments and a high mitochondrial membrane potential which indicates a high level of activity (Wagner et al., 2003).

In axons, but not in the soma of cultured SOD1 motoneurons, mitochondria are more sparsely distributed (De Vos et al., 2007), and *in vivo* mitochondria show more frequent pauses in their movements in pre-symptomatic SOD1 mice (Bilsland et al., 2010). Unfortunately, movement of mitochondria and other membrane-bound organelles has not yet been well studied in the dendrites of SOD1 motoneurons. If the mitochondria are similarly sparse in the dendrites, where most Ca^{2+} channels are located, this could have serious consequences for Ca^{2+} buffering. Spinal motoneurons of SOD1 mice show a significant proliferation in dendritic branches (Amendola and Durand, 2008) and an increased Ca^{2+} PIC (Quinlan et al., 2011), which could make mitochondrial motility in the dendrites more challenging. Without mitochondria to take up Ca^{2+} at the synapses, this would further exacerbate the low Ca^{2+} buffering in vulnerable motoneurons and any increased Ca^{2+} entry with synaptic inputs (Tortarolo et al., 2006). It is also worth noting that the motoneurons that are vulnerable are the largest: the fast, fatiguable alpha motoneurons (Pun et al., 2006, Hegedus et al., 2007, Hegedus et al., 2008). Evidence for further increases size in SOD1 motoneurons is reviewed in the previous chapter by Elbasiouny et al. Perhaps the size of the motoneuron and deficits in transport go hand in hand to produce vulnerability.

Axon transport has been extensively studied and is likely to contribute to ALS and to several neurodegenerative diseases, reviewed by (De Vos et al., 2008). In ALS, both slow and fast axon transport appear to be altered (Zhang et al., 1997, Warita et al., 1999, Williamson and Cleveland, 1999, Kieran et al., 2005, De Vos et al., 2007, Bilsland et al., 2010). Excessive glutamate could cause these deficiencies: high levels of glutamate activate a family of mitogen-activated protein kinases that phosphorylate neurofilaments, thereby decreasing transport (Ackerley et al., 2000, Hiruma et al., 2003, Stevenson et al., 2009). This process can be induced by NMDA or AMPA, blocked by removal of extracellular Ca^{2+}, or reduced by application of riluzole (Hiruma et al., 2003, Stevenson et al., 2009). The protein kinases JNKs, cdk/p35 and p38, which phosphorylate heavy and light chains of kinesin and medium and heavy neurofilament sidearms, may link glutamate neurotransmission and axon transport deficits (Kawasaki et al., 1997, Schwarzschild et al., 1997, Ackerley et al., 2000, Brownlees et al., 2000, Lee et al., 2000). Further suggesting this, p38 has been found to be activated in SOD1 mice and ALS patients (Raoul et al., 2002, Tortarolo et al., 2003, Ackerley et al., 2004). Axon transport deficiencies occur early, with reports of impaired axonal integrity and die-back from the neuromuscular junction occurring weeks in advance of onset of symptoms in SOD1 mice, and appearing in cultured embryonic neurons (Kennel et al., 1996, Zhang et al., 1997, Williamson and Cleveland, 1999, Frey et al., 2000, Fischer et al., 2004, Pun et al., 2006, De Vos et al., 2007, Hegedus et al., 2007, Hegedus et al., 2008, Bilsland et al., 2010). Strengthening these results, transgenic TDP-43 mice show significantly lower levels of expression of heavy and light neurofilaments, though axon transport itself has not yet been assessed (Swarup et al., 2011).

6. Mitochondrial deficiency and energy balance

In motoneurons under normal conditions, the mitochondrial membrane potential powers both the Ca^{2+} uniporter and ATP synthase, so in periods of heavy Ca^{2+} influx, ATP production could be impaired (Mattson et al., 2008, Nguyen et al., 2009). The increased Ca^{2+} influx in SOD1 motoneurons is likely to further impair the function of mitochondria under these conditions. In addition, SOD1 mitochondria appear to be impaired in function under basal conditions (Mattiazzi et al., 2002, Nguyen et al., 2009, Li et al., 2010). Before the onset of symptoms, SOD1 mitochondria show decreased protein import, altered Ca^{2+} sequestering, and an exaggerated response of the electrical gradient of the inner membrane to stimulation-induced Ca^{2+} influx (Damiano et al., 2006, Bilsland et al., 2008, Jaiswal et al., 2009, Nguyen et al., 2009, Li et al., 2010). By the time symptoms appear there is severe damage to mitochondrial membrane potentials, respiration, the electron transport chain and ATP synthesis (Mattiazzi et al., 2002, Jaiswal and Keller, 2009). Another impairment is misfolded SOD1 binding to VDAC1, the general diffusion pore for anions and cations, including Ca^{2+}. Both mitochondrial conductance and the uptake of ADP are thereby reduced, however, this is not observed until after the onset of symptoms (Israelson et al., 2010). Early alterations in SOD1 mitochondria must take place though another mechanism.

In summary, not only are there fewer mitochondria present in the processes of SOD1 neurons (De Vos et al., 2007, Bilsland et al., 2010), but those that are present are impaired in functioning. This is likely to have dire consequences for both Ca^{2+} buffering and ATP production in the large and metabolically-active SOD1 motoneurons.

7. Protein degradation and endoplasmic reticulum stress

Misfolded proteins are degraded through autophagy (Yang and Klionsky, 2010). When the capacity of the cellular machinery in the ER to properly fold proteins is exceeded, cells react with the unfolded protein response (UPR) and signs of ER stress (reviewed by Ron and Walter, 2007). The UPR decreases most protein synthesis in the cell while upregulating synthesis of some ER proteins that assist in proper folding and processing of proteins. Another pathway, known as ER-associated protein degradation (ERAD), helps to clear the ER of misfolded proteins by exporting them to proteasomes where they are broken down (Bernasconi and Molinari, 2011). Proteins to be exported and degraded are marked by ubiquitination, a process in which ubiquitin molecules bind to the protein, tagging it for destruction (Bingol and Sheng, 2011). Normal ER function can be disrupted by blocking the ER-resident proteins from folding properly, inadequate functioning of the ubiquitin-proteosome system, or failure to maintain a high level of Ca^{2+} inside the lumen of the ER (Paschen, 2003).

It is known that mice with the highest expression levels of mutant SOD1 protein have the earliest disease onset (Wong et al., 1995), and that markers for ER stress have been found in the spinal cords of sALS patients (Ilieva et al., 2007, Atkin et al., 2008, Ito et al., 2009). However, recent studies have shed more light on the role of protein degradation and ER stress in the pathology of ALS. In the first study, gene expression patterns from 3 different SOD1 mouse lines all showed an early increase in protein ubiquitination only in those motoneurons that are vulnerable to the disease. This is followed shortly by the UPR and signs of ER stress by P30 in SOD1G93A-high expressor mice (see Fig 1) (Saxena et al., 2009). In another study, cortical motoneurons from SOD1 mutant mice were compared to those from wild type mice that were fed a diet high in branched-chain amino acids (Carunchio et al., 2010). These branched chain amino acids are part of protein supplements that some athletes consume. Like mutant SOD1 neurons, cortical neurons from mice fed the high-protein diet were hyperexcitable compared with neurons from wild type mice on a normal diet. A return to normal levels of excitability after treatment with rapamycin was achieved for both the SOD1 and the amino- acid-supplement-treated cortical neurons (Carunchio et al., 2010). The protein kinase known as the mammalian target of rapamycin (mTOR) serves as an integration point for several cell signaling pathways. As its name suggests, mTOR is inhibited by rapamycin; it also inhibits protein degradation, and promotes increased cell size in some neurons (Lee et al., 2007). These results indicate that promoting autophagy with rapamycin can reduce abnormal excitability and could be beneficial for treatment of the disease (Carunchio et al., 2010). The third, most recent study described a mutation found in 5 different families, located in the gene encoding ubiquilin-2 as a novel genetic cause of fALS (Deng et al., 2011). The function of ubiquilin is to clear certain misfolded proteins during ERAD by shuttling ubiquitinated proteins from the ER to the proteasome, such that loss of ubiquilin leads to ER stress (Kim et al., 2008, Lim et al., 2009). The mutations in ubiquilin-2 found in ALS patients were also found to impair proteosome- mediated protein degradation *in vitro*, suggesting these mutations could be causing similar impairments in the families from whom they were isolated (Deng et al., 2011). Even in sALS patients, ubiquilin-2 was found in abnormal protein aggregates in degenerating neurons, indicating it could play a broad role in both fALS and sALS pathology (Deng et al., 2011). These studies suggest a key role for protein degradation and ER stress in ALS pathology.

In healthy neurons, the resting [Ca^{2+}] in the ER remains high. When ER [Ca^{2+}] drops, the Ca^{2+}-sensing STIM proteins promote Ca^{2+}-channel formation (Luik et al., 2008). Blocking this ER-mediated Ca^{2+}-entry affects neuronal activity and under conditions of chronic hyperexcitability, STIM proteins are upregulated (Steinbeck et al., 2011). Contributions to electrophysiological excitation-mediated Ca^{2+} transients from ER Ca^{2+} release have been documented in motoneurons (Scamps et al., 2004, Jahn et al., 2006). Supporting the possibility that neuronal excitability and neuronal protein processing and ER function could share common pathways, blocking L-type Ca^{2+} channels has been reported to increase autophagy (Williams et al., 2008). To summarize, due to the large role Ca^{2+} plays in cell signaling, (McCue et al., 2010, Pivovarova and Andrews, 2010), even small changes in electrophysiological properties could have broad consequences in cellular function.

8. Non-cell autonomous deficits: Astrocytes and glutamate excitotoxicity

Recent work has shown that the vulnerability of motoneurons is not cell autonomous, and that glia play critical roles in neurodegeneration in SOD1 mice. The involvement of astrocytes and microglia in the disease were elegantly demonstrated in a series of studies using mice with deletable mutant SOD1, mice with a selective knockdown of SOD1, and SOD1/WT chimera mice (Clement et al., 2003, Boillee et al., 2006, Yamanaka et al., 2008, Wang et al., 2009). Simply culturing WT motoneurons on mutant SOD1 astrocytes was sufficient to confer toxicity to motoneurons (Nagai et al., 2007). Glia have this effect on motoneurons through a variety of pathways, including activation of astrocytes, microglia, and T cells shortly after the first signs of pathology appear. The glial response is thought to influence the progression, but not the onset, of the disease (Beers et al., 2006, Boillee et al., 2006, Yamanaka et al., 2008, Wang et al., 2009, Philips and Robberecht, 2011). Presymptomatic involvement of the glia includes a reduction of glial K^+ channel expression shortly before the onset of symptoms (Kaiser et al., 2006) and later in the course of the disease, a reduced expression of astroglial glutamate transporters, GLT1/EAAT2 which mediate glutamate reuptake at synapses and help prevent glutamate excitotoxicity (Bruijn et al., 1997, Bendotti et al., 2001, Warita et al., 2002). Earlier alterations in EAAT2 function are likely due to expression of different splice variants rather than decreased expressions levels (Sasaki et al., 2001, Munch et al., 2002, Ignacio et al., 2005). Some ALS patients also show abnormal splice variants of EAAT2, which could lead to decreased glutamate transport (Rothstein et al., 1992, Maragakis et al., 2004, Lauriat et al., 2007). Stimulation of the expression and transporter activity of EAAT2/GLT1 increases the lifespan of mutant SOD1 mice (Rothstein et al., 2005). An additional, critical function of the glia is regulation of the glutamate receptor's pore-forming GluR2 subunit (Van Damme et al., 2007). The challenges of Ca^{2+} buffering are exacerbated by alterations in the glutamate signaling across disease models of ALS. In SOD1 motoneurons, expression of subunits in the AMPA-type glutamate receptors is shifted from Ca^{2+}-impermeable to Ca^{2+}-permeable (Tortarolo et al., 2006). In TDP mice, levels of RNA that encode proteins involved in synaptic activity, including glutamate receptors, ion channels and voltage gated Ca2+ channels, are altered, with unknown consequences on synaptic transmission (Polymenidou et al., 2011). Lastly, in sALS patients, there is inefficient editing of AMPRA receptor GluR2Q subunit mRNA which also causes a shift from Ca^{2+}-impermeability of the receptors to Ca^{2+}-permeability (Kawahara et al., 2004, Kwak and Kawahara, 2005, Kawahara et al., 2006). Glutamatergic signaling is probably a significant factor in the onset of symptoms since reducing excitatory sensory input delayed the onset of disease in SOD1 mice (Ilieva et al., 2008), and intrathecal administration of the glutamate agonist kainic acid in normal rats produced slow, selective motoneuron death similar to ALS (Sun et al., 2006). If changes in the transmission of glutamate are taking place early enough, it could alter the activity of spinal networks during normal development (Blankenship and Feller, 2010, Landmesser and O'Donovan, 1984, Marder and Rehm, 2005, Gonzalez-Islas and Wenner, 2006). Some evidence for alterations in network activity has been shown in SOD1 hypoglossal motoneurons (van Zundert et al., 2008) and spinal motoneurons (Amendola et al., 2004, Bories et al., 2007) in juvenile mice. After symptom onset, increased network activity has also been shown in the spinal cord (Jiang et al., 2009). However, considering all the documented changes in glutamate-mediated neurotransmission, there has been surprisingly little research into the overall effects on cortical, brainstem and spinal network activity throughout the lifespan of the SOD1 mouse.

9. Future directions

There are many possibilities to explore for new treatments of ALS besides the now-standard drug riluzole (Bellingham, 2011). The neuroinflammation response is a promising approach (Philips and Robberecht, 2011); another could be to manipulate neuromodulatory input to the spinal cord. Serotonin (5HT) and norepinephrine (NE) have potent effects on motoneurons, including increasing PIC amplitude, decreasing input conductance, hyperpolarizing spike threshold, and depolarizing resting potential (Hounsgaard and Kiehn, 1989, Lee and Heckman, 1999, Powers and Binder, 2001, Alaburda et al., 2002, Hultborn et al., 2004, Perrier and Delgado-Lezama, 2005, Heckman et al., 2008). Furthermore, neuromodulators are constantly scaling the level of activation of motoneurons as needed (Heckman et al., 2004). Activation of $5HT_2$ receptors strongly depresses high-voltage-activated Ca^{2+} channels while probably increasing basal $[Ca^{2+}]_I$ by potentiating the Ca^{2+} PIC (Hounsgaard et al., 1988, Bayliss et al., 1995, Hsiao et al., 1998, Ladewig et al., 2004, Li et al., 2007). Both 5HT and dopamine (DA) modulate KIF-5-dependent cellular transport, including transport of mitochondria. Acting through the GSK3 regulator of KIF-5, 5HT is observed to increase transport, while DA decreases it (Chen et al., 2007, Chen et al., 2008). Other neuromodulators, such as nitric oxide, $GABA_B$, and adenosine, could also be worth investigating as modulators of motoneuron synaptic strength, reduction of the Ca^{2+} PIC, and modulation of both high-voltage-activated Ca^{2+} channels and input conductance, respectively (Marks et al., 1993, Mynlieff and Beam, 1994, Li et al., 2004, Moreno-Lopez et al., 2011). Another useful target of neuromodulators that modify Ca^{2+} influx is protein clearance; inhibition of L-type Ca^{2+} channels has been found to increase autophagy (Williams et al., 2008).

10. Conclusions

Factors causing neurodegeneration in ALS are present long before motor function is adversely affected. From research on the animal models of ALS, it is thought that excessive

Ca^{2+} entry, increased motoneuronal size, altered glutamate neurotransmission, astrocyte dysfunction, mitochondrial deficits, failures in axon transport, and problems in protein degradation act in concert and gradually push motoneurons outside the parameters under which they can function properly. The fact that motoneurons are able to remain functioning for as long as they do under adverse conditions suggests that there is a large window of time and intrinsic conditions within which motoneurons can maintain normal function. Hopefully future treatments can target these altered pathways to extend the time motoneuron properties remain within these parameters.

11. References

Ackerley S, Grierson AJ, Banner S, Perkinton MS, Brownlees J, Byers HL, Ward M, Thornhill P, Hussain K, Waby JS, Anderton BH, Cooper JD, Dingwall C, Leigh PN, Shaw CE, Miller CC (2004) p38alpha stress-activated protein kinase phosphorylates neurofilaments and is associated with neurofilament pathology in amyotrophic lateral sclerosis. Mol Cell Neurosci 26:354-364.

Ackerley S, Grierson AJ, Brownlees J, Thornhill P, Anderton BH, Leigh PN, Shaw CE, Miller CC (2000) Glutamate slows axonal transport of neurofilaments in transfected neurons. J Cell Biol 150:165-176.

Alaburda A, Perrier JF, Hounsgaard J (2002) Mechanisms causing plateau potentials in spinal motoneurones. Adv Exp Med Biol 508:219-226.

Alexianu ME, Kozovska M, Appel SH (2001) Immune reactivity in a mouse model of familial ALS correlates with disease progression. Neurology 57:1282-1289.

Amendola J, Durand J (2008) Morphological differences between wild-type and transgenic superoxide dismutase 1 lumbar motoneurons in postnatal mice. J Comp Neurol 511:329-341.

Amendola J, Verrier B, Roubertoux P, Durand J (2004) Altered sensorimotor development in a transgenic mouse model of amyotrophic lateral sclerosis. Eur J Neurosci 20:2822-2826.

Atkin JD, Farg MA, Walker AK, McLean C, Tomas D, Horne MK (2008) Endoplasmic reticulum stress and induction of the unfolded protein response in human sporadic amyotrophic lateral sclerosis. Neurobiol Dis 30:400-407.

Bayliss DA, Umemiya M, Berger AJ (1995) Inhibition of N- and P-type calcium currents and the after-hyperpolarization in rat motoneurones by serotonin. Journal of Physiology 485:635-647.

Beers DR, Henkel JS, Xiao Q, Zhao W, Wang J, Yen AA, Siklos L, McKercher SR, Appel SH (2006) Wild-type microglia extend survival in PU.1 knockout mice with familial amyotrophic lateral sclerosis. Proc Natl Acad Sci U S A 103:16021-16026.

Bellingham MC (2011) A review of the neural mechanisms of action and clinical efficiency of riluzole in treating amyotrophic lateral sclerosis: what have we learned in the last decade? CNS Neurosci Ther 17:4-31.

Bendotti C, Tortarolo M, Suchak SK, Calvaresi N, Carvelli L, Bastone A, Rizzi M, Rattray M, Mennini T (2001) Transgenic SOD1 G93A mice develop reduced GLT-1 in spinal cord without alterations in cerebrospinal fluid glutamate levels. J Neurochem 79:737-746.

Bergmann F, Keller BU (2004) Impact of mitochondrial inhibition on excitability and cytosolic Ca2+ levels in brainstem motoneurones from mouse. J Physiol 555:45-59.

Bernasconi R, Molinari M (2011) ERAD and ERAD tuning: disposal of cargo and of ERAD regulators from the mammalian ER. Curr Opin Cell Biol 23:176-183.

Bilsland LG, Nirmalananthan N, Yip J, Greensmith L, Duchen MR (2008) Expression of mutant SOD1 in astrocytes induces functional deficits in motoneuron mitochondria. J Neurochem 107:1271-1283.

Bilsland LG, Sahai E, Kelly G, Golding M, Greensmith L, Schiavo G (2010) Deficits in axonal transport precede ALS symptoms in vivo. Proc Natl Acad Sci U S A 107:20523-20528.

Bingol B, Sheng M (2011) Deconstruction for reconstruction: the role of proteolysis in neural plasticity and disease. Neuron 69:22-32.

Blankenship AG, Feller MB (2010) Mechanisms underlying spontaneous patterned activity in developing neural circuits. Nat Rev Neurosci 11:18-29.

Boillee S, Yamanaka K, Lobsiger CS, Copeland NG, Jenkins NA, Kassiotis G, Kollias G, Cleveland DW (2006) Onset and progression in inherited ALS determined by motor neurons and microglia. Science 312:1389-1392.

Bories C, Amendola J, Lamotte d'Incamps B, Durand J (2007) Early electrophysiological abnormalities in lumbar motoneurons in a transgenic mouse model of amyotrophic lateral sclerosis. Eur J Neurosci 25:451-459.

Brownlees J, Yates A, Bajaj NP, Davis D, Anderton BH, Leigh PN, Shaw CE, Miller CC (2000) Phosphorylation of neurofilament heavy chain side-arms by stress activated protein kinase-1b/Jun N-terminal kinase-3. J Cell Sci 113 (Pt 3):401-407.

Bruijn LI, Becher MW, Lee MK, Anderson KL, Jenkins NA, Copeland NG, Sisodia SS, Rothstein JD, Borchelt DR, Price DL, Cleveland DW (1997) ALS-linked SOD1 mutant G85R mediates damage to astrocytes and promotes rapidly progressive disease with SOD1-containing inclusions. Neuron 18:327-338.

Byrne S, Walsh C, Lynch C, Bede P, Elamin M, Kenna K, McLaughlin R, Hardiman O (2011) Rate of familial amyotrophic lateral sclerosis: a systematic review and meta-analysis. J Neurol Neurosurg Psychiatry 82:623-627.

Carunchio I, Curcio L, Pieri M, Pica F, Caioli S, Viscomi MT, Molinari M, Canu N, Bernardi G, Zona C (2010) Increased levels of p70S6 phosphorylation in the G93A mouse model of Amyotrophic Lateral Sclerosis and in valine-exposed cortical neurons in culture. Exp Neurol 226:218-230.

Chen S, Owens GC, Crossin KL, Edelman DB (2007) Serotonin stimulates mitochondrial transport in hippocampal neurons. Mol Cell Neurosci 36:472-483.

Chen S, Owens GC, Edelman DB (2008) Dopamine inhibits mitochondrial motility in hippocampal neurons. PLoS One 3:e2804.

Chiu IM, Chen A, Zheng Y, Kosaras B, Tsiftsoglou SA, Vartanian TK, Brown RH, Jr., Carroll MC (2008) T lymphocytes potentiate endogenous neuroprotective inflammation in a mouse model of ALS. Proc Natl Acad Sci U S A 105:17913-17918.

Chiu IM, Phatnani H, Kuligowski M, Tapia JC, Carrasco MA, Zhang M, Maniatis T, Carroll MC (2009) Activation of innate and humoral immunity in the peripheral nervous system of ALS transgenic mice. Proc Natl Acad Sci U S A 106:20960-20965.

Clement AM, Nguyen MD, Roberts EA, Garcia ML, Boillee S, Rule M, McMahon AP, Doucette W, Siwek D, Ferrante RJ, Brown RH, Jr., Julien JP, Goldstein LS, Cleveland DW (2003) Wild-type nonneuronal cells extend survival of SOD1 mutant motor neurons in ALS mice. Science 302:113-117.

Dal Canto MC, Gurney ME (1994) Development of central nervous system pathology in a murine transgenic model of human amyotrophic lateral sclerosis. The American journal of pathology 145:1271-1279.

Dal Canto MC, Gurney ME (1995) Neuropathological changes in two lines of mice carrying a transgene for mutant human Cu,Zn SOD, and in mice overexpressing wild type human SOD: a model of familial amyotrophic lateral sclerosis (FALS). Brain Res 676:25-40.

Damiano M, Starkov AA, Petri S, Kipiani K, Kiaei M, Mattiazzi M, Flint Beal M, Manfredi G (2006) Neural mitochondrial Ca2+ capacity impairment precedes the onset of motor symptoms in G93A Cu/Zn-superoxide dismutase mutant mice. J Neurochem 96:1349-1361.

De Vos KJ, Chapman AL, Tennant ME, Manser C, Tudor EL, Lau KF, Brownlees J, Ackerley S, Shaw PJ, McLoughlin DM, Shaw CE, Leigh PN, Miller CC, Grierson AJ (2007) Familial amyotrophic lateral sclerosis-linked SOD1 mutants perturb fast axonal transport to reduce axonal mitochondria content. Hum Mol Genet 16:2720-2728.

De Vos KJ, Grierson AJ, Ackerley S, Miller CC (2008) Role of axonal transport in neurodegenerative diseases. Annu Rev Neurosci 31:151-173.

Deng HX, Chen W, Hong ST, Boycott KM, Gorrie GH, Siddique N, Yang Y, Fecto F, Shi Y, Zhai H, Jiang H, Hirano M, Rampersaud E, Jansen GH, Donkervoort S, Bigio EH, Brooks BR, Ajroud K, Sufit RL, Haines JL, Mugnaini E, Pericak-Vance MA, Siddique T (2011) Mutations in UBQLN2 cause dominant X-linked juvenile and adult-onset ALS and ALS/dementia. Nature.

Elbasiouny SM, Amendola J, Durand J, Heckman CJ (2010) Evidence from computer simulations for alterations in the membrane biophysical properties and dendritic processing of synaptic inputs in mutant superoxide dismutase-1 motoneurons. J Neurosci In Press.

Fierro L, Llano I (1996) High endogenous calcium buffering in Purkinje cells from rat cerebellar slices. J Physiol 496 (Pt 3):617-625.

Fischer LR, Culver DG, Tennant P, Davis AA, Wang M, Castellano-Sanchez A, Khan J, Polak MA, Glass JD (2004) Amyotrophic lateral sclerosis is a distal axonopathy: evidence in mice and man. Exp Neurol 185:232-240.

Frey D, Schneider C, Xu L, Borg J, Spooren W, Caroni P (2000) Early and selective loss of neuromuscular synapse subtypes with low sprouting competence in motoneuron diseases. J Neurosci 20:2534-2542.

Gonzalez-Islas C, Wenner P (2006) Spontaneous network activity in the embryonic spinal cord regulates AMPAergic and GABAergic synaptic strength. Neuron 49:563-575.

Gowing G, Philips T, Van Wijmeersch B, Audet JN, Dewil M, Van Den Bosch L, Billiau AD, Robberecht W, Julien JP (2008) Ablation of proliferating microglia does not affect motor neuron degeneration in amyotrophic lateral sclerosis caused by mutant superoxide dismutase. J Neurosci 28:10234-10244.

Gurney ME, Pu H, Chiu AY, Dal Canto MC, Polchow CY, Alexander DD, Caliendo J, Hentati A, Kwon YW, Deng HX, et al. (1994) Motor neuron degeneration in mice that express a human Cu,Zn superoxide dismutase mutation. Science 264:1772-1775.

Heckman CJ, Johnson M, Mottram C, Schuster J (2008b) Persistent inward currents in spinal motoneurons and their influence on human motoneuron firing patterns. Neuroscientist 14:264-275.

Heckman CJ, Kuo JJ, Johnson MD (2004) Synaptic integration in motoneurons with hyper-excitable dendrites. Canadian journal of physiology and pharmacology 82:549-555.

Hegedus J, Putman CT, Gordon T (2007) Time course of preferential motor unit loss in the SOD1 G93A mouse model of amyotrophic lateral sclerosis. Neurobiol Dis 28:154-164.

Hegedus J, Putman CT, Tyreman N, Gordon T (2008) Preferential motor unit loss in the SOD1 G93A transgenic mouse model of amyotrophic lateral sclerosis. J Physiol 586:3337-3351.

Hiruma H, Katakura T, Takahashi S, Ichikawa T, Kawakami T (2003) Glutamate and amyloid beta-protein rapidly inhibit fast axonal transport in cultured rat hippocampal neurons by different mechanisms. J Neurosci 23:8967-8977.

Hounsgaard J, Hultborn H, Jespersen B, Kiehn O (1988) Bistability of alpha-motoneurones in the decerebrate cat and in the acute spinal cat after intravenous 5-hydroxytryptophan. J Physiol 405:345-367.

Hounsgaard J, Kiehn O (1989) Serotonin-induced bistability of turtle motoneurones caused by a nifedipine-sensitive calcium plateau potential. J Physiol Lond 414:265-282.

Hsiao CF, Del Negro CA, Trueblood PR, Chandler SH (1998) Ionic basis for serotonin-induced bistable membrane properties in guinea pig trigeminal motoneurons. J Neurophysiol 79:2847-2856.

Hultborn H, Brownstone RB, Toth TI, Gossard JP (2004) Key mechanisms for setting the input-output gain across the motoneuron pool. Prog Brain Res 143:77-95.

Ignacio S, Moore DH, Smith AP, Lee NM (2005) Effect of neuroprotective drugs on gene expression in G93A/SOD1 mice. Ann N Y Acad Sci 1053:121-136.

Ilieva EV, Ayala V, Jove M, Dalfo E, Cacabelos D, Povedano M, Bellmunt MJ, Ferrer I, Pamplona R, Portero-Otin M (2007) Oxidative and endoplasmic reticulum stress interplay in sporadic amyotrophic lateral sclerosis. Brain 130:3111-3123.

Ilieva HS, Yamanaka K, Malkmus S, Kakinohana O, Yaksh T, Marsala M, Cleveland DW (2008) Mutant dynein (Loa) triggers proprioceptive axon loss that extends survival only in the SOD1 ALS model with highest motor neuron death. Proc Natl Acad Sci U S A 105:12599-12604.

Israelson A, Arbel N, Da Cruz S, Ilieva H, Yamanaka K, Shoshan-Barmatz V, Cleveland DW (2010) Misfolded mutant SOD1 directly inhibits VDAC1 conductance in a mouse model of inherited ALS. Neuron 67:575-587.

Ito Y, Yamada M, Tanaka H, Aida K, Tsuruma K, Shimazawa M, Hozumi I, Inuzuka T, Takahashi H, Hara H (2009) Involvement of CHOP, an ER-stress apoptotic mediator, in both human sporadic ALS and ALS model mice. Neurobiol Dis 36:470-476.

Jahn K, Grosskreutz J, Haastert K, Ziegler E, Schlesinger F, Grothe C, Dengler R, Bufler J (2006) Temporospatial coupling of networked synaptic activation of AMPA-type glutamate receptor channels and calcium transients in cultured motoneurons. Neuroscience 142:1019-1029.

Jaiswal MK, Keller BU (2009) Cu/Zn superoxide dismutase typical for familial amyotrophic lateral sclerosis increases the vulnerability of mitochondria and perturbs Ca2+ homeostasis in SOD1G93A mice. Mol Pharmacol 75:478-489.

Jaiswal MK, Zech WD, Goos M, Leutbecher C, Ferri A, Zippelius A, Carri MT, Nau R, Keller BU (2009) Impairment of mitochondrial calcium handling in a mtSOD1 cell culture model of motoneuron disease. BMC Neurosci 10:64.

Jiang M, Schuster JE, Fu R, Siddique T, Heckman CJ (2009) Progressive changes in synaptic inputs to motoneurons in adult sacral spinal cord of a mouse model of amyotrophic lateral sclerosis. J Neurosci 29:15031-15038.

Jiang Z, Rempel J, Li J, Sawchuk MA, Carlin KP, Brownstone RM (1999) Development of L-type calcium channels and a nifedipine-sensitive motor activity in the postnatal mouse spinal cord. Eur J Neurosci 11:3481-3487.

Johnston JA, Dalton MJ, Gurney ME, Kopito RR (2000) Formation of high molecular weight complexes of mutant Cu, Zn-superoxide dismutase in a mouse model for familial amyotrophic lateral sclerosis. Proc Natl Acad Sci U S A 97:12571-12576.

Kaiser M, Maletzki I, Hulsmann S, Holtmann B, Schulz-Schaeffer W, Kirchhoff F, Bahr M, Neusch C (2006) Progressive loss of a glial potassium channel (KCNJ10) in the spinal cord of the SOD1 (G93A) transgenic mouse model of amyotrophic lateral sclerosis. J Neurochem 99:900-912.

Kawahara Y, Ito K, Sun H, Aizawa H, Kanazawa I, Kwak S (2004) Glutamate receptors: RNA editing and death of motor neurons. Nature 427:801.

Kawahara Y, Sun H, Ito K, Hideyama T, Aoki M, Sobue G, Tsuji S, Kwak S (2006) Underediting of GluR2 mRNA, a neuronal death inducing molecular change in sporadic ALS, does not occur in motor neurons in ALS1 or SBMA. Neurosci Res 54:11-14.

Kawasaki H, Morooka T, Shimohama S, Kimura J, Hirano T, Gotoh Y, Nishida E (1997) Activation and involvement of p38 mitogen-activated protein kinase in glutamate-induced apoptosis in rat cerebellar granule cells. J Biol Chem 272:18518-18521.

Kennel PF, Finiels F, Revah F, Mallet J (1996) Neuromuscular function impairment is not caused by motor neurone loss in FALS mice: an electromyographic study. Neuroreport 7:1427-1431.

Kieran D, Hafezparast M, Bohnert S, Dick JR, Martin J, Schiavo G, Fisher EM, Greensmith L (2005) A mutation in dynein rescues axonal transport defects and extends the life span of ALS mice. J Cell Biol 169:561-567.

Kim TY, Kim E, Yoon SK, Yoon JB (2008) Herp enhances ER-associated protein degradation by recruiting ubiquilins. Biochem Biophys Res Commun 369:741-746.

Kuo JJ, Siddique T, Fu R, Heckman CJ (2005) Increased persistent Na+ current and its effect on excitability in motoneurones cultured from mutant SOD1 mice. Journal of Physiology-London 563:843-854.

Kwak S, Kawahara Y (2005) Deficient RNA editing of GluR2 and neuronal death in amyotropic lateral sclerosis. J Mol Med (Berl) 83:110-120.

Ladewig T, Lalley PM, Keller BU (2004) Serotonergic modulation of intracellular calcium dynamics in neonatal hypoglossal motoneurons from mouse. Brain Res 1001:1-12.

Landmesser LT, O'Donovan MJ (1984) Activation patterns of embryonic chick hind limb muscles recorded in ovo and in an isolated spinal cord preparation. J Physiol 347:189-204.

Lauriat TL, Richler E, McInnes LA (2007) A quantitative regional expression profile of EAAT2 known and novel splice variants reopens the question of aberrant EAAT2 splicing in disease. Neurochemistry international 50:271-280.

Lee CH, Inoki K, Guan KL (2007) mTOR pathway as a target in tissue hypertrophy. Annual review of pharmacology and toxicology 47:443-467.

Lee MS, Kwon YT, Li M, Peng J, Friedlander RM, Tsai LH (2000) Neurotoxicity induces cleavage of p35 to p25 by calpain. Nature 405:360-364.

Lee RH, Heckman CJ (1999) Enhancement of bistability in spinal motoneurons in vivo by the noradrenergic alpha1 agonist methoxamine. Journal of neurophysiology 81:2164-2174.

Li Q, Vande Velde C, Israelson A, Xie J, Bailey AO, Dong MQ, Chun SJ, Roy T, Winer L, Yates JR, Capaldi RA, Cleveland DW, Miller TM (2010) ALS-linked mutant superoxide dismutase 1 (SOD1) alters mitochondrial protein composition and decreases protein import. Proc Natl Acad Sci U S A 107:21146-21151.

Li X, Murray K, Harvey PJ, Ballou EW, Bennett DJ (2007) Serotonin facilitates a persistent calcium current in motoneurons of rats with and without chronic spinal cord injury. J Neurophysiol 97:1236-1246.

Li Y, Li X, Harvey PJ, Bennett DJ (2004) Effects of baclofen on spinal reflexes and persistent inward currents in motoneurons of chronic spinal rats with spasticity. J Neurophysiol 92:2694-2703.

Lim PJ, Danner R, Liang J, Doong H, Harman C, Srinivasan D, Rothenberg C, Wang H, Ye Y, Fang S, Monteiro MJ (2009) Ubiquilin and p97/VCP bind erasin, forming a complex involved in ERAD. J Cell Biol 187:201-217.

Lips MB, Keller BU (1998) Endogenous calcium buffering in motoneurones of the nucleus hypoglossus from mouse. J Physiol 511 (Pt 1):105-117.

Luik RM, Wang B, Prakriya M, Wu MM, Lewis RS (2008) Oligomerization of STIM1 couples ER calcium depletion to CRAC channel activation. Nature 454:538-542.

MacAskill AF, Atkin TA, Kittler JT (2010) Mitochondrial trafficking and the provision of energy and calcium buffering at excitatory synapses. Eur J Neurosci 32:231-240.

Macaskill AF, Rinholm JE, Twelvetrees AE, Arancibia-Carcamo IL, Muir J, Fransson A, Aspenstrom P, Attwell D, Kittler JT (2009) Miro1 is a calcium sensor for glutamate receptor-dependent localization of mitochondria at synapses. Neuron 61:541-555.

Mackenzie IR, Rademakers R, Neumann M (2010) TDP-43 and FUS in amyotrophic lateral sclerosis and frontotemporal dementia. Lancet Neurol 9:995-1007.

Maragakis NJ, Dykes-Hoberg M, Rothstein JD (2004) Altered expression of the glutamate transporter EAAT2b in neurological disease. Ann Neurol 55:469-477.

Marder E, Rehm KJ (2005) Development of central pattern generating circuits. Curr Opin Neurobiol 15:86-93.

Marks JD, Donnelly DF, Haddad GG (1993) Adenosine-induced inhibition of vagal motoneuron excitability: receptor subtype and mechanisms. Am J Physiol 264:L124-132.

Mattiazzi M, D'Aurelio M, Gajewski CD, Martushova K, Kiaei M, Beal MF, Manfredi G (2002) Mutated human SOD1 causes dysfunction of oxidative phosphorylation in mitochondria of transgenic mice. J Biol Chem 277:29626-29633.

Mattson MP, Gleichmann M, Cheng A (2008) Mitochondria in neuroplasticity and neurological disorders. Neuron 60:748-766.

McCue HV, Haynes LP, Burgoyne RD (2010) The diversity of calcium sensor proteins in the regulation of neuronal function. Cold Spring Harb Perspect Biol 2:a004085.

Meehan CF, Moldovan M, Marklund SL, Graffmo KS, Nielsen JB, Hultborn H (2010) Intrinsic properties of lumbar motor neurones in the adult G127insTGGG superoxide dismutase-1 mutant mouse in vivo: evidence for increased persistent inward currents. Acta Physiol (Oxf) 200:361-376.

Mironov SL (2007) ADP regulates movements of mitochondria in neurons. Biophys J 92:2944-2952.

Moreno-Lopez B, Sunico CR, Gonzalez-Forero D (2011) NO orchestrates the loss of synaptic boutons from adult "sick" motoneurons: modeling a molecular mechanism. Mol Neurobiol 43:41-66.

Mourelatos Z, Gonatas NK, Stieber A, Gurney ME, Dal Canto MC (1996) The Golgi apparatus of spinal cord motor neurons in transgenic mice expressing mutant Cu,Zn superoxide dismutase becomes fragmented in early, preclinical stages of the disease. Proc Natl Acad Sci U S A 93:5472-5477.

Munch C, Ebstein M, Seefried U, Zhu B, Stamm S, Landwehrmeyer GB, Ludolph AC, Schwalenstocker B, Meyer T (2002) Alternative splicing of the 5'-sequences of the mouse EAAT2 glutamate transporter and expression in a transgenic model for amyotrophic lateral sclerosis. J Neurochem 82:594-603.

Mynlieff M, Beam KG (1994) Adenosine acting at an A1 receptor decreases N-type calcium current in mouse motoneurons. J Neurosci 14:3628-3634.

Nagai M, Re DB, Nagata T, Chalazonitis A, Jessell TM, Wichterle H, Przedborski S (2007) Astrocytes expressing ALS-linked mutated SOD1 release factors selectively toxic to motor neurons. Nat Neurosci 10:615-622.

Neher E (1995) The use of fura-2 for estimating Ca buffers and Ca fluxes. Neuropharmacology 34:1423-1442.

Nguyen KT, Garcia-Chacon LE, Barrett JN, Barrett EF, David G (2009) The Psi(m) depolarization that accompanies mitochondrial Ca2+ uptake is greater in mutant SOD1 than in wild-type mouse motor terminals. Proc Natl Acad Sci U S A 106:2007-2011.

Nishimura AL, Mitne-Neto M, Silva HC, Richieri-Costa A, Middleton S, Cascio D, Kok F, Oliveira JR, Gillingwater T, Webb J, Skehel P, Zatz M (2004) A mutation in the vesicle-trafficking protein VAPB causes late-onset spinal muscular atrophy and amyotrophic lateral sclerosis. American journal of human genetics 75:822-831.

Palecek J, Lips MB, Keller BU (1999) Calcium dynamics and buffering in motoneurones of the mouse spinal cord. J Physiol 520 Pt 2:485-502.

Pardo CA, Xu Z, Borchelt DR, Price DL, Sisodia SS, Cleveland DW (1995) Superoxide dismutase is an abundant component in cell bodies, dendrites, and axons of motor neurons and in a subset of other neurons. Proc Natl Acad Sci U S A 92:954-958.

Paschen W (2003) Endoplasmic reticulum: a primary target in various acute disorders and degenerative diseases of the brain. Cell calcium 34:365-383.

Perrier JF, Delgado-Lezama R (2005) Synaptic release of serotonin induced by stimulation of the raphe nucleus promotes plateau potentials in spinal motoneurons of the adult turtle. J Neurosci 25:7993-7999.

Philips T, Robberecht W (2011) Neuroinflammation in amyotrophic lateral sclerosis: role of glial activation in motor neuron disease. Lancet Neurol 10:253-263.

Pieri M, Carunchio I, Curcio L, Mercuri NB, Zona C (2009) Increased persistent sodium current determines cortical hyperexcitability in a genetic model of amyotrophic lateral sclerosis. Exp Neurol 215:368-379.

Pivovarova NB, Andrews SB (2010) Calcium-dependent mitochondrial function and dysfunction in neurons. The FEBS journal 277:3622-3636.

Polymenidou M, Lagier-Tourenne C, Hutt KR, Huelga SC, Moran J, Liang TY, Ling SC, Sun E, Wancewicz E, Mazur C, Kordasiewicz H, Sedaghat Y, Donohue JP, Shiue L, Bennett CF, Yeo GW, Cleveland DW (2011) Long pre-mRNA depletion and RNA missplicing contribute to neuronal vulnerability from loss of TDP-43. Nat Neurosci 14:459-468.

Powers RK, Binder MD (2001) Input-output functions of mammalian motoneurons. Rev Physiol Biochem Pharmacol 143:137-263.

Pun S, Santos AF, Saxena S, Xu L, Caroni P (2006) Selective vulnerability and pruning of phasic motoneuron axons in motoneuron disease alleviated by CNTF. Nat Neurosci 9:408-419.

Quinlan KA, Schuster JE, Fu R, Siddique T, Heckman CJ (2011) Altered postnatal maturation of electrical properties in spinal motoneurons in a mouse model of amyotrophic lateral sclerosis. J Physiol 589:2245-2260.

Raoul C, Estevez AG, Nishimune H, Cleveland DW, deLapeyriere O, Henderson CE, Haase G, Pettmann B (2002) Motoneuron death triggered by a specific pathway downstream of Fas. potentiation by ALS-linked SOD1 mutations. Neuron 35:1067-1083.

Reaume AG, Elliott JL, Hoffman EK, Kowall NW, Ferrante RJ, Siwek DF, Wilcox HM, Flood DG, Beal MF, Brown RH, Jr., Scott RW, Snider WD (1996) Motor neurons in Cu/Zn superoxide dismutase-deficient mice develop normally but exhibit enhanced cell death after axonal injury. Nat Genet 13:43-47.

Ren K, Ruda MA (1994) A comparative study of the calcium-binding proteins calbindin-D28K, calretinin, calmodulin and parvalbumin in the rat spinal cord. Brain Res Brain Res Rev 19:163-179.

Rintoul GL, Bennett VJ, Papaconstandinou NA, Reynolds IJ (2006) Nitric oxide inhibits mitochondrial movement in forebrain neurons associated with disruption of mitochondrial membrane potential. J Neurochem 97:800-806.

Rintoul GL, Filiano AJ, Brocard JB, Kress GJ, Reynolds IJ (2003) Glutamate decreases mitochondrial size and movement in primary forebrain neurons. J Neurosci 23:7881-7888.

Ron D, Walter P (2007) Signal integration in the endoplasmic reticulum unfolded protein response. Nat Rev Mol Cell Biol 8:519-529.

Rosen DR, Siddique T, Patterson D, Figlewicz DA, Sapp P, Hentati A, Donaldson D, Goto J, O'Regan JP, Deng HX, et al. (1993) Mutations in Cu/Zn superoxide dismutase gene are associated with familial amyotrophic lateral sclerosis. Nature 362:59-62.

Rothstein JD, Martin LJ, Kuncl RW (1992) Decreased glutamate transport by the brain and spinal cord in amyotrophic lateral sclerosis. N Engl J Med 326:1464-1468.

Rothstein JD, Patel S, Regan MR, Haenggeli C, Huang YH, Bergles DE, Jin L, Dykes Hoberg M, Vidensky S, Chung DS, Toan SV, Bruijn LI, Su ZZ, Gupta P, Fisher PB (2005) Beta-lactam antibiotics offer neuroprotection by increasing glutamate transporter expression. Nature 433:73-77.

Sasaki S, Warita H, Abe K, Komori T, Iwata M (2001) EAAT1 and EAAT2 immunoreactivity in transgenic mice with a G93A mutant SOD1 gene. Neuroreport 12:1359-1362.

Saxena S, Cabuy E, Caroni P (2009) A role for motoneuron subtype-selective ER stress in disease manifestations of FALS mice. Nat Neurosci 12:627-636.

Scamps F, Roig A, Boukhaddaoui H, Andre S, Puech S, Valmier J (2004) Activation of P-type calcium channel regulates a unique thapsigargin-sensitive calcium pool in embryonic motoneurons. Eur J Neurosci 19:977-982.

Schwarzschild MA, Cole RL, Hyman SE (1997) Glutamate, but not dopamine, stimulates stress-activated protein kinase and AP-1-mediated transcription in striatal neurons. J Neurosci 17:3455-3466.

Steinbeck JA, Henke N, Opatz J, Gruszczynska-Biegala J, Schneider L, Theiss S, Hamacher N, Steinfarz B, Golz S, Brustle O, Kuznicki J, Methner A (2011) Store-operated calcium entry modulates neuronal network activity in a model of chronic epilepsy. Exp Neurol.

Stevenson A, Yates DM, Manser C, De Vos KJ, Vagnoni A, Leigh PN, McLoughlin DM, Miller CC (2009) Riluzole protects against glutamate-induced slowing of neurofilament axonal transport. Neurosci Lett 454:161-164.

Sukiasyan N, Hultborn H, Zhang M (2009) Distribution of calcium channel Ca(V)1.3 immunoreactivity in the rat spinal cord and brain stem. Neuroscience 159:217-235.

Sun H, Kawahara Y, Ito K, Kanazawa I, Kwak S (2006) Slow and selective death of spinal motor neurons in vivo by intrathecal infusion of kainic acid: implications for AMPA receptor-mediated excitotoxicity in ALS. Journal of neurochemistry 98:782-791.

Swarup V, Phaneuf D, Bareil C, Robertson J, Rouleau GA, Kriz J, Julien JP (2011) Pathological hallmarks of amyotrophic lateral sclerosis/frontotemporal lobar degeneration in transgenic mice produced with TDP-43 genomic fragments. Brain.

Tortarolo M, Grignaschi G, Calvaresi N, Zennaro E, Spaltro G, Colovic M, Fracasso C, Guiso G, Elger B, Schneider H, Seilheimer B, Caccia S, Bendotti C (2006) Glutamate AMPA receptors change in motor neurons of SOD1G93A transgenic mice and their inhibition by a noncompetitive antagonist ameliorates the progression of amytrophic lateral sclerosis-like disease. J Neurosci Res 83:134-146.

Tortarolo M, Veglianese P, Calvaresi N, Botturi A, Rossi C, Giorgini A, Migheli A, Bendotti C (2003) Persistent activation of p38 mitogen-activated protein kinase in a mouse model of familial amyotrophic lateral sclerosis correlates with disease progression. Mol Cell Neurosci 23:180-192.

Turner BJ, Lopes EC, Cheema SS (2003a) Neuromuscular accumulation of mutant superoxide dismutase 1 aggregates in a transgenic mouse model of familial amyotrophic lateral sclerosis. Neurosci Lett 350:132-136.

Turner BJ, Rembach A, Spark R, Lopes EC, Cheema SS (2003b) Opposing effects of low and high-dose clozapine on survival of transgenic amyotrophic lateral sclerosis mice. J Neurosci Res 74:605-613.

Van Damme P, Bogaert E, Dewil M, Hersmus N, Kiraly D, Scheveneels W, Bockx I, Braeken D, Verpoorten N, Verhoeven K, Timmerman V, Herijgers P, Callewaert G, Carmeliet P, Van Den Bosch L, Robberecht W (2007) Astrocytes regulate GluR2 expression in motor neurons and their vulnerability to excitotoxicity. Proc Natl Acad Sci U S A 104:14825-14830.

Van Den Bosch L (2011) Genetic rodent models of amyotrophic lateral sclerosis. Journal of biomedicine & biotechnology 2011:348765.

van Zundert B, Peuscher MH, Hynynen M, Chen A, Neve RL, Brown RH, Jr., Constantine-Paton M, Bellingham MC (2008) Neonatal neuronal circuitry shows hyperexcitable disturbance in a mouse model of the adult-onset neurodegenerative disease amyotrophic lateral sclerosis. J Neurosci 28:10864-10874.

Vanselow BK, Keller BU (2000) Calcium dynamics and buffering in oculomotor neurones from mouse that are particularly resistant during amyotrophic lateral sclerosis (ALS)-related motoneurone disease. J Physiol 525 Pt 2:433-445.

Vinay L, Brocard F, Pflieger JF, Simeoni-Alias J, Clarac F (2000) Perinatal development of lumbar motoneurons and their inputs in the rat. Brain research bulletin 53:635-647.

von Lewinski F, Fuchs J, Vanselow BK, Keller BU (2008) Low Ca2+ buffering in hypoglossal motoneurons of mutant SOD1 (G93A) mice. Neurosci Lett 445:224-228.

von Lewinski F, Keller BU (2005) Mitochondrial Ca2+ buffering in hypoglossal motoneurons from mouse. Neurosci Lett 380:203-208.

Wagner OI, Lifshitz J, Janmey PA, Linden M, McIntosh TK, Leterrier JF (2003) Mechanisms of mitochondria-neurofilament interactions. J Neurosci 23:9046-9058.

Wang L, Sharma K, Grisotti G, Roos RP (2009) The effect of mutant SOD1 dismutase activity on non-cell autonomous degeneration in familial amyotrophic lateral sclerosis. Neurobiol Dis 35:234-240.

Warita H, Itoyama Y, Abe K (1999) Selective impairment of fast anterograde axonal transport in the peripheral nerves of asymptomatic transgenic mice with a G93A mutant SOD1 gene. Brain Res 819:120-131.

Warita H, Manabe Y, Murakami T, Shiote M, Shiro Y, Hayashi T, Nagano I, Shoji M, Abe K (2002) Tardive decrease of astrocytic glutamate transporter protein in transgenic mice with ALS-linked mutant SOD1. Neurological research 24:577-581.

Williams A, Sarkar S, Cuddon P, Ttofi EK, Saiki S, Siddiqi FH, Jahreiss L, Fleming A, Pask D, Goldsmith P, O'Kane CJ, Floto RA, Rubinsztein DC (2008) Novel targets for Huntington's disease in an mTOR-independent autophagy pathway. Nature chemical biology 4:295-305.

Williamson TL, Cleveland DW (1999) Slowing of axonal transport is a very early event in the toxicity of ALS-linked SOD1 mutants to motor neurons. Nat Neurosci 2:50-56.

Wong PC, Pardo CA, Borchelt DR, Lee MK, Copeland NG, Jenkins NA, Sisodia SS, Cleveland DW, Price DL (1995) An adverse property of a familial ALS-linked SOD1 mutation causes motor neuron disease characterized by vacuolar degeneration of mitochondria. Neuron 14:1105-1116.

Xu W, Lipscombe D (2001) Neuronal Ca(V)1.3alpha(1) L-type channels activate at relatively hyperpolarized membrane potentials and are incompletely inhibited by dihydropyridines. J Neurosci 21:5944-5951.

Yamanaka K, Chun SJ, Boillee S, Fujimori-Tonou N, Yamashita H, Gutmann DH, Takahashi R, Misawa H, Cleveland DW (2008) Astrocytes as determinants of disease progression in inherited amyotrophic lateral sclerosis. Nat Neurosci 11:251-253.

Yang Z, Klionsky DJ (2010) Eaten alive: a history of macroautophagy. Nat Cell Biol 12:814-822.

Yi M, Weaver D, Hajnoczky G (2004) Control of mitochondrial motility and distribution by the calcium signal: a homeostatic circuit. J Cell Biol 167:661-672.

Zhang B, Tu P, Abtahian F, Trojanowski JQ, Lee VM (1997) Neurofilaments and orthograde transport are reduced in ventral root axons of transgenic mice that express human SOD1 with a G93A mutation. J Cell Biol 139:1307-1315.

7

Advantages and Pitfalls in Experimental Models Of ALS

Marina Boido[1], Elisa Buschini[1], Antonio Piras[1], Giada Spigolon[1], Valeria Valsecchi[1], Letizia Mazzini[2] and Alessandro Vercelli[1]
[1]*Neuroscience Institute of the Cavalieri Ottolenghi Foundation, University of Turin,*
[2]*ALS Centre, Department of Neurology, Eastern Piedmont University, "Maggiore della Carità" Hospital, Novara*
Italy

1. Introduction

Amyotrophic lateral sclerosis (ALS) is a progressive neurodegenerative disease that targets upper and lower motoneurons (MN) and leads to death in 2-5 years. 5–10% ALS cases are familial (fALS) with a Mendelian pattern of inheritance. The remaining 90% ALS cases are classified as having sporadic disease (sALS). Only in about 30% of fALS mutations in specific genes have been identified, whereas for the others the etiology is unknown. The clinical phenotype of fALS is usually indistinguishable from sALS.

An effective therapy is still lacking, even though many clinical trials have been already conducted. In order to perform preclinical studies to study the etiology and the molecular mechanisms, to design and to test new therapeutic targets and molecules, several *in vitro* and *in vivo* experimental models have been identified, to reproduce the hallmarks of the disease. Such models include transgenic or spontaneously mutated animals as well as *in vitro* preparations, i.e. MN/spinal cord organotypic cultures. Unfortunately, all these models fail to reproduce the complexity of the human disease, even though they represent a very useful tool to investigate several features of the disease.

2. Genetic animal models

To date, at least 13 genes and loci of major effect in fALS have been identified. The most frequent mutations found in fALS consist in mutations in the gene encoding copper/zinc superoxide dismutase 1 (Cu/Zn SOD1), a ubiquitously expressed enzyme that plays a key role in oxygen free radical scavenging. SOD1 catalyzes the dismutation of superoxide (O_2^-) to hydrogen peroxide (Scozzafava & Viezzoli, 1993; Tainer et al., 1982). On average, SOD1 mutations are responsible for about 20% of fALS cases (Deng et al., 1993; Rosen et al., 1993) and 5% of apparently sALS (Andersen et al., 2007). Over 70 different mutations at more than 60 residues throughout SOD1 (153 amino acids) have been linked to fALS (Andersen, 2000). The vast majority of mutations are amino acid substitutions, but a few cause C-terminal truncations of the protein. A spontaneous mutation in SOD1 has also been found in a canine degenerative myelopathy which resembles ALS (Awano et al., 2009).

Recently, mutations in the genes encoding the TAR DNA/RNA-binding protein 43 (TDP-43) (Corrado et al., 2009; Gitcho et al., 2008; Kabashi et al., 2008; Sreedharan et al., 2008; Van Deerlin et al., 2008; Yokoseki et al., 2008) and Fused in sarcoma/Translocated in liposarcoma (FUS/TLS) (Corrado et al., 2010; Kwiatkowski et al., 2009; Vance et al., 2009) have also been identified in approximately 5%-10% typical fALS.

Other genetic causes of rare and/or atypical fALS include mutations in the genes encoding alsin (ALS2; Hadano et al., 2001) and senataxin (ALS4; Chen et al., 2004) in juvenile ALS, spatacsin (ALS5; Orlacchio et al., 2010), vescicle-associated membrane protein B (VAPB; ALS8; Nishimura et al., 2004), angiogenin (ALS9; Greenway et al., 2006), optineurin (ALS12; Maruyama et al., 2010) and dynactin (Puls et al., 2003). Looking for a genotype-phenotype correlation for the different genes, a significant correlation have been demonstrated only for single mutations and considerable intrafamilial phenotypic differences were observed in some families carrying various mutations in the SOD1, TARDBP and FUS genes (Millecamps et al., 2010).

Aiming to unravel the pathogenic mechanisms leading to ALS, several animal models based on genetic mutations in fALS have been created.

2.1 Typical ALS models

2.1.1 SOD1 mutations

The first transgenic mouse model of human fALS was realized by Gurney and colleagues (1994), consisting in overexpressing a dominant "gain-of-function" mutation of the human SOD1. The mutation is characterized by the amino acid substitution at position 93 from glycine to alanine (G93A), which has little effect on the activity of hSOD1. G93A mice express the largest amount of mutant SOD in the brain, and develop neurological changes reminiscent of human MN disorders: they become paralyzed in hindlimbs and die by 5 to 6 months of age. The severity of the disease, in terms of age of onset and death, depends on the number of copies of the transgene. Paralysis is due to spinal MN loss. The pre-symptomatic phase in these mice is characterized by vacuolar degeneration of MNs, leading to the atrophic, neuron-depleted appearance of the anterior horns at later time points (Dal Canto & Gurney, 1994). The end-stage pattern of disease most closely mimics the pathological changes which characterize human ALS, with filamentous inclusions in both neurons and axonal processes (Hirano, 1991). By and large, this is the most used experimental model of ALS. On the other hand, the expression level of mutated SOD1 can vary independently from the number of copies of the transgene, thus modifying the onset and progression of the disease. In fact, the appearance of the first symptoms varies among the animals, in a time window of 1/2 weeks. Afterwards, the progression of the disease is quite fast, and the animals die approximately in one month. In our experience, in order to determine the onset of the symptomatic phase in G93A mice and initiate experimental treatment, we use a battery of motor behavioral tests (Rotarod, Paw Grip Endurance and Neurological tests).

Alternatively, Ripps and coll. (1995) introduced a missense mutation in the mouse SOD1 gene, that switched the glycine at position 86 to an arginine (G86R). The same mutation has been observed in the corresponding amino acid residue (position 85) of some fALS patients (Deng et al., 1993; Rosen, 1993). High expression of this gene in the spinal cord, brain stem and neocortex of transgenic mice is associated with age-related progressive pathological changes of MNs. Moreover, biochemical studies indicate normal total SOD activity in transgenic mice tissues, suggesting that also G86R mutation has no effects on SOD activity. The early symptoms are variable, consisting in either a flaccid or a spastic paralysis of forelimbs/hindlimbs, whereas the time of the onset is very predictable and the progression of the disease extremely rapid: in fact, the disorder progresses from a mild gait abnormality to total paralysis within a 5-days period: animals are healthy at the age of 3 months and dye by 4 months.

The original G85R mutation observed in fALS was introduced in a mouse background by Bruijn and coll. (1997). Low levels of accumulated human G85R are sufficient to cause severe MN disease without altering the protein and activity levels of endogenous SOD1. After an 8 month-latency period, MN loss proceeds nearly synchronously with 40% of large spinal MN axons degenerating in 2 weeks. Moreover, prominent SOD1-containing inclusions in astrocytes appear prior to clinical signs and increase markedly during disease progression, indicating astrocytes as first players in mutant-SOD1 mediated damage. Furthermore, in this mouse model the presence of glial glutamate transporter, the major glutamate transporter in spinal cord, decreases in end-stage G85R mice. This finding is strikingly similar to that observed in patients with sALS (Rothstein et al., 1995), implicating glutamate mediated excitotoxicity as a mechanism to account for the nearly synchronous degeneration of MNs.

Wong and coll. (1995) produced multiple lines of transgenic mice expressing the human G37R SOD1 mutant. These mice, expressing 5 to 14 times normal SOD1 activity levels, develop the clinical phenotype of MN disease. At lower levels of mutant protein accumulation, the pathology is restricted to lower MNs, whereas higher levels cause more severe abnormalities and affect a variety of other neuronal populations (striatum, thalamus, hypothalamus, pyriform cortex), with conspicuous vacuolar degeneration of axons and dendrites even in pre-symptomatic mice. However, vacuolar degeneration is not a well recognized component of MN pathology in human G37R fALS patients. Furthermore, in these mice neurofilamentous accumulations in cell bodies and proximal axons are rarely present, although they are a constant feature of the pathology in SOD1-linked fALS and in sALS (Hirano et al., 1984; Kato et al., 1991).

Wang and coll. (2002) engineered the human SOD1 gene, to encode mutations at the first two of the four histidine residues (46, 48, 63 and 120) that coordinately bind Cu^{2+} in the active site of the enzyme (Parge et al., 1992), as found in a Japanese and an English families, respectively (Aoki et al., 1995; Enayat et al., 1995). The experimental juxtaposition of disease-linked mutations at histidine 46 and 48 (H46R/H48Q) in transgenic mice creates a mutant enzyme with little or no superoxide scavenging ability that induced MN disease (Wang et al., 2003). These mice develop MN disease before 1 year of age, proportionally to the expression level of the transgene. The most prominent pathological feature in the spinal cord from paralyzed mice consists in the accumulation of high molecular weight SOD1 aggregates, and non-native, detergent-insoluble species of mutant protein. Combining the two disease-causing mutations at histidines 46 and 48 with two experimental mutations at histidines 63 and 120 (H63G and H120G), a stable but inactive protein (H46G/H48Q/H63G/H120G or Quad) is obtained: its expression in mice results in a MN disease clinically and pathologically similar to the H46R/H48Q mouse model (Wang et al., 2003).

Among the reported mutations, the hSOD1-D90A is the milder. Homozygous mice develop a fatal MN disease, but the progression is slow. Mice display bladder disturbances similar to those found in human fALS homozygous for this mutation (Jonsson et al., 2006). Transgenic mice accumulate detergent-resistant hSOD1 aggregates in the spinal cord, and hSOD1 inclusions and vacuoles especially in the ventral horns.

In fALS Oki Family a 2 base pair deletion was found at codon 126 of SOD1 gene, causing a frame shift and a premature stop in the protein sequence at codon 131 (Leu126delTT; Nakashima et al., 1995; Pramatarova et al., 1994). The truncated protein lacks important parts for dimer contact and activity site loop (Watanabe et al., 1997). Transgenic mice expressing this mutation display loss of MNs, microglia activation and Lewy body-like hyaline (LBHIs) cytoplasmic inclusions, with a rapid progression to complete paralysis after initial hindlimb paraparesis (Watanabe et al., 2005).

Similarly, mice bearing other two mutations, consisting i) in the insertion of non-native sequence (TGGG) prior to premature termination (SOD1-G127X) (Jonsson et al., 2004) and ii) in a simple C-terminal deletion (SOD1-L126Z) (Wang et al., 2005), develop MN disease, and accumulation of relatively high levels of detergent-insoluble forms of the mutated variants in the spinal cord.

Taken together, transgenic mice bearing mutations on the SOD1 gene represent a good model for the study of human ALS, since they show several features of the disease: behaviorally, for the motor symptoms which can be assessed with standardized tests; morphologically, for the involvement of upper and lower MNs and the cellular alterations leading to death, together with the involvement of astroglia and microglia which make ALS a not cell-autonomous disease. Nevertheless, most clinical trials based on results obtained on SOD1 mice failed to obtain significant effects on disease (Benatar, 2007): it may be argued that SOD1 mice represent a good model for the only fALS, and even that most effective treatments are initiated in mice before the onset of the symptoms, which is not feasible in sALS.

Some experimental manipulations can be difficult to perform in mice for their innate size limitations, such as administration of compounds into the cerebrospinal fluid (CSF) or obtaining sufficient tissue to perform extensive biochemical analyses. Therefore, Nagai and coll. developed a rat model of ALS by expressing a human SOD1 transgene with two ALS-associated mutations: H46R and G93A (2001). Like the murine counterpart, these models reproduce the most common phenotypic features of human ALS. Rats with the highest transgene copy numbers and higher expression of the mutant protein develop a paralytic disorder characterized by MN death together with astrogliosis and microglia activation. In particular, H46R rat pathology is characterized by protein deposition and aggregation, as H46R/H48Q and G85R transgenic mice. Furthermore, H46R rats display a later onset of paralysis and a slower disease progression (24 days) than G93A rats (8 days). The rat model is ideal for drug administration via chronic intrathecal pumps, a strategy used in human ALS clinical trials. Rats can tolerate better than mice immunosuppressive therapy to allow survival of implanted cells. Moreover ALS rats allow CSF access, because their CSF volume is 10-20 fold greater than in the mouse (http://www.axon-neuroscience.at/rat_models_1.php).

ALS models have been engineered also in zebrafish (Lemmens et al., 2007) and in *Caenorhabditis elegans* (Wang et al., 2009). In particular, overexpression of hSOD1-G93A, hSOD1-G37R and hSOD1-A4V in zebrafish induces a very robust axonopathy in the embryos. The major advantages of this model in the zebrafish embryo are i) that spinal motor axons are easily identifiable, ii) that treatment of animals with small compound libraries is more feasible and iii) that drug testing can be performed within 2 days. The *C.*

elegans approach, instead, aims to reveal the primary target of the toxic effect of hSOD1 mutations. In fact, overexpression of the hSOD1-G85R mutant protein leads to severe locomotor defects, associated with macroscopic aggregation in neuronal cell bodies. The mutant protein is unable to fold properly producing neuronal dysfunction at the synaptic level and possibly causing a deficient trafficking of pre-synaptic vesicles.

2.1.2 TDP-43 mutations

Recently, great interest has been raised by studies on TDP-43, a protein implicated in regulation of alternative splicing of mRNA, mRNA stability and transcriptional control. Several different neurodegenerative diseases are characterized by TDP-43 proteinopathies (Wegorzewska et al., 2009; Zhou et al., 2010). For instance, abnormal levels of aggregated TDP-43 are detected in the majority of patients with ALS, frontotemporal lobar dementia (FTLD) and Alzheimer's disease (AD), with ALS and FTLD often associated. Mutations in the TARDBP gene result in neuronal aggregation of abnormal TDP-43 protein in patients dying of MN disease: TDP-43-positive inclusions are present in both sALS and in the syndrome affecting fALS patients with TARDBP mutations, although they are more frequent in the last ones (Sreedharan et al., 2008). The clinical course of patients with TARDBP mutations is similar to that of sALS. Elevated levels of TDP-43 has been found in ALS patients in which the lower MNs were mostly affected (Geser et al., 2011; Noto et al., 2011). Pathological TDP-43 seems to be a less consistent feature of other MN disease phenotypes, such as primary lateral sclerosis and progressive muscular atrophy (Dickson et al., 2007).

Therefore, TDP-43 has been targeted to create animal models of ALS in mice, rats and *Drosophila*. In *Drosophila melanogaster*, the depletion of the TDP homolog results in deficient locomotor activity and defects at neuromuscular junctions (NMJs) (Feiguin et al., 2009). On the other hand, wild-type (WT) TDP-43 overexpression exerts more severe effects on neuromuscular junction architecture, viability and MN vitality (Estes et al., 2011). The neurotoxicity is modulated by the proteasome, the chaperone Hsp70 and the apoptosis pathway (Estes et al., 2011).

Transgenic mice expressing the human mutated TDP-43 gene (A315T and M337V) or the human WT gene (hTDP-43), develop a severe early MN degeneration phenotype, that correlates with TDP-43 levels in spinal cord (Stallings et al., 2010). In particular, TDP-43-A315T mice develop later onset paralysis with cytoplasmic ubiquitin inclusions, gliosis and TDP-43 redistribution and fragmentation (Stallings et al., 2010). Moreover, *in vivo* and also *in vitro* the A315T mutant enhances neurotoxicity and the formation of aberrant TDP-43 species, including protease-resistant fragments (Guo et al., 2011).

Moderate overexpression of hTDP-43 results in TDP-43 truncation, increased cytoplasmic and nuclear ubiquitin levels, intranuclear and cytoplasmic aggregates immunopositive for phosphorylated TDP-43. Furthermore, abnormal juxtanuclear aggregates of mitochondria are observed, accompanied by enhanced levels of Fis1 and phosphorylated DLP1, the key components of the mitochondrial fission machinery. Conversely, a marked reduction in mitofusin 1 expression, which plays an essential role in mitochondrial fusion is observed. Furthermore, hTDP-43 mice show reactive gliosis, axonal and myelin degeneration, gait abnormalities, and early lethality (Xu et al., 2010). Wils and coworkers (2010) confirmed a dose dependent degeneration of cortical and spinal MNs and development of spastic quadriplegia, reminiscent of ALS.

Constitutive and conditional transgenic rat models, overexpressing the hTDP-43-M337V protein develop a widespread neurodegeneration, mostly affecting the motor system. Features of this proteinopathy include the formation of TDP-43 inclusions, cytoplasmic localization of phosphorylated TDP-43, and its fragmentation. The number of MNs is reduced, striated muscles are denervated, astrogliosis and microglial activation are present (Zhou et al., 2010).

Finally, depletion of TDP-43 with antisense oligonucleotide strategy in mouse adult brain alters the expression levels of 601 mRNA (including Fus, Tis, progranulin and other transcripts encoding neurodegenerative disease-associated proteins) and 965 splicing events (e.g. in sortilin, the receptor for progranulin) (Polymenidou et al., 2011). RNAs with the most depleted levels derive from genes with very long introns that encode proteins involved in synaptic activity. The same RNA are altered in ALS patients (Xiao et al., 2011).

Thus far, TDP-43 transgenic mice together with SOD1-G93A mice, represent the ALS model which more closely adheres to human ALS.

Another RNA binding protein, FUS, has been found mutated in both 5% fALS (Lagier-Tourenne & Cleveland, 2009) and 1% sALS (Mackenzie et al., 2010) patients: FUS interacts with TDP-43 (Strong & Volkening, 2011), as shown also in a model of FUS-related neuronal degeneration in *Drosophila* (Lanson et al., 2011). Knocking down either Tardbp or FUS in zebrafish causes a motor phenotype which can be rescued by wild type FUS expression (Kabashi et al., 2011). To our knowledge, there are no transgenic mouse models for studying FUS role in ALS, but studies on TDP-43 mice have shown that this protein and FUS are strictly correlated.

2.2 Rare ALS models

Sequence variants in a number of genes are reported to be associated with ALS. These variations are found in candidate genes or through genome wide association studies. In all cases, it is unclear whether these genes and/or variations play a role in ALS, and these associations remain to be confirmed.

2.2.1 Alsin mutation

Great expectancies have been raised by the discovery of ALS2/alsin, a guanine nucleotide exchange factor (GEF) for the small GTPase Rab5 (Rab5GEF). ALS2 is a novel Rac1 effector, involved in Rac1-activated macropinocytosis and in macropinocytosis-associated endosome fusion and trafficking, and in neurite outgrowth. Therefore, loss of ALS2 may perturb macropinocytosis and/or the following membrane trafficking, which gives rise to neuronal dysfunction in the ALS2-linked MN diseases (Devon et al., 2006; Kunita et al., 2007). In fact, ALS2 loss of function mutations in humans account for several juvenile recessive MN diseases: the juvenile ALS, the primary lateral sclerosis and the infantile-onset ascending hereditary spastic paralysis (Eymard-Pierre et al., 2006; Orban et al., 2007). Furthermore, alsin plays a role in AMPA receptor trafficking, thus providing a novel pathogenic link between ALS2-deficiency and MN degeneration, suggesting a protective role in maintaining the survival of MNs (Lai et al., 2006).

Knocking down of alsin by small interfering RNA in cultured MNs display a reduced apparent size of early endosomes and an increased intracellular accumulation of transferrin and L1 cell adhesion molecule. Moreover, it induces MN death and significantly inhibits axon growth in the surviving ones (Jacquier et al., 2006).

On the other hand, loss of ALS2 in mice does not have a dramatic effect on the survival or function of lower MNs (Cai et al., 2008). On the contrary, ALS2 deficiency causes an upper MN disease that closely resembles a severe form of hereditary spastic paralysis, that is quite distinct from ALS. The hereditary spastic paralysis is characterized by progressive axonal degeneration and slows movement without muscle weakness (Yamanaka et al., 2006). ALS2 -/- mice are more susceptible to oxidative stress compared to WT, although they fail to recapitulate clinical or neuropathological phenotypes consistent with MN disease by 20 months of age (Cai et al., 2005). In addition, the effects of ALS2 ablation strongly depend on the genetic background and sex (Hadano et al., 2010b). Loss of ALS2 in SOD1 mice exacerbates the pathology (Hadano et al., 2010a).

2.2.2 VAPB mutation

A mutation in the vesicle-associated membrane protein-associated protein-B (VAPB) is the cause of a fALS, ALS8 (Nishimura et al., 2004). This mutation is characterized by a proline to serine substitution at position 56 (P56S). The physiological function of VAPB is in part unclear, but it seems involved in bouton formation at the NMJ and in vesicle transport from the endoplasmic reticulum (ER) to the Golgi. Indeed, the protein mainly localizes to the ER compartment and to the junction between intracellular vesicles and cytoskeletal structures (Skehel et al., 2000; Soussan et al., 1999). Transgenic mice expressing the VAPBP56S mutation were created by Tudor and coworkers (2010). These mice develop cytoplasmic TDP-43 accumulations within spinal MNs at 18 months of age, pointing out a possible link between TDP-43 mislocalization and abnormalities in VAPB. Besides, both brain and spinal cord neurons, including MN, show an altered cellular distribution of VAPBP56S with ER-derived aggregates of this protein. Despite this pathological hallmark, the motor function and the MN number in spinal cord are not significantly affected by the mutation, indicating that these animals do not develop overt MN disease, in contrast to mutant SOD1 where low levels of expression can induce aggressive MN disease. The difference between these two ALS models could be related to the late-onset and slowly progressive atypical disease of the vast majority of ALS8 cases.

2.2.3 Cytoskeletal protein mutations: Dynactin, neurofilaments, peripherin, TAU

An increasing number of neurodegenerative diseases are being linked to mutations in genes encoding proteins required for axonal transport and intracellular trafficking (e.g., dynactin). Furthermore, one hallmark of MN degeneration in both affected ALS patients and transgenic mice expressing the SOD1 mutation consists in the accumulation of intermediate filaments (IFs), in particular, the neurofilaments (NFs, the major type of IFs), in the perikarya and axons of MNs.

A missense mutations in a dynactin gene (Dctn1) encoding the p150Glued subunit of dynactin complex has been associated to both fALS and sALS. The dynactin complex consists of at least 10 distinct components, including p150Glued that is the largest subunit: it binds directly to microtubules (MTs) and is required for coordinated anterograde and retrograde organelle movement (Haghnia et al., 2007). The missense mutation occurring in the glycine-rich cytoskeleton-associated protein (CAP-Gly) domain of the p150Glued polypeptide, results in the substitution of serine for glycine at position 59 (G59S), leading to a decreased binding to MTs (Puls et al., 2003). Other missense mutations in Dctn1 have been identified and are linked to ALS, but the specific role of these mutations in the pathogenesis of the disease is unclear (Munch et al., 2005; Munch et al., 2004).

The mouse model expressing human mutant p150Glued dynactin (Thy-1; G59 $p150^{Glued}$) exhibits clinical and pathological hallmarks of MN disease and is characterized phenotypically by slowly progressive muscle weakness. MN degeneration in these mice is associated with abnormalities in intracellular vesicular trafficking, axonal swelling and axon-terminal degeneration. Evidence suggests that autophagic cell death is implicated in the pathogenesis of these mice (Laird et al., 2008). A similar animal model to study the pathogenic mechanism of the G59S mutation *in vivo* is represented by p150Glued G59S knock-in mice. These mice develop a late-onset, slowly progressive MN disease characterized by abnormal accumulation of NFs and synaptic vesicle proteins at the NMJs, loss of MNs, and gait abnormalities (Lai et al., 2007).

LaMonte and coworkers (2002) engineered a targeted disruption of the dynein-dynactin complex in MNs of transgenic mice by overexpression of a subunit of dynactin (dynamitin, p50) that causes the disassembly of the whole complex. Mice overexpressing dynamitin demonstrate a late-onset, slowly progressive MN degenerative disease characterized by muscle weakness, spontaneous trembling, abnormal posture and gait, and deficits in strength and endurance. These mice show MN degeneration and muscle denervation/atrophy. NF accumulations and retrograde transport inhibition observed in these mice confirm the critical role of the axonal transport in the pathogenesis of MN degenerative disease. Whether NF (or more generally IF) accumulations contribute to pathogenesis of human ALS remains unknown; it could simply be the consequence of neuronal dysfunction. However, emerging evidence suggests that sometimes IF aggregates can have detrimental as well as protective effects in MN disease. Transgenic mouse models are used to address whether cytoskeletal changes may contribute to MN disease.

NFs in adult MNs are made by the copolymerization of three proteins, the light (NF-L, 61 kDa), medium (NF-M, 90 kDa) and heavy (NF-H, 115 KDa) NFs. Mice knockout for any of the three NF genes do not develop MN disease, although these deficiencies have several harmful effects: the formation of perikaryal NF accumulations resembling those found in human (Elder et al., 1998a; Elder et al., 1998b; Rao et al., 1998; Zhu et al., 1997). Transgenic mice accumulating NF-L (4-fold the normal level) in the sciatic nerve, also display huge accumulations of NFs in spinal MNs, swollen perikarya, and eccentrically localized nuclei. NF accumulation is associated with some neurodegenerative hallmarks, such as an increased frequency of axonal degeneration, proximal axon swelling, and severe skeletal muscle atrophy (Xu et al., 1993). Also transgenic mice expressing the human NF-H gene (up to 2-fold the levels of the endogenous protein) progressively develop neurological defects and abnormal neurofilamentous swellings by 3-4 months of age (Cote et al., 1993). Transgenic mice expressing a fusion protein in which the carboxyl terminus of the NF-H is replaced by beta-galactosidase accumulates such protein as large filamentous aggregates in perikarya. Axons are not invested with NFs but develop only small calibers (Eyer & Peterson, 1994). Increased expression of NF subunits in all these transgenic mouse models leads to MN dysfunction, in absence of the widespread MN death typical of human ALS.

However, a more severe phenotype is produced by the expression of an assembly-disrupting NF-L mutant having a leucine to proline substitution (NF-L L394P): this mutation causes massive degeneration of spinal MNs accompanied by abnormal accumulations of NFs and severe neurogenic atrophy of skeletal muscles (Lee et al., 1994).

Abnormal NF aggregates are observed in both fALS patients and in SOD1 mice, pointing out that NFs may contribute to SOD1-mediated disease. Mating experiments between SOD1 mice and transgenic mice with deregulated levels of NF proteins were carried out. The overexpression of human NF-H proteins confers an effective protection against the SOD1 mutation, a phenomenon probably due to the ability of NF proteins to chelate calcium. Therefore, these studies show that disorganized NFs can sometimes have noxious effects resulting in neuronopathy. However, there is emerging evidence that in the context of MN disease caused by mutant SOD1, NF proteins may play a protective role (Eyer et al., 1998; Williamson et al., 1998).

Among the IF proteins, also peripherin overexpression in mice determines ALS. Peripherin is a type III neuronal IF protein of 57 kD, found within NF in the majority of IF inclusions (89%) in MNs of ALS patients (Corbo & Hays, 1992; Migheli et al., 1993). In adult rats, peripherin is mostly expressed in autonomic nerves and in peripheral sensory neurons while is barely detectable in spinal MNs (Escurat et al., 1990; Parysek & Goldman, 1988). However, peripherin gene expression is increased up to 300% in spinal MNs after injury of the sciatic nerve (Troy et al., 1990), whereas expression of the other NF proteins is reduced (Muma et al., 1990). Inflammation occurred in injured neurons could explain peripherin upregulation. In fact, peripherin gene expression is upregulated by the inflammatory cytokines interleukin-6 (IL-6) and leukemia inhibitory factor (Djabali et al., 1993; Sterneck et al., 1996). This suggests that peripherin may be part of a general response of MNs to noxious stress and may explain peripherin inclusion bodies in MNs of ALS patients. Beaulieu and coll. (1999) generated two transgenic mice to investigate the potential detrimental effects of peripherin overexpression in MNs, in which the endogenous peripherin gene, inserted with its own promoter or under the control of the Thy1 gene promoters, was overexpressed. Both mouse strains display a late-onset and selective MN disease characterized by the formation of IF inclusions similar to those found in human ALS and in SOD1 mice. Moreover, a deficiency in NF-L protein exacerbates the formation of IF inclusion bodies and the onset of disease precipitates, probably through a deleterious action of the large NF subunits on peripherin organization (Beaulieu et al., 1999).

Cytoskeletal abnormalities reported in ALS involve also MT-associated proteins such as the tau protein, predominantly expressed in neurons. Since tau is required for neurite elaboration in different cell types, a central role in neuronal process outgrowth and integrity is proposed. To date, 30 different intronic and exonic pathogenic mutations have been identified in the human tau gene and have been correlated to several pathological conditions recognized as tauopathies. Among these, exonic tau gene mutations (i.e., P301L and R406W) impair the ability of tau to bind and stabilize MTs as well as to promote their assembly (Hasegawa et al., 1998; Hong et al., 1998). These mutations contribute to the formation of fibrillary tau aggregates (Crowther & Goedert, 2000; Delobel et al., 2002; Vogelsberg-Ragaglia et al., 2000). Transgenic mice expressing the human tau containing the P301L mutation exhibit motor behavioral deficits, with age- and gene-dose-dependent development of neurofibrillary tangles (NFT). This phenotype occurs as early as 6.5 months in hemizygous and 4.5 months in homozygous animals. The spinal cord of both these animals display axonal spheroids, anterior horn cell loss and axonal degeneration in anterior spinal roots. Counts of spinal MNs show a reduction of approximately 48% compared to control animals. Moreover, the expression of P301L mutation results in peripheral neuropathy and skeletal muscle with neurogenic atrophy (Gotz et al., 2001; Lewis et al.,

2000). The specific role of tau in the ALS pathogenesis remains unsettled, but the phenotypical and histological observations in P301L mutant mice suggests that it could be a key molecule in neurodegeneration occurring in ALS.

2.2.4 VEGF

Studies on the vascular endothelial growth factor (VEGF) suggest a novel function for VEGF in the pathogenesis of MN degeneration. VEGF may be involved in spinal cord neuropathy mainly by affecting vascular growth or function. However, VEGF might also affect neural cells directly, but the *in vivo* relevance of such a mechanism has been poorly investigated. To study the potential role of VEGF in MN degeneration, Oosthuyse and coll. (2001) generated a 'knock-in' mouse, in which the hypoxia-response element sequence in the Vegf promoter was deleted. Vegf $^{-/-}$ mice appear healthy until 5 months of age, when they develop symptoms of MN disease, i.e. severe adult-onset muscle weakness due to degeneration of lower MNs, reminiscent of the clinical symptoms and neuropathological signs of ALS. Similarly, VEGF replacement has beneficial effects in SOD1 G93A mice (Lunn et al., 2009). These findings indicate that reduced neural perfusion and maybe also insufficient VEGF-dependent neuroprotection cause MN degeneration (Oosthuyse et al., 2001).

3. Spontaneous mutation models

Since many years, several mouse models bearing spontaneous mutations leading to MN death have been identified: for instance, Wobbler (Duchen & Strich, 1968), Nmd (Cook et al., 1995), Pmn (Schmalbruch et al., 1991), Wasted (Newbery et al., 2005), Loa (Rogers et al., 2001) and Cra (Hrabe de Angelis et al., 2000) mice.

3.1 Wobbler mouse

The Wobbler mouse mutation spontaneously occurred in the breeding stock of Falconer (1956) and was later mapped to the proximal mouse chromosome (Kaupmann et al., 1992). It is the oldest known model of spontaneous MN disease, following a spontaneous recessive mutation in the wobbler (wr) gene, which encodes for the vacuolar-vesicular protein sorting 54 (Vps54) with a missense mutation L967Q. Vps54 mutation has been rarely described in ALS patients (Corrado et al., 2011). The protein is a subunit of the Golgi-associated retrograde protein (GARP) complex, used for fusion of endosome-derived transport vesicles to the trans-Golgi network. This model is considered a good model of MN degeneration, although the molecular mechanisms of the pathology in these mice are still unclear. Duchen and coll. (1968) showed that the progression of disease can be divided into three phases. i) The first, presymptomatic one, during the first 3 weeks after birth, ii) followed by the evolutionary one where the mice show alterations in motor behavior such as fine tremor of the head and slightly unsteady gait. iii) The third phase consists in the stabilization of the disease with the end of the neurodegenerative process. The progression of the disease is variable and leads to progressive denervation of skeletal muscles, determining muscle atrophy especially in the head, neck, shoulders and forelimbs. Limb muscles display different levels of atrophy: distally, atrophy is more severe than proximally, although in this model the hindlimbs are less severely affected. Moreover, there is a final progressive weight loss partially due to nutritional deprivation following muscle atrophy of the face and forelimbs (Boillee et al., 2003). Mice usually live up to 3-4 months, but sometimes the stabilization of the disease can delay their death for longer.

3.2 NMD mouse

Cox and coll. (1998) identified mice carrying 2 independent mutations in the neuromuscular degeneration (Nmd) gene on two alleles: nmd^{j} and nmd^{2j}, leading to a progressive degeneration of spinal MNs and muscular atrophy. The nmd gene produces a ubiquitously expressed DNA helicase/ATPase protein previously described as immunoglobulin S-mu binding protein-2 (Smbp2; Fukita et al., 1993), glial factor 1 (Gf1; Kerr & Khalili, 1991), rat insulin enhancer binding protein 1 (rip1; Shieh et al., 1995) and cardiac transcription factor 1 (Catf1; Sebastiani et al., 1995).

Mutant mice are characterized by a progressive paralysis that initially begins with the hindlimbs. The forelimbs are affected to a variable degree with paralysis, generally evident only toward the latest stages of the disease. Homozygous Nmd mutants can be easily distinguished from their littermate controls at 2 weeks of age by their dorsally contracted hindlimbs and impaired movement. Affected mice rarely survive beyond 4 weeks of age, but the exact cause of death is unclear.

3.3 PMN mouse

Bommel and colleagues (2002) identified animals suffering of a progressive motor neuronopathy (pmn), caused by an autosomal recessive mutation in the tubulin-specific chaperone e gene (tbce). The mutation results from a tryptophan to glycine substitution at position 524 (T524G; Martin et al., 2002). This protein is one of the main cofactors involved in MT stability or polymerization dynamics. These mice between P14 and P20 display a progressive caudal-cranial degeneration of motor axons leading to muscular atrophy, hindlimb paralysis and death in 4 to 6 weeks after birth (Schmalbruch et al., 1991).

Although the pathophysiology of MN death in pmn mice is mainly due to loss of neuromuscular integrity by distal axonopathy rather than alteration of neuron soma (which is instead a common feature in ALS), this model can be considered a good one for MN neurodegeneration.

3.4 WASTED mouse

Wasted (wst) mice bear a spontaneous autosomal mutation that results in the loss of gene encoding the translation factor eEF1A2. From the 3rd week of age they exhibit immunodeficiency and neurological disorders in terms of tremors and disturbance of gait. Subsequently these mice present MN degeneration and hindlimb paralysis.

Moreover, Newbery and coll. (2005) observed reactive gliosis at P19 in the cervical spinal cord with a rostrocaudal gradient, and retraction of MN fibers. Mice develop a rapid neurodegeneration and die around P28. Finally, several studies demonstrated that this model bears increased chromosomal breakage and DNA damage (Shultz et al., 1982).

3.5 LOA and CRA mice

"Legs at odd angles" (Loa) and "Cramping 1" (Cra) mice arose as the result of two independent N-ethyl-N-nitrosourea-(ENU) induced mutagenenesis experiments (Hrabe de Angelis et al., 2000; Rogers et al., 2001).

Loa mouse presents a point mutation that changes phenylalanine to tyrosine at position 580 (F580Y) in the gene encoding the heavy chain of dynein. On the other hand, Cra mice have a substitution from tyrosine to cytosine at position 1055 (Y1055C) in the same gene. Dynein is a motor protein which determines retrograde transport along MTs and this model has been partially used to evaluate the role of dynein in the neuronal migration. However, the disturbance in axonal transport leads to selective MN death, making these mice useful models in ALS studies. Particularly, Loa mice exhibit pathological features similar to human ones, as Lewy body-like inclusions containing SOD1, CDK5 and ubiquitin. However, Ilieva et al., (2008) found no α-MN loss at any age, but a sensory axon deficit of the large proprioceptive (type Ia) axons and the decrease of γ-motor axons innervating muscle spindles. Similarly, Cra mice do not show MN degeneration but rather peripheral sensory neuropathy due to loss of axons in dorsal roots and decrement of large proprioceptive axons (Dupuis et al., 2009).

In conclusion, the pathological features observed in both models do not properly correlate with hALS characteristics. Dynein mutation models will need further investigation, they better represent a model for sensory neuropathy rather than for MN disease.

3.6 Hereditary canine spinal muscular atrophy

Hereditary canine spinal muscular atrophy (HCSMA) is a lower motor neuron disease found in Brittany Spaniels. It shares clinical and pathological features with human ALS (Green et al., 2002). These animals show signs of oxidative stress (Green et al., 2001), but do not have mutations in the SOD1 gene (Green et al., 2002). From the histopathological point of view these animals are characterized by aberrant accumulation of extensively phosphorylated heavy (high molecular weight) neurofilament (NFH) and neurodegeneration (Green et al., 2005).

4. *In vitro* models

Despite *in vivo* models are extremely helpful for studying ALS, when the aim consists in studying the molecular mechanisms of MN death and the role and the involvement of the different cells in the pathological mechanisms, simplified *in vitro* models such as MN and organotypic cultures can be useful, allowing to control the experimental conditions.

4.1 Motoneuron and glia culture

Since the major feature of ALS consists in the progressive loss of upper and lower MNs, cultures of spinal MNs are a valuable tool for studying ALS pathomechanisms. Many authors have developed protocols to isolate MNs from newborn or embryonic murine spinal cord (Berg & Fischbach, 1978; Gingras et al., 2007; Schnaar & Schaffner, 1981), allowing to identify MNs for their size and their Choline Acetyl Transferase (ChAT) activity. However, more recently, Wiese and coll. (2010) have isolated embryonic spinal MNs from rodents using p75 neurotrophin receptor (NTR)-antibody panning step, a technique with low toxicity and high efficiency; in fact, at the embryonic stage, MNs are the only neurons expressing the p75 low-affinity nerve growth factor receptor (Camu & Henderson, 1992). Unlike most studies performed on cultured embryonic spinal MNs, those of cultures of spinal MNs from newborn rodents is less common. In 2004, Anderson and coworkers described a protocol for isolating and culturing neonatal spinal MNs positive to p75NTR and ChAT, in presence of a growth factor cocktail containing glial cell line-derived neurotrophic factor (GDNF), brain-derived neurotrophic factor (BDNF) and ciliary neurotrophic factor (CNTF) (Anderson et al., 2004).

In vitro preparations are age-dependent, since cells or tissues are generally obtained from animals at late embryonic or neonatal stages, but ALS related-alterations or neurodegenerative defects are not yet evident at this early stage. Indeed Avossa and coll. (2006) characterized the alterations in WT and G93A embryonic spinal cord cells analyzing MNs, glial cells, interneurons, distribution of hSOD1, mitochondria, MTs, NFs and synapses. They did not find any substantial difference in all these parameters, excepted for a significant increase in inhibitory synapses compared to excitatory ones in mutant cells. Therefore, it is necessary to use specific molecules or drugs to induce cell death mechanisms in these apparently normal cells.

Since in ALS an imbalance in the glutamatergic system has been described, leading to an excitotoxic environment around MNs (Boillee et al., 2006), an *in vitro* approach can be represented by NMDA exposure. Rothstein and coll. (1993) were the first to use this model, demonstrating that MN degeneration is prevented by non-NMDA glutamate receptor antagonists, consequently used as neuroprotective agents.

Similarly, some authors have proposed that spinal MNs are more vulnerable to AMPA receptor agonists than to NMDA, particularly in spinal cord cultures (Carriedo et al., 1996; Van Damme et al., 2002). In fact, microdialysis perfusion of AMPA agonists in spinal cord reveals a consistent loss of spinal MNs and the consequently paralysis of the hindlimbs, probably due to an increased cytoplasmic Ca^{2+} concentration (Corona & Tapia, 2007).

Finally, it is well-known that also the glia (astrocytes and microglial cells) actively contributes to the death of MNs (Philips & Robberecht, 2011). Glia can be easily obtained and cultured both from embryos/newborns and adults; the first method has been described in 1972 by Booher and Sensenbrenner (1972). Now, concerning astroglia culture, "primary culture", "subculture" and "shaken culture (once or twice)" can be performed (Du et al., 2010), each one with advantages and pitfalls relative to purity of astrocytes, cell viability, expression of glial fibrillary acidic protein (GFAP) and bystin, a protein potentially involved in embryo implantation, which is markedly up-regulated in reactive astrocytes (Fang et al., 2008). Similarly, protocols to isolate microglial cells are easy and reproducible (Ni & Aschner, 2010; Yip et al., 2009), and they have been recently improved by the column-free magnetic separation technology: the cells can be labeled and isolated on the strength of their expression of CD11b, a specific microglial marker, thus allowing to isolate an high number of cells and significantly reducing the animals needed (Gordon et al., 2011).

Cocultures of healthy hMNs with human astrocytes carrying either the WT or mutated SOD1 cDNA have demonstrated the role of astrocytes in ALS disease, since MN number decreased about 50% in the presence of mutant SOD1-expressing astrocytes (Marchetto et al., 2008). This neurotoxicity is probably mediated by the release of soluble factors from astrocytes, finally involving the Bax-dependent death machinery within MNs (Nagai et al., 2007).

4.2 Cell line culture

Due to the technical difficulties in establishing a MN culture for their poor proliferation ability when differentiated, an alternative is represented by the use of a neural hybrid cell line named NSC-34 (neuroblastoma spinal cord), derived from the fusion of neuroblastoma cells with MN enriched spinal cord. These cells perfectly show morphological and physiological properties of primary MNs: extending processes, contacts with cultured myotubes, synthesis and storage of acetylcholine, action potentials and NF proteins (Cashman et al., 1992).

NSC-34 can be transfected with vectors containing mutant forms of hSOD1, allowing to study specific neurodegenerative aspects such as mitochondrial degeneration, NF accumulation or Golgi apparatus disruption (Gomes et al., 2008; Menzies et al., 2002a; Menzies et al., 2002b). This model can also enlighten on the implicated cell death pathways in ALS, i.e. the involvement of MAP kinases (Guo & Bhat, 2007), the interaction between bcl2-A1 and pro-caspase-3 (Iaccarino et al., 2011) or the involvement of kynurenine pathway implicated in the regulatory mechanisms of the immune response (Chen et al., 2011).

In addition, different therapeutic agents have been tested in culture, such as the vascular endothelial growth factor (VEGF) (Kulshreshtha et al., 2011) or the semi-synthetic tetracycline called minocycline (Guo & Bhat, 2007), known for their neuroprotective effects in neurodegeneration models (Orsucci et al., 2009; Storkebaum et al., 2004).

Similarly, other cell lines have been transfected with WT or mutant (G93A) hSOD1 and used for the same purpose: N18TG2 neuroblastoma, the non-neuronal Madin–Darby Canine Kidney (MDCK) (Raimondi et al., 2006) or the mouse embryonic fibroblast NIH3T3 cell lines (Shinder et al., 2001).

The recent finding of human induced pluripotent stem cells (iPSCs) present a novel opportunity for *in vitro* disease modeling. iPSCs can be generated from readily accessible tissue from patients. iPSCs show similar capacity for directed MN differentiation as ESCs (Boulting et al., 2011). iPSCs can be generated from patients, thus carrying the actual mutations associated with the disease and allowing to correlate, any cellular phenotype with the patient's clinical characteristics such as onset, duration, and severity of disease at the time of tissue collection. In 2008, iPSCs were generated from a skin sample from an elderly patient with fALS displaying a SOD1 mutation (Dimos et al., 2008).

4.3 Organotypic cultures

Since ALS is a complex disease originating from an important crosstalk among MNs, glia and muscles (Strong, 2003), a step forward is represented by using organotypic cultures, where the *in vivo* architecture is maintained and MNs as well as neighboring cells (interneurons and glial cells) are preserved. However, this system presents an important limitation, due to the lack of correlation between morphological results and behavioral impairment (as well as for all the *in vitro* preparations) and the isolated slices undergo a series of little traumas (axotomy, deafferentation…) that can unintentionally originate a neuron selection.

Preparations of spinal cord organotypic culture from newborn animals is actually done according the Stoppini's procedure (1991): MNs survive more than 2 months, maintaining their structural and metabolic characteristics and allowing both morphological and electrophysiological experiments. Moreover, these experimental conditions stimulate glial proliferation, reproducing the glial activation observed *in vivo* in ALS patients/animal models (Hall et al., 1998; Vercelli et al., 2008).

As already mentioned, such model requires tissue obtained from embryos or pups, when ALS alterations are not full-blown (Avossa et al., 2006). Therefore, it is possible to use slice cultures obtained from normal animals and to add a glutamate transporter inhibitor (as threohydroxyaspartate (THA) or D,L-threo-B-benzyloxyaspartate), able to induce a chronic glutamate neurotoxicity. This treatment causes selective MNs death, simulating the human ALS neurodegeneration (Bilak et al., 2004; Rothstein et al., 1993). Some authors prepare organotypic spinal slice cultures directly from G93A SOD1 mice and expose them to THA in order to induce loss of MNs (Kosuge et al., 2009).

This *in vitro* model is helpful either for studying specific pathways/organelles or for testing treatments. Particularly, Tolosa and coll. (2008) studied the effects of VEGF on the survival and vulnerability to excitotoxicity of spinal cord MNs treated with THA, demonstrating that this growth factor plays an important role in neuroprotection by activating the phosphatidylinositol 3-kinase/Akt signal transduction pathway. Similarly Kosuge and coworkers (2009) tested the effect of GDNF, showing that threo-hydroxyaspartate -induced MN death was significantly inhibited in G93A mice slice. The pathway of caspase-12 was among the causes of MNs death. Also the anti-convulsant drugs topiramate (Maragakis et al., 2003), valproic acid (Sugai et al., 2004) and lithium (Caldero et al., 2010) were found to significantly prevent MN degeneration in this model.

5. Conclusion

ALS is a devastating neurodegenerative disease the etiology of which is still unclear. Even though the clinical hallmarks are similar, several different genetic and sporadic causes have been found or hypothesized. Experimental models of ALS have been created in transgenic animals, and spontaneously mutated animals affected by MN disease have been identified. Due to the multifactorial causes of the disease, all these models, even though they show motor impairment and neuropathological aspects typical of the human disease, cannot fully address the complexity of the human disease. Nevertheless, they represent useful tools to study the early and late development of the disease from a neuropathological point of view, and the molecular mechanisms involved. The major pitfall of the use of animals models thus far consists in the failure to translate the positive therapeutic outcome in human patients. This might be ascribed to mistakes in both preclinical and clinical research strategy: on one hand, animals, unlike patients, tend to be treated in the early phases of the disease and in any case represent a restricted, uniform population in terms of age, sex and genetic characteristics; on the other hand, patients represent a much more variable population. Therefore, an increasing collaboration between preclinical researchers and clinicians is needed to favor translation from benchside to clinics back and forth.

6. References

Andersen, P.M. (2000). Genetic factors in the early diagnosis of ALS. *Amyotroph Lateral Scler Other Motor Neuron Disord*, 1 Suppl 1, (Mar), pp. (S31-42), 1466-0822 (Print) 1466-0822 (Linking)

Andersen, P.M., Borasio, G.D., Dengler, R., Hardiman, O., Kollewe, K., Leigh, P.N., Pradat, P.F., Silani, V. & Tomik, B. (2007). Good practice in the management of amyotrophic lateral sclerosis: clinical guidelines. An evidence-based review with good practice points. EALSC Working Group. *Amyotroph Lateral Scler*, 8, 4, (Aug), pp. (195-213), 1748-2968 (Print) 1471-180X (Linking)

Anderson, K.N., Potter, A.C., Piccenna, L.G., Quah, A.K., Davies, K.E. & Cheema, S.S. (2004). Isolation and culture of motor neurons from the newborn mouse spinal cord. *Brain Res Brain Res Protoc*, 12, 3, (Feb), pp. (132-136), 1385-299X (Print) 1385-299X (Linking)

Aoki, M., Abe, K., Houi, K., Ogasawara, M., Matsubara, Y., Kobayashi, T., Mochio, S., Narisawa, K. & Itoyama, Y. (1995). Variance of age at onset in a Japanese family with amyotrophic lateral sclerosis associated with a novel Cu/Zn superoxide dismutase mutation. *Ann Neurol*, 37, 5, (May), pp. (676-679), 0364-5134 (Print) 0364-5134 (Linking)

Avossa, D., Grandolfo, M., Mazzarol, F., Zatta, M. & Ballerini, L. (2006). Early signs of motoneuron vulnerability in a disease model system: Characterization of transverse slice cultures of spinal cord isolated from embryonic ALS mice. *Neuroscience*, 138, 4, pp. (1179-1194), 0306-4522 (Print) 0306-4522 (Linking)

Awano, T., Johnson, G.S., Wade, C.M., Katz, M.L., Johnson, G.C., Taylor, J.F., Perloski, M., Biagi, T., Baranowska, I., Long, S., March, P.A., Olby, N.J., Shelton, G.D., Khan, S., O'Brien, D.P., Lindblad-Toh, K. & Coates, J.R. (2009). Genome-wide association analysis reveals a SOD1 mutation in canine degenerative myelopathy that resembles amyotrophic lateral sclerosis. *Proc Natl Acad Sci U S A*, 106, 8, (Feb 24), pp. (2794-2799), 1091-6490 (Electronic) 0027-8424 (Linking)

Beaulieu, J.M., Nguyen, M.D. & Julien, J.P. (1999). Late onset of motor neurons in mice overexpressing wild-type peripherin. *J Cell Biol*, 147, 3, (Nov 1), pp. (531-544), 0021-9525 (Print) 0021-9525 (Linking)

Benatar, M. (2007). Lost in translation: treatment trials in the SOD1 mouse and in human ALS. *Neurobiol Dis*, 26, 1, (Apr), pp. (1-13), 0969-9961 (Print) 0969-9961 (Linking)

Berg, D.K. & Fischbach, G.D. (1978). Enrichment of spinal cord cell cultures with motoneurons. *J Cell Biol*, 77, 1, (Apr), pp. (83-98), 0021-9525 (Print) 0021-9525 (Linking)

Bilak, M., Wu, L., Wang, Q., Haughey, N., Conant, K., St Hillaire, C. & Andreasson, K. (2004). PGE2 receptors rescue motor neurons in a model of amyotrophic lateral sclerosis. *Ann Neurol*, 56, 2, (Aug), pp. (240-248), 0364-5134 (Print) 0364-5134 (Linking)

Boillee, S., Peschanski, M. & Junier, M.P. (2003). The wobbler mouse: a neurodegeneration jigsaw puzzle. *Mol Neurobiol*, 28, 1, (Aug), pp. (65-106), 0893-7648 (Print) 0893-7648 (Linking)

Boillee, S., Vande Velde, C. & Cleveland, D.W. (2006). ALS: a disease of motor neurons and their nonneuronal neighbors. *Neuron*, 52, 1, (Oct 5), pp. (39-59), 0896-6273 (Print) 0896-6273 (Linking)

Bommel, H., Xie, G., Rossoll, W., Wiese, S., Jablonka, S., Boehm, T. & Sendtner, M. (2002). Missense mutation in the tubulin-specific chaperone E (Tbce) gene in the mouse mutant progressive motor neuronopathy, a model of human motoneuron disease. *J Cell Biol*, 159, 4, (Nov 25), pp. (563-569), 0021-9525 (Print) 0021-9525 (Linking)

Booher, J. & Sensenbrenner, M. (1972). Growth and cultivation of dissociated neurons and glial cells from embryonic chick, rat and human brain in flask cultures. *Neurobiology*, 2, 3, pp. (97-105), 0300-8819 (Print) 0300-8819 (Linking)

Boulting, G.L., Kiskinis, E., Croft, G.F., Amoroso, M.W., Oakley, D.H., Wainger, B.J., Williams, D.J., Kahler, D.J., Yamaki, M., Davidow, L., Rodolfa, C.T., Dimos, J.T., Mikkilineni, S., MacDermott, A.B., Woolf, C.J., Henderson, C.E., Wichterle, H. & Eggan, K. (2011). A functionally characterized test set of human induced pluripotent stem cells. *Nat Biotechnol*, 29, 3, (Mar), pp. (279-286), 1546-1696 (Electronic) 1087-0156 (Linking)

Bruijn, L.I., Becher, M.W., Lee, M.K., Anderson, K.L., Jenkins, N.A., Copeland, N.G., Sisodia, S.S., Rothstein, J.D., Borchelt, D.R., Price, D.L. & Cleveland, D.W. (1997). ALS-linked SOD1 mutant G85R mediates damage to astrocytes and promotes rapidly progressive disease with SOD1-containing inclusions. *Neuron*, 18, 2, (Feb), pp. (327-338), 0896-6273 (Print) 0896-6273 (Linking)

Cai, H., Lin, X., Xie, C., Laird, F.M., Lai, C., Wen, H., Chiang, H.C., Shim, H., Farah, M.H., Hoke, A., Price, D.L. & Wong, P.C. (2005). Loss of ALS2 function is insufficient to trigger motor neuron degeneration in knock-out mice but predisposes neurons to oxidative stress. *J Neurosci*, 25, 33, (Aug 17), pp. (7567-7574), 1529-2401 (Electronic) 0270-6474 (Linking)

Cai, H., Shim, H., Lai, C., Xie, C., Lin, X., Yang, W.J. & Chandran, J. (2008). ALS2/alsin knockout mice and motor neuron diseases. *Neurodegener Dis*, 5, 6, pp. (359-366), 1660-2862 (Electronic) 1660-2854 (Linking)

Caldero, J., Brunet, N., Tarabal, O., Piedrafita, L., Hereu, M., Ayala, V. & Esquerda, J.E. (2010). Lithium prevents excitotoxic cell death of motoneurons in organotypic slice cultures of spinal cord. *Neuroscience*, 165, 4, (Feb 17), pp. (1353-1369), 1873-7544 (Electronic) 0306-4522 (Linking)

Camu, W. & Henderson, C.E. (1992). Purification of embryonic rat motoneurons by panning on a monoclonal antibody to the low-affinity NGF receptor. *J Neurosci Methods*, 44, 1, (Aug), pp. (59-70), 0165-0270 (Print) 0165-0270 (Linking)

Carriedo, S.G., Yin, H.Z. & Weiss, J.H. (1996). Motor neurons are selectively vulnerable to AMPA/kainate receptor-mediated injury in vitro. *J Neurosci*, 16, 13, (Jul 1), pp. (4069-4079), 0270-6474 (Print) 0270-6474 (Linking)

Cashman, N.R., Durham, H.D., Blusztajn, J.K., Oda, K., Tabira, T., Shaw, I.T., Dahrouge, S. & Antel, J.P. (1992). Neuroblastoma x spinal cord (NSC) hybrid cell lines resemble developing motor neurons. *Dev Dyn*, 194, 3, (Jul), pp. (209-221), 1058-8388 (Print) 1058-8388 (Linking)

Chen, Y., Brew, B.J. & Guillemin, G.J. (2011). Characterization of the kynurenine pathway in NSC-34 cell line: implications for amyotrophic lateral sclerosis. *J Neurochem*, 118, 5, (Sep), pp. (816-825), 1471-4159 (Electronic) 0022-3042 (Linking)

Chen, Y.Z., Bennett, C.L., Huynh, H.M., Blair, I.P., Puls, I., Irobi, J., Dierick, I., Abel, A., Kennerson, M.L., Rabin, B.A., Nicholson, G.A., Auer-Grumbach, M., Wagner, K., De Jonghe, P., Griffin, J.W., Fischbeck, K.H., Timmerman, V., Cornblath, D.R. & Chance, P.F. (2004). DNA/RNA helicase gene mutations in a form of juvenile amyotrophic lateral sclerosis (ALS4). *Am J Hum Genet*, 74, 6, (Jun), pp. (1128-1135), 0002-9297 (Print) 0002-9297 (Linking)

Cook, S.A., Johnson, K.R., Bronson, R.T. & Davisson, M.T. (1995). Neuromuscular degeneration (nmd): a mutation on mouse chromosome 19 that causes motor neuron degeneration. *Mamm Genome*, 6, 3, (Mar), pp. (187-191), 0938-8990 (Print) 0938-8990 (Linking)

Corbo, M. & Hays, A.P. (1992). Peripherin and neurofilament protein coexist in spinal spheroids of motor neuron disease. *J Neuropathol Exp Neurol*, 51, 5, (Sep), pp. (531-537), 0022-3069 (Print) 0022-3069 (Linking)

Corona, J.C. & Tapia, R. (2007). Ca2+-permeable AMPA receptors and intracellular Ca2+ determine motoneuron vulnerability in rat spinal cord in vivo. *Neuropharmacology*, 52, 5, (Apr), pp. (1219-1228), 0028-3908 (Print) 0028-3908 (Linking)

Corrado, L., Del Bo, R., Castellotti, B., Ratti, A., Cereda, C., Penco, S., Soraru, G., Carlomagno, Y., Ghezzi, S., Pensato, V., Colombrita, C., Gagliardi, S., Cozzi, L., Orsetti, V., Mancuso, M., Siciliano, G., Mazzini, L., Comi, G.P., Gellera, C., Ceroni, M., D'Alfonso, S. & Silani, V. (2010). Mutations of FUS gene in sporadic amyotrophic lateral sclerosis. *J Med Genet*, 47, 3, (Mar), pp. (190-194), 1468-6244 (Electronic) 0022-2593 (Linking)

Corrado, L., Gagliardi, S., Carlomagno, Y., Mennini, T., Ticozzi, N., Mazzini, L., Silani, V., Cereda, C. & D'Alfonso, S. (2011). VPS54 genetic analysis in ALS Italian cohort. *Eur J Neurol*, 18, 4, (Apr), pp. (e41-42), 1468-1331 (Electronic) 1351-5101 (Linking)

Corrado, L., Ratti, A., Gellera, C., Buratti, E., Castellotti, B., Carlomagno, Y., Ticozzi, N., Mazzini, L., Testa, L., Taroni, F., Baralle, F.E., Silani, V. & D'Alfonso, S. (2009). High frequency of TARDBP gene mutations in Italian patients with amyotrophic lateral sclerosis. *Hum Mutat*, 30, 4, (Apr), pp. (688-694), 1098-1004 (Electronic) 1059-7794 (Linking)

Cote, F., Collard, J.F. & Julien, J.P. (1993). Progressive neuronopathy in transgenic mice expressing the human neurofilament heavy gene: a mouse model of amyotrophic lateral sclerosis. *Cell*, 73, 1, (Apr 9), pp. (35-46), 0092-8674 (Print) 0092-8674 (Linking)

Cox, G.A., Mahaffey, C.L. & Frankel, W.N. (1998). Identification of the mouse neuromuscular degeneration gene and mapping of a second site suppressor allele. *Neuron*, 21, 6, (Dec), pp. (1327-1337), 0896-6273 (Print) 0896-6273 (Linking)

Crowther, R.A. & Goedert, M. (2000). Abnormal tau-containing filaments in neurodegenerative diseases. *J Struct Biol*, 130, 2-3, (Jun), pp. (271-279), 1047-8477 (Print) 1047-8477 (Linking)

Dal Canto, M.C. & Gurney, M.E. (1994). Development of central nervous system pathology in a murine transgenic model of human amyotrophic lateral sclerosis. *Am J Pathol*, 145, 6, (Dec), pp. (1271-1279), 0002-9440 (Print) 0002-9440 (Linking)

Delobel, P., Flament, S., Hamdane, M., Delacourte, A., Vilain, J.P. & Buee, L. (2002). Modelling Alzheimer-specific abnormal Tau phosphorylation independently of GSK3beta and PKA kinase activities. *FEBS Lett*, 516, 1-3, (Apr 10), pp. (151-155), 0014-5793 (Print) 0014-5793 (Linking)

Deng, H.X., Hentati, A., Tainer, J.A., Iqbal, Z., Cayabyab, A., Hung, W.Y., Getzoff, E.D., Hu, P., Herzfeldt, B., Roos, R.P. & et al. (1993). Amyotrophic lateral sclerosis and structural defects in Cu,Zn superoxide dismutase. *Science*, 261, 5124, (Aug 20), pp. (1047-1051), 0036-8075 (Print) 0036-8075 (Linking)

Devon, R.S., Orban, P.C., Gerrow, K., Barbieri, M.A., Schwab, C., Cao, L.P., Helm, J.R., Bissada, N., Cruz-Aguado, R., Davidson, T.L., Witmer, J., Metzler, M., Lam, C.K., Tetzlaff, W., Simpson, E.M., McCaffery, J.M., El-Husseini, A.E., Leavitt, B.R. & Hayden, M.R. (2006). Als2-deficient mice exhibit disturbances in endosome trafficking associated with motor behavioral abnormalities. *Proc Natl Acad Sci U S A*, 103, 25, (Jun 20), pp. (9595-9600), 0027-8424 (Print) 0027-8424 (Linking)

Dickson, D.W., Josephs, K.A. & Amador-Ortiz, C. (2007). TDP-43 in differential diagnosis of motor neuron disorders. *Acta Neuropathol*, 114, 1, (Jul), pp. (71-79), 0001-6322 (Print) 0001-6322 (Linking)

Dimos, J.T., Rodolfa, K.T., Niakan, K.K., Weisenthal, L.M., Mitsumoto, H., Chung, W., Croft, G.F., Saphier, G., Leibel, R., Goland, R., Wichterle, H., Henderson, C.E. & Eggan, K. (2008). Induced pluripotent stem cells generated from patients with ALS can be differentiated into motor neurons. *Science*, 321, 5893, (Aug 29), pp. (1218-1221), 1095-9203 (Electronic) 0036-8075 (Linking)

Djabali, K., Zissopoulou, A., de Hoop, M.J., Georgatos, S.D. & Dotti, C.G. (1993). Peripherin expression in hippocampal neurons induced by muscle soluble factor(s). *J Cell Biol*, 123, 5, (Dec), pp. (1197-1206), 0021-9525 (Print) 0021-9525 (Linking)

Du, F., Qian, Z.M., Zhu, L., Wu, X.M., Qian, C., Chan, R. & Ke, Y. (2010). Purity, cell viability, expression of GFAP and bystin in astrocytes cultured by different procedures. *J Cell Biochem*, 109, 1, (Jan 1), pp. (30-37), 1097-4644 (Electronic) 0730-2312 (Linking)

Duchen, L.W. & Strich, S.J. (1968). An hereditary motor neurone disease with progressive denervation of muscle in the mouse: the mutant 'wobbler'. *J Neurol Neurosurg Psychiatry*, 31, 6, (Dec), pp. (535-542), 0022-3050 (Print) 0022-3050 (Linking)

Dupuis, L., Fergani, A., Braunstein, K.E., Eschbach, J., Holl, N., Rene, F., Gonzalez De Aguilar, J.L., Zoerner, B., Schwalenstocker, B., Ludolph, A.C. & Loeffler, J.P. (2009). Mice with a mutation in the dynein heavy chain 1 gene display sensory neuropathy but lack motor neuron disease. *Exp Neurol*, 215, 1, (Jan), pp. (146-152), 1090-2430 (Electronic) 0014-4886 (Linking)

Elder, G.A., Friedrich, V.L., Jr., Bosco, P., Kang, C., Gourov, A., Tu, P.H., Lee, V.M. & Lazzarini, R.A. (1998a). Absence of the mid-sized neurofilament subunit decreases axonal calibers, levels of light neurofilament (NF-L), and neurofilament content. *J Cell Biol*, 141, 3, (May 4), pp. (727-739), 0021-9525 (Print) 0021-9525 (Linking)

Elder, G.A., Friedrich, V.L., Jr., Kang, C., Bosco, P., Gourov, A., Tu, P.H., Zhang, B., Lee, V.M. & Lazzarini, R.A. (1998b). Requirement of heavy neurofilament subunit in the development of axons with large calibers. *J Cell Biol*, 143, 1, (Oct 5), pp. (195-205), 0021-9525 (Print) 0021-9525 (Linking)

Enayat, Z.E., Orrell, R.W., Claus, A., Ludolph, A., Bachus, R., Brockmuller, J., Ray-Chaudhuri, K., Radunovic, A., Shaw, C., Wilkinson, J. & et al. (1995). Two novel mutations in the gene for copper zinc superoxide dismutase in UK families with amyotrophic lateral sclerosis. *Hum Mol Genet*, 4, 7, (Jul), pp. (1239-1240), 0964-6906 (Print) 0964-6906 (Linking)

Escurat, M., Djabali, K., Gumpel, M., Gros, F. & Portier, M.M. (1990). Differential expression of two neuronal intermediate-filament proteins, peripherin and the low-molecular-mass neurofilament protein (NF-L), during the development of the rat. *J Neurosci*, 10, 3, (Mar), pp. (764-784), 0270-6474 (Print) 0270-6474 (Linking)

Estes, P.S., Boehringer, A., Zwick, R., Tang, J.E., Grigsby, B. & Zarnescu, D.C. (2011). Wild-type and A315T mutant TDP-43 exert differential neurotoxicity in a Drosophila model of ALS. *Hum Mol Genet*, 20, 12, (Jun 15), pp. (2308-2321), 1460-2083 (Electronic) 0964-6906 (Linking)

Eyer, J., Cleveland, D.W., Wong, P.C. & Peterson, A.C. (1998). Pathogenesis of two axonopathies does not require axonal neurofilaments. *Nature*, 391, 6667, (Feb 5), pp. (584-587), 0028-0836 (Print) 0028-0836 (Linking)

Eyer, J. & Peterson, A. (1994). Neurofilament-deficient axons and perikaryal aggregates in viable transgenic mice expressing a neurofilament-beta-galactosidase fusion protein. *Neuron*, 12, 2, (Feb), pp. (389-405), 0896-6273 (Print) 0896-6273 (Linking)

Eymard-Pierre, E., Yamanaka, K., Haeussler, M., Kress, W., Gauthier-Barichard, F., Combes, P., Cleveland, D.W. & Boespflug-Tanguy, O. (2006). Novel missense mutation in ALS2 gene results in infantile ascending hereditary spastic paralysis. *Ann Neurol*, 59, 6, (Jun), pp. (976-980), 0364-5134 (Print) 0364-5134 (Linking)

Falconer, D.S. (1956). Wobbler (wr). *Mouse News Letters*, 15, pp. (22),

Fang, D., Li, Z., Zhong-ming, Q., Mei, W.X., Ho, Y.W., Yuan, X.W. & Ya, K. (2008). Expression of bystin in reactive astrocytes induced by ischemia/reperfusion and chemical hypoxia in vitro. *Biochim Biophys Acta*, 1782, 11, (Nov), pp. (658-663), 0006-3002 (Print) 0006-3002 (Linking)

Feiguin, F., Godena, V.K., Romano, G., D'Ambrogio, A., Klima, R. & Baralle, F.E. (2009). Depletion of TDP-43 affects Drosophila motoneurons terminal synapsis and locomotive behavior. *FEBS Lett*, 583, 10, (May 19), pp. (1586-1592), 1873-3468 (Electronic) 0014-5793 (Linking)

Fukita, Y., Mizuta, T.R., Shirozu, M., Ozawa, K., Shimizu, A. & Honjo, T. (1993). The human S mu bp-2, a DNA-binding protein specific to the single-stranded guanine-rich sequence related to the immunoglobulin mu chain switch region. *J Biol Chem*, 268, 23, (Aug 15), pp. (17463-17470), 0021-9258 (Print) 0021-9258 (Linking)

Geser, F., Malunda, J.A., Hurtig, H.I., Duda, J.E., Wenning, G.K., Gilman, S., Low, P.A., Lee, V.M. & Trojanowski, J.Q. (2011). TDP-43 pathology occurs infrequently in multiple system atrophy. *Neuropathol Appl Neurobiol*, 37, 4, (Jun), pp. (358-365), 1365-2990 (Electronic)

Gingras, M., Gagnon, V., Minotti, S., Durham, H.D. & Berthod, F. (2007). Optimized protocols for isolation of primary motor neurons, astrocytes and microglia from embryonic mouse spinal cord. *J Neurosci Methods*, 163, 1, (Jun 15), pp. (111-118), 0165-0270 (Print) 0165-0270 (Linking)

Gitcho, M.A., Baloh, R.H., Chakraverty, S., Mayo, K., Norton, J.B., Levitch, D., Hatanpaa, K.J., White, C.L., 3rd, Bigio, E.H., Caselli, R., Baker, M., Al-Lozi, M.T., Morris, J.C., Pestronk, A., Rademakers, R., Goate, A.M. & Cairns, N.J. (2008). TDP-43 A315T mutation in familial motor neuron disease. *Ann Neurol*, 63, 4, (Apr), pp. (535-538), 1531-8249 (Electronic) 0364-5134 (Linking)

Gomes, C., Palma, A.S., Almeida, R., Regalla, M., McCluskey, L.F., Trojanowski, J.Q. & Costa, J. (2008). Establishment of a cell model of ALS disease: Golgi apparatus disruption occurs independently from apoptosis. *Biotechnol Lett*, 30, 4, (Apr), pp. (603-610), 0141-5492 (Print) 0141-5492 (Linking)

Gordon, R., Hogan, C.E., Neal, M.L., Anantharam, V., Kanthasamy, A.G. & Kanthasamy, A. (2011). A simple magnetic separation method for high-yield isolation of pure primary microglia. *J Neurosci Methods*, 194, 2, (Jan 15), pp. (287-296), 1872-678X (Electronic) 0165-0270 (Linking)

Gotz, J., Chen, F., van Dorpe, J. & Nitsch, R.M. (2001). Formation of neurofibrillary tangles in P301l tau transgenic mice induced by Abeta 42 fibrils. *Science*, 293, 5534, (Aug 24), pp. (1491-1495), 0036-8075 (Print) 0036-8075 (Linking)

Green, S.L., Bouley, D.M., Pinter, M.J., Cork, L.C. & Vatassery, G.T. (2001). Canine motor neuron disease: clinicopathologic features and selected indicators of oxidative stress. *J Vet Intern Med*, 15, 2, (Mar-Apr), pp. (112-119), 0891-6640 (Print) 0891-6640 (Linking)

Green, S.L., Tolwani, R.J., Varma, S., Quignon, P., Galibert, F. & Cork, L.C. (2002). Structure, chromosomal location, and analysis of the canine Cu/Zn superoxide dismutase (SOD1) gene. *J Hered*, 93, 2, (Mar-Apr), pp. (119-124), 0022-1503 (Print) 0022-1503 (Linking)

Green, S.L., Westendorf, J.M., Jaffe, H., Pant, H.C., Cork, L.C., Ostrander, E.A., Vignaux, F. & Ferrell, J.E., Jr. (2005). Allelic variants of the canine heavy neurofilament (NFH) subunit and extensive phosphorylation in dogs with motor neuron disease. *J Comp Pathol*, 132, 1, (Jan), pp. (33-50), 0021-9975 (Print) 0021-9975 (Linking)

Greenway, M.J., Andersen, P.M., Russ, C., Ennis, S., Cashman, S., Donaghy, C., Patterson, V., Swingler, R., Kieran, D., Prehn, J., Morrison, K.E., Green, A., Acharya, K.R., Brown, R.H., Jr. & Hardiman, O. (2006). ANG mutations segregate with familial and 'sporadic' amyotrophic lateral sclerosis. *Nat Genet*, 38, 4, (Apr), pp. (411-413), 1061-4036 (Print) 1061-4036 (Linking)

Guo, G. & Bhat, N.R. (2007). p38alpha MAP kinase mediates hypoxia-induced motor neuron cell death: a potential target of minocycline's neuroprotective action. *Neurochem Res*, 32, 12, (Dec), pp. (2160-2166), 0364-3190 (Print) 0364-3190 (Linking)

Guo, W., Chen, Y., Zhou, X., Kar, A., Ray, P., Chen, X., Rao, E.J., Yang, M., Ye, H., Zhu, L., Liu, J., Xu, M., Yang, Y., Wang, C., Zhang, D., Bigio, E.H., Mesulam, M., Shen, Y., Xu, Q., Fushimi, K. & Wu, J.Y. (2011). An ALS-associated mutation affecting TDP-43 enhances protein aggregation, fibril formation and neurotoxicity. *Nat Struct Mol Biol*, 18, 7, pp. (822-830), 1545-9985 (Electronic) 1545-9985 (Linking)

Gurney, M.E., Pu, H., Chiu, A.Y., Dal Canto, M.C., Polchow, C.Y., Alexander, D.D., Caliendo, J., Hentati, A., Kwon, Y.W., Deng, H.X. & et al. (1994). Motor neuron degeneration in mice that express a human Cu,Zn superoxide dismutase mutation. *Science*, 264, 5166, (Jun 17), pp. (1772-1775), 0036-8075 (Print) 0036-8075 (Linking)

Hadano, S., Hand, C.K., Osuga, H., Yanagisawa, Y., Otomo, A., Devon, R.S., Miyamoto, N., Showguchi-Miyata, J., Okada, Y., Singaraja, R., Figlewicz, D.A., Kwiatkowski, T., Hosler, B.A., Sagie, T., Skaug, J., Nasir, J., Brown, R.H., Jr., Scherer, S.W., Rouleau, G.A., Hayden, M.R. & Ikeda, J.E. (2001). A gene encoding a putative GTPase regulator is mutated in familial amyotrophic lateral sclerosis 2. *Nat Genet*, 29, 2, (Oct), pp. (166-173), 1061-4036 (Print) 1061-4036 (Linking)

Hadano, S., Otomo, A., Kunita, R., Suzuki-Utsunomiya, K., Akatsuka, A., Koike, M., Aoki, M., Uchiyama, Y., Itoyama, Y. & Ikeda, J.E. (2010a). Loss of ALS2/Alsin exacerbates motor dysfunction in a SOD1-expressing mouse ALS model by disturbing endolysosomal trafficking. *PLoS One*, 5, 3, pp. (e9805), 1932-6203 (Electronic) 1932-6203 (Linking)

Hadano, S., Yoshii, Y., Otomo, A., Kunita, R., Suzuki-Utsunomiya, K., Pan, L., Kakuta, S., Iwasaki, Y., Iwakura, Y. & Ikeda, J.E. (2010b). Genetic background and gender effects on gross phenotypes in congenic lines of ALS2/alsin-deficient mice. *Neurosci Res*, 68, 2, (Oct), pp. (131-136), 1872-8111 (Electronic) 0168-0102 (Linking)

Haghnia, M., Cavalli, V., Shah, S.B., Schimmelpfeng, K., Brusch, R., Yang, G., Herrera, C., Pilling, A. & Goldstein, L.S. (2007). Dynactin is required for coordinated bidirectional motility, but not for dynein membrane attachment. *Mol Biol Cell*, 18, 6, (Jun), pp. (2081-2089), 1059-1524 (Print) 1059-1524 (Linking)

Hall, E.D., Oostveen, J.A. & Gurney, M.E. (1998). Relationship of microglial and astrocytic activation to disease onset and progression in a transgenic model of familial ALS. *Glia*, 23, 3, (Jul), pp. (249-256), 0894-1491 (Print) 0894-1491 (Linking)

Hasegawa, M., Smith, M.J. & Goedert, M. (1998). Tau proteins with FTDP-17 mutations have a reduced ability to promote microtubule assembly. *FEBS Lett*, 437, 3, (Oct 23), pp. (207-210), 0014-5793 (Print) 0014-5793 (Linking)

Hirano, A. (1991). Cytopathology of amyotrophic lateral sclerosis. *Adv Neurol*, 56, pp. (91-101), 0091-3952 (Print) 0091-3952 (Linking)

Hirano, A., Nakano, I., Kurland, L.T., Mulder, D.W., Holley, P.W. & Saccomanno, G. (1984). Fine structural study of neurofibrillary changes in a family with amyotrophic lateral sclerosis. *J Neuropathol Exp Neurol*, 43, 5, (Sep), pp. (471-480), 0022-3069 (Print) 0022-3069 (Linking)

Hong, M., Zhukareva, V., Vogelsberg-Ragaglia, V., Wszolek, Z., Reed, L., Miller, B.I., Geschwind, D.H., Bird, T.D., McKeel, D., Goate, A., Morris, J.C., Wilhelmsen, K.C., Schellenberg, G.D., Trojanowski, J.Q. & Lee, V.M. (1998). Mutation-specific functional impairments in distinct tau isoforms of hereditary FTDP-17. *Science*, 282, 5395, (Dec 4), pp. (1914-1917), 0036-8075 (Print) 0036-8075 (Linking)

Hrabe de Angelis, M.H., Flaswinkel, H., Fuchs, H., Rathkolb, B., Soewarto, D., Marschall, S., Heffner, S., Pargent, W., Wuensch, K., Jung, M., Reis, A., Richter, T., Alessandrini, F., Jakob, T., Fuchs, E., Kolb, H., Kremmer, E., Schaeble, K., Rollinski, B., Roscher, A., Peters, C., Meitinger, T., Strom, T., Steckler, T., Holsboer, F., Klopstock, T., Gekeler, F., Schindewolf, C., Jung, T., Avraham, K., Behrendt, H., Ring, J., Zimmer, A., Schughart, K., Pfeffer, K., Wolf, E. & Balling, R. (2000). Genome-wide, large-scale production of mutant mice by ENU mutagenesis. *Nat Genet*, 25, 4, (Aug), pp. (444-447), 1061-4036 (Print) 1061-4036 (Linking)

Iaccarino, C., Mura, M.E., Esposito, S., Carta, F., Sanna, G., Turrini, F., Carri, M.T. & Crosio, C. (2011). Bcl2-A1 interacts with pro-caspase-3: Implications for amyotrophic lateral sclerosis. *Neurobiol Dis*, 43, 3, (Sep), pp. (642-650), 1095-953X (Electronic) 0969-9961 (Linking)

Ilieva, H.S., Yamanaka, K., Malkmus, S., Kakinohana, O., Yaksh, T., Marsala, M. & Cleveland, D.W. (2008). Mutant dynein (Loa) triggers proprioceptive axon loss that extends survival only in the SOD1 ALS model with highest motor neuron death. *Proc Natl Acad Sci U S A*, 105, 34, (Aug 26), pp. (12599-12604), 1091-6490 (Electronic) 0027-8424 (Linking)

Jacquier, A., Buhler, E., Schafer, M.K., Bohl, D., Blanchard, S., Beclin, C. & Haase, G. (2006). Alsin/Rac1 signaling controls survival and growth of spinal motoneurons. *Ann Neurol*, 60, 1, (Jul), pp. (105-117), 0364-5134 (Print) 0364-5134 (Linking)

Jonsson, P.A., Ernhill, K., Andersen, P.M., Bergemalm, D., Brannstrom, T., Gredal, O., Nilsson, P. & Marklund, S.L. (2004). Minute quantities of misfolded mutant superoxide dismutase-1 cause amyotrophic lateral sclerosis. *Brain*, 127, Pt 1, (Jan), pp. (73-88), 0006-8950 (Print) 0006-8950 (Linking)

Jonsson, P.A., Graffmo, K.S., Brannstrom, T., Nilsson, P., Andersen, P.M. & Marklund, S.L. (2006). Motor neuron disease in mice expressing the wild type-like D90A mutant superoxide dismutase-1. *J Neuropathol Exp Neurol*, 65, 12, (Dec), pp. (1126-1136), 0022-3069 (Print) 0022-3069 (Linking)

Kabashi, E., Bercier, V., Lissouba, A., Liao, M., Brustein, E., Rouleau, G.A. & Drapeau, P. (2011). FUS and TARDBP but Not SOD1 Interact in Genetic Models of Amyotrophic Lateral Sclerosis. *PLoS Genet*, 7, 8, (Aug), pp. (e1002214), 1553-7404 (Electronic) 1553-7390 (Linking)

Kabashi, E., Valdmanis, P.N., Dion, P., Spiegelman, D., McConkey, B.J., Vande Velde, C., Bouchard, J.P., Lacomblez, L., Pochigaeva, K., Salachas, F., Pradat, P.F., Camu, W., Meininger, V., Dupre, N. & Rouleau, G.A. (2008). TARDBP mutations in individuals with sporadic and familial amyotrophic lateral sclerosis. *Nat Genet*, 40, 5, (May), pp. (572-574), 1546-1718 (Electronic) 1061-4036 (Linking)

Kato, T., Hirano, A., Manaka, H., Sasaki, H., Katagiri, T., Kawanami, T., Shikama, Y. & Seino, T. (1991). Calcitonin gene-related peptide immunoreactivity in familial amyotrophic lateral sclerosis. *Neurosci Lett*, 133, 2, (Dec 9), pp. (163-167), 0304-3940 (Print) 0304-3940 (Linking)

Kaupmann, K., Simon-Chazottes, D., Guenet, J.L. & Jockusch, H. (1992). Wobbler, a mutation affecting motoneuron survival and gonadal functions in the mouse, maps to proximal chromosome 11. *Genomics*, 13, 1, (May), pp. (39-43), 0888-7543 (Print) 0888-7543 (Linking)

Kerr, D. & Khalili, K. (1991). A recombinant cDNA derived from human brain encodes a DNA binding protein that stimulates transcription of the human neurotropic virus JCV. *J Biol Chem*, 266, 24, (Aug 25), pp. (15876-15881), 0021-9258 (Print) 0021-9258 (Linking)

Kosuge, Y., Sekikawa-Nishida, K., Negi, H., Ishige, K. & Ito, Y. (2009). Characterization of chronic glutamate-mediated motor neuron toxicity in organotypic spinal cord culture prepared from ALS model mice. *Neurosci Lett*, 454, 2, (Apr 24), pp. (165-169), 0304-3940 (Print) 0304-3940 (Linking)

Kulshreshtha, D., Vijayalakshmi, K., Alladi, P.A., Sathyaprabha, T.N., Nalini, A. & Raju, T.R. (2011). Vascular endothelial growth factor attenuates neurodegenerative changes in the NSC-34 motor neuron cell line induced by cerebrospinal fluid of sporadic amyotrophic lateral sclerosis patients. *Neurodegener Dis*, 8, 5, pp. (322-330), 1660-2862 (Electronic) 1660-2854 (Linking)

Kunita, R., Otomo, A., Mizumura, H., Suzuki-Utsunomiya, K., Hadano, S. & Ikeda, J.E. (2007). The Rab5 activator ALS2/alsin acts as a novel Rac1 effector through Rac1-activated endocytosis. *J Biol Chem*, 282, 22, (Jun 1), pp. (16599-16611), 0021-9258 (Print) 0021-9258 (Linking)

Kwiatkowski, T.J., Jr., Bosco, D.A., Leclerc, A.L., Tamrazian, E., Vanderburg, C.R., Russ, C., Davis, A., Gilchrist, J., Kasarskis, E.J., Munsat, T., Valdmanis, P., Rouleau, G.A., Hosler, B.A., Cortelli, P., de Jong, P.J., Yoshinaga, Y., Haines, J.L., Pericak-Vance, M.A., Yan, J., Ticozzi, N., Siddique, T., McKenna-Yasek, D., Sapp, P.C., Horvitz, H.R., Landers, J.E. & Brown, R.H., Jr. (2009). Mutations in the FUS/TLS gene on chromosome 16 cause familial amyotrophic lateral sclerosis. *Science*, 323, 5918, (Feb 27), pp. (1205-1208), 1095-9203 (Electronic) 0036-8075 (Linking)

Lagier-Tourenne, C. & Cleveland, D.W. (2009). Rethinking ALS: the FUS about TDP-43. *Cell*, 136, 6, (Mar 20), pp. (1001-1004), 1097-4172 (Electronic) 0092-8674 (Linking)

Lai, C., Lin, X., Chandran, J., Shim, H., Yang, W.J. & Cai, H. (2007). The G59S mutation in p150(glued) causes dysfunction of dynactin in mice. *J Neurosci*, 27, 51, (Dec 19), pp. (13982-13990), 1529-2401 (Electronic) 0270-6474 (Linking)

Lai, C., Xie, C., McCormack, S.G., Chiang, H.C., Michalak, M.K., Lin, X., Chandran, J., Shim, H., Shimoji, M., Cookson, M.R., Huganir, R.L., Rothstein, J.D., Price, D.L., Wong, P.C., Martin, L.J., Zhu, J.J. & Cai, H. (2006). Amyotrophic lateral sclerosis 2-deficiency leads to neuronal degeneration in amyotrophic lateral sclerosis through altered AMPA receptor trafficking. *J Neurosci*, 26, 45, (Nov 8), pp. (11798-11806), 1529-2401 (Electronic) 0270-6474 (Linking)

Laird, F.M., Farah, M.H., Ackerley, S., Hoke, A., Maragakis, N., Rothstein, J.D., Griffin, J., Price, D.L., Martin, L.J. & Wong, P.C. (2008). Motor neuron disease occurring in a mutant dynactin mouse model is characterized by defects in vesicular trafficking. *J Neurosci*, 28, 9, (Feb 27), pp. (1997-2005), 1529-2401 (Electronic) 0270-6474 (Linking)

LaMonte, B.H., Wallace, K.E., Holloway, B.A., Shelly, S.S., Ascano, J., Tokito, M., Van Winkle, T., Howland, D.S. & Holzbaur, E.L. (2002). Disruption of dynein/dynactin inhibits axonal transport in motor neurons causing late-onset progressive degeneration. *Neuron*, 34, 5, (May 30), pp. (715-727), 0896-6273 (Print) 0896-6273 (Linking)

Lanson, N.A., Jr., Maltare, A., King, H., Smith, R., Kim, J.H., Taylor, J.P., Lloyd, T.E. & Pandey, U.B. (2011). A Drosophila model of FUS-related neurodegeneration reveals genetic interaction between FUS and TDP-43. *Hum Mol Genet*, 20, 13, (Jul 1), pp. (2510-2523), 1460-2083 (Electronic) 0964-6906 (Linking)

Lee, M.K., Marszalek, J.R. & Cleveland, D.W. (1994). A mutant neurofilament subunit causes massive, selective motor neuron death: implications for the pathogenesis of human motor neuron disease. *Neuron*, 13, 4, (Oct), pp. (975-988), 0896-6273 (Print) 0896-6273 (Linking)

Lemmens, R., Van Hoecke, A., Hersmus, N., Geelen, V., D'Hollander, I., Thijs, V., Van Den Bosch, L., Carmeliet, P. & Robberecht, W. (2007). Overexpression of mutant superoxide dismutase 1 causes a motor axonopathy in the zebrafish. *Hum Mol Genet*, 16, 19, (Oct 1), pp. (2359-2365), 0964-6906 (Print) 0964-6906 (Linking)

Lewis, J., McGowan, E., Rockwood, J., Melrose, H., Nacharaju, P., Van Slegtenhorst, M., Gwinn-Hardy, K., Paul Murphy, M., Baker, M., Yu, X., Duff, K., Hardy, J., Corral, A., Lin, W.L., Yen, S.H., Dickson, D.W., Davies, P. & Hutton, M. (2000). Neurofibrillary tangles, amyotrophy and progressive motor disturbance in mice expressing mutant (P301L) tau protein. *Nat Genet*, 25, 4, (Aug), pp. (402-405), 1061-4036 (Print) 1061-4036 (Linking)

Lunn, J.S., Sakowski, S.A., Kim, B., Rosenberg, A.A. & Feldman, E.L. (2009). Vascular endothelial growth factor prevents G93A-SOD1-induced motor neuron degeneration. *Dev Neurobiol*, 69, 13, (Nov), pp. (871-884), 1932-846X (Electronic) 1932-8451 (Linking)

Mackenzie, I.R., Rademakers, R. & Neumann, M. (2010). TDP-43 and FUS in amyotrophic lateral sclerosis and frontotemporal dementia. *Lancet Neurol*, 9, 10, (Oct), pp. (995-1007), 1474-4465 (Electronic) 1474-4422 (Linking)

Maragakis, N.J., Jackson, M., Ganel, R. & Rothstein, J.D. (2003). Topiramate protects against motor neuron degeneration in organotypic spinal cord cultures but not in G93A SOD1 transgenic mice. *Neurosci Lett*, 338, 2, (Feb 27), pp. (107-110), 0304-3940 (Print) 0304-3940 (Linking)

Marchetto, M.C., Muotri, A.R., Mu, Y., Smith, A.M., Cezar, G.G. & Gage, F.H. (2008). Non-cell-autonomous effect of human SOD1 G37R astrocytes on motor neurons derived from human embryonic stem cells. *Cell Stem Cell*, 3, 6, (Dec 4), pp. (649-657), 1875-9777 (Electronic)

Martin, N., Jaubert, J., Gounon, P., Salido, E., Haase, G., Szatanik, M. & Guenet, J.L. (2002). A missense mutation in Tbce causes progressive motor neuronopathy in mice. *Nat Genet*, 32, 3, (Nov), pp. (443-447), 1061-4036 (Print) 1061-4036 (Linking)

Maruyama, H., Morino, H., Ito, H., Izumi, Y., Kato, H., Watanabe, Y., Kinoshita, Y., Kamada, M., Nodera, H., Suzuki, H., Komure, O., Matsuura, S., Kobatake, K., Morimoto, N., Abe, K., Suzuki, N., Aoki, M., Kawata, A., Hirai, T., Kato, T., Ogasawara, K., Hirano, A., Takumi, T., Kusaka, H., Hagiwara, K., Kaji, R. & Kawakami, H. (2010). Mutations of optineurin in amyotrophic lateral sclerosis. *Nature*, 465, 7295, (May 13), pp. (223-226), 1476-4687 (Electronic) 0028-0836 (Linking)

Menzies, F.M., Cookson, M.R., Taylor, R.W., Turnbull, D.M., Chrzanowska-Lightowlers, Z.M., Dong, L., Figlewicz, D.A. & Shaw, P.J. (2002a). Mitochondrial dysfunction in a cell culture model of familial amyotrophic lateral sclerosis. *Brain*, 125, Pt 7, (Jul), pp. (1522-1533), 0006-8950 (Print) 0006-8950 (Linking)

Menzies, F.M., Grierson, A.J., Cookson, M.R., Heath, P.R., Tomkins, J., Figlewicz, D.A., Ince, P.G. & Shaw, P.J. (2002b). Selective loss of neurofilament expression in Cu/Zn superoxide dismutase (SOD1) linked amyotrophic lateral sclerosis. *J Neurochem*, 82, 5, (Sep), pp. (1118-1128), 0022-3042 (Print) 0022-3042 (Linking)

Migheli, A., Pezzulo, T., Attanasio, A. & Schiffer, D. (1993). Peripherin immunoreactive structures in amyotrophic lateral sclerosis. *Lab Invest*, 68, 2, (Feb), pp. (185-191), 0023-6837 (Print) 0023-6837 (Linking)

Millecamps, S., Salachas, F., Cazeneuve, C., Gordon, P., Bricka, B., Camuzat, A., Guillot-Noel, L., Russaouen, O., Bruneteau, G., Pradat, P.F., Le Forestier, N., Vandenberghe, N., Danel-Brunaud, V., Guy, N., Thauvin-Robinet, C., Lacomblez, L., Couratier, P., Hannequin, D., Seilhean, D., Le Ber, I., Corcia, P., Camu, W., Brice, A., Rouleau, G., LeGuern, E. & Meininger, V. (2010). SOD1, ANG, VAPB, TARDBP, and FUS mutations in familial amyotrophic lateral sclerosis: genotype-phenotype correlations. *J Med Genet*, 47, 8, (Aug), pp. (554-560), 1468-6244 (Electronic) 0022-2593 (Linking)

Muma, N.A., Hoffman, P.N., Slunt, H.H., Applegate, M.D., Lieberburg, I. & Price, D.L. (1990). Alterations in levels of mRNAs coding for neurofilament protein subunits during regeneration. *Exp Neurol*, 107, 3, (Mar), pp. (230-235), 0014-4886 (Print) 0014-4886 (Linking)

Munch, C., Rosenbohm, A., Sperfeld, A.D., Uttner, I., Reske, S., Krause, B.J., Sedlmeier, R., Meyer, T., Hanemann, C.O., Stumm, G. & Ludolph, A.C. (2005). Heterozygous

R1101K mutation of the DCTN1 gene in a family with ALS and FTD. *Ann Neurol*, 58, 5, (Nov), pp. (777-780), 0364-5134 (Print) 0364-5134 (Linking)

Munch, C., Sedlmeier, R., Meyer, T., Homberg, V., Sperfeld, A.D., Kurt, A., Prudlo, J., Peraus, G., Hanemann, C.O., Stumm, G. & Ludolph, A.C. (2004). Point mutations of the p150 subunit of dynactin (DCTN1) gene in ALS. *Neurology*, 63, 4, (Aug 24), pp. (724-726), 1526-632X (Electronic) 0028-3878 (Linking)

Nagai, M., Aoki, M., Miyoshi, I., Kato, M., Pasinelli, P., Kasai, N., Brown, R.H., Jr. & Itoyama, Y. (2001). Rats expressing human cytosolic copper-zinc superoxide dismutase transgenes with amyotrophic lateral sclerosis: associated mutations develop motor neuron disease. *J Neurosci*, 21, 23, (Dec 1), pp. (9246-9254), 1529-2401 (Electronic) 0270-6474 (Linking)

Nagai, M., Re, D.B., Nagata, T., Chalazonitis, A., Jessell, T.M., Wichterle, H. & Przedborski, S. (2007). Astrocytes expressing ALS-linked mutated SOD1 release factors selectively toxic to motor neurons. *Nat Neurosci*, 10, 5, (May), pp. (615-622), 1097-6256 (Print) 1097-6256 (Linking)

Nakashima, K., Watanabe, Y., Kuno, N., Nanba, E. & Takahashi, K. (1995). Abnormality of Cu/Zn superoxide dismutase (SOD1) activity in Japanese familial amyotrophic lateral sclerosis with two base pair deletion in the SOD1 gene. *Neurology*, 45, 5, (May), pp. (1019-1020), 0028-3878 (Print) 0028-3878 (Linking)

Newbery, H.J., Gillingwater, T.H., Dharmasaroja, P., Peters, J., Wharton, S.B., Thomson, D., Ribchester, R.R. & Abbott, C.M. (2005). Progressive loss of motor neuron function in wasted mice: effects of a spontaneous null mutation in the gene for the eEF1 A2 translation factor. *J Neuropathol Exp Neurol*, 64, 4, (Apr), pp. (295-303), 0022-3069 (Print) 0022-3069 (Linking)

Ni, M. & Aschner, M. (2010). Neonatal rat primary microglia: isolation, culturing, and selected applications. *Curr Protoc Toxicol*, Chapter 12, (Feb), pp. (Unit 12 17), 1934-9262 (Electronic) 1934-9254 (Linking)

Nishimura, A.L., Mitne-Neto, M., Silva, H.C., Richieri-Costa, A., Middleton, S., Cascio, D., Kok, F., Oliveira, J.R., Gillingwater, T., Webb, J., Skehel, P. & Zatz, M. (2004). A mutation in the vesicle-trafficking protein VAPB causes late-onset spinal muscular atrophy and amyotrophic lateral sclerosis. *Am J Hum Genet*, 75, 5, (Nov), pp. (822-831), 0002-9297 (Print) 0002-9297 (Linking)

Noto, Y., Shibuya, K., Sato, Y., Kanai, K., Misawa, S., Sawai, S., Mori, M., Uchiyama, T., Isose, S., Nasu, S., Sekiguchi, Y., Fujimaki, Y., Kasai, T., Tokuda, T., Nakagawa, M. & Kuwabara (2011)., S. Elevated CSF TDP-43 levels in amyotrophic lateral sclerosis: specificity, sensitivity, and a possible prognostic value. *Amyotroph Lateral Scler*, 12, 2, (Mar), pp. (140-143), 1471-180X (Electronic) 1471-180X (Linking)

Oosthuyse, B., Moons, L., Storkebaum, E., Beck, H., Nuyens, D., Brusselmans, K., Van Dorpe, J., Hellings, P., Gorselink, M., Heymans, S., Theilmeier, G., Dewerchin, M., Laudenbach, V., Vermylen, P., Raat, H., Acker, T., Vleminckx, V., Van Den Bosch, L., Cashman, N., Fujisawa, H., Drost, M.R., Sciot, R., Bruyninckx, F., Hicklin, D.J., Ince, C., Gressens, P., Lupu, F., Plate, K.H., Robberecht, W., Herbert, J.M., Collen, D. & Carmeliet, P. (2001). Deletion of the hypoxia-response element in the vascular endothelial growth factor promoter causes motor neuron degeneration. *Nat Genet*, 28, 2, (Jun), pp. (131-138), 1061-4036 (Print) 1061-4036 (Linking)

Orban, P., Devon, R.S., Hayden, M.R. & Leavitt, B.R. (2007). Chapter 15 Juvenile amyotrophic lateral sclerosis. *Handb Clin Neurol*, 82, pp. (301-312), 0072-9752 (Print) 0072-9752 (Linking)

Orlacchio, A., Babalini, C., Borreca, A., Patrono, C., Massa, R., Basaran, S., Munhoz, R.P., Rogaeva, E.A., St George-Hyslop, P.H., Bernardi, G. & Kawarai, T. (2010). SPATACSIN mutations cause autosomal recessive juvenile amyotrophic lateral sclerosis. *Brain*, 133, Pt 2, (Feb), pp. (591-598), 1460-2156 (Electronic) 0006-8950 (Linking)

Orsucci, D., Calsolaro, V., Mancuso, M. & Siciliano, G. (2009). Neuroprotective effects of tetracyclines: molecular targets, animal models and human disease. *CNS Neurol Disord Drug Targets*, 8, 3, (Jun), pp. (222-231), 1996-3181 (Electronic) 1871-5273 (Linking)

Parge, H.E., Hallewell, R.A. & Tainer, J.A. (1992). Atomic structures of wild-type and thermostable mutant recombinant human Cu,Zn superoxide dismutase. *Proc Natl Acad Sci U S A*, 89, 13, (Jul 1), pp. (6109-6113), 0027-8424 (Print) 0027-8424 (Linking)

Parysek, L.M. & Goldman, R.D. (1988). Distribution of a novel 57 kDa intermediate filament (IF) protein in the nervous system. *J Neurosci*, 8, 2, (Feb), pp. (555-563), 0270-6474 (Print) 0270-6474 (Linking)

Philips, T. & Robberecht, W. (2011). Neuroinflammation in amyotrophic lateral sclerosis: role of glial activation in motor neuron disease. *Lancet Neurol*, 10, 3, (Mar), pp. (253-263), 1474-4465 (Electronic) 1474-4422 (Linking)

Polymenidou, M., Lagier-Tourenne, C., Hutt, K.R., Huelga, S.C., Moran, J., Liang, T.Y., Ling, S.C., Sun, E., Wancewicz, E., Mazur, C., Kordasiewicz, H., Sedaghat, Y., Donohue, J.P., Shiue, L., Bennett, C.F., Yeo, G.W. & Cleveland, D.W. (2011). Long pre-mRNA depletion and RNA missplicing contribute to neuronal vulnerability from loss of TDP-43. *Nat Neurosci*, 14, 4, (Apr), pp. (459-468), 1546-1726 (Electronic) 1097-6256 (Linking)

Pramatarova, A., Goto, J., Nanba, E., Nakashima, K., Takahashi, K., Takagi, A., Kanazawa, I., Figlewicz, D.A. & Rouleau, G.A. (1994). A two basepair deletion in the SOD 1 gene causes familial amyotrophic lateral sclerosis. *Hum Mol Genet*, 3, 11, (Nov), pp. (2061-2062), 0964-6906 (Print) 0964-6906 (Linking)

Puls, I., Jonnakuty, C., LaMonte, B.H., Holzbaur, E.L., Tokito, M., Mann, E., Floeter, M.K., Bidus, K., Drayna, D., Oh, S.J., Brown, R.H., Jr., Ludlow, C.L. & Fischbeck, K.H. (2003). Mutant dynactin in motor neuron disease. *Nat Genet*, 33, 4, (Apr), pp. (455-456), 1061-4036 (Print) 1061-4036 (Linking)

Raimondi, A., Mangolini, A., Rizzardini, M., Tartari, S., Massari, S., Bendotti, C., Francolini, M., Borgese, N., Cantoni, L. & Pietrini, G. (2006). Cell culture models to investigate the selective vulnerability of motoneuronal mitochondria to familial ALS-linked G93ASOD1. *Eur J Neurosci*, 24, 2, (Jul), pp. (387-399), 0953-816X (Print) 0953-816X (Linking)

Rao, M.V., Houseweart, M.K., Williamson, T.L., Crawford, T.O., Folmer, J. & Cleveland, D.W. (1998). Neurofilament-dependent radial growth of motor axons and axonal organization of neurofilaments does not require the neurofilament heavy subunit (NF-H) or its phosphorylation. *J Cell Biol*, 143, 1, (Oct 5), pp. (171-181), 0021-9525 (Print) 0021-9525 (Linking)

Ripps, M.E., Huntley, G.W., Hof, P.R., Morrison, J.H. & Gordon, J.W. (1995). Transgenic mice expressing an altered murine superoxide dismutase gene provide an animal model of amyotrophic lateral sclerosis. *Proc Natl Acad Sci U S A*, 92, 3, (Jan 31), pp. (689-693), 0027-8424 (Print) 0027-8424 (Linking)

Rogers, D.C., Peters, J., Martin, J.E., Ball, S., Nicholson, S.J., Witherden, A.S., Hafezparast, M., Latcham, J., Robinson, T.L., Quilter, C.A. & Fisher, E.M. (2001). SHIRPA, a protocol for behavioral assessment: validation for longitudinal study of neurological dysfunction in mice. *Neurosci Lett*, 306, 1-2, (Jun 22), pp. (89-92), 0304-3940 (Print) 0304-3940 (Linking)

Rosen, D.R. (1993). Mutations in Cu/Zn superoxide dismutase gene are associated with familial amyotrophic lateral sclerosis. *Nature*, 364, 6435, (Jul 22), pp. (362), 0028-0836 (Print) 0028-0836 (Linking)

Rosen, D.R., Siddique, T., Patterson, D., Figlewicz, D.A., Sapp, P., Hentati, A., Donaldson, D., Goto, J., O'Regan, J.P., Deng, H.X. & et al. (1993). Mutations in Cu/Zn superoxide dismutase gene are associated with familial amyotrophic lateral sclerosis. *Nature*, 362, 6415, (Mar 4), pp. (59-62), 0028-0836 (Print) 0028-0836 (Linking)

Rothstein, J.D., Jin, L., Dykes-Hoberg, M. & Kuncl, R.W. (1993). Chronic inhibition of glutamate uptake produces a model of slow neurotoxicity. *Proc Natl Acad Sci U S A*, 90, 14, (Jul 15), pp. (6591-6595), 0027-8424 (Print) 0027-8424 (Linking)

Rothstein, J.D., Van Kammen, M., Levey, A.I., Martin, L.J. & Kuncl, R.W. (1995). Selective loss of glial glutamate transporter GLT-1 in amyotrophic lateral sclerosis. *Ann Neurol*, 38, 1, (Jul), pp. (73-84), 0364-5134 (Print) 0364-5134 (Linking)

Schmalbruch, H., Jensen, H.J., Bjaerg, M., Kamieniecka, Z. & Kurland, L. (1991). A new mouse mutant with progressive motor neuronopathy. *J Neuropathol Exp Neurol*, 50, 3, (May), pp. (192-204), 0022-3069 (Print) 0022-3069 (Linking)

Schnaar, R.I. & Schaffner, A.E. (1981). Separation of cell types from embryonic chicken and rat spinal cord: characterization of motoneuron-enriched fractions. *J Neurosci*, 1, 2, (Feb), pp. (204-217), 0270-6474 (Print) 0270-6474 (Linking)

Scozzafava, A. & Viezzoli, M.S. (1993). The role of the active site amino acid residues on the catalytic activity of Cu2Zn2SOD. *Mol Chem Neuropathol*, 19, 1-2, (May-Jun), pp. (193-204), 1044-7393 (Print) 1044-7393 (Linking)

Sebastiani, G., Durocher, D., Gros, P., Nemer, M. & Malo, D. (1995). Localization of the Catf1 transcription factor gene to mouse chromosome 19. *Mamm Genome*, 6, 2, (Feb), pp. (147-148), 0938-8990 (Print) 0938-8990 (Linking)

Shieh, S.Y., Stellrecht, C.M. & Tsai, M.J. (1995). Molecular characterization of the rat insulin enhancer-binding complex 3b2. Cloning of a binding factor with putative helicase motifs. *J Biol Chem*, 270, 37, (Sep 15), pp. (21503-21508), 0021-9258 (Print) 0021-9258 (Linking)

Shinder, G.A., Lacourse, M.C., Minotti, S. & Durham, H.D. (2001). Mutant Cu/Zn-superoxide dismutase proteins have altered solubility and interact with heat shock/stress proteins in models of amyotrophic lateral sclerosis. *J Biol Chem*, 276, 16, (Apr 20), pp. (12791-12796), 0021-9258 (Print) 0021-9258 (Linking)

Shultz, L.D., Sweet, H.O., Davisson, M.T. & Coman, D.R. (1982). 'Wasted', a new mutant of the mouse with abnormalities characteristic to ataxia telangiectasia. *Nature*, 297, 5865, (Jun 3), pp. (402-404), 0028-0836 (Print) 0028-0836 (Linking)

Skehel, P.A., Fabian-Fine, R. & Kandel, E.R. (2000). Mouse VAP33 is associated with the endoplasmic reticulum and microtubules. *Proc Natl Acad Sci U S A*, 97, 3, (Feb 1), pp. (1101-1106), 0027-8424 (Print) 0027-8424 (Linking)

Soussan, L., Burakov, D., Daniels, M.P., Toister-Achituv, M., Porat, A., Yarden, Y. & Elazar, Z. (1999). ERG30, a VAP-33-related protein, functions in protein transport mediated by COPI vesicles. *J Cell Biol*, 146, 2, (Jul 26), pp. (301-311), 0021-9525 (Print) 0021-9525 (Linking)

Sreedharan, J., Blair, I.P., Tripathi, V.B., Hu, X., Vance, C., Rogelj, B., Ackerley, S., Durnall, J.C., Williams, K.L., Buratti, E., Baralle, F., de Belleroche, J., Mitchell, J.D., Leigh, P.N., Al-Chalabi, A., Miller, C.C., Nicholson, G. & Shaw, C.E. (2008). TDP-43 mutations in familial and sporadic amyotrophic lateral sclerosis. *Science*, 319, 5870, (Mar 21), pp. (1668-1672), 1095-9203 (Electronic) 0036-8075 (Linking)

Stallings, N.R., Puttaparthi, K., Luther, C.M., Burns, D.K. & Elliott, J.L. (2010). Progressive motor weakness in transgenic mice expressing human TDP-43. *Neurobiol Dis*, 40, 2, (Nov), pp. (404-414), 1095-953X (Electronic) 0969-9961 (Linking)

Sterneck, E., Kaplan, D.R. & Johnson, P.F. (1996). Interleukin-6 induces expression of peripherin and cooperates with Trk receptor signaling to promote neuronal differentiation in PC12 cells. *J Neurochem*, 67, 4, (Oct), pp. (1365-1374), 0022-3042 (Print) 0022-3042 (Linking)

Stoppini, L., Buchs, P.A. & Muller, D. (1991). A simple method for organotypic cultures of nervous tissue. *J Neurosci Methods*, 37, 2, (Apr), pp. (173-182), 0165-0270 (Print) 0165-0270 (Linking)

Storkebaum, E., Lambrechts, D. & Carmeliet, P. (2004). VEGF: once regarded as a specific angiogenic factor, now implicated in neuroprotection. *Bioessays*, 26, 9, (Sep), pp. (943-954), 0265-9247 (Print) 0265-9247 (Linking)

Strong, M.J. (2003). The basic aspects of therapeutics in amyotrophic lateral sclerosis. *Pharmacol Ther*, 98, 3, (Jun), pp. (379-414), 0163-7258 (Print) 0163-7258 (Linking)

Strong, M.J. & Volkening, K. (2011). TDP-43 and FUS/TLS: Sending a complex message about messenger RNA in Amyotrophic Lateral Sclerosis? *FEBS J*, (Aug 2), 1742-4658 (Electronic) 1742-464X (Linking)

Sugai, F., Yamamoto, Y., Miyaguchi, K., Zhou, Z., Sumi, H., Hamasaki, T., Goto, M. & Sakoda, S. (2004). Benefit of valproic acid in suppressing disease progression of ALS model mice. *Eur J Neurosci*, 20, 11, (Dec), pp. (3179-3183), 0953-816X (Print) 0953-816X (Linking)

Tainer, J.A., Getzoff, E.D., Beem, K.M., Richardson, J.S. & Richardson, D.C. (1982). Determination and analysis of the 2 A-structure of copper, zinc superoxide dismutase. *J Mol Biol*, 160, 2, (Sep 15), pp. (181-217), 0022-2836 (Print) 0022-2836 (Linking)

Tolosa, L., Mir, M., Asensio, V.J., Olmos, G. & Llado, J. (2008). Vascular endothelial growth factor protects spinal cord motoneurons against glutamate-induced excitotoxicity via phosphatidylinositol 3-kinase. *J Neurochem*, 105, 4, (May), pp. (1080-1090), 1471-4159 (Electronic) 0022-3042 (Linking)

Troy, C.M., Muma, N.A., Greene, L.A., Price, D.L. & Shelanski, M.L. (1990). Regulation of peripherin and neurofilament expression in regenerating rat motor neurons. *Brain Res*, 529, 1-2, (Oct 8), pp. (232-238), 0006-8993 (Print) 0006-8993 (Linking)

Tudor, E.L., Galtrey, C.M., Perkinton, M.S., Lau, K.F., De Vos, K.J., Mitchell, J.C., Ackerley, S., Hortobagyi, T., Vamos, E., Leigh, P.N., Klasen, C., McLoughlin, D.M., Shaw, C.E. & Miller, C.C. (2010). Amyotrophic lateral sclerosis mutant vesicle-associated membrane protein-associated protein-B transgenic mice develop TAR-DNA-binding protein-43 pathology. *Neuroscience*, 167, 3, (May 19), pp. (774-785), 1873-7544 (Electronic) 0306-4522 (Linking)

Van Damme, P., Van Den Bosch, L., Van Houtte, E., Callewaert, G. & Robberecht, W. (2002). GluR2-dependent properties of AMPA receptors determine the selective vulnerability of motor neurons to excitotoxicity. *J Neurophysiol*, 88, 3, (Sep), pp. (1279-1287), 0022-3077 (Print) 0022-3077 (Linking)

Van Deerlin, V.M., Leverenz, J.B., Bekris, L.M., Bird, T.D., Yuan, W., Elman, L.B., Clay, D., Wood, E.M., Chen-Plotkin, A.S., Martinez-Lage, M., Steinbart, E., McCluskey, L., Grossman, M., Neumann, M., Wu, I.L., Yang, W.S., Kalb, R., Galasko, D.R., Montine, T.J., Trojanowski, J.Q., Lee, V.M., Schellenberg, G.D. & Yu, C.E. (2008). TARDBP mutations in amyotrophic lateral sclerosis with TDP-43 neuropathology: a genetic and histopathological analysis. *Lancet Neurol*, 7, 5, (May), pp. (409-416), 1474-4422 (Print) 1474-4422 (Linking)

Vance, C., Rogelj, B., Hortobagyi, T., De Vos, K.J., Nishimura, A.L., Sreedharan, J., Hu, X., Smith, B., Ruddy, D., Wright, P., Ganesalingam, J., Williams, K.L., Tripathi, V., Al-Saraj, S., Al-Chalabi, A., Leigh, P.N., Blair, I.P., Nicholson, G., de Belleroche, J., Gallo, J.M., Miller, C.C. & Shaw, C.E. (2009). Mutations in FUS, an RNA processing protein, cause familial amyotrophic lateral sclerosis type 6. *Science*, 323, 5918, (Feb 27), pp. (1208-1211), 1095-9203 (Electronic) 0036-8075 (Linking)

Vercelli, A., Mereuta, O.M., Garbossa, D., Muraca, G., Mareschi, K., Rustichelli, D., Ferrero, I., Mazzini, L., Madon, E. & Fagioli, F. (2008). Human mesenchymal stem cell transplantation extends survival, improves motor performance and decreases neuroinflammation in mouse model of amyotrophic lateral sclerosis. *Neurobiol Dis*, 31, 3, (Sep), pp. (395-405), 1095-953X (Electronic) 0969-9961 (Linking)

Vogelsberg-Ragaglia, V., Bruce, J., Richter-Landsberg, C., Zhang, B., Hong, M., Trojanowski, J.Q. & Lee, V.M. (2000). Distinct FTDP-17 missense mutations in tau produce tau aggregates and other pathological phenotypes in transfected CHO cells. *Mol Biol Cell*, 11, 12, (Dec), pp. (4093-4104), 1059-1524 (Print) 1059-1524 (Linking)

Wang, F.C., Bouquiaux, O., De Pasqua, V. & Delwaide, P.J. (2002). Changes in motor unit numbers in patients with ALS: a longitudinal study using the adapted multiple point stimulation method. *Amyotroph Lateral Scler Other Motor Neuron Disord*, 3, 1, (Mar), pp. (31-38), 1466-0822 (Print) 1466-0822 (Linking)

Wang, J., Farr, G.W., Hall, D.H., Li, F., Furtak, K., Dreier, L. & Horwich, A.L. (2009). An ALS-linked mutant SOD1 produces a locomotor defect associated with aggregation and synaptic dysfunction when expressed in neurons of Caenorhabditis elegans. *PLoS Genet*, 5, 1, (Jan), pp. (e1000350), 1553-7404 (Electronic) 1553-7390 (Linking)

Wang, J., Slunt, H., Gonzales, V., Fromholt, D., Coonfield, M., Copeland, N.G., Jenkins, N.A. & Borchelt, D.R. (2003). Copper-binding-site-null SOD1 causes ALS in transgenic mice: aggregates of non-native SOD1 delineate a common feature. *Hum Mol Genet*, 12, 21, (Nov 1), pp. (2753-2764), 0964-6906 (Print) 0964-6906 (Linking)

Wang, J., Xu, G., Li, H., Gonzales, V., Fromholt, D., Karch, C., Copeland, N.G., Jenkins, N.A. & Borchelt, D.R. (2005). Somatodendritic accumulation of misfolded SOD1-L126Z in motor neurons mediates degeneration: alphaB-crystallin modulates aggregation. *Hum Mol Genet*, 14, 16, (Aug 15), pp. (2335-2347), 0964-6906 (Print) 0964-6906 (Linking)

Watanabe, Y., Kuno, N., Kono, Y., Nanba, E., Ohama, E., Nakashima, K. & Takahashi, K. (1997). Absence of the mutant SOD1 in familial amyotrophic lateral sclerosis (FALS) with two base pair deletion in the SOD1 gene. *Acta Neurol Scand*, 95, 3, (Mar), pp. (167-172), 0001-6314 (Print) 0001-6314 (Linking)

Watanabe, Y., Yasui, K., Nakano, T., Doi, K., Fukada, Y., Kitayama, M., Ishimoto, M., Kurihara, S., Kawashima, M., Fukuda, H., Adachi, Y., Inoue, T. & Nakashima, K. (2005). Mouse motor neuron disease caused by truncated SOD1 with or without C-terminal modification. *Brain Res Mol Brain Res*, 135, 1-2, (Apr 27), pp. (12-20), 0169-328X (Print) 0169-328X (Linking)

Wegorzewska, I., Bell, S., Cairns, N.J., Miller, T.M. & Baloh, R.H. (2009). TDP-43 mutant transgenic mice develop features of ALS and frontotemporal lobar degeneration. *Proc Natl Acad Sci U S A*, 106, 44, (Nov 3), pp. (18809-18814), 1091-6490 (Electronic) 0027-8424 (Linking)

Wiese, S., Herrmann, T., Drepper, C., Jablonka, S., Funk, N., Klausmeyer, A., Rogers, M.L., Rush, R. & Sendtner, M. (2010). Isolation and enrichment of embryonic mouse motoneurons from the lumbar spinal cord of individual mouse embryos. *Nat Protoc*, 5, 1, pp. (31-38), 1750-2799 (Electronic) 1750-2799 (Linking)

Williamson, T.L., Bruijn, L.I., Zhu, Q., Anderson, K.L., Anderson, S.D., Julien, J.P. & Cleveland, D.W. (1998). Absence of neurofilaments reduces the selective vulnerability of motor neurons and slows disease caused by a familial amyotrophic lateral sclerosis-linked superoxide dismutase 1 mutant. *Proc Natl Acad Sci U S A*, 95, 16, (Aug 4), pp. (9631-9636), 0027-8424 (Print) 0027-8424 (Linking)

Wils, H., Kleinberger, G., Janssens, J., Pereson, S., Joris, G., Cuijt, I., Smits, V., Ceuterick-de Groote, C., Van Broeckhoven, C. & Kumar-Singh, S. (2010). TDP-43 transgenic mice develop spastic paralysis and neuronal inclusions characteristic of ALS and frontotemporal lobar degeneration. *Proc Natl Acad Sci U S A*, 107, 8, (Feb 23), pp. (3858-3863), 1091-6490 (Electronic) 0027-8424 (Linking)

Wong, P.C., Pardo, C.A., Borchelt, D.R., Lee, M.K., Copeland, N.G., Jenkins, N.A., Sisodia, S.S., Cleveland, D.W. & Price, D.L. (1995). An adverse property of a familial ALS-linked SOD1 mutation causes motor neuron disease characterized by vacuolar degeneration of mitochondria. *Neuron*, 14, 6, (Jun), pp. (1105-1116), 0896-6273 (Print) 0896-6273 (Linking)

Xiao, S., Sanelli, T., Dib, S., Sheps, D., Findlater, J., Bilbao, J., Keith, J., Zinman, L., Rogaeva, E. & Robertson, J. (2011). RNA targets of TDP-43 identified by UV-CLIP are deregulated in ALS. *Mol Cell Neurosci*, 47, 3, (Jul), pp. (167-180), 1095-9327 (Electronic) 1044-7431 (Linking)

Xu, Y.F., Gendron, T.F., Zhang, Y.J., Lin, W.L., D'Alton, S., Sheng, H., Casey, M.C., Tong, J., Knight, J., Yu, X., Rademakers, R., Boylan, K., Hutton, M., McGowan, E., Dickson,

D.W., Lewis, J. & Petrucelli, L. (2010). Wild-type human TDP-43 expression causes TDP-43 phosphorylation, mitochondrial aggregation, motor deficits, and early mortality in transgenic mice. *J Neurosci*, 30, 32, (Aug 11), pp. (10851-10859), 1529-2401 (Electronic) 0270-6474 (Linking)

Xu, Z., Cork, L.C., Griffin, J.W. & Cleveland, D.W. (1993). Increased expression of neurofilament subunit NF-L produces morphological alterations that resemble the pathology of human motor neuron disease. *Cell*, 73, 1, (Apr 9), pp. (23-33), 0092-8674 (Print) 0092-8674 (Linking)

Yamanaka, K., Miller, T.M., McAlonis-Downes, M., Chun, S.J. & Cleveland, D.W. (2006). Progressive spinal axonal degeneration and slowness in ALS2-deficient mice. *Ann Neurol*, 60, 1, (Jul), pp. (95-104), 0364-5134 (Print) 0364-5134 (Linking)

Yip, P.K., Kaan, T.K., Fenesan, D. & Malcangio, M. (2009). Rapid isolation and culture of primary microglia from adult mouse spinal cord. *J Neurosci Methods*, 183, 2, (Oct 15), pp. (223-237), 1872-678X (Electronic) 0165-0270 (Linking)

Yokoseki, A., Shiga, A., Tan, C.F., Tagawa, A., Kaneko, H., Koyama, A., Eguchi, H., Tsujino, A., Ikeuchi, T., Kakita, A., Okamoto, K., Nishizawa, M., Takahashi, H. & Onodera, O. (2008). TDP-43 mutation in familial amyotrophic lateral sclerosis. *Ann Neurol*, 63, 4, (Apr), pp. (538-542), 1531-8249 (Electronic) 0364-5134 (Linking)

Zhou, H., Huang, C., Chen, H., Wang, D., Landel, C.P., Xia, P.Y., Bowser, R., Liu, Y.J. & Xia, X.G. (2010). Transgenic rat model of neurodegeneration caused by mutation in the TDP gene. *PLoS Genet*, 6, 3, (Mar), pp. (e1000887), 1553-7404 (Electronic) 1553-7390 (Linking)

Zhu, Q., Couillard-Despres, S. & Julien, J.P. (1997). Delayed maturation of regenerating myelinated axons in mice lacking neurofilaments. *Exp Neurol*, 148, 1, (Nov), pp. (299-316), 0014-4886 (Print) 0014-4886 (Linking)

Part 2

Signalling Pathways and Molecular Pathophysiology

8

Mutant Cu/Zn-Superoxide Dismutase Induced Mitochondrial Dysfunction in Amyotrophic Lateral Sclerosis

Jari Koistinaho and Gundars Goldsteins
A.I.Virtanen Institute for Molecular Sciences, University of Eastern Finland, Finland

1. Introduction

Mutations in Cu/Zn superoxide dismutase (SOD1) gene are linked to the motor neuron death in familial amyotrophic lateral sclerosis (FALS). More than 100 missense mutations have been described to cause the disease and are distributed throughout the whole 153 amino acid sequence of SOD1 molecule (Valentine et al., 2005; Boillée et al., 2006). Mutant SOD1 molecules can be grouped according to their biochemical characteristics into wild type-like proteins, that bind metal ions and possess enzymatic dismutase activity (e.g. G93A-SOD1 and G37R-SOD1), and mutant molecules with impaired metal binding capacity, which have significantly reduced dismutase activity (e.g. G85R-SOD1) (Valentine et al., 2005). Therefore, the toxicity of mutant SOD1 is not thought to be mediated by a lack of dismutase activity, but rather by gain of one or more detrimental functions.

The exact nature of the toxic gain of function for mutant SOD1 has not been identified yet. Most of the studies demonstrate a link between the disease pathology and increased oxidative stress. Augmented generation of free radicals and reactive oxygen species (ROS) is thought to be a major contributor to the destruction of motor neurons (Beckman et al., 1994; Wiedau-Pazos et al., 1996; Estévez et al., 1999).

The suggested toxic mechanisms include aberrant mutant SOD1 enzymatic activities (Beckman et al., 1993; Wiedau-Pazos et al., 1996) as well as destabilized SOD1 protein misfolding, causing enhanced aggregation of SOD1 or pathological interaction of SOD1 with other proteins (Stathopulos et al., 2003; Liu et al., 2004).

In a number of studies mitochondrial localization of mutant SOD1 has been implicated in ALS pathogenesis (Liu et al., 2004; Vijayvergiya et al., 2005; Bergemalm et al., 2006; Deng et al., 2006; Ferri et al., 2006) and increased recruitment of mutant SOD1 into mitochondria in the spinal cord might be a reason for death of motor neurons in some forms of familial ALS. However, the detailed mechanisms for toxicity of the mitochondria resident mutant SOD1 are not entirely clear yet. Here we review the current state of the art in the studies on mitochondrial toxicity of SOD1 in ALS.

2. Factors controlling SOD1 translocation to mitochondria and SOD1 activity in mitochondrial intermembrane space

Although the majority of SOD1 is present in the cytosol (Okado-Matsumoto & Fridovich, 2001), a fraction of SOD1 is translocated into the mitochondrial intermembrane space (IMS)

(Sturtz et al., 2001; Higgins et al., 2002). Since SOD1 does not contain mitochondrial targeting sequence, the true physiological function of SOD1 in the IMS remains mostly enigmatic.

In mammalian cells the mitochondrial localization of SOD1 is regulated by the folding state of this enzyme, depending on the intracellular distribution of copper chaperone for SOD1 (CCS), which in turn is regulated by oxygen concentration. Redox status of the cysteine residues in human SOD1 is critical for its retention in mitochondria. The cysteine residues form intramolecular disulphide bonds and interact with CCS (Kawamata & Manfredi, 2008). This regulation appears to be impaired for SOD1 mutants, which can lead to misfolding and aggregation of mutant SOD1 and eventually result in SOD1 accumulation inside the mitochondria. In animal models the mitochondrial association of mutant SOD1 is apparent even before the disease onset (Liu et al., 2004), indicating a causative link of mitochondrial SOD1 to the initiation of pathology.

Even though SOD1 has been suggested to be an important part of the mitochondrial superoxide scavenging system, as previously demonstrated in the yeast (Sturtz et al., 2001) and rat (Iñarrea et al., 2005) mitochondrion IMS, SOD1 activity is kept under redox control in this compartment and undergoes activation upon increased hydroperoxide concentration (Iñarrea et al., 2005).

There are 4 cysteines in the human SOD1 molecule, located at 6, 57, 111 and 144 position of the sequence. The intramolecular disulphide bridge between Cys57 and Cys146 is required for the proper tertiary and quaternary structure and enzymatic activity of SOD1 (Arnesano et al., 2004). Diminished copper loading and reduced intramolecular disulphide bound has been thought to be responsible for increased aggregation potential of G93A and D90A mutant SOD1 (Jonsson et al., 2006).

The maturation and activation of SOD1 in the cytosol is controlled by a number of factors and can be divided in several principal steps. Upon post-translational activation, an SOD1 monomer binds a Zn^{2+} ion. Next ,CCS transiently binds to SOD1 monomer and inserts a Cu^{2+} ion in the molecule (Culotta et al., 1997; Casareno et al., 1998). After the dissociation of SOD1 from CCS, oxidative formation of disulphide bounds takes place (Arnesano et al., 2004; Ding & Dokholyan, 2008), which is followed by dimerisation yielding an active SOD1 molecule (Vonk et al., 2010).

Active SOD1 dimers are not capable of entering mitochondria, in contrast to disulphide reduced apo-SOD1. According to the model proposed (Kawamata & Manfredi, 2008; Reddehase et al., 2009), CCS is first imported into mitochondria by interaction with Mia40, an IMS component critical for protein import to mitochondria. The CCS-Mia40 complex is formed through an intermolecular disulphide bound (Fig. 1.). Further disulphide rearrangement generates oxidized CCS, preventing its escape from the IMS. The activation of SOD1 in IMS is thought to be similar to the activation of SOD1 in cytosol, where SOD1 binds to CCS in the presence of Cu^{2+} ions and oxygen generating an active enzyme retained in IMS (Leitch et al., 2009).

Surprisingly, CCS overexpression in G93A-SOD1 mouse, a widely used transgenic mouse model of ALS, produces severe mitochondrial pathology and accelerates disease course (Son et al., 2007). According to the model above, the potentiation of mutant SOD1 toxicity by CCS overexpression can be explained by the CCS-mediated increase in SOD1 mitochondrial import, leading to enhanced SOD1 aggregation.

In contrast to the model of CCS-dependent activation of mitochondrial SOD1, a number of recent studies suggest that SOD1 in the IMS of intact mitochondria is mostly inactive and an oxidative modification of its critical thiol groups is necessary for the activation (Iñarrea et al., 2005, 2011; Goldsteins et al., 2008). This activation, at least partly, depends on protein disulphide isomerase (PDI) activity (Iñarrea et al., 2005). On the other hand, the toxicity of mutant SOD1 is not correlated with its aggregation potential but with the ability to form active dimeric molecules (Witan et al., 2008). These findings are in concert with a concept that mitochondrial dysfunction and cell damage are paradoxically induced by SOD1-mediated hydroperoxide production in the IMS (Goldsteins et al., 2008).

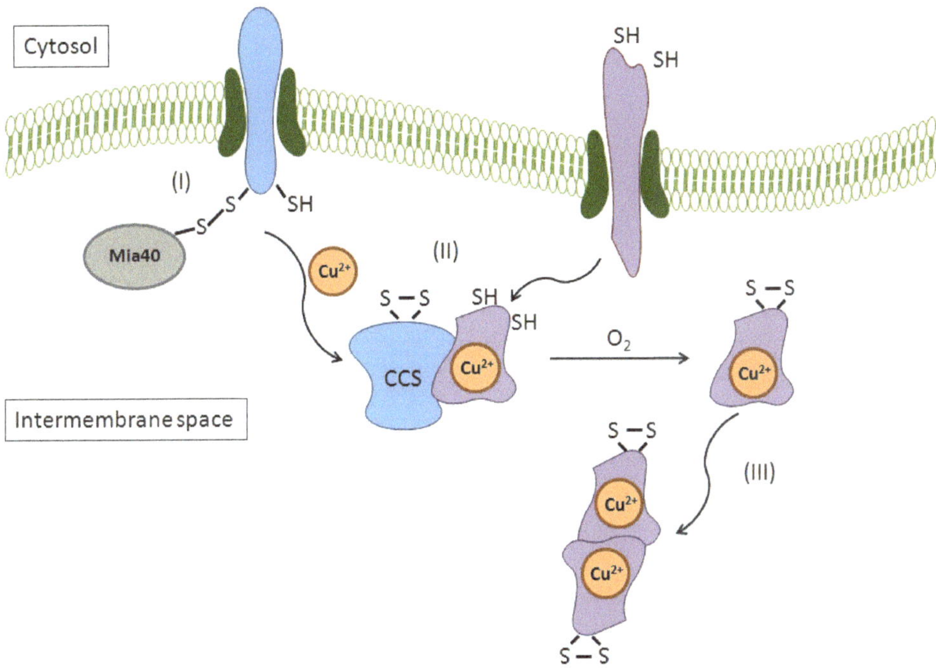

Fig. 1. Import and activation of SOD1 in IMS. CCS is imported into mitochondria through formation of a complex with Mia40 (I). Disulphide-reduced SOD1 monomer enters IMS and acquires copper ion (Cu^{2+}) with a help of CCS (II). Formation of intramolecular disulphide bound and dimerisation of SOD1 creates an active SOD1 molecule retained in IMS (III).

3. Proposed mechanisms for mutant SOD1 toxicity in mitochondria

Mitochondrial abnormalities and degeneration of motor neurons are early signs of ALS disease (Wong et al., 1995; Dal Canto & Gurney, 1997; Kong & Xu, 1998). They also represent pathological hallmarks in mutant SOD1 transgenic animal models for FALS as well as in patients with sporadic ALS (Kong & Xu, 1998; Mattiazzi et al., 2002; Manfredi & Xu, 2005). Mitochondrial toxicity may thus be an important factor in the degeneration of motor neurons. The pathology, demonstrated in sporadic ALS cases includes mitochondrial aggregates, mitochondrion swelling and increased calcium levels in mitochondria (Atsumi, 1981; Siklós et al., 1996). In G93A-SOD1 transgenic mice the disease onset is associated with a remarkable increase of vacuolated mitochondria in motor neurons (Kong & Xu, 1998). It has been proposed that formation of vacuoles originates from the expansion of mitochondrial IMS and degeneration of mitochondrial matrix (Jaarsma et al., 2001; Bendotti et al., 2001; Higgins et al., 2003; Xu et al., 2004).

Currently, there is no consensus on how mutant SOD1 causes mitochondrial pathology. The proposed mechanisms for mitochondrial toxicity of mutant SOD1 are summarized in Table 1. Among other toxic mechanisms reduced activities of respiratory complexes (Browne et al., 1998), mitochondrial depolarization and impaired calcium homeostasis (Kruman et al., 1999) have been demonstrated in the spinal cord of G93A-SOD1 mice. The observed dysfunctions of mitochondria might be caused by the recruitment of mutant SOD1, which has been shown to be selective to spinal cord mitochondria (Stathopulos et al., 2003; Liu et al., 2004; Pasinelli et al., 2004).

TOXIC MECHANISM	REFERENCES
Aggregate accumulation in mitochondria	(Higgins et al., 2002; Vande Velde et al., 2008)
Aberrant mutant SOD1 enzymatic activities, causing ROS production	(Estévez et al., 1999; Elliott, 2001)
Impaired energy metabolism	(Siciliano et al., 2001; Mattiazzi et al., 2002)
Impaired Ca^{2+} buffering	(Jaiswal & Keller, 2009; Grosskreutz et al., 2010)
Gain in pro-apoptotic function	(Pasinelli et al., 2004)
Interfering with mitochondrial protein import	(Liu et al., 2004)
Increased hydroperoxide production in IMS	(Goldsteins et al., 2008)

Table 1. Proposed mechanisms for mitochondrial toxicity of mutant SOD1

Among the proposed mechanisms, impairment of mitochondrial calcium buffering capacity has been shown in motor neurons of transgenic ALS mice (Damiano et al., 2006). On the other hand, ATP levels have been reported to be diminished in spinal cords of mutant SOD1 mouse model (Mattiazzi et al., 2002). Another view to the mitochondrial toxicity of mutant SOD1 was brought up by Vande Velde et al., who demonstrated that misfolded mutant SOD1 damages mitochondria by its deposition onto the cytoplasmic side of the outer membrane of spinal cord mitochondria (Vande Velde et al., 2008).

Other studies have demonstrated that the increased dismutase activity in rodent ALS models expressing mutant SOD1 paradoxically boosts the production of toxic ROS in the IMS (Goldsteins et al., 2008). It was shown that in a G93A-SOD1 rat model of ALS, the stability and quaternary structure of mutant SOD1 are lost most prominently in the spinal cord already several weeks before the onset of the disease (Ahtoniemi et al., 2008). These results suggest that destabilization of mutant SOD1 is associated with its increased binding to the inner mitochondrial membrane and elevated ROS production in the IMS. (Liu et al., 2004; Kirkinezos et al., 2005; Ahtoniemi et al., 2008).

Importantly, it was also recently demonstrated, that disulphide-reduced apo-SOD1 can rapidly initiate SOD1 fibrillation upon physiological conditions, suggesting that such disulphide-reduced apo-SOD1 may act as a seed for the amyloid like aggregates originating from the destabilized and folding intermediates of mutant SOD1 (Chattopadhyay et al., 2008).

Despite of rather different mechanisms proposed for the toxic properties of mutant SOD1 in mitochondria, most of the recent studies document that mitochondrial dysfunction results in increased ROS production (Beretta et al., 2003). Mitochondria isolated from the neural tissue (brain, spinal cord) have distinct metabolic properties regarding the extent of ROS produced upon oxidation of respiratory substrates (Panov et al., 2011). Especially in G93A-SOD1 transgenic rats, brain and spinal cord mitochondria generate 5-7 fold more ROS than mitochondria of corresponding wild-type tissues. Particularly, the spinal cord mitochondria produce two times more hydroperoxide than brain mitochondria of the same animals (Panov et al., n.d.)

Analysis of mitochondrial morphology in G37R and G85R-SOD1 transgenic mice has revealed that somal mitochondria become shorter and rounder in both dismutase active and inactive mutant SOD1 mouse lines. In contrast, axonal mitochondria in G37R-SOD1 animals shift from elongated tubular mitochondria to punctate mitochondria, while in G85R-SOD1 mice the mitochondria have been reported to show an increase in length (Vande Velde et al., 2011). These changes in mitochondrial shape and distribution were characteristic prior to ALS disease onset and support the notion of early mitochondrial pathology in ALS.

4. SOD1 catalyzes increased hydroperoxide production in IMS

The growing body of evidence provides support to the concept that superoxide dismutation in IMS may cause an increased hydroperoxide production with toxic consequences. Mitochondria are the major intracellular source of superoxide, the primary ROS, where superoxide anion radical is generated by one electron reduction of oxygen.

The two major pathways of superoxide production in mitochondria are autooxidation or complex III catalyzed oxidation of ubisemiquinone (Muller et al., 2004) and complex I catalyzed reduction of oxygen through reversed electron flow in the respiratory chain (Fig. 2.) (Liu et al., 2002). The produced superoxide anion radical has ability to actively react with a number of cellular targets leading to the loss of their proper function. The main detoxifying mechanism for superoxide instead of reverse oxidation of superoxide to oxygen, includes dismutation to hydroperoxide and oxygen.

Besides SOD1, there are other dedicated enzymes catalyzing this dismutation reaction. In mitochondria Mn-superoxide dismutase (SOD2), which is found in the mitochondrial matrix, scavenges superoxide in this compartment. Extracellular superoxide dismutase (SOD3) is secreted into the extracellular space and protects tissues against excess of superoxide (Zelko et al., 2002). In the IMS superoxide is produced presumably by complex III (Fig. 2.) (Muller et al., 2004). Unlike hydroperoxide, which freely diffuses through the membranes, superoxide cannot cross the mitochondrial inner membrane. In the matrix SOD2 converts superoxide to hydroperoxide, which in turn is reduced to water by the matrix glutathione peroxidase (Inoue et al., 2003). Homozygous SOD2 knockout mice are neonatally lethal (Li et al., 1995), whereas deletion of SOD1 gene does not have apparent motor neuron disease phenotype (Maier & Chan, 2002).

In IMS the fate of superoxide is determined by SOD1 and cytochrome c, which is present there in millimolar concentrations (Forman & Azzi, 1997; van Beek-Harmsen & van der Laarse, 2005). Cytochrome c is a heme containing protein, which functions as an electron carrier between complex III and cytochrome oxidase in the respiratory chain. Cytocrome c can also efficiently oxidize superoxide to oxygen. In this respect, cytochrome c can function as an efficient antioxidant, scavenging superoxide without production of secondary ROS (Fig. 2. reaction II), in contrast to SOD1, which produces hydroperoxide (Fig. 2, reaction III) (Pereverzev et al., 2003). However, cytochrome c has also a potential to catalyze oxidation by hydroperoxide. Upon this reaction, hydroperoxide oxidizes the prosthetic heme in the cytochrome c molecule to oxoferryl heme, forming so-called peroxidase compound I-type intermediate, a highly reactive oxidant that is able to react with a number of intracellular targets including proteins, nucleic acids and lipids, causing cell damage (Fig. 3) (Lawrence et al., 2003). Cytochrome c peroxidase activity is controlled by the coordination state of heme iron, particularly by the sulphur ligand of methionine-80 (Met-80), which can be easily displaced by hydroperoxide (Barr et al., 1996; Qian et al., 2002). The peroxidase activity of cytochrome c may increase by unfolding and post-translational modifications, such as proteolytic cleavage, nitration and oxidation (Diederix et al., 2002; Everse & Coates, 2005; Jang & Han, 2006).

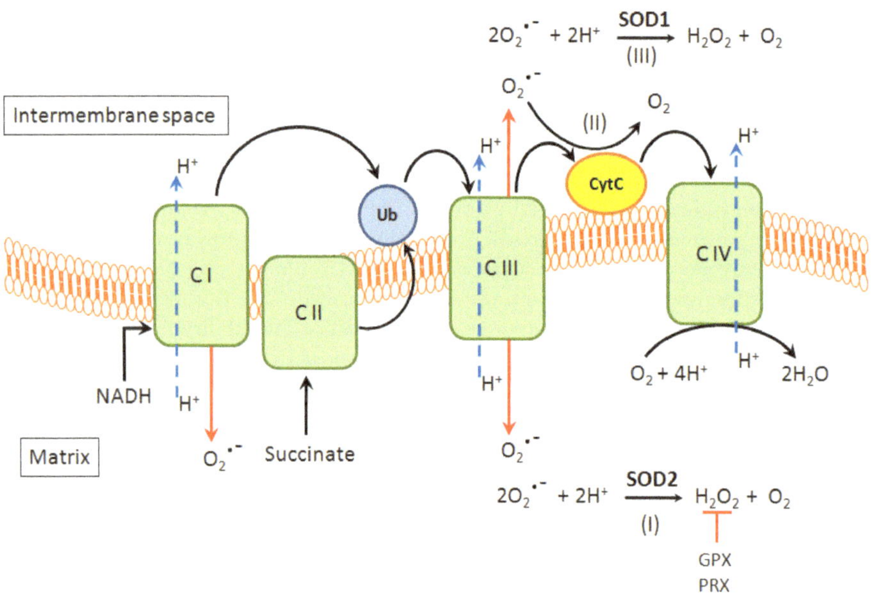

Fig. 2. Mitochondrial production and clearance of superoxide. Upon respiration superoxide is inevitably generated predominantly at respiratory complexes CI and CIII. The superoxide released to the matrix is dismutated by mitochondrial SOD2 (I) and the hydroperoxide produced is cleared by glutathione peroxidase and peroxyredoxins. Most of the superoxide released in IMS is generated at respiratory complex CIII. Oxidized form of cytochrome c, present in the IMS at high concentration can exercise clean clearance of superoxide by its oxidation to oxygen (II). An alternative dismutation catalyzed by SOD1 results in increased hydroperoxide generation in the IMS (III).

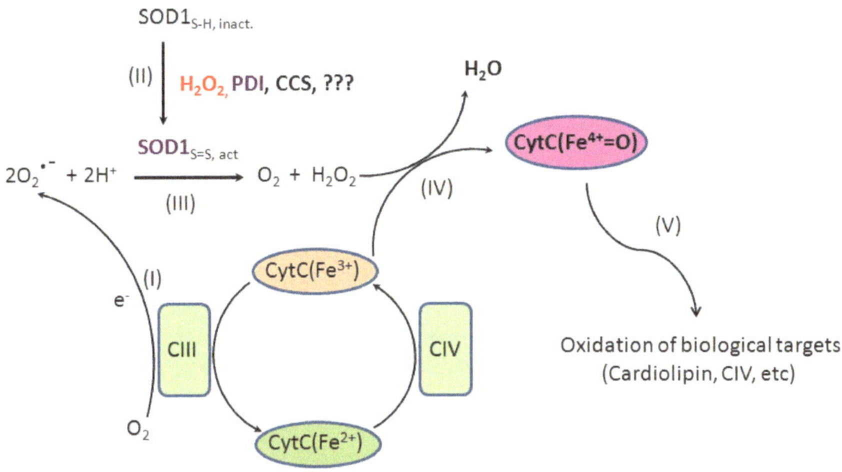

Fig. 3. Deleterious role of superoxide dismutase in the mitochondrial intermembrane space. Superoxide (O2·-) is released in IMS by one electron reduction of oxygen at a site in the inner membrane (I). Cu/Zn Superoxide dismutase (SOD1) in IMS is activated by oxidation of cysteine thiols, leading to formation of intramolecular S=S bounds (II). SOD1 produces hydroperoxide (H_2O_2) by dismutating superoxide (III). Hydroperoxide oxydizes cytochrome c (CytC) to oxoferryl-CytC (CytC(Fe^{4+}=O)), an exceptionally strong oxidant (IV), able to oxidize a number of vital biological targets (V).

We have recently proposed a model, where upon mitochondrial stress SOD1 may compete with cytochrome c for superoxide in the IMS and generate hydroperoxide, which then could react with cytochrome c and form peroxidase compound I-type intermediate, eventually leading to a deleterious increase in ROS production and cellular injury (Fig. 2) (Goldsteins et al., 2008). According to this model the SOD1-catalyzed superoxide dismutation in the IMS causes paradoxically augmented ROS production.

The data obtained demonstrate that inhibition of electron transfer at the level of complex III leads to SOD1 activation in the IMS, resulting in increased hydroperoxide production and, consequently, cytochrome c-catalyze peroxidation (Goldsteins et al., 2008). This could trigger a vicious circle where oxidative damage to mitochondrial respiratory components leads to further ROS production and peroxidation. Indeed, we have demonstrated that inhibition of mitochondrial respiration at the level of complex III causes SOD1-dependent ROS production and apoptotic death of isolated blood lymphocytes. In contrast, mitochondria isolated from SOD1 knockout mice do not show increased ROS production upon mitochondrial stress. Moreover, accumulation of mutant human G93A-SOD1 in the IMS that is observed in the tg animal models of ALS, leads to elevated SOD1 activity and increased cytochrome c-catalyzed oxidation in the IMS.

Our proposed model provides also an explanation for observations in other neurodegenerative disorders that elevated SOD1 activity worsens the pathology instead of the expected protective effect. For instance, immature mouse brains overexpressing SOD1 show an increased propensity for injury and accumulate more hydroperoxide after hypoxia-ischemia than wt mouse brains (Fullerton et al., 1998). Also, elevation of SOD1 increases acoustic trauma from noise exposure in some models (Endo et al., 2005). Impotantly, mice deficient in SOD1 have been reported to be resistant to acetaminophen toxicity (Lei et al., 2006). Even though SOD1 as a cytosolic antioxidant protects against mitochondrial dysfunction in a mouse model of transient focal cerebral ischemia (Fujimura et al., 2000), SOD1 deficiency, rather than overexpression, is associated with enhanced recovery and attenuated activation of NF-kappaB after brain trauma in mice (Beni et al., 2006).

This apparent discrepancy concerning the role of SOD1 in cellular injury can be explained by the model introduced, showing that increased SOD1 activity in the IMS paradoxically produces peroxides which are converted to highly toxic ROS. This view is further supported by an observation in mouse model of genetic disorder ataxia-telangiectasia, where elevated levels of SOD1 exacerbate the phenotype of neurodegeneration (Peter et al., 2001). It is also of interest that SOD1 overexpression and high tissue dismutase activity may potentiate atherogenesis in fat-fed atherosclerosis-susceptible mice (Tribble et al., 1997). The evidence about deleterious role of increased SOD1 expression has been most recently complemented by studies demonstrating that overexpression of SOD1 in retina leads to increased hydroperoxide levels and accelerated damage of cone cells (Usui et al., n.d.).

The key component for the SOD1-derived hydroperoxide toxicity in IMS is cytochrome c. Previous studies, including electron paramagnetic resonance (EPR) studies (Barr et al., 1996; Svistunenko, 2005; Belikova et al., 2006; Basova et al., 2007) have demonstrated that the reaction of cytochrome c with hydroperoxide results in formation of oxoferryl cytochrome c (peroxidase compound I-type intermediate) and corresponding protein-derived tyrosyl radical, which is highly reactive and has a potential to oxidize proteins, DNA, and lipids, as well as endogenous antioxidants such as glutathione, NADH, and ascorbate (Lawrence et al., 2003) (Fig. 3). In particular, oxidation of cardiolipin, a phospholipid which is in complex with cytochrome c on the surface of the inner mitochondrial membrane, causes the release of proapoptotic factors from mitochondria (Kagan et al., 2005; Belikova et al., 2006). This leads to a scenario where the hydroperoxide produced by increased SOD1 activity in the IMS, would thus serve as a substrate for cardiolipin-bound cytochrome c and consequently switch on very early proapoptotic processes, inducing consecutive programmed cell death. Additionally, upon increased hydroperoxide levels cytochrome c peroxidase activity may cause NADH oxidation producing a radical, which in turn donates an electron to oxygen augmenting superoxide formation (Velayutham et al., 2011).

The toxicity based on the dismutase activity of mutant SOD1 in the IMS might also be true even for dismutase inactive mutant SOD1 proteins. In human FALS SOD1 mutations are dominantly inherited resulting in the presence of both wild type and mutant SOD1 subunits in each cell. Thus, dismutase activity lacking G85R-SOD1 can form active heterodimers with wt SOD1 molecules. In mice the co-expression of human mutant and wt SOD1 accelerated disease (Jaarsma et al., 2000; Fukada et al., 2001; Deng et al., 2006). Importantly, unaffected A4V-SOD1 mutant mice developed the disease only when mated with human wt SOD1 overexpressing mice (Deng et al., 2006). It was also shown recently that the toxicity of mutant SOD1 dimers is not correlated with their capacity to form protein aggregates but rather with their dismutase activity (Witan et al., 2008).

5. Conclusion

Until now, several pathological mechanisms have been demonstrated how mutant SOD1 induces mitochondrial dysfunction in FALS models. Among them, the emerging evidence indicates that the SOD1-dependant hydroperoxide production in mitochondrial IMS may fuel the cytochrome c-catalyzed peroxidation and play a key role in oxidation of biological targets in the IMS. Thus, SOD1 activity and factors leading to its increase in this compartment can be regarded as deleterious mechanisms to the mitochondria and the cell. Increased SOD1 activity causing elevated hydroperoxide production in the IMS may be one of general mechanism in neurodegeneration.

At the moment it is not clear how mutations in SOD1 directly affect hydroperoxide production in IMS. One possibility may be the already demonstrated increased mitochondrial import for mutant molecules in neurons of ALS models. Another possible mechanism is linked to less strict dismutase activity control. Altogether, we hypothesize that the mutant SOD1 may gain toxic features because the proper control mechanism for its dismutase activity in mitochondrial IMS may be lost. In conclusion, we suggest that SOD1 activity in the IMS is a relevant therapeutic target for ALS and other neurodegenerative diseases involving mitochondrial pathogenesis.

6. Acknowledgment

For the construction of figures, elements from www.motifolio.com Free PowerPoint Diagrams were used.

The authors were supported by the Sigrid Juselius Foundation, Finland.

7. References

Ahtoniemi, T., Jaronen, M., Keksa-Goldsteine, V., Goldsteins, G. & Koistinaho, J. (2008). Mutant SOD1 from spinal cord of G93A rats is destabilized and binds to inner mitochondrial membrane. *Neurobiol Dis*, Vol.32, No.3, (December 2008), pp. 479-485.

Arnesano, F., Banci, L., Bertini, I., Martinelli, M., Furukawa, Y. & O'Halloran, T.V. (2004). The unusually stable quaternary structure of human Cu,Zn-superoxide dismutase 1 is controlled by both metal occupancy and disulfide status. *J Biol Chem*, Vol.279, No.46, (November 2004), pp. 47998-48003.

Atsumi, T. (1981). The ultrastructure of intramuscular nerves in amyotrophic lateral sclerosis. *Acta Neuropathol*, Vol.55, No.3, (1981), pp. 193-198.

Barr, D.P., Gunther, M.R., Deterding, L.J., Tomer, K.B. & Mason, R.P. (1996). ESR spin-trapping of a protein-derived tyrosyl radical from the reaction of cytochrome c with hydrogen peroxide. *J Biol Chem*, Vol.271, No.26, (1996), pp. 15498-503.

Basova, L.V., Kurnikov, I.V., Wang, L., Ritov, V.B., Belikova, N.A., Vlasova, I., Pacheco, A.A., Winnica, D.E., Peterson, J., Bayir, H., Waldeck, D.H. & Kagan, V.E. (2007). Cardiolipin switch in mitochondria: shutting off the reduction of cytochrome c and turning on the peroxidase activity. *Biochemistry*, Vol.46, No.11, (2007), pp. 3423-34.

Beckman, J.S., Carson, M., Smith, C.D. & Koppenol, W.H. (1993). ALS, SOD and peroxynitrite. *Nature*, Vol.364, No.6438, (August 1993), pp. 584.

Beckman, J.S., Chen, J., Crow, J.P. & Ye, Y.Z. (1994). Reactions of nitric oxide, superoxide and peroxynitrite with superoxide dismutase in neurodegeneration. *Prog Brain Res*, Vol.103, (1994), pp. 371-380.

van Beek-Harmsen, B.J. & van der Laarse, W.J. (2005). Immunohistochemical determination of cytosolic cytochrome C concentration in cardiomyocytes. *J Histochem Cytochem*, Vol.53, No.7, (2005), pp. 803-7.

Belikova, N.A., Vladimirov, Y.A., Osipov, A.N., Kapralov, A.A., Tyurin, V.A., Potapovich, M.V., Basova, L.V., Peterson, J., Kurnikov, I.V. & Kagan, V.E. (2006). Peroxidase Activity and Structural Transitions of Cytochrome c Bound to Cardiolipin-Containing Membranes. *Biochemistry*, Vol.45, No.15, (2006), pp. 4998-5009.

Bendotti, C., Calvaresi, N., Chiveri, L., Prelle, A., Moggio, M., Braga, M., Silani, V. & De Biasi, S. (2001). Early vacuolization and mitochondrial damage in motor neurons of FALS mice are not associated with apoptosis or with changes in cytochrome oxidase histochemical reactivity. *J Neurol Sci*, Vol.191, No.1-2, (October 2001), pp. 25-33.

Beni, S.M., Tsenter, J., Alexandrovich, A.G., Galron-Krool, N., Barzilai, A., Kohen, R., Grigoriadis, N., Simeonidou, C. & Shohami, E. (2006). CuZn-SOD deficiency, rather than overexpression, is associated with enhanced recovery and attenuated activation of NF-kappaB after brain trauma in mice. *J Cereb Blood Flow Metab*, Vol.26, No.4, (2006), pp. 478-90.

Beretta, S., Sala, G., Mattavelli, L., Ceresa, C., Casciati, A., Ferri, A., Carrì, M.T. & Ferrarese, C. (2003). Mitochondrial dysfunction due to mutant copper/zinc superoxide dismutase associated with amyotrophic lateral sclerosis is reversed by N-acetylcysteine. *Neurobiol Dis*, Vol.13, No.3, (August 2003), pp. 213-221.

Bergemalm, D., Jonsson, P.A., Graffmo, K.S., Andersen, P.M., Brännström, T., Rehnmark, A. & Marklund, S.L. (2006). Overloading of stable and exclusion of unstable human superoxide dismutase-1 variants in mitochondria of murine amyotrophic lateral sclerosis models. *J Neurosci*, Vol.26, No.16, (April 2006), pp. 4147-4154.

Boillée, S., Vande Velde, C. & Cleveland, D.W. (2006). ALS: a disease of motor neurons and their nonneuronal neighbors. *Neuron*, Vol.52, No.1, (October 2006), pp. 39-59.

Browne, S.E., Bowling, A.C., Baik, M.J., Gurney, M., Brown, R.H., Jr & Beal, M.F. (1998). Metabolic dysfunction in familial, but not sporadic, amyotrophic lateral sclerosis. *J Neurochem*, Vol.71, No.1, (July 1998), pp. 281-287.

Dal Canto, M.C. & Gurney, M.E. (1997). A low expressor line of transgenic mice carrying a mutant human Cu,Zn superoxide dismutase (SOD1) gene develops pathological changes that most closely resemble those in human amyotrophic lateral sclerosis. *Acta Neuropathol*, Vol.93, No.6, (June 1997), pp. 537-550.

Casareno, R.L.B., Waggoner, D. & Gitlin, J.D. (1998). The Copper Chaperone CCS Directly Interacts with Copper/Zinc Superoxide Dismutase. *Journal of Biological Chemistry*, Vol.273, No.37, (1998), pp. 23625 -23628.

Chattopadhyay, M., Durazo, A., Sohn, S.H., Strong, C.D., Gralla, E.B., Whitelegge, J.P. & Valentine, J.S. (2008). Initiation and elongation in fibrillation of ALS-linked superoxide dismutase. *Proc Natl Acad Sci U S A*, Vol.105, No.48, (December 2008), pp. 18663-18668.

Culotta, V.C., Klomp, L.W.J., Strain, J., Casareno, R.L.B., Krems, B. & Gitlin, J.D. (1997). The Copper Chaperone for Superoxide Dismutase. *Journal of Biological Chemistry*, Vol.272, No.38, (1997), pp. 23469 -23472.

Damiano, M., Starkov, A.A., Petri, S., Kipiani, K., Kiaei, M., Mattiazzi, M., Flint Beal, M. & Manfredi, G. (2006). Neural mitochondrial Ca2+ capacity impairment precedes the onset of motor symptoms in G93A Cu/Zn-superoxide dismutase mutant mice. *J Neurochem*, Vol.96, No.5, (March 2006), pp. 1349-1361.

Deng, H.-X., Shi, Y., Furukawa, Y., Zhai, H., Fu, R., Liu, E., Gorrie, G.H., Khan, M.S., Hung, W.-Y., Bigio, E.H., Lukas, T., Dal Canto, M.C., O'Halloran, T.V. & Siddique, T. (2006). Conversion to the amyotrophic lateral sclerosis phenotype is associated with intermolecular linked insoluble aggregates of SOD1 in mitochondria. *Proc Natl Acad Sci U S A*, Vol.103, No.18, (May 2006), pp. 7142-7147.

Diederix, R.E., Ubbink, M. & Canters, G.W. (2002). Peroxidase activity as a tool for studying the folding of c-type cytochromes. *Biochemistry*, Vol.41, No.43, (2002), pp. 13067-77.

Ding, F. & Dokholyan, N.V. (2008). Dynamical roles of metal ions and the disulfide bond in Cu, Zn superoxide dismutase folding and aggregation. *Proceedings of the National Academy of Sciences*, Vol.105, No.50, (December 2008), pp. 19696 -19701.

Elliott, J.L. (2001). Zinc and copper in the pathogenesis of amyotrophic lateral sclerosis. *Prog Neuropsychopharmacol Biol Psychiatry*, Vol.25, No.6, (August 2001), pp. 1169-1185.

Endo, T., Nakagawa, T., Iguchi, F., Kita, T., Okano, T., Sha, S.-H., Schacht, J., Shiga, A., Kim, T.-S. & Ito, J. (2005). Elevation of superoxide dismutase increases acoustic trauma from noise exposure. *Free Radic Biol Med*, Vol.38, No.4, (February 2005), pp. 492-498.

Estévez, A.G., Crow, J.P., Sampson, J.B., Reiter, C., Zhuang, Y., Richardson, G.J., Tarpey, M.M., Barbeito, L. & Beckman, J.S. (1999). Induction of nitric oxide-dependent apoptosis in motor neurons by zinc-deficient superoxide dismutase. *Science*, Vol.286, No.5449, (December 1999), pp. 2498-2500.

Everse, J. & Coates, P.W. (2005). Role of peroxidases in Parkinson disease: a hypothesis. *Free Radic Biol Med*, Vol.38, No.10, (2005), pp. 1296-310.

Ferri, A., Cozzolino, M., Crosio, C., Nencini, M., Casciati, A., Gralla, E.B., Rotilio, G., Valentine, J.S. & Carrì, M.T. (2006). Familial ALS-superoxide dismutases associate with mitochondria and shift their redox potentials. *Proc Natl Acad Sci U S A*, Vol.103, No.37, (September 2006), pp. 13860-13865.

Forman, H.J. & Azzi, A. (1997). On the virtual existence of superoxide anions in mitochondria: thoughts regarding its role in pathophysiology. *Faseb J*, Vol.11, No.5, (1997), pp. 374-5.

Fujimura, M., Morita-Fujimura, Y., Noshita, N., Sugawara, T., Kawase, M. & Chan, P.H. (2000). The cytosolic antioxidant copper/zinc-superoxide dismutase prevents the early release of mitochondrial cytochrome c in ischemic brain after transient focal cerebral ischemia in mice. *J Neurosci*, Vol.20, No.8, (2000), pp. 2817-24.

Fukada, K., Nagano, S., Satoh, M., Tohyama, C., Nakanishi, T., Shimizu, A., Yanagihara, T. & Sakoda, S. (2001). Stabilization of mutant Cu/Zn superoxide dismutase (SOD1) protein by coexpressed wild SOD1 protein accelerates the disease progression in familial amyotrophic lateral sclerosis mice. *Eur J Neurosci*, Vol.14, No.12, (December 2001), pp. 2032-2036.

Fullerton, H.J., Ditelberg, J.S., Chen, S.F., Sarco, D.P., Chan, P.H., Epstein, C.J. & Ferriero, D.M. (1998). Copper/zinc superoxide dismutase transgenic brain accumulates hydrogen peroxide after perinatal hypoxia ischemia. *Ann Neurol*, Vol.44, No.3, (September 1998), pp. 357-364.

Furukawa, Y. & O'Halloran, T.V. (2006). Posttranslational modifications in Cu,Zn-superoxide dismutase and mutations associated with amyotrophic lateral sclerosis. *Antioxid Redox Signal*, Vol.8, No.5-6, (June 2006), pp. 847-867.

Goldsteins, G., Keksa-Goldsteine, V., Ahtoniemi, T., Jaronen, M., Arens, E., Akerman, K., Chan, P.H. & Koistinaho, J. (2008). Deleterious role of superoxide dismutase in the mitochondrial intermembrane space. *J Biol Chem*, Vol.283, No.13, (March 2008), pp. 8446-8452.

Grosskreutz, J., Van Den Bosch, L. & Keller, B.U. (2010). Calcium dysregulation in amyotrophic lateral sclerosis. *Cell Calcium*, Vol.47, No.2, (February 2010), pp. 165-174.

Higgins, C.M.J., Jung, C. & Xu, Z. (2003). ALS-associated mutant SOD1G93A causes mitochondrial vacuolation by expansion of the intermembrane space and by involvement of SOD1 aggregation and peroxisomes. *BMC Neurosci*, Vol.4, (July 2003), pp. 16.

Higgins, C.M.J., Jung, C., Ding, H. & Xu, Z. (2002). Mutant Cu, Zn superoxide dismutase that causes motoneuron degeneration is present in mitochondria in the CNS. *J Neurosci*, Vol.22, No.6, (March 2002), pp. RC215.

Iñarrea, P., Casanova, A., Alava, M.A., Iturralde, M. & Cadenas, E. (2011). Melatonin and steroid hormones activate intermembrane Cu,Zn-superoxide dismutase by means of mitochondrial cytochrome P450. *Free Radic Biol Med*, Vol.50, No.11, (June 2011), pp. 1575-1581.

Iñarrea, P., Moini, H., Rettori, D., Han, D., Martínez, J., García, I., Fernández-Vizarra, E., Iturralde, M. & Cadenas, E. (2005). Redox activation of mitochondrial intermembrane space Cu,Zn-superoxide dismutase. *Biochem J*, Vol.387, No.Pt 1, (April 2005), pp. 203-209.

Inoue, M., Sato, E.F., Nishikawa, M., Park, A.M., Kira, Y., Imada, I. & Utsumi, K. (2003). Mitochondrial generation of reactive oxygen species and its role in aerobic life. *Curr Med Chem*, Vol.10, No.23, (2003), pp. 2495-505.

Jaarsma, D., Haasdijk, E.D., Grashorn, J.A., Hawkins, R., van Duijn, W., Verspaget, H.W., London, J. & Holstege, J.C. (2000). Human Cu/Zn superoxide dismutase (SOD1) overexpression in mice causes mitochondrial vacuolization, axonal degeneration, and premature motoneuron death and accelerates motoneuron disease in mice expressing a familial amyotrophic lateral sclerosis mutant SOD1. *Neurobiol Dis*, Vol.7, No.6 Pt B, (December 2000), pp. 623-643.

Jaarsma, D., Rognoni, F., van Duijn, W., Verspaget, H.W., Haasdijk, E.D. & Holstege, J.C. (2001). CuZn superoxide dismutase (SOD1) accumulates in vacuolated mitochondria in transgenic mice expressing amyotrophic lateral sclerosis-linked SOD1 mutations. *Acta Neuropathol*, Vol.102, No.4, (October 2001), pp. 293-305.

Jaiswal, M.K. & Keller, B.U. (2009). Cu/Zn superoxide dismutase typical for familial amyotrophic lateral sclerosis increases the vulnerability of mitochondria and perturbs Ca2+ homeostasis in SOD1G93A mice. *Mol Pharmacol*, Vol.75, No.3, (March 2009), pp. 478-489.

Jang, B. & Han, S. (2006). Biochemical properties of cytochrome c nitrated by peroxynitrite. *Biochimie*, Vol.88, No.1, (2006), pp. 53-8.

Jonsson, P.A., Graffmo, K.S., Andersen, P.M., Brännström, T., Lindberg, M., Oliveberg, M. & Marklund, S.L. (2006). Disulphide-reduced superoxide dismutase-1 in CNS of transgenic amyotrophic lateral sclerosis models. *Brain*, Vol.129, No.Pt 2, (February 2006), pp. 451-464.

Kagan, V.E., Tyurin, V.A., Jiang, J., Tyurina, Y.Y., Ritov, V.B., Amoscato, A.A., Osipov, A.N., Belikova, N.A., Kapralov, A.A., Kini, V., Vlasova, I., Zhao, Q., Zou, M., Di, P., Svistunenko, D.A., Kurnikov, I.V. & Borisenko, G.G. (2005). Cytochrome c acts as a cardiolipin oxygenase required for release of proapoptotic factors. *Nat Chem Biol*, Vol.1, No.4, (2005), pp. 223-32.

Kawamata, H. & Manfredi, G. (2008). Different regulation of wild-type and mutant Cu,Zn superoxide dismutase localization in mammalian mitochondria. *Hum Mol Genet*, Vol.17, No.21, (November 2008), pp. 3303-3317.

Kirkinezos, I.G., Bacman, S.R., Hernandez, D., Oca-Cossio, J., Arias, L.J., Perez-Pinzon, M.A., Bradley, W.G. & Moraes, C.T. (2005). Cytochrome c association with the inner mitochondrial membrane is impaired in the CNS of G93A-SOD1 mice. *J Neurosci*, Vol.25, No.1, (January 2005), pp. 164-172.

Kong, J. & Xu, Z. (1998). Massive mitochondrial degeneration in motor neurons triggers the onset of amyotrophic lateral sclerosis in mice expressing a mutant SOD1. *J Neurosci*, Vol.18, No.9, (May 1998), pp. 3241-3250.

Kruman, I.I., Pedersen, W.A., Springer, J.E. & Mattson, M.P. (1999). ALS-linked Cu/Zn-SOD mutation increases vulnerability of motor neurons to excitotoxicity by a mechanism involving increased oxidative stress and perturbed calcium homeostasis. *Exp Neurol*, Vol.160, No.1, (November 1999), pp. 28-39.

Lawrence, A., Jones, C.M., Wardman, P. & Burkitt, M.J. (2003). Evidence for the role of a peroxidase compound I-type intermediate in the oxidation of glutathione, NADH, ascorbate, and dichlorofluorescin by cytochrome c/H2O2. Implications for oxidative stress during apoptosis. *J Biol Chem*, Vol.278, No.32, (2003), pp. 29410-9.

Lei, X.G., Zhu, J.H., McClung, J.P., Aregullin, M. & Roneker, C.A. (2006). Mice deficient in Cu,Zn-superoxide dismutase are resistant to acetaminophen toxicity. *Biochem J*, Vol.399, No.3, (2006), pp. 455-61.

Leitch, J.M., Yick, P.J. & Culotta, V.C. (2009). The right to choose: multiple pathways for activating copper,zinc superoxide dismutase. *J Biol Chem*, Vol.284, No.37, (September 2009), pp. 24679-24683.

Li, Y., Huang, T.-T., Carlson, E.J., Melov, S., Ursell, P.C., Olson, J.L., Noble, L.J., Yoshimura, M.P., Berger, C., Chan, P.H., Wallace, D.C. & Epstein, C.J. (1995). Dilated cardiomyopathy and neonatal lethality in mutant mice lacking manganese superoxide dismutase. *Nat Genet*, Vol.11, No.4, (December 1995), pp. 376-381.

Liu, J., Lillo, C., Jonsson, P.A., Vande Velde, C., Ward, C.M., Miller, T.M., Subramaniam, J.R., Rothstein, J.D., Marklund, S., Andersen, P.M., Brännström, T., Gredal, O., Wong, P.C., Williams, D.S. & Cleveland, D.W. (2004). Toxicity of familial ALS-linked SOD1 mutants from selective recruitment to spinal mitochondria. *Neuron*, Vol.43, No.1, (July 2004), pp. 5-17.

Liu, Y., Fiskum, G. & Schubert, D. (2002). Generation of reactive oxygen species by the mitochondrial electron transport chain. *J Neurochem*, Vol.80, No.5, (2002), pp. 780-7.

Maier, C.M. & Chan, P.H. (2002). Role of superoxide dismutases in oxidative damage and neurodegenerative disorders. *Neuroscientist*, Vol.8, No.4, (August 2002), pp. 323-334.

Manfredi, G. & Xu, Z. (2005). Mitochondrial dysfunction and its role in motor neuron degeneration in ALS. *Mitochondrion*, Vol.5, No.2, (April 2005), pp. 77-87.

Mattiazzi, M., D'Aurelio, M., Gajewski, C.D., Martushova, K., Kiaei, M., Beal, M.F. & Manfredi, G. (2002). Mutated human SOD1 causes dysfunction of oxidative phosphorylation in mitochondria of transgenic mice. *J Biol Chem*, Vol.277, No.33, (August 2002), pp. 29626-29633.

Muller, F.L., Liu, Y. & Van Remmen, H. (2004). Complex III releases superoxide to both sides of the inner mitochondrial membrane. *J Biol Chem*, Vol.279, No.47, (2004), pp. 49064-73.

Okado-Matsumoto, A. & Fridovich, I. (2001). Subcellular distribution of superoxide dismutases (SOD) in rat liver: Cu,Zn-SOD in mitochondria. *J Biol Chem*, Vol.276, No.42, (October 2001), pp. 38388-38393.

Panov, A.V., Kubalik, N., Zinchenko, N., Ridings, D.M., Radoff, D.A., Hemendinger, R., Brooks, B.R. & Bonkovsky, H.L. (2011). Metabolic and functional differences between brain and spinal cord mitochondria underlie different predisposition to pathology. *Am J Physiol Regul Integr Comp Physiol*, Vol.300, No.4, (April 2011), pp. R844-854.

Panov, A., Kubalik, N., Zinchenko, N., Hemendinger, R., Dikalov, S. & Bonkovsky, H.L. (n.d.). Respiration and ROS production in brain and spinal cord mitochondria of transgenic rats with mutant G93a Cu/Zn-superoxide dismutase gene. *Neurobiology of Disease*, In Press

Pasinelli, P., Belford, M.E., Lennon, N., Bacskai, B.J., Hyman, B.T., Trotti, D. & Brown, R.H., Jr (2004). Amyotrophic lateral sclerosis-associated SOD1 mutant proteins bind and aggregate with Bcl-2 in spinal cord mitochondria. *Neuron*, Vol.43, No.1, (July 2004), pp. 19-30.

Pereverzev, M.O., Vygodina, T.V., Konstantinov, A.A. & Skulachev, V.P. (2003). Cytochrome c, an ideal antioxidant. *Biochem Soc Trans*, Vol.31, No.Pt 6, (2003), pp. 1312-5.

Peter, Y., Rotman, G., Lotem, J., Elson, A., Shiloh, Y. & Groner, Y. (2001). Elevated Cu/Zn-SOD exacerbates radiation sensitivity and hematopoietic abnormalities of Atm-deficient mice. *EMBO J*, Vol.20, No.7, (April 2001), pp. 1538-1546.

Qian, S.Y., Chen, Y.R., Deterding, L.J., Fann, Y.C., Chignell, C.F., Tomer, K.B. & Mason, R.P. (2002). Identification of protein-derived tyrosyl radical in the reaction of cytochrome c and hydrogen peroxide: characterization by ESR spin-trapping, HPLC and MS. *Biochem J*, Vol.363, No.Pt 2, (2002), pp. 281-8.

Reddehase, S., Grumbt, B., Neupert, W. & Hell, K. (2009). The disulfide relay system of mitochondria is required for the biogenesis of mitochondrial Ccs1 and Sod1. *J Mol Biol*, Vol.385, No.2, (January 2009), pp. 331-338.

Siciliano, G., Pastorini, E., Pasquali, L., Manca, M.L., Iudice, A. & Murri, L. (2001). Impaired oxidative metabolism in exercising muscle from ALS patients. *J Neurol Sci*, Vol.191, No.1-2, (October 2001), pp. 61-65.

Siklós, L., Engelhardt, J., Harati, Y., Smith, R.G., Joó, F. & Appel, S.H. (1996). Ultrastructural evidence for altered calcium in motor nerve terminals in amyotropic lateral sclerosis. *Ann Neurol*, Vol.39, No.2, (February 1996), pp. 203-216.

Son, M., Puttaparthi, K., Kawamata, H., Rajendran, B., Boyer, P.J., Manfredi, G. & Elliott, J.L. (2007). Overexpression of CCS in G93A-SOD1 mice leads to accelerated neurological deficits with severe mitochondrial pathology. *Proc Natl Acad Sci U S A*, Vol.104, No.14, (April 2007), pp. 6072-6077.

Stathopulos, P.B., Rumfeldt, J.A.O., Scholz, G.A., Irani, R.A., Frey, H.E., Hallewell, R.A., Lepock, J.R. & Meiering, E.M. (2003). Cu/Zn superoxide dismutase mutants associated with amyotrophic lateral sclerosis show enhanced formation of aggregates in vitro. *Proc Natl Acad Sci U S A*, Vol.100, No.12, (June 2003), pp. 7021-7026.

Sturtz, L.A., Diekert, K., Jensen, L.T., Lill, R. & Culotta, V.C. (2001). A fraction of yeast Cu,Zn-superoxide dismutase and its metallochaperone, CCS, localize to the intermembrane space of mitochondria. A physiological role for SOD1 in guarding against mitochondrial oxidative damage. *J Biol Chem*, Vol.276, No.41, (October 2001), pp. 38084-38089.

Svistunenko, D.A. (2005). Reaction of haem containing proteins and enzymes with hydroperoxides: the radical view. *Biochim Biophys Acta*, Vol.1707, No.1, (2005), pp. 127-55.

Tribble, D.L., Gong, E.L., Leeuwenburgh, C., Heinecke, J.W., Carlson, E.L., Verstuyft, J.G. & Epstein, C.J. (1997). Fatty streak formation in fat-fed mice expressing human copper-zinc superoxide dismutase. *Arterioscler Thromb Vasc Biol*, Vol.17, No.9, (September 1997), pp. 1734-1740.

Usui, S., Oveson, B.C., Iwase, T., Lu, L., Lee, S.Y., Jo, Y.-J., Wu, Z., Choi, E.-Y., Samulski, R.J. & Campochiaro, P.A. (n.d.). Overexpression of SOD in retina: Need for increase in H2O2-detoxifying enzyme in same cellular compartment. *Free Radical Biology and Medicine*, In Press

Valentine, J.S., Doucette, P.A. & Zittin Potter, S. (2005). Copper-zinc superoxide dismutase and amyotrophic lateral sclerosis. *Annu Rev Biochem*, Vol.74, (2005), pp. 563-593.

Vande Velde, C., McDonald, K.K., Boukhedimi, Y., McAlonis-Downes, M., Lobsiger, C.S., Bel Hadj, S., Zandona, A., Julien, J.-P., Shah, S.B. & Cleveland, D.W. (2011). Misfolded SOD1 Associated with Motor Neuron Mitochondria Alters Mitochondrial Shape and Distribution Prior to Clinical Onset. *PLoS ONE*, Vol.6, No.7, (2011), pp. e22031.

Vande Velde, C., Miller, T.M., Cashman, N.R. & Cleveland, D.W. (2008). Selective association of misfolded ALS-linked mutant SOD1 with the cytoplasmic face of mitochondria. *Proc Natl Acad Sci U S A*, Vol.105, No.10, (March 2008), pp. 4022-4027.

Velayutham, M., Hemann, C. & Zweier, J.L. (2011). Removal of H(2)O(2) and generation of superoxide radical: Role of cytochrome c and NADH. *Free Radic Biol Med*, Vol.51, No.1, (July 2011), pp. 160-170.

Wiedau-Pazos, M., Goto, J.J., Rabizadeh, S., Gralla, E.B., Roe, J.A., Lee, M.K., Valentine, J.S. & Bredesen, D.E. (1996). Altered reactivity of superoxide dismutase in familial amyotrophic lateral sclerosis. *Science*, Vol.271, No.5248, (January 1996), pp. 515-518.

Vijayvergiya, C., Beal, M.F., Buck, J. & Manfredi, G. (2005). Mutant superoxide dismutase 1 forms aggregates in the brain mitochondrial matrix of amyotrophic lateral sclerosis mice. *J Neurosci*, Vol.25, No.10, (March 2005), pp. 2463-2470.

Witan, H., Kern, A., Koziollek-Drechsler, I., Wade, R., Behl, C. & Clement, A.M. (2008). Heterodimer formation of wild-type and amyotrophic lateral sclerosis-causing mutant Cu/Zn-superoxide dismutase induces toxicity independent of protein aggregation. *Hum Mol Genet*, Vol.17, No.10, (May 2008), pp. 1373-1385.

Wong, P.C., Pardo, C.A., Borchelt, D.R., Lee, M.K., Copeland, N.G., Jenkins, N.A., Sisodia, S.S., Cleveland, D.W. & Price, D.L. (1995). An adverse property of a familial ALS-linked SOD1 mutation causes motor neuron disease characterized by vacuolar degeneration of mitochondria. *Neuron*, Vol.14, No.6, (June 1995), pp. 1105-1116.

Vonk, W.I.M., Wijmenga, C., Berger, R., van de Sluis, B. & Klomp, L.W.J. (2010). Cu,Zn Superoxide Dismutase Maturation and Activity Are Regulated by COMMD1. *Journal of Biological Chemistry*, Vol.285, No.37, (2010), pp. 28991 -29000.

Xu, Z., Jung, C., Higgins, C., Levine, J. & Kong, J. (2004). Mitochondrial degeneration in amyotrophic lateral sclerosis. *J Bioenerg Biomembr*, Vol.36, No.4, (August 2004), pp. 395-399.

Zelko, I.N., Mariani, T.J. & Folz, R.J. (2002). Superoxide dismutase multigene family: a comparison of the CuZn-SOD (SOD1), Mn-SOD (SOD2), and EC-SOD (SOD3) gene structures, evolution, and expression. *Free Radic Biol Med*, Vol.33, No.3, (2002), pp. 337-49.

9

Role of Mitochondrial Dysfunction in Motor Neuron Degeneration in ALS

Luz Diana Santa-Cruz, Uri Nimrod Ramírez-Jarquín and Ricardo Tapia
División de Neurociencias, Instituto de Fisiología Celular, Universidad Nacional Autónoma de México, México, D.F., México

1. Introduction

Amyotrophic lateral sclerosis (ALS), which was described since 1869 by Jean Martin Charcot, is a devastating neurodegenerative disease characterized by the selective and progressive loss of upper and lower motor neurons of the cerebral cortex, brainstem and the spinal cord. Progressive motor neuron loss causes muscle weakness, spasticity and fasciculation, eventually paralysis and finally death by respiratory failure 3 to 5 years after diagnosis. ALS worldwide prevalence is about 2 to 8 people per 100,000, and presents two important differences with respect to other neurogenerative diseases: the cognitive process is not affected and is not merely the result of aging because may occur at young ages (Chancellor & Warlow, 1992; Huisman et al., 2011). Two forms of ALS are known, the familial type (FALS), associated with genetic mutations, mainly in the gene encoding superoxide dismutase 1 (SOD1, enzyme responsible for superoxide dismutation to oxygen and hydrogen peroxide), and the sporadic form (SALS), of unknown origin. FALS represents only about 5-10% of cases (Rosen et al., 1993; Rowland & Shneider, 2001), and SALS comprises the remaining 90%. Despite having different origins, both ALS types develop similar histopathological and clinical characteristics.

2. Mechanisms of motor neuron death in ALS

After one hundred fifty years since the first ALS description of the disease, the cause of motor neuron degeneration remains unknown, but progress in neuroscience and clinical research has identified several mechanisms that seem to be involved in the cell death process, such as glutamate-mediated excitotoxicity, inflammatory events, axonal transport deficits, oxidative stress, mitochondrial dysfunction and energy failure.

2.1 Excitotoxicity

Based on the reduction of glutamate transporter-1 (GLT1 in rodents and excitatory amino acid transporter 2 or EAAT2 in human) content detected post-mortem in motor cortex and spinal cord of ALS patients (Rothstein et al., 1992; Rothstein et al., 1995) and on the increase of glutamate concentration in the cerebrospinal fluid (CSF) of about 40% of ALS patients (Shaw et al., 1995b; Spreux-Varoquaux et al., 2002), one proposed mechanism to explain motor neuron death in ALS is glutamate-mediated excitotoxicity. This hypothesis has been generally accepted, although some data from our laboratory do not support it because a chronic increase in extracellular glutamate due to glutamate transport inhibition in the spinal cord in vivo was innocuous for motor neurons (Tovar-y-Romo et al., 2009b). However, overactivation of glutamate ionotropic receptors by agonists leads to neuronal death by augmenting the influx of Ca^{2+} into motor neurons. Experimental models in vivo have shown that of three major glutamate ionotropic receptor types, NMDA (N-methyl-D-aspartate), kainate and AMPA (α-amino-3-hydroxy-5-isoxazolepropionate), the Ca^{2+}-permeable AMPA receptor seems to be particularly involved in motor neuron death, because the selective blockade of Ca^{2+}-permeable AMPA receptors or the chelation of intracellular Ca^{2+} prevents the motor neuron loss and the consequent paralysis induced by the infusion of AMPA into the rat lumbar spinal cord (Corona & Tapia, 2004, 2007; Tovar-y-Romo et al., 2009a). The Ca^{2+} permeability of this receptor is governed by the presence of the GluR2 subunit and its edition in the Q/R (glutamine/arginine) site of the second transmembrane domain (Burnashev et al., 1992; Corona & Tapia, 2007; Hollmann et al., 1991; Hume et al., 1991).

Increases in cytoplasmic Ca^{2+} concentration can be buffered by mitochondria, but when maintained for prolonged periods can cause mitochondrial swelling and dysfunction. These alterations are associated with deficits in mitochondrial ATP synthesis and energetic failure (this topic will be discussed later). The energetic deficits have been mainly associated with cell death process similar to necrosis (Kroemer et al., 2009; Martin, 2010). On the other hand, mitochondrial damage has also been linked to the release of proapoptotic factors such as cytochrome c and apoptosis-inducing factor (Martin et al., 2009). Cytochrome c involvement has been stressed because of its role in triggering the caspases pathway, which leads to apoptotic cellular death. In the cytoplasm cytochrome c promotes the formation of the apoptosome complex and activates caspase-3. The necrosis and apoptosis pathways are illustrated in Fig. 1.

2.2 Axonal transport deficits

Because of the structural and functional characteristics of motor neuron axons, the role of axonal transport is essential for the communication between the neuronal soma and the periphery, as well as for the anterograde and retrograde dispersive distribution of cargo intracellular structures such as vesicles or organelles. Changes in the speed of anterograde and retrograde transport (Breuer & Atkinson, 1988; Breuer et al., 1987; Sasaki & Iwata, 1996), as well as neurofilament disorganization and accumulation of mitochondria, vesicles and smooth endoplasmic reticulum have been described in peripheral nerves of ALS patients (Hirano et al., 1984a, b; Sasaki & Iwata, 1996). These alterations in axonal transport have been observed also in transgenic models of FALS, which have allowed the study of their progression and the molecular machinery involved (Bilsland et al., 2010; Brunet et al., 2009; Collard et al., 1995; De Vos et al., 2007; Ligon et al., 2005; Perlson et al., 2009; Pun et al., 2006; Tateno et al., 2009; Warita et al., 1999; Williamson & Cleveland, 1999). In mutant SOD1 (mSOD1) rodents, some motor proteins such as: dynein, dynactin, kinesin, myosin, actin, and microtubules and neurofilaments are affected by mSOD1 aggregates (Breuer & Atkinson, 1988; Breuer et al., 1987; Collard et al., 1995; Ligon et al., 2005; Sasaki & Iwata, 1996; Williamson & Cleveland, 1999; Zhang et al., 2007).

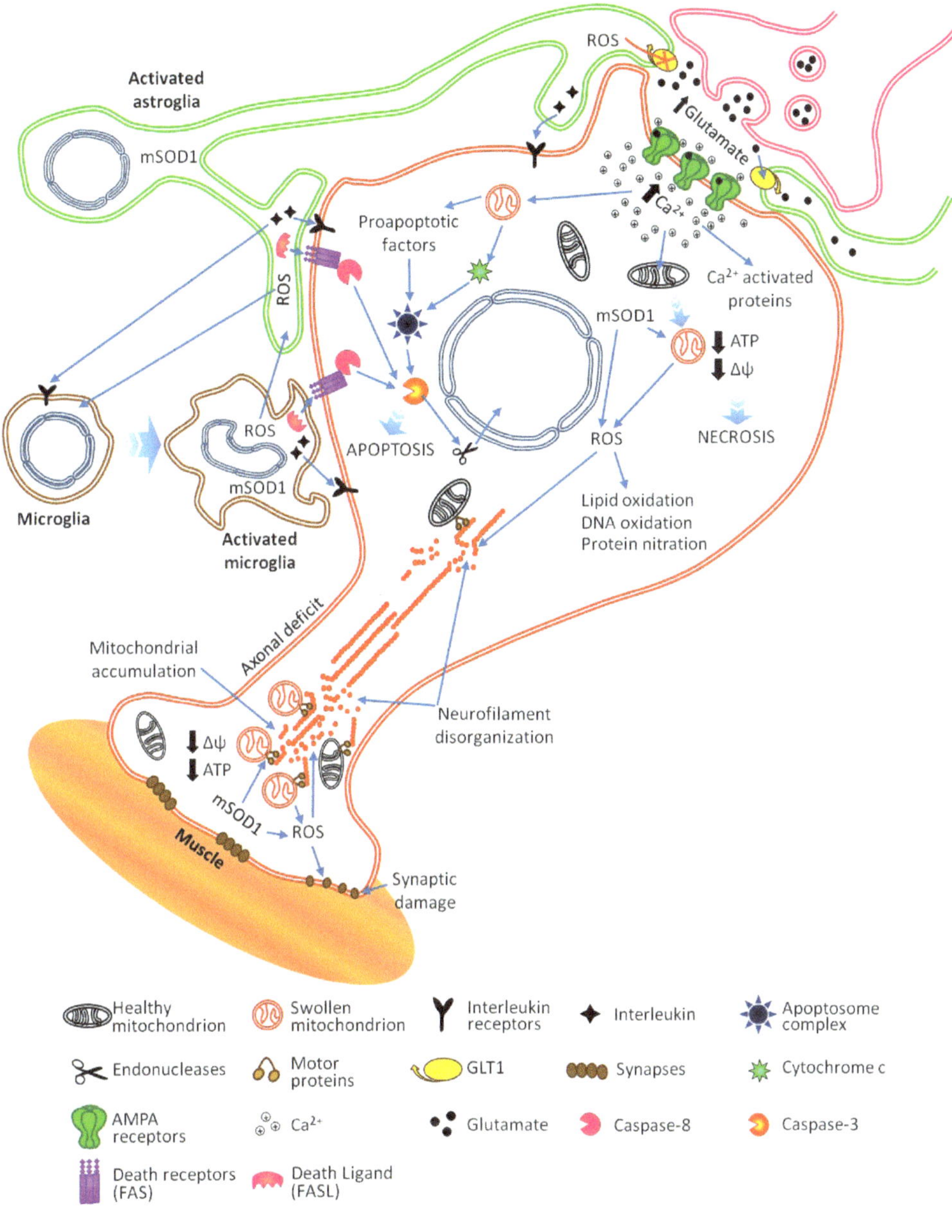

Fig. 1. Scheme of the main proposed mechanisms involved in motor neuron death. Description in the text.

These deficits may affect the renewal of organelles in the axon terminals of motor neurons, leading to accumulation of damaged mitochondria or autophagosomes, increased ROS production, disruption of microtubule formation and stability (Julien & Mushynski, 1998), as well as damage of presynaptic structure such as swelling of axon terminals (Komatsu et al., 2007). Accumulation of damaged mitochondria may result in energetic failure (Liu et al., 2004; Martin et al., 2009; Menzies et al., 2002a, b; Pasinelli et al., 2004; Wong et al., 1995; Zhu et al., 2002) and in the release of proapoptotic factors (Pasinelli et al., 2004) (Fig. 1, bottom left). These alterations may be involved in the distal neurophaty and impairment of muscular reinnervation observed in ALS.

2.3 Oxidative stress

Another mechanism implicated in motor neuron degeneration in ALS that involves both motor neurons and non-neuronal cells is oxidative stress. Reactive oxygen species (ROS) arise in cells as aerobic metabolism by-products, mostly due to the leakage of electrons from the mitochondrial respiratory chain, resulting in an incomplete reduction of molecular oxygen during the oxidative phosphorylation, generating the superoxide radical anion ($O_2^{\bullet -}$). The $O_2^{\bullet -}$ anion reacts quickly with the nitric oxide radical ($NO^{\bullet}$, produced by nitric oxide synthase, NOS) to form peroxynitrite ($ONOO^-$). Meanwhile, the product of $O_2^{\bullet -}$ dismutation, H_2O_2, slowly decomposes to form the highly reactive hydroxyl radical ($^{\bullet}OH$). Both $ONOO^-$ and $^{\bullet}OH$ are highly reactive and can damage proteins, membranes and DNA by oxidation. Cellular mechanisms to combat the constant production of free radicals are: 1) enzymes such as SOD, catalase and peroxidase, which catalytically remove reactive species; 2) reducing agents synthesized in vivo, such as glutathione, α-keto acids, lipoic acid and coenzyme Q, and compounds obtained from the diet, such as ascorbate (vitamin C) and α-tocopherol (vitamin E); and 3) chaperone heat shock proteins which remove or facilitate repair of damaged proteins. Oxidative stress arises from an imbalance between ROS production and its control mechanisms.

The involvement of oxidative stress in ALS pathogenesis is supported by abundant evidence that has been reported in both SALS and FALS patients, where several indicators of increased oxidative damage have been found: 1) In postmortem central nervous system (CNS) tissue samples (mainly spinal cord) these markers include oxidized DNA (Ferrante et al., 1997b; Fitzmaurice et al., 1996), lipid peroxidation (Siciliano et al., 2002), protein glycoxidation (Shibata et al., 2001), elevated protein carbonylation (Ferrante et al., 1997b; Shaw et al., 1995a), and increased protein tyrosine nitration; remarkably, nitrotyrosine immunoreactivity was more densely detected in motor neurons (Abe et al., 1995; Abe et al., 1997; Beal et al., 1997; Ferrante et al., 1997a). 2) Oxidation markers in CSF, plasma and blood from living ALS patients during the course of the disease have also been described. The most relevant are oxidized DNA (Bogdanov et al., 2000; Ihara et al., 2005), hydroxyl and ascorbate free radicals (Ihara et al., 2005), lipid peroxidation (Baillet et al., 2010; Bogdanov et al., 2000; Bonnefont-Rousselot et al., 2000; Ihara et al., 2005; Oteiza et al., 1997; Simpson et al., 2004; Smith et al., 1998), and a remarkable elevation of 3-nitrotyrosine levels in CSF (Tohgi et al., 1999). However, in other study, 3-nitroyrosine was not different between the CSF of ALS patients and control subjects (Ryberg et al., 2004). Increased oxidative damage to proteins, lipids and DNA has also been demonstrated in CNS tissue of transgenic mouse model of FALS expressing mSOD1 (Andrus et al., 1998; Casoni et al., 2005; Liu et al., 1999; Liu et al., 1998; Poon et al., 2005).

Mitochondria, ROS and glutamate-induced excitotoxicity are closely related and this is relevant in ALS, because the mitochondrion is the main oxygen consumer and it is also the main producer of ROS. These species can be produced in neurons and in non-neuronal cells and can cause failure in the glutamate uptake system of both motor neurons and astroglia (Rao et al., 2003; Trotti et al., 1996, 1998; Volterra et al., 1994; Zagami et al., 2009). This may contribute to an excitotoxic condition due to increased concentration of extracellular glutamate. ROS production and its effects on motor neurons and non-neuronal cells are illustrated in Fig. 1.

2.4 Inflammation

A mechanism of non-cell-autonomous death associated with motor neuron degeneration in both FALS and SALS is the participation of non-neuronal cells in inflammatory events (Boillee et al., 2006a; Boillee et al., 2006b; Hall et al., 1998; Yamanaka et al., 2008; Yang et al., 2011). The main histopathological feature of inflammation is the proliferation of reactive astrogliosis and of activated microglial cells, associated with alterations in their cellular functions, such as glutamate reuptake failure and release of proapoptotic and proinflammatory factors (Sanagi et al., 2010; Sargsyan et al., 2005; Sofroniew, 2005). Molecules associated with inflammatory process, such as interleukins 6, 12, 15, 17A, 23, C4d and C3d complement proteins, as well as tumor necrosis factor-alpha, have been found in blood and CSF from ALS patients (Almer et al., 2002; Fiala et al., 2010; Henkel et al., 2004; Kawamata et al., 1992; McGeer et al., 1991; Moreau et al., 2005; Rentzos et al., 2010a, b). The finding of increased levels of granzymes A, B in serum (Ilzecka, 2011) and decrease in cytochrome c levels in the CSF (Ilzecka, 2007), suggests an apoptotic process in human disease. The proliferation of activated non-neuronal cells has been associated with the disease severity (Clement et al., 2003). Nevertheless, alteration in their functions may be more important than their proliferation (Lepore et al., 2008). In experimental models of FALS (mSOD1) it has been attempted to prevent the motor neuron loss through the use of drugs with anti-inflammatory properties, such as minocycline (Keller et al., 2010; Kriz et al., 2002; Neymotin et al., 2009; Van Den Bosch et al., 2002; Zhu et al., 2002). This drug was effective in delaying the motor neurons loss when given prior to the symptoms onset, but when given at late stages it exaggerated the neuroinflammatory response and accelerated the progression of the symptoms (Keller et al., 2010). In this transgenic ALS model, apoptosis processes can be triggered by non-neuronal cells through the extrinsic apoptotic pathway, via the release from activated glial cells of several death ligands (for example FasL) that bind to their respective death receptor (Fas) and trigger the cleavage of caspase-8 (Locatelli et al., 2007; Petri et al., 2006; Raoul et al., 2006) (Fig. 1).

3. Mitochondrial dysfunction in ALS and in experimental motor neuron degeneration

A convergent point of the deleterious mechanisms discussed above is the mitochondrion. This organelle is the main energy producer in eukaryotic cells and plays a fundamental role in normal cell physiology. Among the functions mitochondria carry out, besides ATP synthesis, intracellular Ca^{2+}buffering has been recognized as another relevant factor for the protection against deleterious processes such as oxidative stress, excitotoxicity and necrotic and apoptotic death, thus playing a central role in neuronal survival.

Mitochondria are closely related to necrotic and apoptotic processes, which are the main cellular death mechanisms. During necrosis, mitochondria undergo rapid swelling and lysis. Although apoptosis is an energy-dependent active process, sometimes mitochondrial morphological alterations are associated with the intrinsic-apoptosis pathway. Furthermore, it is now recognized that apoptosis and necrosis are not two mutually exclusive processes, but they can occur simultaneously or one preceding the other (Kroemer et al., 2009; Martin, 2010; Martin et al., 2009; Shrivastava & Vivekanandhan, 2011).

As the organelle responsible for energy production in the cell, mitochondria possess the enzymatic machinery to catalyze the oxidation of various substrates generated inside and outside mitochondria, including pyruvate trough pyruvate dehydrogenase, fatty acids through β-oxidation, and carbon chains from amino acids. Energy is obtained by oxidation of all these biomolecules to finally CO_2 and H_2O through the tricarboxylic acid cycle and the respiratory chain. The tricarboxylic acid cycle is the converging point because the carbon skeletons of carbohydrates and fatty acids are metabolized to yield the acetyl group of acetyl-Coenzyme A, and many of the carbons of the amino acid skeleton also enter the cycle via its conversion to some cycle intermediates. The reducing equivalents generated in the tricarboxylic acid cycle reactions reduce pyridine and flavin nucleotides to NADH and $FADH_2$. These electron transporters enter the respiratory chain, where electron flux through various redox carriers and centers in the enzyme complexes located in the inner mitochondrial membrane finally reduces O_2 to H_2O; this flux is coupled to ATP synthesis through oxidative phosphorylation.

The energy released by the electron flux through respiratory chain complexes is used to pump protons through the inner mitochondrial membrane, producing an alkaline and negatively charged mitochondrial matrix, as compared to the intermembrane space, thus creating a proton gradient. This proton gradient generates an electrochemical potential called proton-motive force (Δp), which supplies the energy to ATP synthase for ATP synthesis from ADP and inorganic phosphate. The Δp depends mainly on the mitochondrial transmembrane potential ($\Delta\psi_m$), which is the electric potential (negative inside), but it also depends on the transmembrane pH gradient (ΔpH), which is the chemical potential (alkaline inside). Energy stored in the proton gradient can also transport solutes against concentration gradient across the membrane. The $\Delta\psi_m$ is a central parameter that controls three fundamental and highly relevant cellular processes for neuronal survival: ATP synthesis, mitochondrial Ca^{2+} sequestration, and mitochondrial ROS generation. On the other hand, $\Delta\psi_m$ is controlled by substrate availability, ATP demand, respiratory chain capacity, mitochondrial proton conductance, and mitochondrial Ca^{2+} sequestration (Nicholls & Budd, 2000). Therefore, mitochondrial bioenergetic status is crucial for controlling the susceptibility of neurons to chronic or acute stress and also in determining cellular fate (survival, apoptosis or necrosis).

Owing to the great relevance of mitochondria, their morphological, ultrastructural and functional characteristics have been studied in ALS patients. Deficits in respiratory chain complexes I and IV activities have been detected in the spinal cord and skeletal muscle (Borthwick et al., 1999; Crugnola et al., 2010; Vielhaber et al., 2000; Wiedemann et al., 2002; Wiedemann et al., 1998), and a temporal study of mitochondrial respiratory function in skeletal muscle in SALS demonstrated that respiratory complex IV activity is progressively altered as the disease develops (Echaniz-Laguna et al., 2006). Some cases of ALS have been described as a mitochondriopathy (Finsterer, 2002, 2003) including a mitochondrial DNA mutation in the gene encoding subunit I of the mitochondrial respiratory chain complex IV (Comi et al., 1998). The electron transport chain proteins FAD synthetase, riboflavin kinase, cytochrome C1, and succinate dehydrogenase complex subunit B expression were significantly decreased in some ALS patients (Lin et al., 2009).

In the mSOD1 mice or cell culture familial ALS model, complexes I, II and IV of the electron transport chain exhibit decreased enzyme activities, even at early stages of the disease (Jung et al., 2002; Mattiazzi et al., 2002; Menzies et al., 2002a,b). In G93A-SOD1 mice the association of cytochrome c with the inner mitochondrial membrane was reduced and there was a significant decrease in respiratory chain complex IV (Kirkinezos et al., 2005). SOD-containing aggregates (Higgins et al., 2002; Jaarsma et al., 2001; Pasinelli et al., 2004) and decreased oxygen consumption, lack of ADP-dependent respiratory control, and decreased membrane potential (Cassina et al., 2008), were observed in mitochondria from spinal cord of transgenic mSOD1 rodents.

In neuronal cultures, glutamate-mediated excitotoxicity caused significant changes in mitochondrial function, such as decline in ATP levels, mitochondrial transmembrane potential collapse, decreased mitochondrial and cellular oxygen consumption, and oxidative phosphorylation uncoupling, all these events preceding cell death (Ankarcrona et al., 1995; Atlante et al., 1996; Maus et al., 1999; Monje et al., 2001). There is a link between excitotoxicity-induced intracellular Ca^{2+} overload and the collapse of $\Delta\psi_m$, since intracellular Ca^{2+} increase and its accumulation in mitochondria are sufficient to induce prominent and persistent depolarization, leading to mitochondrial dysfunction and to neuronal death in vitro (Schinder et al., 1996; White & Reynolds, 1996).

Few studies on excitotoxicity have been carried out in vivo. In our laboratory we have developed two experimental models of spinal motor neurons degeneration by overactivation of AMPA receptors, both by infusing AMPA directly in the lumbar spinal cord of rats. In the first one AMPA is administered through microdialysis cannulas during short time periods (Corona & Tapia, 2004) and in the other AMPA is infused chronically during several days, using osmotic minipumps (Tovar-y-Romo et al., 2007). These models reproduce the main histopathological features of ALS: loss of lumbar motor neurons, astroglial activation and motor deficits that progresses to complete paralysis of the rear limbs. The main difference between the two models is the time required for the occurrence of motor neuron degeneration and the development of the paralysis. AMPA perfusion by microdialysis causes a rapid loss of motor neuron and paralysis, occurring within the initial 12 hours, while chronic AMPA infusion with osmotic minipumps triggers a progressive motor neuron loss and motor deficits throughout three to four days. For these reasons, the microdialysis model is defined as an acute model and the minipumps model as a chronic model of spinal motor neuron degeneration by excitotoxicity (Tovar-y-Romo et al., 2009a). The most important feature of both models is that motor neuron loss occurs without the influence of a genetic factor and thus presumably can be used to study the mechanisms that may be involved in motor neuron loss occurring in SALS, which accounts for over 90% of ALS cases.

We have recently assessed mitochondrial function in our acute model of spinal excitotoxic motor neuron degeneration, by studying mitochondrial oxygen consumption and transmembrane potential in mitochondria isolated from the lumbar spinal cord of rats perfused with AMPA. The AMPA-treated group showed decreased oxygen consumption, ADP-dependent respiratory control and transmembrane potential, as compared to control rats perfused only with Krebs-Ringer medium (Santa-Cruz and Tapia, in preparation). These results suggest that mitochondrial dysfunction plays a crucial role in spinal motoneuron degeneration induced by overactivation of AMPA receptors in vivo. These mechanisms could be involved in ALS motoneuron degeneration.

3.1 Ca^{2+}, mitochondria and motor neuron degeneration

Under physiological conditions, Ca^{2+} participates as intracellular messenger in many normal cellular functions, such as cell growth, differentiation, signal transduction, membrane excitability regulation, exocytosis and synaptic activity. Cytoplasmic Ca^{2+} concentration in resting neurons is maintained at low concentrations (~100 nM), 10,000 times lower than extracellular space concentration. To achieve this, neurons possess specialized homeostatic mechanisms, such as regulation of Ca^{2+} input and output, Ca^{2+} binding proteins, mitochondrial and endoplasmic reticulum storage, and Ca^{2+}-ATPases. Moreover, neurons not only control intracellular Ca^{2+} levels, but also its location in the cell by means of complex interactions among Ca^{2+} input, output, buffering and internal storage. Under physiological conditions, these processes maintain spatial and temporal location of Ca^{2+}, so that multiple Ca^{2+}-regulated signaling pathways can take place independently within the same cell.

Excessive intracellular Ca^{2+} concentration damages neurons through several mechanisms, including mitochondrial damage, energy metabolism deficit, toxic ROS generation, membrane depolarization, and activation of lytic enzymes such as proteases, lipases, phosphatases and endonucleases. Intracellular Ca^{2+} accumulation also stimulates ROS production through NOS activation and the conversion of xanthine dehydrogenase to xanthine oxidase through proteases activation. All these events eventually produce membrane destruction and neuronal death (Arundine & Tymianski, 2003; Shaw, 1999).

Intracellular Ca^{2+} regulation is an expensive process from the energy point of view. Ca^{2+} is extruded from the cell and sequestered into the endoplasmic reticulum through active transport using Ca^{2+}-ATPases, and it is also removed by secondary active transport using the Na^+/Ca^{2+} exchanger, which activates Na^+/K^+-ATPases to take out Na^+. Mitochondria also play a critical role in the regulation of cytosolic Ca^{2+} concentration, since they sequester this cation through a Ca^{2+} uniporter located in the inner mitochondrial membrane and driven by the electric potential (Nicholls, 1985). To prevent a potentially lethal Ca^{2+} accumulation in mitochondrial matrix, there is an output system that exchanges Na^+/Ca^{2+}, besides a mitochondrial Na^+/H^+ transporter that extrudes Na^+, so that ion flux under a constant Ca^{2+} entrance to mitochondria involves a sequential transfer of Ca^{2+}, Na^+ and H^+, the latter driven by the respiratory chain (Crompton & Heid, 1978; Nicholls & Budd, 2000). When Ca^{2+} concentration surpasses a certain critical point, under physiological phosphate concentration an osmotically inactive and rapidly dissociable Ca^{2+}-phosphate complex is formed in the mitochondrial matrix, so that mitochondria work as efficient buffers of extramitochondrial Ca^{2+} by accumulating this cation (Becker et al., 1980; Nicholls, 1978). Apparently, this organelle acts as a temporary Ca^{2+} store during high cytoplasmic concentrations peaks, as suggested by the kinetics of mitochondrial Ca^{2+} transport; because the Ca^{2+}-phosphate complex is rapidly dissociable, mitochondria can release Ca^{2+} back to the cytoplasm when its concentration decreases below the critical point. As long as mitochondria are polarized, cytosolic Ca^{2+} accumulates within the mitochondrial matrix through the Ca^{2+} uniporter. Mitochondrial Ca^{2+} uptake is driven by $\Delta\psi_m$, so it will compete with ATP synthase for proton gradient, in such a way that Ca^{2+} uptake could dominate due to the fact that ATP synthesis requires a thermodynamic threshold for $\Delta\psi_m$, while Ca^{2+} transport can proceed at much lower $\Delta\psi_m$ and excessive Ca^{2+} concentrations reduce $\Delta\psi_m$ dramatically. When Ca^{2+} concentration does not recover below the critical point, excessive Ca^{2+} overload in the mitochondrial matrix can lead to mitochondrial swelling, loss of respiratory control, increased mitochondrial ROS generation, $\Delta\psi_m$ collapse (depolarization) diminished ATP synthesis, and Ca^{2+} release from the mitochondrial matrix caused by inner mitochondrial membrane permeabilization through the mitochondrial permeability transition pore (MPTP, a large protein complex forming a non-selective pore through the inner mitochondrial membrane) (Al-Nasser & Crompton, 1986; Nicholls & Budd, 2000; Peng & Jou, 2010). When mitochondrion depolarizes, accumulated Ca^{2+} goes back into the cytoplasm, either through the Ca^{2+} uniporter, the Na^+/Ca^{2+} exchanger, or through the MPTP. Since Δp depends mainly on $\Delta\psi_m$, its collapse causes Δp collapse, which results not only in halting ATP synthesis but also in a rapid cytoplasmic ATP hydrolysis because ATP synthase catalytic function reverses in an attempt to restore Δp.

In motor neurons, the damage produced by these alterations may be enhanced because they do not have sufficient mitochondrial Ca^{2+}-buffering capacity, due in part to a lower mitochondrial density per volume compared to non-motor neurons (Grosskreutz et al., 2007). In addition, other buffering mechanisms are deficient in spinal and cortical motor neurons because they lack the Ca^{2+}-binding proteins calbindin D-28K and parvalbumin. This may explain why other motor neurons that express these proteins, such as those located in oculomotor and Onuf's nuclei, are not usually affected in ALS (Alexianu et al., 1994; Celio, 1990; Ince et al., 1993; Palecek et al., 1999). For all these reasons, mitochondrial Ca^{2+} overload plays a key role in glutamatergic excitotoxicity (Nicholls et al., 2003), given that overactivation of Ca^{2+}-permeable AMPA receptors, which are abundant in spinal motor neurons, confers to these cells a special vulnerability to AMPA receptor-mediated excitotoxicity (Corona & Tapia, 2007; Grosskreutz et al., 2010). AMPA exposure to spinal motor neuron cultures results in an intracellular Ca^{2+} concentration increase that triggers mitochondrial Ca^{2+} overload, depolarization and ROS generation (Carriedo et al., 2000). So, there is abundant evidence that suggest that mitochondrial damage, probably related to Ca^{2+} homeostasis disturbances, is involved in SALS and FALS (Manfredi & Xu, 2005; Menzies et al., 2002a; Swerdlow et al., 1998; von Lewinski & Keller, 2005).

3.2 Energy deficits

Due to the large size of motor neurons and their long processes reaching muscles, they have an expensive energy cost and this renders them very vulnerable to energy deficits. Much of the ATP demand in neurons is used in the ion pumping through plasma membrane to maintain membrane potential. Thus, Na^+/K^+-ATPase is the most demanding ATP process in neurons (Scott & Nicholls, 1980) in order to expel Na^+ excess resulting from excitation. Intracellular Ca^{2+} regulation by Ca-ATPases is also highly energy consuming, as previously discussed.

There is abundant evidence both in vitro and in vivo that any restriction in the ability of the cell to generate ATP can exacerbate or even induce glutamatergic excitotoxicity. The energy-linked excitotoxic hypothesis (Beal et al., 1993; Greene & Greenamyre, 1996; Novelli et al., 1988) proposes that the correlation between excitotoxic damage and energy restriction is due to plasma membrane depolarization. Diminished ATP levels cause a decrease in Na^+/K^+-ATPase and Ca^{2+}-ATPase functions, lessening Na^+ and Ca^{2+} removal. This triggers plasma

membrane depolarization and as a consequence Ca^{2+} enters the cell through voltage-dependent Ca^{2+}channels and glutamate is released to the extracellular space by exocytosis. This in turn activates Ca^{2+} influx through the NMDA receptor, which is also voltage-dependent. Further, under energetic failure conditions, glutamate transporters operate in reverse because Na^{+}/K^{+} electrochemical gradient collapse due to ATP decrease, resulting in diminished glutamate uptake and non-vesicular glutamate release into extracellular space (Jabaudon et al., 2000; Longuemare & Swanson, 1995).
The observation that inhibition of mitochondrial respiratory chain complexes activity can induce pathological changes similar to those observed in some neurodegenerative diseases in specific CNS regions has generated great interest. Association among glutamatergic excitotoxicity and bioenergetic limitation has been proposed for Alzheimer, Parkinson, Huntington's disease and ALS (Beal, 1998), and in many cases specific respiratory chain complexes are involved. In organotypic spinal cord cultures, motor neurons are selectively vulnerable to chronic mitochondrial blockade by inhibitors of mitochondrial respiratory chain complex II and complex IV and this motor neuron degeneration displays structural changes similar to those seen following excitotoxicity (Brunet et al., 2009; Kaal et al., 2000).
In our acute model of excitotoxic motor neuron degeneration previously described (Corona & Tapia, 2004, 2007) we have demonstrated the importance of Ca^{2+}-permeable AMPA receptors and of intracellular Ca^{2+} overload in motor neuron death process. Using this model, we aimed to study the importance of energy deficits and oxidative stress in AMPA-induced degeneration. With this purpose, we assessed the potential neuroprotection of various energy substrates and antioxidants at different concentrations, co-perfusing them with AMPA in the rat lumbar spinal cord. We observed protection at different degrees depending on the concentration of each compound, but in general antioxidants only partially protected, while various energy substrates prevented the AMPA-induced motor impairment and the spinal motor neuron loss (Santa-Cruz and Tapia, in preparation). These findings suggest that intracellular Ca^{2+} overload in vivo disrupts mitochondrial energy metabolism. On the other hand, energy substrates can directly prevent $\Delta\psi_m$ collapse and thus prevent mitochondrial dysfunction. Because one of the factors that control $\Delta\psi_m$ is substrate availability, excess mitochondrial substrates administered exogenously can stimulate respiratory chain and increase oxidative phosphorylation, maintaining the electrochemical proton gradient and thus preventing the collapse of ATP synthesis.

3.3 Oxidative stress

Since mitochondria are the organelles where oxidative phosphorylation is accomplished, they consume about 98 % of the cell oxygen requirement and constitute a major site for intracellular ROS production. Some steps along mitochondrial oxygen reduction pathway have the potential to produce, and indeed generate free radicals, due to the fact that electron flux along respiratory chain may have leakage of electrons to oxygen. The intermediate radical ubisemiquinone, involved in the transfer of electrons through respiratory complexes III and I, can grant an electron to oxygen, forming the superoxide radical $O_2^{\bullet-}$, a powerful oxidant and a very reactive intermediate (Turrens et al., 1985) that must be rapidly removed by antioxidant enzymes to avoid its lethal effects. About 0.1-4% of the O_2 used by actively respiring mitochondria is converted to $O_2^{\bullet-}$. Nevertheless, respiratory chain enzymes defects or other mitochondrial perturbations could be responsible of an excessive mitochondrial

ROS production, triggering or increasing cellular injure. Among them, mitochondrial Ca^{2+} overload resulting from NMDA, AMPA or kainate receptor overactivation (Carriedo et al., 1998; Carriedo et al., 2000; Dugan et al., 1995) increases ROS production (Dykens, 1994; Peng & Jou, 2010); thus, an initial excitotoxic event might also contribute to increased oxidative stress.

In addition, it is important to consider that mitochondria are not only ROS producers but also that they are a susceptible target of them. Thereby, in a pathologic situation where an increased ROS production occurs initially, oxidative damage to mitochondrial lipids, nucleic acids and proteins can reduce mitochondrial respiration, disturb normal function and seriously damage this organelle (Lenaz et al., 2002). Furthermore, mitochondrial DNA is more susceptible to oxidative damage than nuclear DNA, due to its close location next to an important ROS production site, to the lack of protective histones and to less effective repair mechanisms, as compared to the nuclear DNA (Richter et al., 1988). Mitochondrial redox status also influences the opening of the MPTP, since it is enhanced by oxidative stress in isolated mitochondria (Saxena et al., 1995).

4. Mitochondrial structural damage in ALS and experimental motor neuron degeneration

The death process involved in the motor neuron loss characteristic of ALS is not yet fully understood. Several functional alterations present in both human disease and experimental models have been reviewed in the previous sections, but several studies have shown also morphological and ultrastructural changes in motor neurons that may be associated with apoptosis and/or necrosis.

Postmortem examination of ALS patients tissues has revealed morphological and ultrastructural abnormalities in mitochondria. Atypical mitochondrial aggregates were found in skeletal muscle subsarcolemmal region and in intramuscular axons (Afifi et al., 1966; Atsumi, 1981), and morphological abnormalities were also detected in proximal axons, as well as dense clusters of mitochondria in the ventral horn of spinal cord SALS patients (Hirano et al., 1984a; b; Sasaki & Iwata, 1996). Giant mitochondria with intramitochondrial inclusions were observed in the liver of some ALS patients and these alterations were disease specific (Nakano et al., 1987). Further, mitochondria with increased volume and with high Ca^{2+} concentration were found in motor nerve terminals in muscle biopsies of alive ALS patients, which were not observed in patients with other neuropathies or in control subjects (Siklos et al., 1996). Ultrastructural damage of mitochondria, characterized by swelling and rounding, was recently described in platelets of ALS patients (Shrivastava & Vivekanandhan, 2011; Shrivastava et al., 2011a,b).

The main problem with pathological studies in human ALS is the difficulty in determining whether the alterations observed are a cause or a consequence of the disease. This highlights the importance of developing experimental models of motor neuron death to study the temporal progress of the morphological changes, including the alterations of mitochondrial structure. With this objective, we have recently studied the ultrastructural changes of mitochondria in both our acute and chronic models of spinal motor neuron death described above. In the acute model we observed motor neurons with mitochondrial swelling as soon as 2 h after AMPA perfusion, followed in a few hours by the rupture of mitochondrial, nuclear and plasma membranes, which led to total neuronal disruption. These ultrastructural alterations are characteristic of a necrotic process. In contrast, in the chronic model we observed by day one swelling of the endoplasmic reticulum and only later progressive alterations in mitochondrial internal and external membranes that generated mitochondrial swelling. So, the initial mitochondrial integrity might indicate an apoptotic process, although motor neurons eventually probably die by a slow necrotic process (Fig. 2; Ramírez-Jarquín and Tapia, in preparation). The mitochondrial swelling observed in both models may be associated with energy failure, which as discussed above causes ATP depletion, oxidative stress and inflammatory events, leading to cell death.

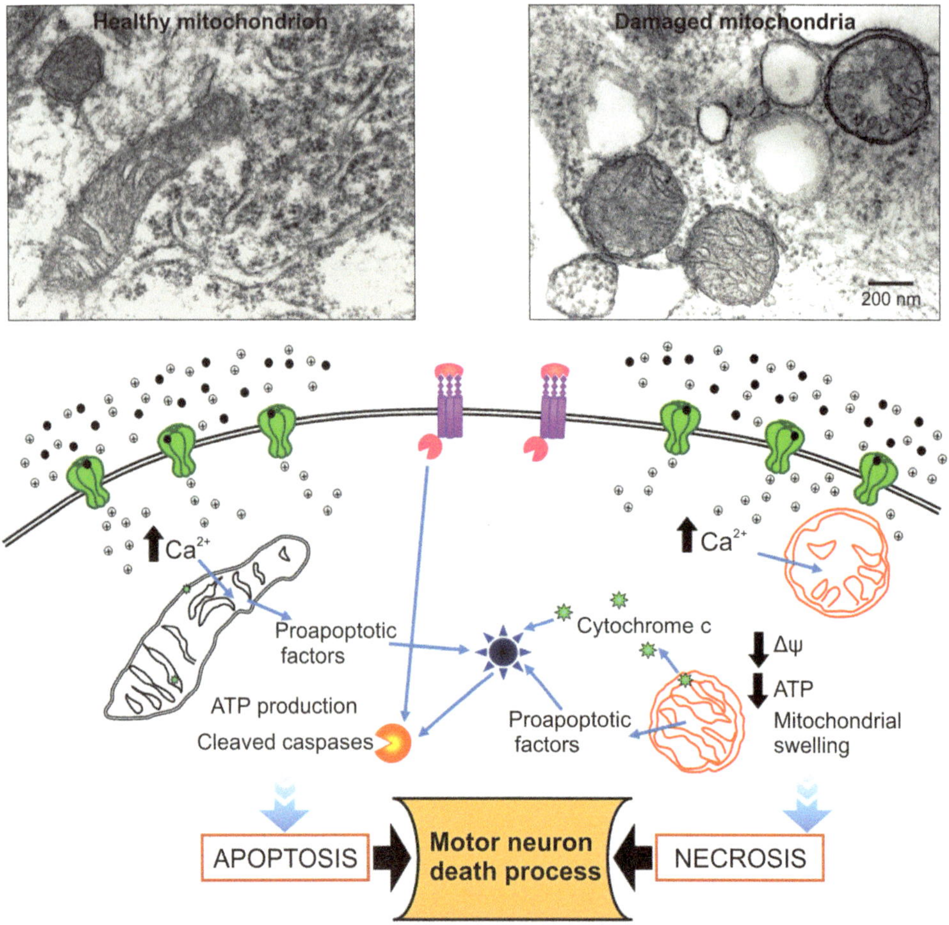

Fig. 2. Role of mitochondrial damage in motor neuron excitotoxicity. The electron-micrographs show normal mitochondria and endoplasmic reticulum in a spinal motor neuron of a control rat (left), and swollen mitochondria with altered cristae observed 2 h after perfusion of AMPA by microdialysis (right) (Ramírez-Jarquín and Tapia, unpublished). Bottom: proposal of the involvement of mitochondrial damage in the apoptosis and necrosis processes leading to motor neuron death. The symbols are the same as in Fig. 1. Description in the text.

The mitochondrial damage seen in our models is similar to those observed in the human disease and also in muscle and spinal cord of mSOD1 rodent models, namely mitochondrial fragmentation, enlargement, vacuolization, rearrangement of the cristae and swelling (Bendotti et al., 2001; Kong & Xu, 1998; Martin et al., 2009; Menzies et al., 2002b; Wong et al., 1995). The observed rearrangement of the inner membrane to form small vacuoles has been associated with an alteration in the MPTP permeability and also with the trigger of intrinsic-apoptosis pathway by release of proapoptotic factors, such as cytochrome c (Bendotti et al., 2001; Martin, 2010; Martin et al., 2009; Ohta et al., 2008) followed by the cleavage of caspases (Li et al., 2000; Pasinelli et al., 2000) Fig. 2 illustrates the ultrastructural mitochondrial damage and shows a schematic representation of the mechanisms associated with these alterations.

5. Conclusions

Altogether the foregoing data suggest that mitochondrial respiratory chain damage is a relevant event in ALS pathogenesis, although it is still unknown if mitochondrial abnormalities are the cause of the disease process or if they are consequence of neuronal degeneration, However, it is clear from the evidence reviewed here that mitochondria definitely play a central role in determining the fate of motor neurons and in their degeneration process. This evidence comes from studies in several tissues of ALS patients, both from biopsies or from postmortem observations, and from direct measurements of mitochondrial function in experimental models of motor neuron degeneration, both in vitro and in vivo. These experiments clearly point to energy deficits and disruption of Ca^{2+} homeostasis and axonal transport.

Integrity of the mitochondria morphology and structure is pivotal for their function and for cellular health. It is interesting that similar structural alterations have been observed in ALS tissues and in in vitro and in vivo models of motor neuron degeneration, including transgenic mSOD1 rodents and excitotoxicity. Clearly, this damage can be associated with the mitochondrial functional deficits, which trigger deleterious process resulting in cellular death by apoptosis, necrosis or a combination of these mechanisms. Although there is biochemical evidence of an apoptotic process involving the mitochondria, no ultrastructural evidence of classic apoptosis, such as apoptotic bodies, has been found. Rather, mitochondrial swelling and membrane disruption are frequently observed, suggesting the predominance of a necrotic process.

The evidence for a role of calcium homeostasis disruption in the induction of neuronal death is vast, and the involvement of mitochondria in this mechanism seems determinant. The advances in the elucidation of this process should help to understand the importance of the preservation of mitochondrial structure and function, which hopefully can lead to the design of preventive and therapeutic measures for ALS.

6. Acknowledgement

This work and the authors' experiments cited were supported by Dirección General del Personal Académico, Universidad Nacional Autónoma de México, (project IN215610) and Consejo Nacional de Ciencia y Tecnología (CONACYT), México (project 128229). L.D.S.C. and U.N.R.J. are recipients of a scholarship from CONACYT.

7. References

Abe, K., Pan, L. H., Watanabe, M., Kato, T. & Itoyama, Y. (1995). Induction of nitrotyrosine-like immunoreactivity in the lower motor neuron of amyotrophic lateral sclerosis. *Neuroscience letters,* Vol.199, No.2, (October 1995), pp. 152-154, ISSN 0304-3940.

Abe, K., Pan, L. H., Watanabe, M., Konno, H., Kato, T. & Itoyama, Y. (1997). Upregulation of protein-tyrosine nitration in the anterior horn cells of amyotrophic lateral sclerosis. *Neurological research,* Vol.19, No.2, (April 1997), pp. 124-128, ISSN 0161-6412.

Afifi, A. K., Aleu, F. P., Goodgold, J. & MacKay, B. (1966). Ultrastructure of atrophic muscle in amyotrophic lateral sclerosis. *Neurology,* Vol.16, No.5, (May 1996), pp. 475-481, ISSN 0028-3878.

Al-Nasser, I. & Crompton, M. (1986). The reversible Ca2+-induced permeabilization of rat liver mitochondria. *The Biochemical journal,* Vol.239, No.1, (October 1986), pp. 19-29, ISSN 0264-6021.

Alexianu, M. E., Ho, B. K., Mohamed, A. H., La Bella, V., Smith, R. G. & Appel, S. H. (1994). The role of calcium-binding proteins in selective motoneuron vulnerability in amyotrophic lateral sclerosis. *Annals of neurology,* Vol.36, No.6, (December 1994), pp. 846-858, ISSN 0364-5134

Almer, G., Teismann, P., Stevic, Z., Halaschek-Wiener, J., Deecke, L., Kostic, V. & Przedborski, S. (2002). Increased levels of the pro-inflammatory prostaglandin PGE2 in CSF from ALS patients. *Neurology,* Vol.58, No.8, (April 2002), pp. 1277-1279, ISSN 0028-3878.

Andrus, P. K., Fleck, T. J., Gurney, M. E. & Hall, E. D. (1998). Protein oxidative damage in a transgenic mouse model of familial amyotrophic lateral sclerosis. *Journal of neurochemistry,* Vol.71, No.5, (November 1998), pp. 2041-2048, ISSN 0022-3042.

Ankarcrona, M., Dypbukt, J. M., Bonfoco, E., Zhivotovsky, B., Orrenius, S., Lipton, S. A. & Nicotera, P. (1995). Glutamate-induced neuronal death: a succession of necrosis or apoptosis depending on mitochondrial function. *Neuron,* Vol.15, No.4, (October 1995), pp. 961-973, ISSN 0896-6273.

Arundine, M. & Tymianski, M. (2003). Molecular mechanisms of calcium-dependent neurodegeneration in excitotoxicity. *Cell calcium,* Vol.34, No.4-5, (October-November 2003), pp. 325-337, ISSN 0143-4160.

Atlante, A., Gagliardi, S., Minervini, G. M., Marra, E., Passarella, S. & Calissano, P. (1996). Rapid uncoupling of oxidative phosphorylation accompanies glutamate toxicity in rat cerebellar granule cells. *Neuroreport,* Vol.7, No.15-17, (November 1996), pp. 2519-2523, ISSN 0959-4965.

Atsumi, T. (1981). The ultrastructure of intramuscular nerves in amyotrophic lateral sclerosis. *Acta neuropathologica,* Vol.55, No.3, pp. 193-198, ISSN 0001-6322.

Baillet, A., Chanteperdrix, V., Trocme, C., Casez, P., Garrel, C. & Besson, G. (2010). The role of oxidative stress in amyotrophic lateral sclerosis and Parkinson's disease. *Neurochemical research,* Vol.35, No.10, (October 2010), pp. 1530-1537, ISSN 1573-6903 (Electronic), 0364-3190 (Linking).

Beal, M. F. (1998). Mitochondrial dysfunction in neurodegenerative diseases. *Biochimica et biophysica acta,* Vol.1366, No.1-2, (August 1998), pp. 211-223, ISSN 0006-3002.

Beal, M. F., Hyman, B. T. & Koroshetz, W. (1993). Do defects in mitochondrial energy metabolism underlie the pathology of neurodegenerative diseases? *Trends in neurosciences,* Vol.16, No.4, (April 1993), pp. 125-131, ISSN 0166-2236.

Beal, M. F., Ferrante, R. J., Browne, S. E., Matthews, R. T., Kowall, N. W. & Brown, R. H., Jr. (1997). Increased 3-nitrotyrosine in both sporadic and familial amyotrophic lateral sclerosis. *Annals of neurology,* Vol.42, No.4, (October 1997), pp. 644-654, ISSN 0364-5134.

Becker, G. L., Fiskum, G. & Lehninger, A. L. (1980). Regulation of free Ca2+ by liver mitochondria and endoplasmic reticulum. *The Journal of biological chemistry,* Vol.255, No.19, (October 1980), pp. 9009-9012, ISSN 0021-9258.

Bendotti, C., Calvaresi, N., Chiveri, L., Prelle, A., Moggio, M., Braga, M., Silani, V. & De Biasi, S. (2001). Early vacuolization and mitochondrial damage in motor neurons of FALS mice are not associated with apoptosis or with changes in cytochrome oxidase histochemical reactivity. *Journal of the neurological sciences,* Vol.191, No.1-2, (October 2001), pp. 25-33, ISSN 0022-510X.

Bilsland, L. G., Sahai, E., Kelly, G., Golding, M., Greensmith, L. & Schiavo, G. (2010). Deficits in axonal transport precede ALS symptoms in vivo. *Proceedings of the National Academy of Sciences of the United States of America,* Vol.107, No.47, (November 2010), pp. 20523-20528, ISSN 1091-6490 (Electronic), 0027-8424 (Linking).

Bogdanov, M., Brown, R. H., Matson, W., Smart, R., Hayden, D., O'Donnell, H., Flint Beal, M. & Cudkowicz, M. (2000). Increased oxidative damage to DNA in ALS patients. *Free radical biology & medicine,* Vol.29, No.7, (October 2000), pp. 652-658, ISSN 0891-5849.

Boillee, S., Vande Velde, C. & Cleveland, D. W. (2006a). ALS: a disease of motor neurons and their nonneuronal neighbors. *Neuron,* Vol.52, No.1, (October 2006), pp. 39-59, ISSN 0896-6273.

Boillee, S., Yamanaka, K., Lobsiger, C. S., Copeland, N. G., Jenkins, N. A., Kassiotis, G., Kollias, G. & Cleveland, D. W. (2006b). Onset and progression in inherited ALS determined by motor neurons and microglia. *Science (New York, N.Y,* Vol.312, No.5778, (June 2006), pp. 1389-1392, ISSN 1095-9203 (Electronic), 0036-8075 (Linking).

Bonnefont-Rousselot, D., Lacomblez, L., Jaudon, M., Lepage, S., Salachas, F., Bensimon, G., Bizard, C., Doppler, V., Delattre, J. & Meininger, V. (2000). Blood oxidative stress in amyotrophic lateral sclerosis. *Journal of the neurological sciences,* Vol.178, No.1, (September 2000), pp. 57-62, ISSN 0022-510X.

Borthwick, G. M., Johnson, M. A., Ince, P. G., Shaw, P. J. & Turnbull, D. M. (1999). Mitochondrial enzyme activity in amyotrophic lateral sclerosis: implications for the role of mitochondria in neuronal cell death. *Annals of neurology,* Vol.46, No.5, (November 1999), pp. 787-790, ISSN 0364-5134.

Breuer, A. C. & Atkinson, M. B. (1988). Fast axonal transport alterations in amyotrophic lateral sclerosis (ALS) and in parathyroid hormone (PTH)-treated axons. *Cell motility and the cytoskeleton,* Vol.10, No.1-2, pp. 321-330, ISSN 0886-1544.

Breuer, A. C., Lynn, M. P., Atkinson, M. B., Chou, S. M., Wilbourn, A. J., Marks, K. E., Culver, J. E. & Fleegler, E. J. (1987). Fast axonal transport in amyotrophic lateral sclerosis: an intra-axonal organelle traffic analysis. *Neurology,* Vol.37, No.5, (May 1987), pp. 738-748, ISSN 0028-3878.

Brunet, N., Tarabal, O., Esquerda, J. E. & Caldero, J. (2009). Excitotoxic motoneuron degeneration induced by glutamate receptor agonists and mitochondrial toxins in organotypic cultures of chick embryo spinal cord. *The Journal of comparative neurology,* Vol.516, No.4, (October 2009), pp. 277-290, ISSN 1096-9861 (Electronic), 0021-9967 (Linking).

Burnashev, N., Monyer, H., Seeburg, P. H. & Sakmann, B. (1992). Divalent ion permeability of AMPA receptor channels is dominated by the edited form of a single subunit. *Neuron,* Vol.8, No.1, (January 1992), pp. 189-198, ISSN 0896-6273.

Carriedo, S. G., Yin, H. Z., Sensi, S. L. & Weiss, J. H. (1998). Rapid Ca2+ entry through Ca2+-permeable AMPA/Kainate channels triggers marked intracellular Ca2+ rises and consequent oxygen radical production. *J Neurosci,* Vol.18, No.19, (October 1998), pp. 7727-7738, ISSN 0270-6474.

Carriedo, S. G., Sensi, S. L., Yin, H. Z. & Weiss, J. H. (2000). AMPA exposures induce mitochondrial Ca(2+) overload and ROS generation in spinal motor neurons in vitro. *J Neurosci,* Vol.20, No.1, (January 2000), pp. 240-250, ISSN 1529-2401 (Electronic), 0270-6474 (Linking).

Casoni, F., Basso, M., Massignan, T., Gianazza, E., Cheroni, C., Salmona, M., Bendotti, C. & Bonetto, V. (2005). Protein nitration in a mouse model of familial amyotrophic lateral sclerosis: possible multifunctional role in the pathogenesis. *The Journal of biological chemistry,* Vol.280, No.16, (April 2005), pp. 16295-16304, ISSN 0021-9258.

Cassina, P., Cassina, A., Pehar, M., Castellanos, R., Gandelman, M., de Leon, A., Robinson, K. M., Mason, R. P., Beckman, J. S., Barbeito, L. & Radi, R. (2008). Mitochondrial dysfunction in SOD1G93A-bearing astrocytes promotes motor neuron degeneration: prevention by mitochondrial-targeted antioxidants. *J Neurosci,* Vol.28, No.16, (April 2008), pp. 4115-4122, ISSN 1529-2401 (Electronic), 0270-6474 (Linking).

Celio, M. R. (1990). Calbindin D-28k and parvalbumin in the rat nervous system. *Neuroscience,* Vol.35, No.2, pp. 375-475, ISSN 0306-4522.

Chancellor, A. M. & Warlow, C. P. (1992). Adult onset motor neuron disease: worldwide mortality, incidence and distribution since 1950. *Journal of neurology, neurosurgery, and psychiatry,* Vol.55, No.12, (December 1992), pp. 1106-1115, ISSN 0022-3050 (Print), 0022-3050 (Linking).

Clement, A. M., Nguyen, M. D., Roberts, E. A., Garcia, M. L., Boillee, S., Rule, M., McMahon, A. P., Doucette, W., Siwek, D., Ferrante, R. J., Brown, R. H., Jr., Julien, J. P., Goldstein, L. S. & Cleveland, D. W. (2003). Wild-type nonneuronal cells extend survival of SOD1 mutant motor neurons in ALS mice. *Science (New York, N.Y,* Vol.302, No.5642, (October 2003), pp. 113-117, ISSN 1095-9203 (Electronic), 0036-8075 (Linking).

Collard, J. F., Cote, F. & Julien, J. P. (1995). Defective axonal transport in a transgenic mouse model of amyotrophic lateral sclerosis. *Nature,* Vol.375, No.6526, (May 1995), pp. 61-64, ISSN 0028-0836.

Comi, G. P., Bordoni, A., Salani, S., Franceschina, L., Sciacco, M., Prelle, A., Fortunato, F., Zeviani, M., Napoli, L., Bresolin, N., Moggio, M., Ausenda, C. D., Taanman, J. W. & Scarlato, G. (1998). Cytochrome c oxidase subunit I microdeletion in a patient with motor neuron disease. *Annals of neurology*, Vol.43, No.1, (January 1998), pp. 110-116, ISSN 0364-5134.

Corona, J. C. & Tapia, R. (2004). AMPA receptor activation, but not the accumulation of endogenous extracellular glutamate, induces paralysis and motor neuron death in rat spinal cord in vivo. *Journal of neurochemistry*, Vol.89, No.4, (May 2004), pp. 988-997, ISSN 0022-3042.

Corona, J. C. & Tapia, R. (2007). Ca2+-permeable AMPA receptors and intracellular Ca2+ determine motoneuron vulnerability in rat spinal cord in vivo. *Neuropharmacology*, Vol.52, No.5, (April 2007), pp. 1219-1228, ISSN 0028-3908.

Crompton, M. & Heid, I. (1978). The cycling of calcium, sodium, and protons across the inner membrane of cardiac mitochondria. *European journal of biochemistry / FEBS*, Vol.91, No.2, (November 1978), pp. 599-608, ISSN 0014-2956.

Crugnola, V., Lamperti, C., Lucchini, V., Ronchi, D., Peverelli, L., Prelle, A., Sciacco, M., Bordoni, A., Fassone, E., Fortunato, F., Corti, S., Silani, V., Bresolin, N., Di Mauro, S., Comi, G. P. & Moggio, M. (2010). Mitochondrial respiratory chain dysfunction in muscle from patients with amyotrophic lateral sclerosis. *Archives of neurology*, Vol.67, No.7, (July 2010), pp. 849-854, ISSN 1538-3687 (Electronic), 0003-9942 (Linking).

De Vos, K. J., Chapman, A. L., Tennant, M. E., Manser, C., Tudor, E. L., Lau, K. F., Brownlees, J., Ackerley, S., Shaw, P. J., McLoughlin, D. M., Shaw, C. E., Leigh, P. N., Miller, C. C. & Grierson, A. J. (2007). Familial amyotrophic lateral sclerosis-linked SOD1 mutants perturb fast axonal transport to reduce axonal mitochondria content. *Human molecular genetics*, Vol.16, No.22, (November 2007), pp. 2720-2728, ISSN 0964-6906 (Print), 0964-6906 (Linking).

Dugan, L. L., Sensi, S. L., Canzoniero, L. M., Handran, S. D., Rothman, S. M., Lin, T. S., Goldberg, M. P. & Choi, D. W. (1995). Mitochondrial production of reactive oxygen species in cortical neurons following exposure to N-methyl-D-aspartate. *J Neurosci*, Vol.15, No.10, (October 1995), pp. 6377-6388, ISSN 0270-6474.

Dykens, J. A. (1994). Isolated cerebral and cerebellar mitochondria produce free radicals when exposed to elevated CA2+ and Na+: implications for neurodegeneration. *Journal of neurochemistry*, Vol.63, No.2, (August 1994), pp. 584-591, ISSN 0022-3042.

Echaniz-Laguna, A., Zoll, J., Ponsot, E., N'Guessan, B., Tranchant, C., Loeffler, J. P. & Lampert, E. (2006). Muscular mitochondrial function in amyotrophic lateral sclerosis is progressively altered as the disease develops: a temporal study in man. *Experimental neurology*, Vol.198, No.1, (March 2006), pp. 25-30, ISSN 0014-4886.

Ferrante, R. J., Shinobu, L. A., Schulz, J. B., Matthews, R. T., Thomas, C. E., Kowall, N. W., Gurney, M. E. & Beal, M. F. (1997a). Increased 3-nitrotyrosine and oxidative damage in mice with a human copper/zinc superoxide dismutase mutation. *Annals of neurology*, Vol.42, No.3, (September 1997), pp. 326-334, ISSN 0364-5134.

Ferrante, R. J., Browne, S. E., Shinobu, L. A., Bowling, A. C., Baik, M. J., MacGarvey, U., Kowall, N. W., Brown, R. H., Jr. & Beal, M. F. (1997b). Evidence of increased oxidative damage in both sporadic and familial amyotrophic lateral sclerosis. *Journal of neurochemistry,* Vol.69, No.5, (November 1997), pp. 2064-2074, ISSN 0022-3042.

Fiala, M., Chattopadhay, M., La Cava, A., Tse, E., Liu, G., Lourenco, E., Eskin, A., Liu, P. T., Magpantay, L., Tse, S., Mahanian, M., Weitzman, R., Tong, J., Nguyen, C., Cho, T., Koo, P., Sayre, J., Martinez-Maza, O., Rosenthal, M. J. & Wiedau-Pazos, M. (2010). IL-17A is increased in the serum and in spinal cord CD8 and mast cells of ALS patients. *Journal of neuroinflammation,* Vol.7, pp. 76, ISSN 1742-2094.

Finsterer, J. (2002). Mitochondriopathy as a differential diagnosis of amyotrophic lateral sclerosis. *Amyotroph Lateral Scler Other Motor Neuron Disord,* Vol.3, No.4, (December 2002), pp. 219-224, ISSN 1466-0822.

Finsterer, J. (2003). Mitochondriopathy mimicking amyotrophic lateral sclerosis. *The neurologist,* Vol.9, No.1, (January 2003), pp. 45-48, ISSN 1074-7931.

Fitzmaurice, P. S., Shaw, I. C., Kleiner, H. E., Miller, R. T., Monks, T. J., Lau, S. S., Mitchell, J. D. & Lynch, P. G. (1996). Evidence for DNA damage in amyotrophic lateral sclerosis. *Muscle & nerve,* Vol.19, No.6, (June 1996), pp. 797-798, ISSN 0148-639X.

Greene, J. G. & Greenamyre, J. T. (1996). Bioenergetics and glutamate excitotoxicity. *Progress in neurobiology,* Vol.48, No.6, (April 1996), pp. 613-634, ISSN 0301-0082.

Grosskreutz, J., Van Den Bosch, L. & Keller, B. U. (2010). Calcium dysregulation in amyotrophic lateral sclerosis. *Cell calcium,* Vol.47, No.2, (February 2010), pp. 165-174, ISSN 1532-1991 (Electronic), 0143-4160 (Linking).

Grosskreutz, J., Haastert, K., Dewil, M., Van Damme, P., Callewaert, G., Robberecht, W., Dengler, R. & Van Den Bosch, L. (2007). Role of mitochondria in kainate-induced fast Ca2+ transients in cultured spinal motor neurons. *Cell calcium,* Vol.42, No.1, (July 2007), pp. 59-69, ISSN 0143-4160.

Hall, E. D., Oostveen, J. A. & Gurney, M. E. (1998). Relationship of microglial and astrocytic activation to disease onset and progression in a transgenic model of familial ALS. *Glia,* Vol.23, No.3, (July 1998), pp. 249-256, ISSN 0894-1491.

Henkel, J. S., Engelhardt, J. I., Siklos, L., Simpson, E. P., Kim, S. H., Pan, T., Goodman, J. C., Siddique, T., Beers, D. R. & Appel, S. H. (2004). Presence of dendritic cells, MCP-1, and activated microglia/macrophages in amyotrophic lateral sclerosis spinal cord tissue. *Annals of neurology,* Vol.55, No.2, (February 2004), pp. 221-235, ISSN 0364-5134.

Higgins, C. M., Jung, C., Ding, H. & Xu, Z. (2002). Mutant Cu, Zn superoxide dismutase that causes motoneuron degeneration is present in mitochondria in the CNS. *J Neurosci,* Vol.22, No.6, (March 2002), pp. RC215, ISSN 1529-2401 (Electronic), 0270-6474 (Linking).

Hirano, A., Donnenfeld, H., Sasaki, S. & Nakano, I. (1984a). Fine structural observations of neurofilamentous changes in amyotrophic lateral sclerosis. *Journal of neuropathology and experimental neurology,* Vol.43, No.5, (September 1984), pp. 461-470, ISSN 0022-3069.

Hirano, A., Nakano, I., Kurland, L. T., Mulder, D. W., Holley, P. W. & Saccomanno, G. (1984b). Fine structural study of neurofibrillary changes in a family with amyotrophic lateral sclerosis. *Journal of neuropathology and experimental neurology,* Vol.43, No.5, (September 1984), pp. 471-480, ISSN 0022-3069.

Hollmann, M., Hartley, M. & Heinemann, S. (1991). Ca2+ permeability of KA-AMPA--gated glutamate receptor channels depends on subunit composition. *Science (New York, N.Y,* Vol.252, No.5007, (May 1991), pp. 851-853, ISSN 0036-8075.

Huisman, M. H., de Jong, S. W., van Doormaal, P. T., Weinreich, S. S., Schelhaas, H. J., van der Kooi, A. J., de Visser, M., Veldink, J. H. & van den Berg, L. H. (2011). Population based epidemiology of amyotrophic lateral sclerosis using capture-recapture methodology. *Journal of neurology, neurosurgery, and psychiatry,* (May 2011), pp., ISSN 1468-330X (Electronic), 0022-3050 (Linking).

Hume, R. I., Dingledine, R. & Heinemann, S. F. (1991). Identification of a site in glutamate receptor subunits that controls calcium permeability. *Science (New York, N.Y,* Vol.253, No.5023, (August 1991), pp. 1028-1031, ISSN 0036-8075.

Ihara, Y., Nobukuni, K., Takata, H. & Hayabara, T. (2005). Oxidative stress and metal content in blood and cerebrospinal fluid of amyotrophic lateral sclerosis patients with and without a Cu, Zn-superoxide dismutase mutation. *Neurological research,* Vol.27, No.1, (January 2005), pp. 105-108, ISSN 0161-6412.

Ilzecka, J. (2007). Decreased cerebrospinal fluid cytochrome c levels in patients with amyotrophic lateral sclerosis. *Scandinavian journal of clinical and laboratory investigation,* Vol.67, No.3, pp. 264-269, ISSN 0036-5513.

Ilzecka, J. (2011). Granzymes A and B levels in serum of patients with amyotrophic lateral sclerosis. *Clinical biochemistry,* Vol.44, No.8-9, (June 2011), pp. 650-653, ISSN 1873-2933 (Electronic), 0009-9120 (Linking).

Ince, P., Stout, N., Shaw, P., Slade, J., Hunziker, W., Heizmann, C. W. & Baimbridge, K. G. (1993). Parvalbumin and calbindin D-28k in the human motor system and in motor neuron disease. *Neuropathology and applied neurobiology,* Vol.19, No.4, (August 1993), pp. 291-299, ISSN 0305-1846.

Jaarsma, D., Rognoni, F., van Duijn, W., Verspaget, H. W., Haasdijk, E. D. & Holstege, J. C. (2001). CuZn superoxide dismutase (SOD1) accumulates in vacuolated mitochondria in transgenic mice expressing amyotrophic lateral sclerosis-linked SOD1 mutations. *Acta neuropathologica,* Vol.102, No.4, (October 2001), pp. 293-305, ISSN 0001-6322.

Jabaudon, D., Scanziani, M., Gahwiler, B. H. & Gerber, U. (2000). Acute decrease in net glutamate uptake during energy deprivation. *Proceedings of the National Academy of Sciences of the United States of America,* Vol.97, No.10, (May 2000), pp. 5610-5615, ISSN 0027-8424.

Julien, J. P. & Mushynski, W. E. (1998). Neurofilaments in health and disease. *Progress in nucleic acid research and molecular biology,* Vol.61, pp. 1-23, ISSN 0079-6603.

Jung, C., Higgins, C. M. & Xu, Z. (2002). Mitochondrial electron transport chain complex dysfunction in a transgenic mouse model for amyotrophic lateral sclerosis. *Journal of neurochemistry,* Vol.83, No.3, (November 2002), pp. 535-545, ISSN 0022-3042.

Kaal, E. C., Vlug, A. S., Versleijen, M. W., Kuilman, M., Joosten, E. A. & Bar, P. R. (2000). Chronic mitochondrial inhibition induces selective motoneuron death in vitro: a new model for amyotrophic lateral sclerosis. *Journal of neurochemistry,* Vol.74, No.3, (March 2000), pp. 1158-1165, ISSN 0022-3042.

Kawamata, T., Akiyama, H., Yamada, T. & McGeer, P. L. (1992). Immunologic reactions in amyotrophic lateral sclerosis brain and spinal cord tissue. *The American journal of pathology,* Vol.140, No.3, (March 1992), pp. 691-707, ISSN 0002-9440.

Keller, A. F., Gravel, M. & Kriz, J. (2010). Treatment with minocycline after disease onset alters astrocyte reactivity and increases microgliosis in SOD1 mutant mice. *Experimental neurology,* Vol.228, No.1, (March 2010), pp. 69-79, ISSN 1090-2430 (Electronic), 0014-4886 (Linking).

Kirkinezos, I. G., Bacman, S. R., Hernandez, D., Oca-Cossio, J., Arias, L. J., Perez-Pinzon, M. A., Bradley, W. G. & Moraes, C. T. (2005). Cytochrome c association with the inner mitochondrial membrane is impaired in the CNS of G93A-SOD1 mice. *J Neurosci,* Vol.25, No.1, (January 2005), pp. 164-172, ISSN 1529-2401 (Electronic), 0270-6474 (Linking).

Komatsu, M., Wang, Q. J., Holstein, G. R., Friedrich, V. L., Jr., Iwata, J., Kominami, E., Chait, B. T., Tanaka, K. & Yue, Z. (2007). Essential role for autophagy protein Atg7 in the maintenance of axonal homeostasis and the prevention of axonal degeneration. *Proceedings of the National Academy of Sciences of the United States of America,* Vol.104, No.36, (September 2007), pp. 14489-14494, ISSN 0027-8424.

Kong, J. & Xu, Z. (1998). Massive mitochondrial degeneration in motor neurons triggers the onset of amyotrophic lateral sclerosis in mice expressing a mutant SOD1. *J Neurosci,* Vol.18, No.9, (May 1), pp. 3241-3250, ISSN 0270-6474.

Kriz, J., Nguyen, M. D. & Julien, J. P. (2002). Minocycline slows disease progression in a mouse model of amyotrophic lateral sclerosis. *Neurobiology of disease,* Vol.10, No.3, (August 2002), pp. 268-278, ISSN 0969-9961.

Kroemer, G., Galluzzi, L., Vandenabeele, P., Abrams, J., Alnemri, E. S., Baehrecke, E. H., Blagosklonny, M. V., El-Deiry, W. S., Golstein, P., Green, D. R., Hengartner, M., Knight, R. A., Kumar, S., Lipton, S. A., Malorni, W., Nunez, G., Peter, M. E., Tschopp, J., Yuan, J., Piacentini, M., Zhivotovsky, B. & Melino, G. (2009). Classification of cell death: recommendations of the Nomenclature Committee on Cell Death 2009. *Cell death and differentiation,* Vol.16, No.1, (January 2009), pp. 3-11, ISSN 1476-5403 (Electronic), 1350-9047 (Linking).

Lenaz, G., Bovina, C., D'Aurelio, M., Fato, R., Formiggini, G., Genova, M. L., Giuliano, G., Merlo Pich, M., Paolucci, U., Parenti Castelli, G. & Ventura, B. (2002). Role of mitochondria in oxidative stress and aging. *Annals of the New York Academy of Sciences,* Vol.959, (April 2002), pp. 199-213, ISSN 0077-8923.

Lepore, A. C., Dejea, C., Carmen, J., Rauck, B., Kerr, D. A., Sofroniew, M. V. & Maragakis, N. J. (2008). Selective ablation of proliferating astrocytes does not affect disease outcome in either acute or chronic models of motor neuron degeneration. *Experimental neurology,* Vol.211, No.2, (June 2008), pp. 423-432, ISSN 1090-2430 (Electronic), 0014-4886 (Linking).

Li, M., Ona, V. O., Guegan, C., Chen, M., Jackson-Lewis, V., Andrews, L. J., Olszewski, A. J., Stieg, P. E., Lee, J. P., Przedborski, S. & Friedlander, R. M. (2000). Functional role of caspase-1 and caspase-3 in an ALS transgenic mouse model. *Science (New York, N.Y,* Vol.288, No.5464, (April 2000), pp. 335-339, ISSN 0036-8075.

Ligon, L. A., LaMonte, B. H., Wallace, K. E., Weber, N., Kalb, R. G. & Holzbaur, E. L. (2005). Mutant superoxide dismutase disrupts cytoplasmic dynein in motor neurons. *Neuroreport,* Vol.16, No.6, (April 2005), pp. 533-536, ISSN 0959-4965.

Lin, J., Diamanduros, A., Chowdhury, S. A., Scelsa, S., Latov, N. & Sadiq, S. A. (2009). Specific electron transport chain abnormalities in amyotrophic lateral sclerosis. *Journal of neurology,* Vol.256, No.5, (May 2009), pp. 774-782, ISSN 1432-1459 (Electronic), 0340-5354 (Linking).

Liu, D., Wen, J., Liu, J. & Li, L. (1999). The roles of free radicals in amyotrophic lateral sclerosis: reactive oxygen species and elevated oxidation of protein, DNA, and membrane phospholipids. *Faseb J,* Vol.13, No.15, (December 1999), pp. 2318-2328, ISSN 0892-6638.

Liu, J., Lillo, C., Jonsson, P. A., Vande Velde, C., Ward, C. M., Miller, T. M., Subramaniam, J. R., Rothstein, J. D., Marklund, S., Andersen, P. M., Brannstrom, T., Gredal, O., Wong, P. C., Williams, D. S. & Cleveland, D. W. (2004). Toxicity of familial ALS-linked SOD1 mutants from selective recruitment to spinal mitochondria. *Neuron,* Vol.43, No.1, (July 2004), pp. 5-17, ISSN 0896-6273.

Liu, R., Althaus, J. S., Ellerbrock, B. R., Becker, D. A. & Gurney, M. E. (1998). Enhanced oxygen radical production in a transgenic mouse model of familial amyotrophic lateral sclerosis. *Annals of neurology,* Vol.44, No.5, (November 1998), pp. 763-770, ISSN 0364-5134.

Locatelli, F., Corti, S., Papadimitriou, D., Fortunato, F., Del Bo, R., Donadoni, C., Nizzardo, M., Nardini, M., Salani, S., Ghezzi, S., Strazzer, S., Bresolin, N. & Comi, G. P. (2007). Fas small interfering RNA reduces motoneuron death in amyotrophic lateral sclerosis mice. *Annals of neurology,* Vol.62, No.1, (July 2007), pp. 81-92, ISSN 0364-5134.

Longuemare, M. C. & Swanson, R. A. (1995). Excitatory amino acid release from astrocytes during energy failure by reversal of sodium-dependent uptake. *Journal of neuroscience research,* Vol.40, No.3, (February 1995), pp. 379-386, ISSN 0360-4012.

Manfredi, G. & Xu, Z. (2005). Mitochondrial dysfunction and its role in motor neuron degeneration in ALS. *Mitochondrion,* Vol.5, No.2, (April 2005), pp. 77-87, ISSN 1567-7249.

Martin, L. J. (2010). Mitochondrial and Cell Death Mechanisms in Neurodegenerative Diseases. *Pharmaceuticals (Basel, Switzerland),* Vol.3, No.4, pp. 839-915, ISSN 1424-8247.

Martin, L. J., Gertz, B., Pan, Y., Price, A. C., Molkentin, J. D. & Chang, Q. (2009). The mitochondrial permeability transition pore in motor neurons: involvement in the pathobiology of ALS mice. *Experimental neurology,* Vol.218, No.2, (August 2009), pp. 333-346, ISSN 1090-2430 (Electronic), 0014-4886 (Linking).

Mattiazzi, M., D'Aurelio, M., Gajewski, C. D., Martushova, K., Kiaei, M., Beal, M. F. & Manfredi, G. (2002). Mutated human SOD1 causes dysfunction of oxidative phosphorylation in mitochondria of transgenic mice. *The Journal of biological chemistry,* Vol.277, No.33, (August, 2002), pp. 29626-29633, ISSN 0021-9258.

Maus, M., Marin, P., Israel, M., Glowinski, J. & Premont, J. (1999). Pyruvate and lactate protect striatal neurons against N-methyl-D-aspartate-induced neurotoxicity. *The European journal of neuroscience,* Vol.11, No.9, (September 1999), pp. 3215-3224, ISSN 0953-816X.

McGeer, P. L., McGeer, E. G., Kawamata, T., Yamada, T. & Akiyama, H. (1991). Reactions of the immune system in chronic degenerative neurological diseases. *The Canadian journal of neurological sciences,* Vol.18, No.3 Suppl, (August 1991), pp. 376-379, ISSN 0317-1671.

Menzies, F. M., Ince, P. G. & Shaw, P. J. (2002a). Mitochondrial involvement in amyotrophic lateral sclerosis. *Neurochemistry international,* Vol.40, No.6, (May 2002), pp. 543-551, ISSN 0197-0186.

Menzies, F. M., Cookson, M. R., Taylor, R. W., Turnbull, D. M., Chrzanowska-Lightowlers, Z. M., Dong, L., Figlewicz, D. A. & Shaw, P. J. (2002b). Mitochondrial dysfunction in a cell culture model of familial amyotrophic lateral sclerosis. *Brain,* Vol.125, No.Pt 7, (July 2002), pp. 1522-1533, ISSN 0006-8950.

Monje, M. L., Phillips, R. & Sapolsky, R. (2001). Calbindin overexpression buffers hippocampal cultures from the energetic impairments caused by glutamate. *Brain research,* Vol.911, No.1, (August 2001), pp. 37-42, ISSN 0006-8993.

Moreau, C., Devos, D., Brunaud-Danel, V., Defebvre, L., Perez, T., Destee, A., Tonnel, A. B., Lassalle, P. & Just, N. (2005). Elevated IL-6 and TNF-alpha levels in patients with ALS: inflammation or hypoxia? *Neurology,* Vol.65, No.12, (December 2005), pp. 1958-1960, ISSN 1526-632X (Electronic), 0028-3878 (Linking).

Nakano, Y., Hirayama, K. & Terao, K. (1987). Hepatic ultrastructural changes and liver dysfunction in amyotrophic lateral sclerosis. *Archives of neurology,* Vol.44, No.1, (January 1987), pp. 103-106, ISSN 0003-9942.

Neymotin, A., Petri, S., Calingasan, N. Y., Wille, E., Schafer, P., Stewart, C., Hensley, K., Beal, M. F. & Kiaei, M. (2009). Lenalidomide (Revlimid) administration at symptom onset is neuroprotective in a mouse model of amyotrophic lateral sclerosis. *Experimental neurology,* Vol.220, No.1, (November 2009), pp. 191-197, ISSN 1090-2430 (Electronic), 0014-4886 (Linking).

Nicholls, D. G. (1978). The regulation of extramitochondrial free calcium ion concentration by rat liver mitochondria. *Biochem J,* Vol.176, No.2, (November 1978), pp. 463-474, ISSN 0264-6021.

Nicholls, D. G. (1985). A role for the mitochondrion in the protection of cells against calcium overload? *Progress in brain research,* Vol.63, pp. 97-106, ISSN 0079-6123.

Nicholls, D. G. & Budd, S. L. (2000). Mitochondria and neuronal survival. *Physiological reviews,* Vol.80, No.1, (January 2000), pp. 315-360, ISSN 0031-9333.

Nicholls, D. G., Vesce, S., Kirk, L. & Chalmers, S. (2003). Interactions between mitochondrial bioenergetics and cytoplasmic calcium in cultured cerebellar granule cells. *Cell calcium,* Vol.34, No.4-5, (October-November 2003), pp. 407-424, ISSN 0143-4160.

Novelli, A., Reilly, J. A., Lysko, P. G. & Henneberry, R. C. (1988). Glutamate becomes neurotoxic via the N-methyl-D-aspartate receptor when intracellular energy levels are reduced. *Brain research,* Vol.451, No.1-2, (June 1988), pp. 205-212, ISSN 0006-8993.

Ohta, Y., Kamiya, T., Nagai, M., Nagata, T., Morimoto, N., Miyazaki, K., Murakami, T., Kurata, T., Takehisa, Y., Ikeda, Y., Asoh, S., Ohta, S. & Abe, K. (2008). Therapeutic benefits of intrathecal protein therapy in a mouse model of amyotrophic lateral sclerosis. *Journal of neuroscience research,* Vol.86, No.13, (October 2008), pp. 3028-3037, ISSN 1097-4547 (Electronic), 0360-4012 (Linking).

Oteiza, P. I., Uchitel, O. D., Carrasquedo, F., Dubrovski, A. L., Roma, J. C. & Fraga, C. G. (1997). Evaluation of antioxidants, protein, and lipid oxidation products in blood from sporadic amyotrophic lateral sclerosis patients. *Neurochemical research,* Vol.22, No.4, (April 1997), pp. 535-539, ISSN 0364-3190.

Palecek, J., Lips, M. B. & Keller, B. U. (1999). Calcium dynamics and buffering in motoneurones of the mouse spinal cord. *The Journal of physiology,* Vol.520 Pt 2, (October 1999), pp. 485-502, ISSN 0022-3751.

Pasinelli, P., Houseweart, M. K., Brown, R. H., Jr. & Cleveland, D. W. (2000). Caspase-1 and -3 are sequentially activated in motor neuron death in Cu,Zn superoxide dismutase-mediated familial amyotrophic lateral sclerosis. *Proceedings of the National Academy of Sciences of the United States of America,* Vol.97, No.25, (December 2000), pp. 13901-13906, ISSN 0027-8424.

Pasinelli, P., Belford, M. E., Lennon, N., Bacskai, B. J., Hyman, B. T., Trotti, D. & Brown, R. H., Jr. (2004). Amyotrophic lateral sclerosis-associated SOD1 mutant proteins bind and aggregate with Bcl-2 in spinal cord mitochondria. *Neuron,* Vol.43, No.1, (July 2004), pp. 19-30, ISSN 0896-6273.

Peng, T. I. & Jou, M. J. (2010). Oxidative stress caused by mitochondrial calcium overload. *Annals of the New York Academy of Sciences,* Vol.1201, (July 2010), pp. 183-188, ISSN 1749-6632 (Electronic), 0077-8923 (Linking).

Perlson, E., Jeong, G. B., Ross, J. L., Dixit, R., Wallace, K. E., Kalb, R. G. & Holzbaur, E. L. (2009). A switch in retrograde signaling from survival to stress in rapid-onset neurodegeneration. *J Neurosci,* Vol.29, No.31, (August 2009), pp. 9903-9917, ISSN 1529-2401 (Electronic), 0270-6474 (Linking).

Petri, S., Kiaei, M., Wille, E., Calingasan, N. Y. & Flint Beal, M. (2006). Loss of Fas ligand-function improves survival in G93A-transgenic ALS mice. *Journal of the neurological sciences,* Vol.251, No.1-2, (December 2006), pp. 44-49, ISSN 0022-510X.

Poon, H. F., Hensley, K., Thongboonkerd, V., Merchant, M. L., Lynn, B. C., Pierce, W. M., Klein, J. B., Calabrese, V. & Butterfield, D. A. (2005). Redox proteomics analysis of oxidatively modified proteins in G93A-SOD1 transgenic mice--a model of familial amyotrophic lateral sclerosis. *Free radical biology & medicine,* Vol.39, No.4, (August 2005), pp. 453-462, ISSN 0891-5849.

Pun, S., Santos, A. F., Saxena, S., Xu, L. & Caroni, P. (2006). Selective vulnerability and pruning of phasic motoneuron axons in motoneuron disease alleviated by CNTF. *Nature neuroscience,* Vol.9, No.3, (March 2006), pp. 408-419, ISSN 1097-6256.

Rao, S. D., Yin, H. Z. & Weiss, J. H. (2003). Disruption of glial glutamate transport by reactive oxygen species produced in motor neurons. *J Neurosci,* Vol.23, No.7, (April 2003), pp. 2627-2633, ISSN 1529-2401 (Electronic), 0270-6474 (Linking).

Raoul, C., Buhler, E., Sadeghi, C., Jacquier, A., Aebischer, P., Pettmann, B., Henderson, C. E. & Haase, G. (2006). Chronic activation in presymptomatic amyotrophic lateral sclerosis (ALS) mice of a feedback loop involving Fas, Daxx, and FasL. *Proceedings of the National Academy of Sciences of the United States of America,* Vol.103, No.15, (April 2006), pp. 6007-6012, ISSN 0027-8424.

Rentzos, M., Rombos, A., Nikolaou, C., Zoga, M., Zouvelou, V., Dimitrakopoulos, A., Alexakis, T., Tsoutsou, A., Samakovli, A., Michalopoulou, M. & Evdokimidis, I. (2010a). Interleukin-15 and interleukin-12 are elevated in serum and cerebrospinal fluid of patients with amyotrophic lateral sclerosis. *European neurology,* Vol.63, No.5, pp. 285-290, ISSN 1421-9913 (Electronic), 0014-3022 (Linking).

Rentzos, M., Rombos, A., Nikolaou, C., Zoga, M., Zouvelou, V., Dimitrakopoulos, A., Alexakis, T., Tsoutsou, A., Samakovli, A., Michalopoulou, M. & Evdokimidis, J. (2010b). Interleukin-17 and interleukin-23 are elevated in serum and cerebrospinal fluid of patients with ALS: a reflection of Th17 cells activation? *Acta neurologica Scandinavica,* Vol.122, No.6, (December 2010), pp. 425-429, ISSN 1600-0404 (Electronic), 0001-6314 (Linking).

Richter, C., Park, J. W. & Ames, B. N. (1988). Normal oxidative damage to mitochondrial and nuclear DNA is extensive. *Proceedings of the National Academy of Sciences of the United States of America,* Vol.85, No.17, (September 1988), pp. 6465-6467, ISSN 0027-8424.

Rosen, D. R., Siddique, T., Patterson, D., Figlewicz, D. A., Sapp, P., Hentati, A., Donaldson, D., Goto, J., O'Regan, J. P., Deng, H. X. & et al. (1993). Mutations in Cu/Zn superoxide dismutase gene are associated with familial amyotrophic lateral sclerosis. *Nature,* Vol.362, No.6415, (March 1993), pp. 59-62, ISSN 0028-0836.

Rothstein, J. D., Martin, L. J. & Kuncl, R. W. (1992). Decreased glutamate transport by the brain and spinal cord in amyotrophic lateral sclerosis. *The New England journal of medicine,* Vol.326, No.22, (May 1992), pp. 1464-1468, ISSN 0028-4793.

Rothstein, J. D., Van Kammen, M., Levey, A. I., Martin, L. J. & Kuncl, R. W. (1995). Selective loss of glial glutamate transporter GLT-1 in amyotrophic lateral sclerosis. *Annals of neurology,* Vol.38, No.1, (July 1995), pp. 73-84, ISSN 0364-5134.

Rowland, L. P. & Shneider, N. A. (2001). Amyotrophic lateral sclerosis. *The New England journal of medicine,* Vol.344, No.22, (May 2001), pp. 1688-1700, ISSN 0028-4793.

Ryberg, H., Soderling, A. S., Davidsson, P., Blennow, K., Caidahl, K. & Persson, L. I. (2004). Cerebrospinal fluid levels of free 3-nitrotyrosine are not elevated in the majority of patients with amyotrophic lateral sclerosis or Alzheimer's disease. *Neurochemistry international,* Vol.45, No.1, (July 2004), pp. 57-62, ISSN 0197-0186.

Sanagi, T., Yuasa, S., Nakamura, Y., Suzuki, E., Aoki, M., Warita, H., Itoyama, Y., Uchino, S., Kohsaka, S. & Ohsawa, K. (2010). Appearance of phagocytic microglia adjacent to motoneurons in spinal cord tissue from a presymptomatic transgenic rat model of amyotrophic lateral sclerosis. *Journal of neuroscience research,* Vol.88, No.12, (September 2010), pp. 2736-2746, ISSN 1097-4547 (Electronic), 0360-4012 (Linking).

Sargsyan, S. A., Monk, P. N. & Shaw, P. J. (2005). Microglia as potential contributors to motor neuron injury in amyotrophic lateral sclerosis. *Glia,* Vol.51, No.4, (September 2005), pp. 241-253, ISSN 0894-1491.

Sasaki, S. & Iwata, M. (1996). Impairment of fast axonal transport in the proximal axons of anterior horn neurons in amyotrophic lateral sclerosis. *Neurology,* Vol.47, No.2, (August 1996), pp. 535-540, ISSN 0028-3878.

Saxena, K., Henry, T. R., Solem, L. E. & Wallace, K. B. (1995). Enhanced induction of the mitochondrial permeability transition following acute menadione administration. *Archives of biochemistry and biophysics,* Vol.317, No.1, (February 1995), pp. 79-84, ISSN 0003-9861.

Scott, I. D. & Nicholls, D. G. (1980). Energy transduction in intact synaptosomes. Influence of plasma-membrane depolarization on the respiration and membrane potential of internal mitochondria determined in situ. *Biochem J,* Vol.186, No.1, (January 1980), pp. 21-33, ISSN 0264-6021.

Schinder, A. F., Olson, E. C., Spitzer, N. C. & Montal, M. (1996). Mitochondrial dysfunction is a primary event in glutamate neurotoxicity. *J Neurosci,* Vol.16, No.19, (October 1996), pp. 6125-6133, ISSN 0270-6474.

Shaw, P. J. (1999). Calcium, glutamate, and amyotrophic lateral sclerosis: more evidence but no certainties. *Annals of neurology,* Vol.46, No.6, (December 1999), pp. 803-805, ISSN 0364-5134.

Shaw, P. J., Ince, P. G., Falkous, G. & Mantle, D. (1995a). Oxidative damage to protein in sporadic motor neuron disease spinal cord. *Annals of neurology,* Vol.38, No.4, (October 1995), pp. 691-695, ISSN 0364-5134.

Shaw, P. J., Forrest, V., Ince, P. G., Richardson, J. P. & Wastell, H. J. (1995b). CSF and plasma amino acid levels in motor neuron disease: elevation of CSF glutamate in a subset of patients. *Neurodegeneration,* Vol.4, No.2, (June 1995), pp. 209-216, ISSN 1055-8330.

Shibata, N., Nagai, R., Uchida, K., Horiuchi, S., Yamada, S., Hirano, A., Kawaguchi, M., Yamamoto, T., Sasaki, S. & Kobayashi, M. (2001). Morphological evidence for lipid peroxidation and protein glycoxidation in spinal cords from sporadic amyotrophic lateral sclerosis patients. *Brain research,* Vol.917, No.1, (October 2001), pp. 97-104, ISSN 0006-8993.

Shrivastava, M. & Vivekanandhan, S. (2011). An insight into ultrastructural and morphological alterations of platelets in neurodegenerative diseases. *Ultrastructural pathology,* Vol.35, No.3, (May 2011), pp. 110-116, ISSN 1521-0758 (Electronic), 0191-3123 (Linking).

Shrivastava, M., Das, T. K., Behari, M., Pati, U. & Vivekanandhan, S. (2011a). Ultrastructural variations in platelets and platelet mitochondria: a novel feature in amyotrophic lateral sclerosis. *Ultrastructural pathology,* Vol.35, No.2, (April 2011), pp. 52-59, ISSN 1521-0758 (Electronic), 0191-3123 (Linking).

Shrivastava, M., Vivekanandhan, S., Pati, U., Behari, M. & Das, T. K. (2011b). Mitochondrial perturbance and execution of apoptosis in platelet mitochondria of patients with amyotrophic lateral sclerosis. *The International journal of neuroscience,* Vol.121, No.3, (March 2011), pp. 149-158, ISSN 1563-5279 (Electronic), 0020-7454 (Linking).

Siciliano, G., D'Avino, C., Del Corona, A., Barsacchi, R., Kusmic, C., Rocchi, A., Pastorini, E. & Murri, L. (2002). Impaired oxidative metabolism and lipid peroxidation in exercising muscle from ALS patients. *Amyotroph Lateral Scler Other Motor Neuron Disord,* Vol.3, No.2, (June 2002), pp. 57-62, ISSN 1466-0822.

Siklos, L., Engelhardt, J., Harati, Y., Smith, R. G., Joo, F. & Appel, S. H. (1996). Ultrastructural evidence for altered calcium in motor nerve terminals in amyotropic lateral sclerosis. *Annals of neurology,* Vol.39, No.2, (February 1996), pp. 203-216, ISSN 0364-5134.

Simpson, E. P., Henry, Y. K., Henkel, J. S., Smith, R. G. & Appel, S. H. (2004). Increased lipid peroxidation in sera of ALS patients: a potential biomarker of disease burden. *Neurology,* Vol.62, No.10, (May 2004), pp. 1758-1765, ISSN 1526-632X (Electronic), 0028-3878 (Linking).

Smith, R. G., Henry, Y. K., Mattson, M. P. & Appel, S. H. (1998). Presence of 4-hydroxynonenal in cerebrospinal fluid of patients with sporadic amyotrophic lateral sclerosis. *Annals of neurology,* Vol.44, No.4, (October 1998), pp. 696-699, ISSN 0364-5134.

Sofroniew, M. V. (2005). Reactive astrocytes in neural repair and protection. *Neuroscientist,* Vol.11, No.5, (October 2005), pp. 400-407, ISSN 1073-8584.

Spreux-Varoquaux, O., Bensimon, G., Lacomblez, L., Salachas, F., Pradat, P. F., Le Forestier, N., Marouan, A., Dib, M. & Meininger, V. (2002). Glutamate levels in cerebrospinal fluid in amyotrophic lateral sclerosis: a reappraisal using a new HPLC method with coulometric detection in a large cohort of patients. *Journal of the neurological sciences,* Vol.193, No.2, (January 2002), pp. 73-78, ISSN 0022-510X.

Swerdlow, R. H., Parks, J. K., Cassarino, D. S., Trimmer, P. A., Miller, S. W., Maguire, D. J., Sheehan, J. P., Maguire, R. S., Pattee, G., Juel, V. C., Phillips, L. H., Tuttle, J. B., Bennett, J. P., Jr., Davis, R. E. & Parker, W. D., Jr. (1998). Mitochondria in sporadic amyotrophic lateral sclerosis. *Experimental neurology,* Vol.153, No.1, (September 1998), pp. 135-142, ISSN 0014-4886.

Tateno, M., Kato, S., Sakurai, T., Nukina, N., Takahashi, R. & Araki, T. (2009). Mutant SOD1 impairs axonal transport of choline acetyltransferase and acetylcholine release by sequestering KAP3. *Human molecular genetics,* Vol.18, No.5, (March 2009), pp. 942-955, ISSN 1460-2083 (Electronic), 0964-6906 (Linking).

Tohgi, H., Abe, T., Yamazaki, K., Murata, T., Ishizaki, E. & Isobe, C. (1999). Remarkable increase in cerebrospinal fluid 3-nitrotyrosine in patients with sporadic amyotrophic lateral sclerosis. *Annals of neurology,* Vol.46, No.1, (July 1999), pp. 129-131, ISSN 0364-5134.

Tovar-y-Romo, L. B., Zepeda, A. & Tapia, R. (2007). Vascular endothelial growth factor prevents paralysis and motoneuron death in a rat model of excitotoxic spinal cord neurodegeneration. *Journal of neuropathology and experimental neurology,* Vol.66, No.10, (October 2007), pp. 913-922, ISSN 0022-3069.

Tovar-y-Romo, L. B., Santa-Cruz, L. D. & Tapia, R. (2009a). Experimental models for the study of neurodegeneration in amyotrophic lateral sclerosis. *Molecular neurodegeneration,* Vol.4, pp. 31, ISSN 1750-1326.

Tovar-y-Romo, L. B., Santa-Cruz, L. D., Zepeda, A. & Tapia, R. (2009b). Chronic elevation of extracellular glutamate due to transport blockade is innocuous for spinal motoneurons in vivo. *Neurochemistry international,* Vol.54, No.3-4, (March-April 2009), pp. 186-191, ISSN 1872-9754 (Electronic), 0197-0186 (Linking).

Trotti, D., Danbolt, N. C. & Volterra, A. (1998). Glutamate transporters are oxidant-vulnerable: a molecular link between oxidative and excitotoxic neurodegeneration?

Trends in pharmacological sciences, Vol.19, No.8, (August 1998), pp. 328-334, ISSN 0165-6147.

Trotti, D., Rossi, D., Gjesdal, O., Levy, L. M., Racagni, G., Danbolt, N. C. & Volterra, A. (1996). Peroxynitrite inhibits glutamate transporter subtypes. *The Journal of biological chemistry,* Vol.271, No.11, (March 1996), pp. 5976-5979, ISSN 0021-9258.

Turrens, J. F., Alexandre, A. & Lehninger, A. L. (1985). Ubisemiquinone is the electron donor for superoxide formation by complex III of heart mitochondria. *Archives of biochemistry and biophysics,* Vol.237, No.2, (March 1985), pp. 408-414, ISSN 0003-9861.

Van Den Bosch, L., Tilkin, P., Lemmens, G. & Robberecht, W. (2002). Minocycline delays disease onset and mortality in a transgenic model of ALS. *Neuroreport,* Vol.13, No.8, (June 2002), pp. 1067-1070, ISSN 0959-4965.

Vielhaber, S., Kunz, D., Winkler, K., Wiedemann, F. R., Kirches, E., Feistner, H., Heinze, H. J., Elger, C. E., Schubert, W. & Kunz, W. S. (2000). Mitochondrial DNA abnormalities in skeletal muscle of patients with sporadic amyotrophic lateral sclerosis. *Brain,* Vol.123, (July 2000), pp. 1339-1348, ISSN 0006-8950.

Volterra, A., Trotti, D. & Racagni, G. (1994). Glutamate uptake is inhibited by arachidonic acid and oxygen radicals via two distinct and additive mechanisms. *Molecular pharmacology,* Vol.46, No.5, (November 1994), pp. 986-992, ISSN 0026-895X.

von Lewinski, F. & Keller, B. U. (2005). Ca2+, mitochondria and selective motoneuron vulnerability: implications for ALS. *Trends in neurosciences,* Vol.28, No.9, (September 2005), pp. 494-500, ISSN 0166-2236.

Warita, H., Itoyama, Y. & Abe, K. (1999). Selective impairment of fast anterograde axonal transport in the peripheral nerves of asymptomatic transgenic mice with a G93A mutant SOD1 gene. *Brain research,* Vol.819, No.1-2, (February 1999), pp. 120-131, ISSN 0006-8993.

White, R. J. & Reynolds, I. J. (1996). Mitochondrial depolarization in glutamate-stimulated neurons: an early signal specific to excitotoxin exposure. *J Neurosci,* Vol.16, No.18, (September 1996), pp. 5688-5697, ISSN 0270-6474.

Wiedemann, F. R., Manfredi, G., Mawrin, C., Beal, M. F. & Schon, E. A. (2002). Mitochondrial DNA and respiratory chain function in spinal cords of ALS patients. *Journal of neurochemistry,* Vol.80, No.4, (February 2002), pp. 616-625, ISSN 0022-3042.

Wiedemann, F. R., Winkler, K., Kuznetsov, A. V., Bartels, C., Vielhaber, S., Feistner, H. & Kunz, W. S. (1998). Impairment of mitochondrial function in skeletal muscle of patients with amyotrophic lateral sclerosis. *Journal of the neurological sciences,* Vol.156, No.1, pp. 65-72, ISSN 0022-510X.

Williamson, T. L. & Cleveland, D. W. (1999). Slowing of axonal transport is a very early event in the toxicity of ALS-linked SOD1 mutants to motor neurons. *Nature neuroscience,* Vol.2, No.1, (January 1999), pp. 50-56, ISSN 1097-6256.

Wong, P. C., Pardo, C. A., Borchelt, D. R., Lee, M. K., Copeland, N. G., Jenkins, N. A., Sisodia, S. S., Cleveland, D. W. & Price, D. L. (1995). An adverse property of a familial ALS-linked SOD1 mutation causes motor neuron disease characterized by vacuolar degeneration of mitochondria. *Neuron,* Vol.14, No.6, (June 1995), pp. 1105-1116, ISSN 0896-6273.

Yamanaka, K., Chun, S. J., Boillee, S., Fujimori-Tonou, N., Yamashita, H., Gutmann, D. H., Takahashi, R., Misawa, H. & Cleveland, D. W. (2008). Astrocytes as determinants of disease progression in inherited amyotrophic lateral sclerosis. *Nature neuroscience*, Vol.11, No.3, (March 2008), pp. 251-253, ISSN 1097-6256.

Yang, W. W., Sidman, R. L., Taksir, T. V., Treleaven, C. M., Fidler, J. A., Cheng, S. H., Dodge, J. C. & Shihabuddin, L. S. (2011). Relationship between neuropathology and disease progression in the SOD1(G93A) ALS mouse. *Experimental neurology*, Vol.227, No.2, (February 2011), pp. 287-295, ISSN 1090-2430 (Electronic), 0014-4886 (Linking).

Zagami, C. J., Beart, P. M., Wallis, N., Nagley, P. & O'Shea, R. D. (2009). Oxidative and excitotoxic insults exert differential effects on spinal motoneurons and astrocytic glutamate transporters: Implications for the role of astrogliosis in amyotrophic lateral sclerosis. *Glia*, Vol.57, No.2, (January 2009), pp. 119-135, ISSN 1098-1136 (Electronic), 0894-1491 (Linking).

Zhang, F., Strom, A. L., Fukada, K., Lee, S., Hayward, L. J. & Zhu, H. (2007). Interaction between familial amyotrophic lateral sclerosis (ALS)-linked SOD1 mutants and the dynein complex. *The Journal of biological chemistry*, Vol.282, No.22, (June 2007), pp. 16691-16699, ISSN 0021-9258.

Zhu, S., Stavrovskaya, I. G., Drozda, M., Kim, B. Y., Ona, V., Li, M., Sarang, S., Liu, A. S., Hartley, D. M., Wu, D. C., Gullans, S., Ferrante, R. J., Przedborski, S., Kristal, B. S. & Friedlander, R. M. (2002). Minocycline inhibits cytochrome c release and delays progression of amyotrophic lateral sclerosis in mice. *Nature*, Vol.417, No.6884, (May 2002), pp. 74-78, ISSN 0028-0836.

10

Role of Neuronal Mitochondrial Metabolic Phenotype in Pathogenesis of ALS

Alexander Panov[1, 3], Nury Steuerwald[1], Valentin Vavilin[2], Svetlana Dambinova[3] and Herbert L. Bonkovsky[1]
[1]Cannon Research Center, Carolinas Medical Center, Charlotte, NC,
[2]Institute of Molecular Biology and Biophysics, Novosibirsk,
[3]Laboratory of Brain Biomarkers, WellStar College of Health & Human Services, Kennesaw State University, Kennesaw, GA,
[1,3]USA
[2]Russia

1. Introduction

Amyotrophic lateral sclerosis (ALS) is one of the group of diseases of the central nerve system (CNS), which are characterized by progressive loss of structure and function of neurons in different regions of brain or spinal cord. Therefore, these diseases are collectively designated as "Neurodegenerative Diseases" (NDDs). Usually the loss of specific functions precedes the death of affected neurons, and the related clinical features depend on localization and degree of neurodegeneration. NDDs include such diseases as Alzheimer's, Parkinson's, Huntington's, spinocerebellar ataxias, and ALS. In spite of differences in predominant localization of neurodegeneration and clinical features, there are many parallels among different neurodegenerative disorders. These include involvement of mitochondrial dysfunctions, increased oxidative stress, and atypical protein assemblies (Backman et al., 2006).

Amyotrophic lateral sclerosis (ALS) refers to several adult-onset conditions characterized by progressive degeneration of motor neurons. "Amyotrophic" refers to the muscle atrophy, weakness, and fasciculation (spontaneous contraction affecting a small number of muscle fibers) that signify disease of the lower motor neurons. There are two forms of this fatal disease: sporadic, with no known genetic component, and familial, which make up about 10% of all ALS cases (Rowland & Schneider, 2001; Martin et al., 2009). Among the familial cases, approximately 20% are caused by dominantly inherited mutations in the Cu/Zn superoxide dismutase (*SOD1*) gene, with more than 100 known mutations (reviewed in Bruijn et al., 2004). So far, there is very little information that links familial and sporadic cases of the disease. One established fact, based on studies of patients and transgenic animals, is that mitochondria dysfunction is an early manifestation. However, it is unclear whether mitochondrial dysfunctions are the primary pathogenic mechanism, or the result of some other proximate pathogenic mechanism.

Although the cases associated with mutations in the *SOD1* gene comprise only about 2% of all ALS cases, understandably, transgenic animals bearing mutated *SOD1* gene became the major targets for research on pathogenesis of ALS (Bendotti and Carri, 2004; Bruijn et al., 2004; Matsumoto et al., 2006). Of these, a transgenic mouse carrying the G93A (Gly-93 → Ala) mutant human *SOD1* gene was the first described (Gurney et al., 1994). This animal model of ALS was used all over the world because it closely recapitulates clinical and histopathological features of the human disease (Matsumoto et al., 2006).

Researchers from Wyeth, John Hopkins and Harvard in collaboration with ALS Association as part of its Lou Gehrig Challenge Initiative established the SOD1G93A mutant rat line. Taconic (Germantown, NY) established a production colony in 2002, which was sponsored by grant funding from ALS Association. The original publication on this strain (tgSOD1) reported disease onset around 115 days of age, with rapid disease progression thereafter (Howland et al., 2002). Taconic has maintained a colony since 2002. In our recent work (Panov et al., 2011b) we presented data obtained in 2007 on 45 tgSOD1 animals obtained from 9 separate simultaneous isolations of BM and SCM. We studied respiration and reactive oxygen species production by mitochondria isolated from the brains (tgBM) and spinal cords (tgSCM), of such rats and the results obtained were highly reproducible (Panov et al., 2011b). Beginning late in 2008 and in 2009 we encountered difficulties in reproducing the results obtained in 2007. Moreover, we have found that the transgenic rat line did not develop symptoms of the disease at age of more than 200 days even though the mutated gene was evident in DNA samples from tails and ears. In 2010 we received information from Taconic (Germantown, NY) that changes in features can be attributed to a variable phenotype in this model, "which may be due to in part to both the outbred nature of the background strain as well as to possible copy number variation of the transgene" (Information Letter from Taconic). Whether these phenotypic changes were associated with the decline of the level to which the transgene was expressed is impossible to conclude because, in the rats studied in 2007, neither Taconic company, nor our lab quantified the expression of the mutated SOD1 gene or protein. Nevertheless, our comparative studies of metabolic properties of BM and SCM suggest that potentially the loss of morbidity could be explained by different patterns of substrates metabolism and associated ROS generation in BM and SCM studied in 2007 and 2010.

In 2008 we found that BM and SCM isolated from the wild type Sprague Dawley rats began to show metabolic features that were different from those described earlier for the same strain of the wild type and tgSOD1 rats (Panov et al., 2009, 2011a). In this work we present a comparison of metabolic phenotypes and the substrate-dependent ROS generation in the wild type and transgenic rats with mutant G93A Cu/Zn-superoxide dismutase gene isolated in 2007 and 2010. We conclude that the shift in mitochondrial metabolic phenotype, which resulted in a dramatic decrease in ROS production by tgBM and tgSCM, may have contributed to the significant loss of morbidity of the established tgSOD1 rat line. This could result from the breeding method of the transgenic animals, when males bearing the dominant mutated *SOD1* gene were mated with the wild type females. Because mitochondrial DNA has maternal inheritance (Wallace, 2001), the resulting progeny has the mitochondrial phenotype of females, and thus the mutated SOD1 protein was acting on mitochondria with different metabolism that resulted in much lower rates of ROS production. We conclude that mitochondria are the key players in the pathogenesis of ALS.

We suggest a hypothesis, which links together pathogenic mechanisms of sporadic and familial forms of ALS. Our hypothesis is based on results obtained in experiments on animals, which showed that between species and even within one species there may exist different phenotypes of mitochondrial metabolism. Neuronal mitochondria of some phenotypes may produce very large amounts of superoxide radical, which is dismutated to hydrogen peroxide (H_2O_2). High levels of H_2O_2 may damage the extramitochondrial isoform of superoxide dismutase (SOD1). The oxidatively damaged proteins lose Cu and Zn from the hem centers, and the demetallated protein enters mitochondrial membranes, further increases ROS production by a mechanism similar to that described for cholesterol-β-D-glucoside and fitosterol glucosides (Panov et al., 2010b), causes mitochondrial dysfunctions, and finally the death of neurons. These are sporadic cases of ALS associated with disorders of mitochondrial metabolism. The familial cases with mutations in the *SOD1* gene have basically the same mechanism of motor neuron death, but, because mutated SOD1 protein is exceptionally sensitive to oxidative damage, the loss of Cu and Zn may occur at relatively low levels of H_2O_2 formation by neuronal mitochondria. The predominant involvement of spinal cord can be accounted for by metabolic and structural features of spinal cord and SCM, which were published elsewhere (Panov et al., 2011a, 2011b).

2. General characterization of mitochondria in ALS

Clinical features of ALS, a severe neuromuscular degenerative disease, were described by Charcot in 1874 (Rowland & Shneider, 2001). Since that time clinical definitions (Shook and Pioro, 2009) and pathological features of the disease have been greatly expanded, aided in no small measure by advances in genetics of the disease (Rowland & Shneider, 2001) and development of transgenic animal models of ALS (Bendotti & Carri, 2004; Matsumoto et al., 2006; Howland et al., 2002). However, the etiology and pathogenesis of the disease remain poorly understood.

Clinical and experimental evidence showed that ALS is a systemic disease, with particular vulnerability of motor neurons due to some unique properties (Martin et al., 2007; von Lewinski & Keller, 2005; Panov et al., 2011a). Many ALS patients are hypermetabolic, an early and persistent phenomenon (Bouteloup et al., 2009, Desport et al., 2005). Muscular mitochondrial function in amyotrophic lateral sclerosis is progressively altered in ALS patients (Echaniz-Laguna et al., 2006, Krasnianski et al., 2005), and subtle ultrastructural changes of hepatocytes and liver dysfunction have also been described in biopsy specimens from ALS patients (Nakano et al., 1987). Significant changes were also found in skeletal muscle mitochondria of transgenic SOD1 (tgSOD1) animals (Dupuis et al., 2009, Krasnianski et al., 2005). It was suggested that increased ROS generation by skeletal muscle mitochondria (Muller et al., 2007) or mitochondrial uncoupling (Dupuis et al., 2009) may be primarily responsible for the loss of neuromuscular junctions and secondary distal degeneration of motor neurons in SOD1 mice. This is an interesting and important alternative hypothesis, which requires a more detailed and critical discussion.

The paper by Muller et al. (2007) presents data on generation of ROS by skeletal muscle mitochondria (SMM) from two lines of transgenic mice bearing different mutations in SOD1 gene, SOD1 knockout mice, and mice with denervated muscle. The authors concluded that "enhanced generation of mitochondrial ROS may be a common factor in the mechanism underlying denervation-induced atrophy". The authors suggested also that increased ROS generation in ALS mutant model may also cause the loss of neuro-muscular junctions, and thus initiate the loss of motor neurons. There are, however, experimental facts, which oppose this conclusion. Muller et al (2007) isolated skeletal muscle mitochondria using a protease nagarse for digestion of the tissue. With the nagarse method, more than 90% of mitochondria are interfibrillar. Without the protease the yields of subsarcolemmal mitochondria are very low (A. Panov, unpublished observations). ROS generated *in situ* by interfibrillar mitochondria are unlikely to gain access to the sarcolemmal membrane where the neuro-muscular junctions are located. This is because superoxide radical has difficulty to leave mitochondria (Panov et al. 2005). Besides, both superoxide radicals and H_2O_2 are substrates for the antioxidant enzymes in the cytoplasm, such as SOD1, catalase, etc. Rather, it is more likely that increased ROS act locally to cause damage to interfibrillar mitochondria, particularly to mtDNA, and thus cause muscle atrophy. Data presented by Muller et al. (2007) do not show direct damage to neuromuscular junctions by increased ROS. Therefore this issue requires further study. There is also a quantitative aspect of ROS generation presented by Muller et al. (2007). A comparison of the rates of ROS production by skeletal muscle mitochondria (SMM) (Figure 1 in Muller et al., 2007) and brain (BM) and spinal cord mitochondria (SCM) (see Fig. 7 in Panov et al., 2011a) shows that BM and SCM generate several times more ROS than SMM. Therefore, it is more likely that the causes of degeneration of motor neurons in ALS are associated with primary pathological processes in neurons rather than in muscle.

Dupuis et al. (2009) also concluded that "a muscle restricted mitochondrial defect is sufficient to generate motor neuron degeneration". The authors based their conclusion on mitochondrial dysfunctions observed in animals with overexpression of uncoupling protein 1 (UCP1). Overexpression of UCP1 results in deenergization of the mitochondria due to increased conductivity of the inner membrane for protons. This condition results in complete inhibition of ROS production associated with the energy-dependent reverse electron transport. The major consequence of overexpression of UCP1 is inhibition of ATP production and suppression of functions, which depend on mitochondrial ATP levels. Because in neuronal tissue reverse electron transport is the major source of ROS production (Panov et al. 2007, 2009), and increased ROS generation is one of the leading pathogenic pathways in ALS, the mechanism proposed by Dupius et al. (2009), although interesting, probably has little to do with neurodegeneration in ALS.

It was hypothesized that sporadic and familial forms of ALS may share some final pathogenic mechanisms (Bendotti & Carri, 2004; von Lewinski & Keller, 2005). Several pathogenic factors have been proposed (reviewed in Bruijn et al., 2004): glutamate excitotoxicity (Heath & Shaw, 2002); mitochondrial dysfunction (Dupuis et al., 2009); increased production of reactive oxygen species (ROS) (reviewed in Barber & Shaw, 2010) and nitroxyradicals (NO^- and $ONOO^-$) (Martin et al., 2007); deregulation of Ca^{2+} homeostasis and triggering of permeability transition of mitochondria (von Lewinski and Keller, 2005; Martin et al., 2009; Morota et al., 2007); induction of pro-apoptotic pathways (Przedborski, 2004); misfolding and intracellular accumulation of mutant SOD1 (Tateno et al., 2004), including in brain and spinal mitochondria (Liu et al., 2004; Higgins et al., 2002); mutant SOD1-induced conformational changes in Bcl-2 (Pedrini et al., 2010) and VDAC1 (porin)

(Israelson et al., 2010); and abnormal axonal transport (Magrane & Manfredi, 2009). However, almost all of these proposed pathogenic mechanisms directly or indirectly involve mitochondria. The major problem in searching for alternative pathogenic mechanisms, in case of severe mitochondrial disability, is that practically all cellular and organ functions depend on energy and thus also become disturbed (Gershoni et al., 2009). Therefore, it is of paramount importance to precisely understand the nature and causes of mitochondrial dysfunctions, and whether they are early or late events in disease evolution.

In the majority of studies of ALS, the mitochondrial abnormalities were assessed using morphological methods, which showed swollen brain and spinal mitochondria with dilated cristae, and vacuoles in matrix (Sasaki et al., 2004, Jaarsma et al., 2006). It was suggested that vacuolization may depend on accumulation amount, rather than from toxic property, of mutant SOD1 (Jaarsma, 2006). Morphologic methods, including quantitative histochemistry, and immunological methods, showed that both in ALS patients and tgSOD1 animals, the activities of respiratory chain complexes were diminished (Jung et al., 2002), and that the spinal cord mitochondria are predisposed to opening of the Ca^{2+}-dependent permeability transition pores (mPTP), which trigger death of motor neurons (Martin et al., 2009). There is a large body of evidence that spinal cords in tgSOD1 animals are subjected to increased oxidative and nitrative stress, as indicated by accumulation of protein carbonyls and nitrated proteins (Martin et al., 2007, 2009). These data also demonstrated that mitochondria are involved early in the pathogenesis of ALS (Martin et al., 2007, 2009). Recently, Panov et al. (2011b) provided direct evidence that isolated mitochondria from the brain and spinal cord of tgSOD1 rats generate significantly more reactive oxygen species (ROS) as compared with mitochondria from wild type animals.

Morphological, histochemical and immunological methods provided important information about involvement of mitochondria in the pathology, however they do not tell us what caused the changes in mitochondrial morphology. Relatively few studies were performed on isolated BM and SCM mitochondria from control (Sullivan et al., 2004, Panov et al., 2011a), tgSOD1 animals (Kirkinezos et al., 2005, Damiano et al., 2006, Fischer et al., 2011, Panov et al., 2011b), Wobbler mice (Dave et al., 2003, Xu et al., 2001), or *mnd* mice, which spontaneously develop motor neuron pathology (Bertamini et al., 2002). In their pioneering work, Sullivan et al (2004) have shown that normal SCM have lower respiratory activity, lower threshold for calcium-induced mitochondrial permeability transition, and a higher degree of superoxide radical production (determined with dehydroethidium) and lipid peroxidation as compared with BM. However, the dehydroethidium method does not identify the origin of superoxide radical. Studies of isolated mitochondria from tgSOD1 mice showed that BM and SCM had decreased rates of respiration associated with the loss of complex IV activity (Kirkinezos et al., 2005). Very early in the course of the disease, the mitochondrial Ca^{2+} loading capacity was significantly diminished as compared with the age-matched control mice (Damiano et al., 2006). Respiratory activities were also diminished in SCM of Wobbler mice (Dave et al., 2003, Xu et al., 2001) and mice with motor neuron degeneration disease (Bertamini et al., 2002).

A comparative study of isolated normal and tgSOD1 brain and spinal cord mitochondria was published recently by Panov et al. (2011a, b), and the unique metabolic features of BM and SCM were described (see also Panov et al, 2009). Normal SCM produced significantly more ROS than BM, and this was associated with the succinate-dependent reverse electron transport (Panov et al. 2011a). A rather unexpected finding was that BM and SCM isolated

from presymptomatic tgSOD1 rats showed almost normal rates of oxidative phosphorylation. Panov et all. (2011b) purified mitochondria in a Percoll gradient, and thus eliminated damaged mitochondria. This resulted in significantly lower yields of mitochondria per 1 gram of tissue of tgSOD1 rats: the yields were diminished by 27% for the brain and by 58% for spinal cord as compared with the normal Sprague Dawley rats (Panov et al., 2011b). Avossa et al. (2006) used immunocytochemistry and electron microscopy techniques to compare wild type and G93A spinal cord tissues after 14 days of growth under standard *in vitro* conditions. Wild type and mutant cultures displayed no differences in the analyzed parameters as well as in the number of motor neurons, and there were no signs of mitochondria vacuolization or protein aggregate formation in G93A ventral horns. Together, the results of Panov et al. (2011b) and Avossa et al. (2006) suggest that in tgSOD1 rats the BM and SCM are primarily normal but suffer from some pathological events, which rapidly deteriorate mitochondria and cause death of neurons.
In order to better understand the metabolic events involved in putative pathological mechanisms of neurodegeneration, we have to discuss the distinctive features of brain and spinal cord energy metabolism and their mitochondria.

3. General features of neuronal energy metabolism

Neuronal cells are strictly aerobic and require large quantities of ATP produced at high rate in order to function normally. Humans brain constitutes only 2% of the body's weight, but accounts for 20% of its resting O_2 metabolism (Attwell & Laughlin, 2001). However, even in humans, heart and kidney consume significantly more oxygen per unit of the organ's mass than the brain (Rolfe & Brown, 1997). In rats, liver, kidney and heart consume correspondingly 2, 3 and 3.9 times more oxygen than the brain (Rolfe & Brown, 1997). Thus it is not the necessity for the high rate of oxidative metabolism that is unique for the central nerve system, but how the oxidative metabolism is organized in neuronal cells.
Cortical tissue is composed mainly of two types of cells: the nerve cells (or neurons) and the neuroglial cells (or glia). Glial cells greatly outnumber the neurons (Abeles, 1991; Attwell & Laughlin, 2001; Stolzenburg et al., 1989). Glial cells do not directly take part in the interactions between neurons, but play an important role in maintaining neuronal metabolism and in directing the development and growth of the brain. The classical categorization of neurons was based mainly on morphology of the cell body and its dendritic tree, and to a lesser extent on the morphology of the axon and its branches (Abeles, 1991).
There are two main categories of the cortical cells according to their physiological effects on each other: excitatory and inhibitory cells. Excitatory cells release transmitters (glutamate) at their synaptic ends that, on contact with the postsynaptic membrane, create ion currents that depolarize the postsynaptic cell. Inhibitory cells release transmitters, such as γ-aminobutyric acid (GABA), that tend to hyperpolarize the postsynaptic cell or to increase the conductance of the postsynaptic membrane to chloride, thereby diminishing the effects of the depolarizing currents generated by the excitatory synapses. Excitatory synapses dominate the brain's grey matter because excitatory neurons outnumber inhibitory cells by a factor of 9 to 1, and 90% of synapses release glutamate (Abeles, 1991; Braitenberg & Schüz, 1998). The distribution of mitochondria points to these glutamatergic synapses as the major users of metabolic energy (Wong-Riley, 1989; Attwell & Laughlin, 2001).
More than 80% of neuronal mitochondria are located in the dendrites and axonal terminals (Wong-Riley, 1989; Attwell & Laughlin, 2001). With high synaptic density of 8 x 10^8 per 1

mm^3 in all cortices (the density of synapses is not very much different among species) it is clear that in the brain most energy expenditures are associated with synaptic activity, where most mitochondria are located (Abeles, 1991). The close spacing of terminals along axons (5 μm, implying a diffusion time of only 25 milliseconds) make terminal and axonal mitochondria functionally indistinguishable (Attwell & Laughlin, 2001).

Neurons communicate by means of signals that lead to depolarization of their excitable membranes. The degree of depolarization of the dendritic or soma membranes is determined by complex interactions between excitatory and inhibitory transmitters. The depolarization spreads to the axon, leading to release of an excitatory or inhibitory transmitter at the axonal endings of the cell, thus allowing information to be transferred to the next cell. When impulses are propagated, the cell loses K^+ and gains Na^+, and in order to preserve excitability the cell must extrude Na^+ and accumulate K^+, using metabolic energy derived from oxidative metabolism (Abeles, 1991). Postsynaptic ion fluxes (Na^+, K^+, Cl^-) and presynaptic Ca^{2+} influx consume in grey matter approximately 75% of the brain's energy (Abeles, 1991; Attwell & Laughlin, 2001). Because depolarization and restoration of ionic composition across the neuronal membrane occur in the millisecond scale, neuronal mitochondria must provide large quantities of ATP in a very short time. This distribution of energy use reflects the fact that a chemical synapse is an amplifier: for each glutamate released approximately 100 ions enter the postsynaptic terminal (Abeles, 1991). The rest (25%) of the brain's energy is used for the basic "housekeeping" functions, such as maintenance of pH gradients, asymmetrical distributions of phospholipids in membrane bilayers, protein synthesis (about 2%), anaplerotic functions and recycling of glutamate from synaptic clefts (Attwell & Laughlin, 2001). It was suggested that white and grey matter require similar amounts of energy on basic (nonsignaling) cellular activities (Attwell & Laughlin, 2001).

It is widely accepted that nerve tissues of adult mammals use glucose as the major source of energy. To fully understand the specifics of energy metabolism in brain, it is important to take into account that, in dendrites and synaptic terminals, there is limited space for glycolytic enzymes that would provide mitochondria with enough pyruvate derived from glucose. Therefore, neurons cannot be functionally and metabolically regarded without astroglia. Astrocytes provide neurons with lactate, as the major source of energy, replenish the neuronal pool of glutamine and recycle glutamate (Ebert et al., 2003; Pellerin et al., 2007; Suzuki et al., 2011). Of the total energy consumed by the brain, approximately 80% of energy expenditure is satisfied by oxidation of glucose and 20% by oxidation of fatty acids (Ebert et al., 2003). As we will see later, neurons also oxidize significant amounts of glutamate and GABA as a source of energy. The neurotransmitter GABA is formed from glutamate by the action of glutamate decarboxylase. It appears that glutamine serves as the precursor for glutamate and GABA. Therefore, the pool of glutamine must be constantly replenished in anaplerotic reactions, which occur predominantly in astroglia.

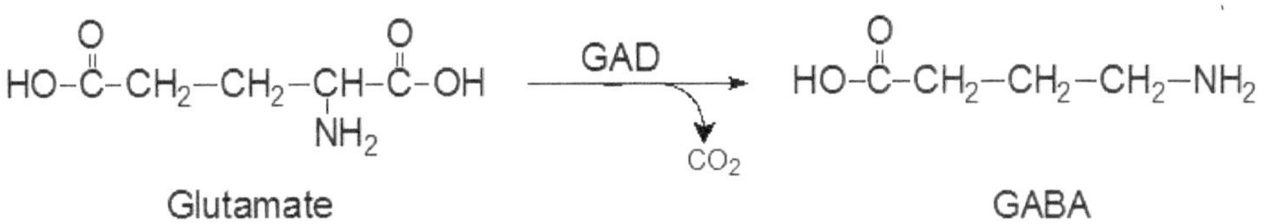

Fig. 1. Formation of GABA from glutamate. GAD – glutamate decarboxylase.

Because anaplerotic functions of astrocytes require energy, oxidation of fatty acids occurs in glial mitochondria (Ebert et al., 2003) providing energy and saving glucose for production of lactate in aerobic glycolysis and α-ketoglutarate for synthesis *de novo* neuromediators glutamate and GABA (Waagepetersen et al., 1999; Ebert et al., 2003). Glutamine synthetase is an astrocyte-specific enzyme (Norenberg & Martinez-Hernandez, 1979), and during octanoate oxidation in astrocytes most of the anaplerotic flux in brain is occurring in the TCA cycle associated with glutamine production (Ebert et al., 2003). In order to fulfill the task of metabolic provision of neuronal functions there are several mechanisms that ensure functional and metabolic compartmentalization and complementation between neurons and astroglia, which thus exclude competition for energy substrates. Neuronal mitochondria do not possess the full range activity of β-oxidation enzymes, whereas glial mitochondria readily oxidize fatty acids (Ebert et al., 2003). On the other hand, glial mitochondria do not have active glutamate-aspartate translocase (Berkich et al., 2007), which is the key enzyme of the malate aspartate shuttle and the major pathway for oxidation of glutamate by neuronal mitochondria. Thus astrocytes do not utilize glutamate as a respiratory substrate. The distribution of lactate dehydrogenase isoforms between glial cells and neurons promotes aerobic glycolysis in astroglia and utilization of lactate by neurons as the major respiratory substrate (Pellerin et al., 2007).

4. In activated neurons mitochondria utilize a mixture of substrates

Mitochondria are devices for burning hydrogen producing water and releasing energy, a large part of which is accumulated as electrochemical transmembrane potential ($\Delta\mu_H+$) (Mitchell, 1977; Nicholls, 2008). $\Delta\mu_H+$ is utilized for production of ATP, and other useful work in the mitochondria and cell. Therefore lactate, which has additional hydrogen, as compared with pyruvate, has higher energetic value for neuronal mitochondria. In the cytosol of a neuron, lactate is oxidized to pyruvate in the reaction catalyzed by lactate dehydrogenase (LDH): NAD^+ + Lactate → NADH + H^+ + Pyruvate. Pyruvate is transported into mitochondria and metabolized.

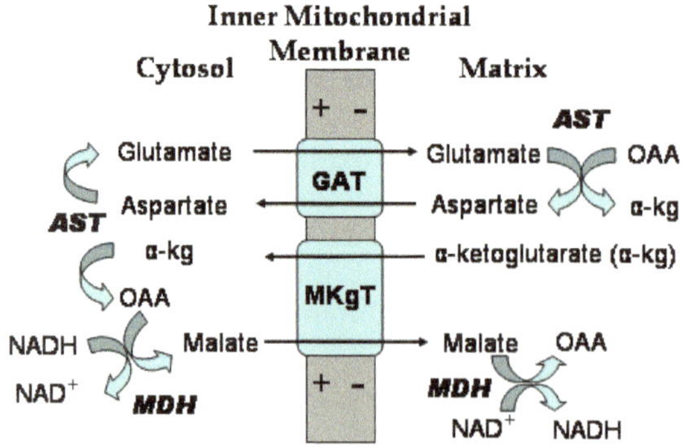

Abbreviations: AST – aspartate aminotransferase; GAT – glutamate-aspartate transporter, MDH – malate dehydrogenase; MKgT – malate- α -ketoglutarate transporter; OAA – oxaloacetate

Fig. 2. **The malate aspartate shuttle.** In a cell with respiring energized mitochondria the malate aspartate shuttle serves for transport and oxidation of hydrogen from cytosolic NADH to mitochondrial respiratory chain. The process is unidirectional because GAT is electrogenic and the matrix NADH is rapidly oxidized by respiratory chain.

In order to rapidly oxidize lactate to pyruvate, the cytosolic NADH must be oxidized back to NAD^+. In neurons the task of reoxidation of the cytosolic NADH and transport of hydrogen into mitochondria occur via a number of functionally coupled cytosolic and mitochondrial enzymes, which form the malate-aspartate shuttle (MAS) (Figure 2). Glutamate is a necessary component of MAS. Because nonsynaptic and presynaptic neuronal mitochondria effectively oxidize glutamate (Yudkoff et al. 1994), neuronal cells constantly have to replenish the cytosolic pool of glutamate.

Until recently, it was generally accepted that most of the glutamate is rapidly removed from the synaptic cleft by glutamate transporters EAAT1 (GLT-1) and EAAT2 (GLAST) located on presynaptic termini and glial cells (Furness et al., 2008). However, recent data show that a significant fraction of glutamate is rapidly bound and transported by the glutamate transporter isoform, EAAT4, located juxtasynaptically in the membranes of spines and dendrites (Auger & Attwell., 2000; Brasnjo& Otis., 2004). EAAT4 protein was found to be omnipresent throughout the fore- and midbrain (Massie et al., 2008). These data suggest that postsynaptic transport of glutamate into nerve terminals, where mitochondria are located (Abeles, 1991), may occur in all brain regions. According to calculations of Brasnjo and Otis (2004), in a single synapse EAAT4 bind and transport postsynaptically about $1.3 \pm 0.1 \times 10^6$ glutamate molecules. In the brain, on average, 1 mm^3 of tissue contains 1×10^8 synapses (Abeles, 1991; Nicholls, 1993). Because of the high density of synaptic contacts, the neuronal cells may be exposed to mediators released from hundreds of firing synapses. Thus in a narrow space of spines and dendrites several million glutamate molecules postsynaptically transported from synaptic boutons may create local cytosolic concentration of glutamate in a low mM range. Consequently, neuronal mitochondria, particularly those located at the axonal or dendritic synaptic junctions may temporarily metabolize, in addition to pyruvate, some amounts of glutamate (Yudkoff et al. 1994; Panov et al. 2009). Besides, GABA is also transported postsynaptically where it is catabolized in mitochondria to succinate (Tillakaratne et al., 1995).

As we have mentioned, for rapid conversion of lactate to pyruvate, postsynaptic neurons must receive a certain amount of glutamate to fuel MAS to recycle cytosolic NAD^+ (Berkich et al., 2007). Importantly, the activity of the brain mitochondrial isoform of aspartate glutamate transporter is controlled by Ca^{2+} (Pardo et al., 2006). Therefore increased neuronal activity through small changes in the extramitochondrial Ca^{2+} activates MAS, whereas increased mitochondrial Ca^{2+} activates mitochondrial respiration (Nicholls, 2009).

There is evidence (Yudkoff et al., 1994), that in the presence of glutamate + pyruvate, the tricarboxylic acid (TCA) cycle in brain mitochondria operates as two coupled cycles: one (cycle A) leads from α-KG to OAA, and another (cycle B) from OAA to a-KG that includes the citrate synthase reaction (see figure 3). According to Yudkoff et al. (1994), the flux of substrates through cycle A is 3-5-fold faster than that through the cycle B. Thus, with pyruvate + glutamate + malate, activation of α-ketoglutarate dehydrogenase complex (α-KGDHC) and succinate dehydrogenase (SDH) may significantly increase the rates of the tricarboxylic acid cycle (TCA) cycle and respiratory chain in state 3 and state 3U (Fig. 3). A high turnover of cycle A with activated SDH would increase reverse electron transport (RET) and the associated ROS production.

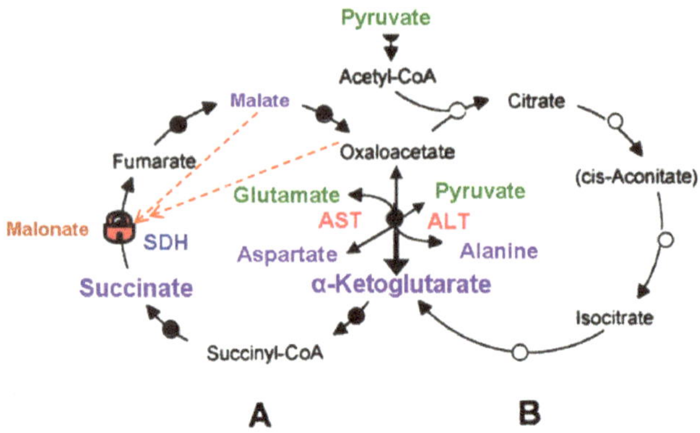

Abbreviations: ALT - alanine aminotransferase; AST -aspartate aminotransferase; SDH - succinate dehydrogenase (Complex II).

Fig. 3. **The tricarboxylic acid cycle in the presence of pyruvate and glutamate operates as two coupled cycles A and B**. In the presence of glutamate and/or pyruvate as substrates high activities of AST and ALT may "short-circuit" oxaloacetate and α-ketoglutarate, thus converting the "normal" TCA cycle into two independently operating cycles A and B. Malonate is a quasi-irreversible inhibitor of SDH, whereas oxaloacetate (OAA) is a competitive but strong inhibitor. SDH has similar affinities for succinate and malate, but oxidation of malate results in formation of OAA on the enzyme's active center, which makes malate a strong inhibitor of SDH.

Thus in activated neurons mitochondria may oxidize simultaneously glutamate, pyruvate, and metabolites of the TCA cycle, such as malate, and succinate. Postsynaptically transported GABA is catabolized in mitochondria to succinate (Tillakaratne et al., 1995). Under these conditions, brain (BM) and spinal cord (SCM) mitochondria significantly increase the rate of oxidative phosphorylation and the succinate-dependent production of ROS (Panov et al., 2009, 2011a). With glutamate + pyruvate + malate as substrates, increased production of ATP and ROS was associated with dramatic increase in the matrix concentration of α-ketoglutarate (Balasz, 1965a) due to increased activities of mitochondrial aminotransferases AST and ALT (Fig. 3). Under these conditions glutamate dehydrogenase (GLDH) does not participate in production of α-KG (Balasz, 1965b). Since AST and ALT are present in great excess, compared with the respiration rate, the oxaloacetate (OAA) formed is continuously removed by the transamination reactions. Balazs (1965b) concluded that a competition takes place between the α-KGDHC and GLDH, probably for NAD+, resulting in preferential oxidation of α-oxoglutarate.

5. Distinctive properties of ROS generation in brain and spinal cord mitochondria

In neuronal tissue mitochondria are the major source of ROS production (Stowe & Camara, 2009), which is indispensable feature of aerobic metabolism. It is generally accepted that during oxidation of the NAD-dependent substrates the limiting step is at the NADH-dehydrogenase site of Complex I (see Panov et al. 2007, 2009). With succinate as a substrate, production of ROS is significantly higher, because Complex II, which is also part of the TCA cycle - succinate dehydrogenase (SDH), feeds electrons into the mitochondrial pool of CoQ_{10} (ubiquinone, Q). The reduced ubiquinone (QH_2) in its turn reduces the sites on Complex I that can generate superoxide radicals at high rate. This process, known as reverse electron transport, is energy-dependent and inhibited by rotenone. Some researchers deny the significance of succinate in ROS production on the pretext that succinate concentration is too low in mitochondria (Starkov, 2008; Stowe & Camara, 2009; Zoccarato et al., 2007). As we have shown recently, however, brain and spinal cord mitochondria may produce succinate even in the presence of pyruvate + malate (Panov et al., 2009) , and as we show in this article (see Fig. 6) even with glutamate + malate a large part of ROS production may be associated with oxidation of succinate. However a particularly large production of the succinate-dependent ROS was observed in the presence of glutamate + pyruvate + malate (Panov et al., 2009, 2011a, 2011b). With these substrates the increased succinate oxidation was caused by a dramatic increase in mitochondrial α-ketoglutarate due to high activities of aminotransferases (Balasz, 1965a, 1965b). Besides, GABA is catabolized with formation of succinate in postsynaptic mitochondria (Tillakaratne et al. 1995). Thus, in the excited neurons succinate is an indispensable mitochondrial metabolite. In this paper we provide evidence that ROS generation associated with the succinate-dependent reverse electron transport is a subject for phenotypic variations.

Another objection to the importance of reverse electron transport (RET) in ROS generation argues that, because RET is energy-dependent, in the functioning cell the diminished mitochondrial energization will inhibit production of ROS (Starkov, 2008). The latter objection is valid for the most perpetually functioning organs, such as heart, kidney and liver. But it is only partially applicable to brain and spinal cord where a very large number of mitochondria are located at axonal and dendritic junctions (Wong-Riley, 1989). At the narrow spaces of synaptic junctions there is no other task for mitochondria beside provision of ATP for restoration of ionic composition in excited synapses. If the neurons are not excited, mitochondria become fully energized and produce ROS at high rate. Therefore axonal and synaptic junctions, including neuro muscular junctions, are particularly vulnerable to oxidative damage if neurons are not excited for some reason.

Another possible reason why the succinate-dependent ROS production was underrated could be the fact that most researchers use "classical" mixtures of substrates, such as glutamate + malate, pyruvate + malate, succinate alone, or, very often, in the presence of rotenone.

Figure 4 shows a representative experiment with the BM and SCM isolated in 2007 from tg SOD1 rats. One can see that with glutamate + malate, the rate of ROS production, measured as H_2O_2, there were no differences between tgBM and tgSCM, wtBM or wtSCM (not shown). With pyruvate + malate as substrates, tgSCM generated significantly more ROS than tgBM (see Fig. 5). This was because SCM in general oxidize succinate at higher rate than BM, presumably due to the lower intrinsic inhibition of SDH by oxaloacetate (Panov et al., 2011a). However, when tgBM and tgSCM oxidized a mixture of glutamate + pyruvate + malate, there was a several-fold increase in ROS production. TgSCM produced much more ROS than tgBM (Fig. 4, see also Fig. 6 in Panov et al., 2011b). Thus the usage of physiologically relevant mixtures of substrates is far more informative for understanding the role of mitochondria in pathogenesis of diseases, than the "classical" approach.

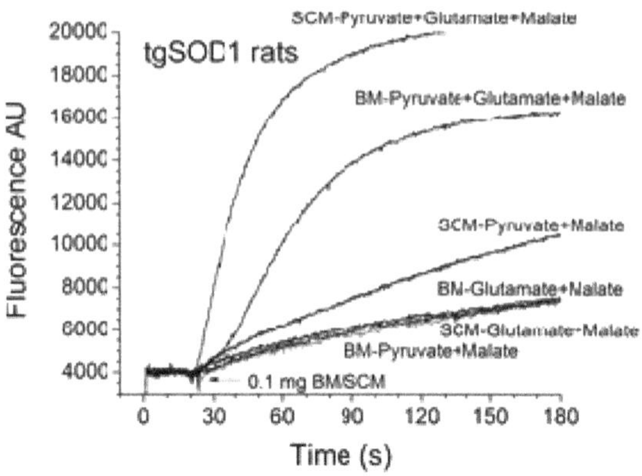

Fig. 4. **Production of ROS by brain and spinal cord mitochondria from tgSOD1 rats.** Mitochondrial production of ROS was registered as H_2O_2 by Amplex red method (Panov et al., 2009).

We suggested the following metabolic scenario for the neuronal mitochondria located at synaptic junctions. During neuronal activity, the postsynaptic mitochondria are exposed to increased levels of pyruvate and glutamate, which enhance ATP production due to specific interactions between the glutamate transforming enzymes and the TCA cycle enzymes. This effect of the substrate mixtures is specific for the BM, and SCM (Panov et al., 2009, 2011a). As soon as activation of a synapse comes to an end, transport of glutamate from the synaptic cleft would also stop. As a result, activation of respiration induced by the simultaneous presence of glutamate and pyruvate will also end because glutamate becomes exhausted. Thus the neuromediator glutamate controls energy metabolism in brain not only at the level of astrocytes by enhancing production of lactate, but also at the level of neurons by controlling the activity of MAS and specific interactions between aminotransferases.

In the absence of neuronal activation, SDH (Complex II) in the postsynaptic mitochondria is inhibited by OAA (Panov et al. 2010a). The physiological significance of this inhibition is to prevent excessive ROS production associated with reverse electron transport. This is particularly important for neurons because with pyruvate, which is the major mitochondrial substrate in resting neurons (Pellerin et al., 1994; Hertz, 2004), there is a substantial production of succinate and thus a possibility of increased RET-dependent ROS production (see Fig. 5A, 5B; Panov et al. 2009, 2011a, 2011b). During increased neuronal activity glutamate and pyruvate temporarily release the inhibition of SDH. Increased ATP production (state 3) prevents generation of ROS (Starkov, 2008; Votyakova & Reynolds, 2001). Because SCM in general oxidize succinate at higher rates than BM, due to lower intrinsic inhibition of SDH, they are more vulnerable to oxidative stress than BM (Panov et al., 2011a, 2011b).

Activation of oxidative phosphorylation and increased ROS generation with pyruvate + glutamate + malate was observed only with BM and SCM (Panov et al., 2009, 2011a). However, activation of succinate oxidation by pyruvate and glutamate may be a common phenomenon for mitochondria from many organs. Our experiments with mitochondria from different organs and different species of rats and mice, and with one species (Sprague Dawley) of rats over period of 6 years, have shown that mitochondrial metabolism is a subject to phenotypic variations between species and in one species with time (Panov et al., 2010). Below we describe how changes in mitochondrial metabolism of BM and SCM of wild type Sprague Dawley rats affected mitochondrial dysfunctions in tgSOD1 rats in 2007 and 2010.

6. Differences between BM and SCM isolated in 2007 and 2010 in the rates of ROS production with different substrates

ROS production by mitochondria strongly depends on the metabolic state of the mitochondria, type of substrates, and is also tissue-specific (Kwong, Sohal, 1998; Muller et al., 2008, Panov et al., 2007). There are two types of ROS production by mitochondria – energy-dependent and non-energy-dependent (Panov et al., 2007). The energy-dependent ROS production is associated with the reverse electron transport (Kwong, Sohal, 1998; Muller et al., 2008, Panov et al., 2007). ROS production, which does not depend on energization and the metabolic state of the mitochondria may occur on complexes I, II and III and depends on the presence of inhibitors of the electron transport (Kwong, Sohal, 1998; Panov et al., 2007; St-Pierre et al. 2002). In the absence of respiratory inhibitors the rate of the non-energy dependent ROS production is relatively slow (Panov et al., 2007). We have shown that in BM and SCM the major source of ROS correlates with the reverse electron transport, which occurs during oxidation of succinate (Kwong, Sohal, 1998; Panov et al., 2007, 2009, 2011a, b), fatty acids (Panov et al., 2010c), or α-glycerophosphate (Tretter et al., 2007). Thus respiration rates in State 4 in the well coupled mitochondria oxidizing succinate correlates with the rates of ROS production (Panov et al., 2007, 2011a). Therefore changes in the rates of ROS production presented in Figure 4 closely reflect metabolic pattern of the mitochondria. Another reason why we do not present respiratory data is that in 2010 we had limited number of tgSOD1 rats, which precluded obtaining statistically significant data with all substrates and their mixtures.

In our studies on mitochondrial dysfunctions in the rat model of ALS (tgSOD1), we used as a reference control Sprague Dawley rats from Taconic (Germantown, NY). In the years of 2005-2007 we have discovered, that in this strain both BM and SCM had a unique metabolic attribute, which was absent in mitochondria from other organs: during simultaneous oxidation of pyruvate + glutamate + malate the rates of oxidative phosphorylation and the State 4 ROS production were significantly higher than with either glutamate or pyruvate alone (Panov 2009, 2011a). This substrate mixture corresponded to the metabolic situation in activated neurons (Panov et al., 2009). Addition of malonate, a potent inhibitor of SDH, attenuated the rates of respiration and ROS production with pyruvate + malate and glutamate + pyruvate + malate to the level with glutamate + malate.

With succinate as a substrate, ROS production was several times higher than with glutamate + pyruvate + malate, and was further increased in the presence of glutamate + pyruvate (Fig. 5A, 5B). The stimulation of the succinate-supported State 4 respiration and ROS production by glutamate and pyruvate was attributed to removal of endogenous oxaloacetate, which inhibits succinate dehydrogenase (SDH) (Panov et al. 2009, 2010). SCM from the control rats produced significantly more ROS than BM, particularly with the succinate containing substrate mixtures (Figure 5A, 5B; see also Panov et al. 2009, 2011a). We have concluded that in BM the activity of SDH was primordially inhibited by endogenous oxaloacetate (Panov 2009, 2010). This intrinsic inhibition of SDH by oxaloacetate was less evident in SCM, and therefore SCM produced more ROS with substrate mixtures that produced or contained succinate (Panov 2011a). The described above metabolic features of BM and SCM were consistently observed in the wild type and tgSOD1 rats during period of 2005 - 2007 years (Panov et al. 2009, 2011a, 2011b).

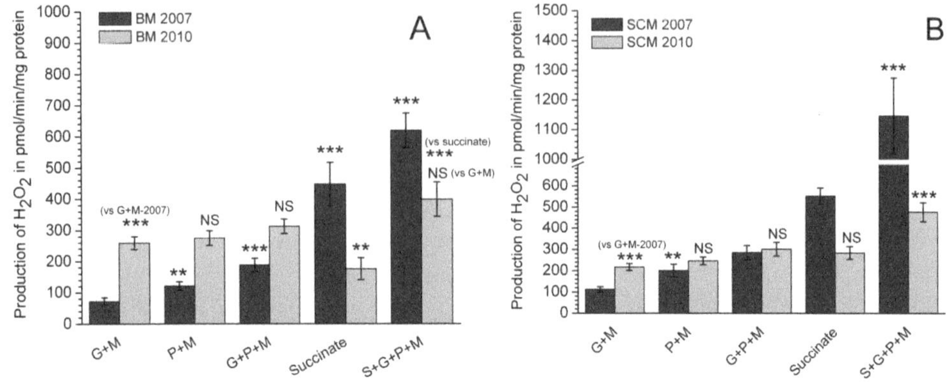

A. Brain mitochondria; **B.** Spinal cord mitochondria. Dark grey - wild type rats in 2007, light gray - wild type rats in 2010. Mitochondria were incubated in a medium containing: 125 mM KCl, 10 mM MOPS, pH 7.2, 2 mM $MgCl_2$, 2 mM KH_2PO_4, 10 mM NaCl, 1 mM EGTA, 0.7 mM $CaCl_2$. At a Ca^{2+}/EGTA ratio of 0.7, the free [Ca^{2+}] is close to 1 μM as determined using Fura-2. The substrate concentrations were: 5 mM succinate without rotenone, 5 mM glutamate, 2.5 mM pyruvate, and 2 mM malate. (Panov et al. 2009, 2011a, b). The results are presented as Mean ± SE, n = 3, and show the rates of ROS production in pmol H_2O_2 /minute/mg mitochondrial protein. Additions: 5 μM Amplex red, 1 U of horse radish peroxidase, 50 U of superoxide dismutase (Sigma), 0.05 mg mitochondria, glutamate 5 mM + malate 2 mM (G + M); pyruvate 2.5 mM + malate 2 mM (P + M); glutamate 5 mM + pyruvate 2.5 mM + malate 2 mM (G + P + M); succinate 5 mM (S); succinate 5 mM + glutamate 5 mM + pyruvate 2.5 mM + malate 2 mM (S + G + P + M). Statistics: ** $p < 0.01$; *** $p < 0.001$. For each year the data were compared with the rates of ROS production with glutamate + malate.

Fig. 5. **Comparison of ROS production by wild type brain and spinal cord mitochondria, isolated in 2007 and 2010, oxidizing different substrates and substrate mixtures.**

In 2008 we observed that BM and SCM from the wild type rats displayed a metabolic pattern that was different from the one described above. To highlight the differences in metabolic features of BM and SCM, we present data restricted to 2007, when significant mitochondrial dysfunctions in tgBM and tgSCM were observed as described in (Panov et al. 2011b), and 2010, when the tgSOD1 rat line failed to develop the disease features, and mitochondria showed little or no dysfunction as compared with the corresponding wild type animals. The related metabolic properties of the BM and SCM isolated from wild type animals in 2007 are presented and compared with those of 2010 in figures 5A and 5B.

Figure 5A compares ROS production by WT-BM isolated in 2007 and 2010. Of notice, the rate of ROS production by WT-BM isolated in 2010 was 3.5 fold higher than WT-BM isolated in 2007. However, in 2010 there was no differences in State 4 respiration (not shown) and ROS production (Fig. 5A) when BM oxidized glutamate + malate, pyruvate + malate or glutamate + pyruvate + malate. In contrast to WT-BM isolated in 2007, the much higher basic rate of ROS production supported by glutamate + malate in 2010 was inhibited by malonate to the level close to that in 2007 (Fig. 6). Similarly, in 2010 malonate inhibited ROS production in BM oxidizing glutamate + pyruvate + malate (Fig. 6) and pyruvate (not shown).

In contrast to WT-BM isolated in 2007, the WT-BM isolated in 2010 produced ROS supported by succinate at much lower rates than with glutamate + pyruvate + malate (Fig. 5A). Addition of glutamate + pyruvate + malate to the WT-BM -2010 oxidizing succinate stimulated ROS production only to the level with glutamate + malate (Fig. 5A). Similar metabolic features were also observed with the WT-SCM isolated in 2010, although the differences from 2007 WT-SCM were smaller than for the BM (Fig 5B). It is important to note that in 2010 WT-SCM generated ROS with different substrates at the same levels as WT-BM, whereas in 2007 the WT-SCM generated significantly more ROS than the corresponding WT-BM (Fig. 5A and 5B. Note the scale difference between the figures).

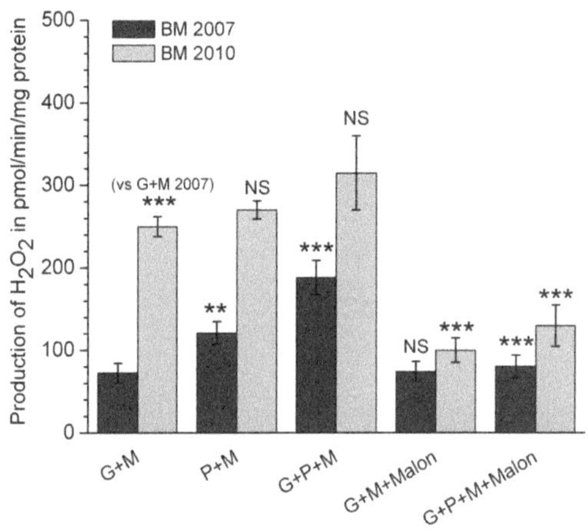

Incubation conditions and designations as described in Fig. 5. Malonate 5 mM was added before mitochondria. Dark gray - BM isolated in 2007, light gray columns - BM isolated in 2010. Statistics: *** $p < 0.001$, NS - not significant difference. The dark columns and grey columns were compared with the corresponding column representing ROS production with glutamate and malate, taken as 100%.

Fig. 6. Effect of malonate on ROS production by wild type brain mitochondria, isolated in 2007 and 2010, oxidizing glutamate + malate, pyruvate + malate, and glutamate + pyruvate + malate.

The sensitivity of the State 4 ROS production supported by either pyruvate or glutamate to malonate (Fig, 6; Panov et al. 2009) demonstrates that at least with BM and SCM both glutamate and pyruvate cannot be regarded as "pure complex I substrates", as is commonly accepted. In BM and SCM during oxidation of glutamate or pyruvate, and particularly when glutamate and pyruvate are present simultaneously, significant amounts of α-ketoglutarate can be formed in transaminase reactions, which is further converted to succinate (Balasz, 1965; Panov et al. 2009).

7. Effects of metabolic phenotype on ROS production by tgBM and tgSCM

Figure 7A shows generation of ROS by tgBM and tgSCM isolated from tgSOD1 rats in 2007, and figure 7B presents corresponding results for tgBM and tgSCM isolated from tgSOD1 rats in 2010. The figures clearly show that in spite of higher basic ROS production with glutamate and pyruvate by BM and SCM in 2010 (Fig. 5A and 5B), the overall rates of ROS generation with physiologically relevant substrate mixture - glutamate + pyruvate + malate were 5 times lower for tgBM and 10 times for tgSCM , when compared with transgenic mitochondria in 2007 (Fig. 7A and 7B).

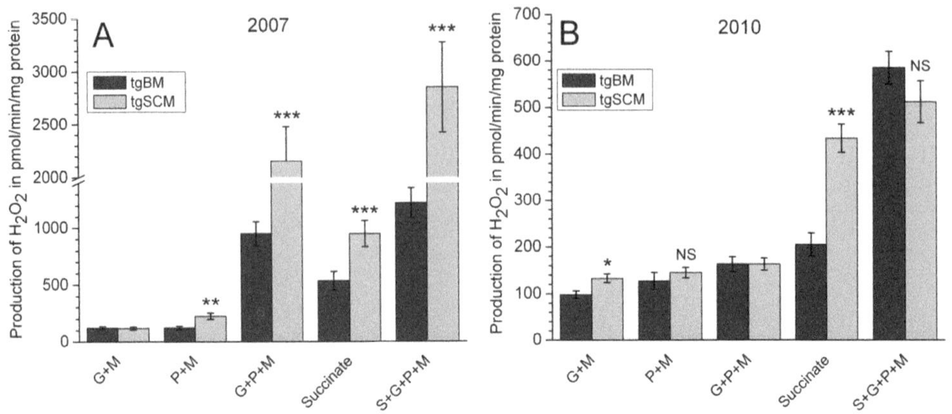

A. 2007; **B.** 2010. Dark grey - brain mitochondria, light gray - spinal cord mitochondria. Incubation conditions as in Fig. 5. Statistics: * $p < 0.05$; ** $p < 0.01$; *** $p < 0.001$. The data for tgSCM were compared with the corresponding results for tgBM.

Fig. 7. **Generation of ROS by brain and spinal cord mitochondria from tgSOD1 rats, isolated in 2007 and 2010, oxidizing various substrates.**

Similar multiple-fold differences in ROS production existed also with succinate and succinate containing substrate mixtures (Figs. 7A, 7B). In tgBM and tgSCM, the increases in ROS generation were substrate specific and depended on activity of SDH. These results led us to conclusion that changes in the metabolic phenotype of neuronal mitochondria, which occurred in 2008, resulted in a dramatic decrease in production of ROS in tgSOD1 rats.

8. Hydrogen peroxide is the major species to cause oxidative stress in tgSOD1 mitochondria

One of the distinctions of BM and SCM is a very high activity of MnSOD (SOD2) (Panov et al., 2009, 2011a, 2011b), which is distinct from the heart and skeletal muscle mitochondria (Muller et al., 2008). Even at very high rates of ROS production, such as shown in Figures 4 and 5A, 5B, addition of external SOD did not increase fluorescence of resorufin. The high activity of SOD2 means that BM and SCM effectively eliminate superoxide radicals from the matrix by converting them to H_2O_2. Therefore, we suggest that the major damaging factor in tgSOD1 motor neurons is H_2O_2. It was shown that H_2O_2 can interact with Cu,Zn-SOD (SOD1) resulting in peroxidase activity of SOD1 (Liochev, Fridovich, 2004), formation of strong oxidant $CO_3^{\bullet -}$ radical (reviewed in Valentine et al., 2005), enzyme inactivation, release of Cu^{2+}, protein oxidation and aggregation (Ramirez et al., 2009, Durer et al., 2009). At this point, the damaging effects of H_2O_2 will be increased dramatically because Cu^{2+} ions are several orders more active than Fe^{2+} in Fenton-like reaction with H_2O_2 (Dikalov et al., 2004), which will produce hydroxyl radical-like species and further drive lipid peroxidation, protein damage and promote mitochondrial dysfunction. Loss of metals by mutant SOD1 leads to formation of amyloid-like aggregates (Durer et al., 2009). Mutations in SOD1 amplify reactions with H_2O_2, increase the lifetime of incorrectly folded states, and if exposed to even mild oxidative stress, incorrect disulfide links form and stabilize larger aggregates that may be resistant to the degradation by the quality control machinery of the cell, and thus increase association with mitochondria (Field et al., 2003; Furukawa, O'Halloran, 2008).

9. Proposed mechanisms of increased ROS production in tgSOD1 mitochondria

There is strong evidence that tgSOD1 selectively binds to the outer (Vande Velde et al., 2008) and inner mitochondrial membranes (Liu et al., 2004; Ahtoniemi et al., 2008). Mutant SOD1 protein associated with mitochondria forms cross-linked oligomers and causes a shift in the redox state of respiratory components (Ferri et al., 2006). We propose a mechanism by which tgSOD1 might increase generation of ROS associated with reverse electron transport. The hypothesis is based on our recently published data on the effects of cholesterol β-D-glucoside and cycad phytosterol glucosides on ROS generation by BM (Panov et al., 2010b). These compounds are neurotoxic and suspected as the cause of the cluster of neurodegenerative disorders in the western Pacific termed amyotrophic lateral sclerosis-parkinsonism dementia complex (ALS-PDC) (Wilson et al., 2002). When added *in vitro* to mitochondria, cholesterol β-D-glucoside increased ROS production, which was specifically dependent on activity of SDH. Cholesterol β-D-glucoside is known to diminish the surface area of the membranes and thus affect the activity of the membrane's enzymes (Deliconstantinos et al., 1989). Here we suggest, that tgSOD1 upon its interaction with the mitochondria may change physical-chemical properties of the membranes and increase the rate of reverse electron transport in a way similar to that of cholesterol β-D-glucoside.

10. Oxidative stress increases sensitivity of mitochondria to Ca^{2+}-dependent excitotoxicity

Increased oxidative stress makes mitochondria more sensitive to the Ca^{2+}-induced permeability transition, which may initiate apoptotic or necrotic cell death (Halestrap et al., 2000; Nicholls, 2008b, 2009). Mitochondria from tgSOD1 animals have high sensitivity to the deleterious effects of calcium (Martin et al., 2009). SCM are particularly sensitive to calcium overload (Sullivan et al., 2004, Panov et al., 2011a). This scenario becomes very likely to occur in tgSOD1 animals in view of the fact that spinal cord tissue contains 8 times more calcium than brain tissue (Panov et al., 2011a). We estimated that when normalized for 1 gram of tissue, BM could sequester several times more Ca^{2+} than was available in the whole tissue. SCM, on the other hand, could sequester only approximately 20% of the total spinal cord tissue Ca^{2+} (Panov et al., 2011a). We suggest that the high content of Ca^{2+} is necessary to hold together the sheets of myelin, which protects the neurons. We have shown recently that increased oxidative stress promotes demyelination in brains of OXYS rats with genetically accelerated aging, which was ameliorated by feeding of animals with malate (Kolosova et al. 2011). Underwood et al. (2010), using magnetic resonance imaging, have shown signs of demyelination in the lumbar spinal cord of ALS-affected SOD1 mice, which were limited to white matter tracts arising from the motor neurons, whereas sensory white matter fibers were preserved. Damages to myelin sheets of motor neurons may evidently release large amounts of calcium. The tissue calcium content in the spinal cord from presymptomatic tgSOD1 rats was diminished by 26% (Panov et al., 2011b). Thus, oxidatively damaged mitochondria may encounter increased amounts of Ca^{2+} released during demyelination and undergo permeability transition. Halestrap (2005) has pointed out that when mitochondria massively undergo permeability transition, the cells will die by necrosis, which was documented Martin et al.(2009) for ALS animals.

11. Conclusions

The results presented by us in this and other papers (Panov et al., 2009, 20011a, 2011b) lead us to suggest the role of the brain and spinal cord mitochondria in the loss of motor neurons in ALS. We hypothesize that increased oxidative stress associated with specific metabolic phenotypes, which promote reverse electron transport due to reduction of the membrane pool of ubiquinone by succinate (Panov et al., 2009, 2011a, 2011b) or fatty acids (Panov et al., 2010c), is a prerequisite for cases of sporadic ALS. The energy-dependent reverse electron transport is a way of dissipation of the mitochondrial membrane potential, which increases the rate of resting mitochondrial respiration. In mammals, the standard metabolic rate depends on the intrinsic (in state 4) mitochondrial proton conductivity (Rolfe & Brown , 1997). Therefore in patients with ALS hypermetabolism could be associated with the systemically increased dissipation of mitochondrial membrane potential. The specific vulnerability of motor neurons in ALS is, more likely than not, associated with the specific features of spinal cord described in Panov et al. (2011a, 2011b).

Normally, SCM produce significantly more ROS than BM when oxidizing physiologically relevant mixture of neuromediator glutamate and the tricarboxylic acid cycle substrates pyruvate, succinate and malate. Mutated SOD1 is extremely sensitive to the damaging effect of H_2O_2, which in tgBM and tgSCM were dramatically increased. This results in demetallation of mSOD1 and association with mitochondria, thus changing the physical properties of the mitochondrial membranes and further enhancing production of ROS. Increased oxidative stress initiates damage to myelin and released the tissue calcium. Finally, oxidatively damaged mitochondria undergo the Ca^{2+}-induced permeability transition, and motor neurons die by apoptotic or necrotic pathway. Thus, mitochondria are early and directly involved in the pathogenesis of ALS. We suggest that sporadic ALS is preferentially acquired by individuals with the mitochondrial metabolic phenotype, that promotes very high levels of ROS production. In individuals with mutated SOD1 gene, the abnormal SOD1 protein has high sensitivity to deleterious effect of H_2O_2 and the disease may develop even at normal levels of ROS production.

12. Proposals for future studies

The results and the hypothesis presented in this article highlight the importance to consider determination of metabolic phenotypes together with the disease mechanisms when working with patients or animal models of the ALS.

13. Acknowledgements

The authors thank the Carolinas HealthCare Foundation and Carolinas ALS Research Fund for financial support of this study. The authors thank Dr. Richelle Hemendinger and Dr.

Nataliya Kubalik for testing in 2010 the tgSOD1 rats for the time of development of ALS symptoms.

14. References

Abeles, Moshe. *Corticonics: Neural Circuits of the Cerebral Cortex*. Cambridge Univ. Press, 1991 ISBN 0521374766

Ahtoniemi, T., Jaronen, M., Keksa-Goldsteine, V., Goldsteins, G., & Koistinaho, J. (2008) Mutant SOD1 from spinal cord of G93A rats is destabilized and binds to inner mitochondrial membrane. *Neurobiol. Dis.* 32 (3), 479-485

Attwell D., & Laughlin S.B. (2001) An energy budget for signaling in the grey matter of the brain. *J Cereb Blood Flow Metab.* 21, 1133-1145

Auger, C. & Attwell, D. (2000) Fast removal of synaptic glutamate by postsynaptic transporters. *Neuron.* 28 (2), 547-558

Avossa, D., Grandolfo, M., Mazzarol, F., Zatta, M. & Ballerini, L. (2006) Early signs of motoneuron vulnerability in a disease model system: Characterization of transverse slice cultures of spinal cord isolated from embryonic ALS mice. *Neuroscience.* 138 (4), 1179-1194

Bacman, S.R., Bradley, W.G. and Moraes, C.T. (2006) Mitochondrial involvement in amyotrophic lateral sclerosis: Trigger or target? *Mol. Neurobiol.* 33 (2), 113-131

Balazs, R. (1965) Control of glutamate metabolism. The effect of pyruvate. *J. Neurochem.* 12, 63-76

Balazs R. (1965) Control of glutamate oxidation in brain and liver mitochondrial systems. *Biochem. J.* 95, 497-508

Barber, S. C. & Shaw, P.J. (2010) Oxidative stress in ALS: key role in motor neuron injury and therapeutic target. *Free Radic. Biol. Med.* 48(5), 629-641

Bendotti, C., & Carri, M.T. (2004) Lessons from models of SOD1-linked familial ALS. *Trends Mol. Med.* 10 (8), 393-400

Berkich, D. A., Ola, M.S., Cole, J., Sweatt, A.J., Hutson, S.M., & LaNoue, K.F. (2007) Mitochondrial transport proteins of the brain. *J. Neurosci. Res.* 85 (15), 3367-3677

Bertamini, M., Marzani, B., Guarneri, R., Guarneri, P., Bigini, P., Mennini, T. & Curti, D. (2002) Mitochondrial oxidative metabolism in motor neuron degeneration (mnd) mouse central nervous system. *Eur. J. Neurosci.* 16 (12), 2291-2296

Bouteloup, C., Desport, J.C., Clavelou, P., Guy, N., Derumeaux-Burel, H., Ferrier, A. & Couratier, P. (2009) Hypermetabolism in ALS patients: an early and persistent phenomenon. *J. Neurol.* 256 (8), 1236-1242

Braitenberg, V., & Schüz, A. (1998) *Cortex: statistics and geometry of neuronal connectivity*, 2nd ed. Berlin: Springer.

Brasnjo, G., & Otis, T.S. (2004) Isolation of glutamate transport-coupled charge flux and estimation of glutamate uptake at the climbing fiber-purkinje cell synapse. *Proc. Natl. Acad. Sci. USA.* 101, 6273-6278

Bruijn, L.I., Miller, T.M., & Cleveland, D.W. (2004) Unraveling the mechanisms involved in motor neuron degeneration in ALS. *Annu. Rev. Neurosci.* 27, 723-749

Damiano, M., Starkov, A.A., Petri, S., Kipiani, K., Kiaei, M., Mattiazzi, M., Beal, F. M., & Manfredi, G. (2006) Neural mitochondrial Ca capacity impairment precedes the onset of motor symptoms in G93A Cu/Zn-superoxide dismutase mutant mice. *J. Neurochem.* 96, 1349-1361

Dave, K.R., Bradley, W.G., & Perez-Pinzon, M.A. (2003) Early mitochondrial dysfunction occurs in motor cortex and spinal cord at the onset of disease in the Wobbler mouse. *Exp Neurol*. 182, 412-420

Deliconstantinos, G, Kopeikina, L, &Villiotou, V. 1989. Evoked effects of cholesterol binding on integral proteins and lipid fluidity of dog brain synaptosomal plasma membranes. *Biochem. Cell. Biol*. 67 (1), 16-24

Desport, J. C., Torny, F., Lacoste, M., Preux, P.M. & Couratier, P. (2005). Hypermetabolism in ALS: correlations with clinical and paraclinical parameters. Neurodegener. Dis. 2 (3-4), 202-207

Dikalov, S. I., Vitek, M.P. & Mason, R.P. (2004). Cupric-amyloid beta peptide complex stimulates oxidation of ascorbate and generation of hydroxyl radical. *Free Radic. Biol. Med*. 36 (3), 340-347

Dupuis, L., Gonzalez de Aguilar, J.L., Echaniz-Laguna, A., Eschbach, J., Rene, F., Oudart, H., Halter, B., Huze, C., Schaeffer, L., Bouillaud, F., & Loeffler, J.P. (2009) Muscle mitochondrial uncoupling dismantles neuromuscular junction and triggers distal degeneration of motor neurons. *PLoS One*. 4 (4), e5390

Durer, Z.A.O., Cohlberg, J.A., Dinh, P., Padua, S., Ehrenclou, K., Downes, S., Tan, J.K., Nakano, Y., Bowman, C.J., Hoskins, J.L., Kwon, C., Mason, A.Z., Rodriguez, J.A., Doucette, P.A., Shaw, B.F., & Valentine, J.S. (2009) Loss of Metal Ions, Disulfide Reduction and Mutations Related to Familial ALS Promote Formation of Amyloid-Like Aggregates from Superoxide Dismutase. *PLoS One*. 4 (3), e5004

Ebert, D., Haller, R.G. & Walton, M.E. (2003) Energy contribution of octanoate to intact rat brain metabolism measured by 13C nuclear magnetic resonance spectroscopy. *J. Neurosci*. 23 (13), 5928-5935

Echaniz-Laguna, A., Zoll, J., Ponsot, E., N'Guessan, B., Tranchant, C., Loeffler, J.P. & Lampert, E. (2006) Muscular mitochondrial function in amyotrophic lateral sclerosis is progressively altered as the disease develops: a temporal study in man. *Exp. Neurol*. 198 (1), 25-30

Field, L. S., Y. Furukawa, T. V. O'Halloran and V. C. Culotta (2003). Factors controlling the uptake of yeast copper/zinc superoxide dismutase into mitochondria. *J. Biol. Chem*. 278 (30), 28052-28059

Fischer, L.R., Igoudjil, A., Magrané, J., Li, Y., Hansen, J.M., Manfredi, G., Glass, J.D. (2011) SOD1 targeted to the mitochondrial intermembrane space prevents motor neuropathy in the Sod1 knockout mouse. *Brain*. 134 (Pt 1),196-209

Furness, D. N., Dehnes, Y., Akhtar, A.Q., Rossi, D.J., Hamann, M., Grutle, N.J., Gundersen, V., Holmseth, S., Lehre, K.P., Ullensvang, K., Wojewodzic, M., Zhou, Y., Attwell, D. & Danbolt, D.C. (2008) A quantitative assessment of glutamate uptake into hippocampal synaptic terminals and astrocytes: New insights into a neuronal role for excitatory amino acid transporter 2 (EAAT2). *Neuroscience*. 157 (1), 80-94

Furukawa, Y. & O'Halloran, T.V. (2006) Posttranslational modifications in Cu,Zn-superoxide dismutase and mutations associated with amyotrophic lateral sclerosis. *Antioxid Redox Signal*. 8 (5-6), 847-867

Gershoni, M., Templeton, A.R. & Mishmar, D. (2009) Mitochondrial bioenergetics as a major motive force of speciation. *Bioessays*. 31 (6), 642-650

Gurney, M.E., Pu, H., Chiu, A.Y., Dal Canto, M.C., Polchow, C.Y., Alexander, D.D., Caliendo, J., Hentati, A., Kwon, Y.W., & Deng, H.X. (1994) Motor neuron degeneration in mice that express a human Cu,Zn superoxide dismutase mutation. *Science*. 264 (5166), 1772-1775

Halestrap, A.P., Doran, E., Gillespie, J,P.,b & O'Toole, A. (2000) Mitochondria and cell death. *Biochem. Soc. Trans.* 28 (2), 170-177.

Halestrap, H. A pore way to die. (2005) *Nature*. 434, 578-579

Heath P.R. & Shaw P.J. (2002) Update on the glutamatergic neurotransmitter system and the role of excitotoxicity in amyotrophic lateral sclerosis. *Muscle Nerve*. 26, 438-458

Hertz, L. (2004) Intercellular metabolic compartmentation in the brain: past, present and future. *Neurochem Int.* 45, (2-3), 285-296

Higgins C.M., Jung C., Ding H. & Xu Z. (2002) Mutant Cu, Zn superoxide dismutase that causes motoneuron degeneration is present in mitochondria in the CNS. *J. Neurosci.* 22, RC215

Howland, D.S., Liu, J., She, Y., Goad, B., Maragakis, N.J., Kim, B., Erickson, J., Kulik, J., DeVito, L., Psaltis, G., DeGennaro, L.J., Cleveland, D.W., Rothstein, J.D. (2002) Focal loss of the glutamate transporter EAAT2 in a transgenic rat model of SOD1 mutant-mediated amyotrophic lateral sclerosis (ALS). *Proc. Natl. Acad. Sci. USA*. 99, 1604-1609.

Israelson, A., Arbel, N., Da Cruz, S., Illeva, H., Yamanaka, K., Shoshan-Barmatz, V. & Cleveland, D.W. (2010) Misfolded mutant SOD1 directly inhibits VDAC1 conductance in a mouse model inherited ALS. *Neuron*, 67, 575-587

Jaarsma D. (2006) Swelling and vacuolisation of mitochondria in transgenic sod1-als mice: A consequence of supranormal sod1 expression? *Mitochondrion*. 6 (1), 48-49

Jung, C., Higgins, C.M.J. & Xu, Z. (2002) A quantitative histochemical assay for activities of mitochondrial electron transport chain complexes in mouse spinal cord sections. *J. Neurosci. Methods*. 114 (2), 165-172

Kirkinezos, I. G., Bacman, S.R., Hernandez, D., Oca-Cossio, J., Arias, L.J., Perez-Pinzon, M.A., Bradley, W.G. & Moraes, C.T. (2005) Cytochrome c association with the inner mitochondrial membrane is impaired in the CNS of G93A-SOD1 mice. *J. Neurosci.* 25, 164-172

Kolosova, N.G., Akulov, A.E., Stefanova, N.A., Moshkin, M.P., Savelov, A.A., Koptyug, I.V., Panov, A.V. & Vavilin, V.A. (2011) Effect of malate on development of rotenone-induced brain changes in Wistar and OXYS rats: An MRI study. *Doklady Biol. Sci.* 437, 1-4

Krasnianski, A., Deschauer, M., Neudecker, S., Gellerich, F.N., Muller, T., Schoser, B.G., Krasnianski, M. & Zierz, S. (2005) Mitochondrial changes in skeletal muscle in amyotrophic lateral sclerosis and other neurogenic atrophies. *Brain*. 128 (Pt 8), 1870-1876

Kwong, L.K. & Sohal, R.S. (1998) Substrate and site specificity of hydrogen peroxide generation in mouse mitochondria. *Arch. Biochem. Biophys.* 350 (1), 118-126

Liochev, S. I. & Fridovich, I. (2004) CO2 enhanced peroxidase activity of SOD1: the effects of pH. *Free Radic. Biol. Med.* 36 (11), 1444-1447

Liu, J., Lillo, C., Jonsson, P.A., Vande Velde, C., Ward, C.M., Miller, T.M., Subramaniam, J.R., Rothstein, J.D., Marklund, S., Andersen, P.M., Brannstrom, T., Gredal, O., Wong, P.C., Williams, D.S. & Cleveland, D.W. (2004) Toxicity of familial ALS-linked SOD1 mutants from selective recruitment to spinal mitochondria. *Neuron*. 43, 5-17

Magrane, J. & Manfredi, G. (2009) Mitochondrial function, morphology, and axonal transport in amyotrophic lateral sclerosis. *Antioxidants & Redox Signaling*. 11 (7), 1615-1626

Martin, L.J., Liu, Z., Chen, K., Price, A.C., Pan, Y., Swaby, J.A. & Golden, W.C. 2007. Motor neuron degeneration in amyotrophic lateral sclerosis mutant superoxide dismutase-1 transgenic mice: mechanisms of mitochondriopathy and cell death. *J. Comp. Neurol.* 500 (1), 20-46

Martin, L.J., Gertz, B., Pan, Y., Price, A.C., Molkentin, J.D. & Chang, Q. (2009) The mitochondrial permeability transition pore in motor neurons: Involvement in the pathobiology of ALS mice. *Experim. Neurol.* 218 (2), 333-346

Massie, A., Cnops, L., Smolders, I., McCullumsmith, R., Kooijman, R., Kwak, S., Arckens, L. & Michotte, Y. (2008) High-affinity Na+/K+-dependent glutamate transporter EAAT4 is expressed throughout the rat fore- and midbrain. *J Comp Neurol.* 511 (2), 155-172

Matsumoto, A., Okada, Y., Nakamichi, M., Nakamura, M., Toyama, Y., Sobue, G., Nagai, M., Aoki, M., Itoyama, Y. & Okano, H. (2006) Disease progression of human SOD1 (G93A) transgenic ALS model rats. *J. Neurosci. Res.* 83 (1), 119-133

Mitchell, P. (1977) Vectorial chemiosmotic processes. *Ann. Rev. Biochem.* 46, 996-1005

Morota, S.; Hansson, M.J.; Ishii, N.; Kudo, Y.; Elmer, E.; Uchino, H. (2007) Spinal cord mitochondria display lower calcium retention capacity compared with brain mitochondria without inherent differences in sensitivity to cyclophilin D inhibition. *J Neurochem.* 103 (5), 2066-2076, 2007

Muller, F.L., Liu, Y., Abdul-Ghani, M.A., Lustgarten, M.S., Bhattacharya, A., Jang, Y.C. & Van Remmen, H. (2008) High rates of superoxide production in skeletal-muscle mitochondria respiring on both complex I- and complex II-linked substrates. *Biochem. J.* 409 (2), 491-499.

Muller, F.L.; Song, W.; Jang, Y.C.; Liu, Y.; Sabia, M.; Richardson, A. & Van Remmen, H. (2007) Denervation-induced skeletal muscle atrophy is associated with increased mitochondrial ROS production. *Am. J. Physiol. Regul. Integr. Comp. Physiol.* 293, 3, R1159-R1168

Nakano, Y., Hirayama, K. & Terao, K. (1987) Hepatic ultrastructural changes and liver dysfunction in amyotrophic lateral sclerosis. *Arch. Neurol.* 44 (1), 103-106

Nicholls, D. G. (1993). The glutamatergic nerve terminal. *Eur. J. Biochem.* 212 (3), 613-631

Nicholls, D. G. (2008) Oxidative stress and energy crises in neuronal dysfunction. *Ann. N. Y. Acad. Sci.* 1147, 53-60

Nicholls, D. G. (2008) Forty years of Mitchell's proton circuit: From little grey books to little grey cells. *Biochim. Biophys. Acta.* 1777 (7-8), 550-556

Nicholls, D. G. (2009) Mitochondrial calcium function and dysfunction in the central nervous system. *Biochim. Biophys. Acta.* 1787 (11), 1416-142

Norenberg, M. D. & Martinez-Hernandez, A. (1979) Fine structural localization of glutamine synthetase in astrocytes of rat brain. *Brain Res.* 161 (2), 303-310

Panov, A., Dikalov, S., Shalbuyeva, N., Hemendinger, R., Greenamyre, J.T. & Rosenfeld, J. (2007) Species and tissue specific relationships between mitochondrial permeability transition and generation of ROS in brain and liver mitochondria of rats and mice. *Am. J. Physiol. Cell. Physiol.* 292 (2), C708-C718

Panov, A., Schonfeld, O., Dikalov, S., Hemendinger, R., Bonkovsky, H.L. & Brooks, B.R. (2009) The neuromediator glutamate, through specific substrate interactions, enhances mitochondrial ATP production and reactive oxygen species generation in nonsynaptic brain mitochondria. *J. Biol. Chem.* 284 (21), 14448-14456.

Panov, A.V., Vavilin, V.A., Lyalkhovich, V.V., Brooks, B.R., Bonkovsky, H.L. (2010a) Effects of defatted bovine serum albumin on respiratory activities of brain and liver mitochondria from C57Bl/6G mice and Sprague Dawley rats. *Bull. Exp. Biol. Med.* 149 (2), 187-190

Panov, A., Kubalik, N., Brooks, B.R. & Shaw, C.A. (2010b) In vitro effects of cholesterol β-D-glucoside, cholesterol and cycad phytosterol glucosides on respiration and reactive oxygen species generation in brain mitochondria. *J. Membr. Biol.* 237, 71-77

Panov, A., Kubalik, N., & Brooks, B.R. (2010c) Effects of palmitoyl carnitine on brain, spinal cord and heart mitochondria from wild type and transgenic SOD1 rats. 21st International Symposium on ALS/MND, Orlando 11-13 December, 2010. *Amyotrophic Lateral Sclerosis.* 11 (Suppl. 1), 115

Panov, A.V., Kubalik, N., Zinchenko, N., Hemendinger R., Brooks B.R. & Bonkovsky, H.L. (2011a) Metabolic and functional differences between brain and spinal cord mitochondria underlie different predisposition to pathology. *Am. J. Physiol. Regul. Integr. Comp. Physiol.* 300 (4), R844-R854

Panov, A., Kubalik, N., Zinchenko, N., Hemendinger, R., Dikalov, S. & Bonkovsky, H.L. (2011b) Respiration and ROS production in brain and spinal cord mitochondria of transgenic rats with mutant G93A Cu/Zn-Superoxide dismutase gene. *Neurobiol. Dis.* 44, 53-62

Pardo, B., Contreras, L., Serrano, A., Ramos, M., Kobayashi, K., Iijima, M., Saheki, T. & Satrustegui, J. (2006). Essential role of aralar in the transduction of small ca2+ signals to neuronal mitochondria. *J. Biol. Chem.* 281 (2), 1039-1047

Pedrini, S., Sau, D., Guareschi, S., Bogush, M., Brown, R.H., Jr., Naniche, N., Kia, A., Trotti, D. & Pasinelli, P. (2010) ALS-linked mutant SOD1 damages mitochondria by promoting conformational changes in Bcl-2. *Hum. Mol. Genet.* 19 (15), 2974-2986

Pellerin, L., Bouzier-Sore, A.K., Aubert, A., Serres, S., Merle, M., Costalat, R. & Magistretti, P.J. (2007) Activity-dependent regulation of energy metabolism by astrocytes: an update. *Glia.* 55 (12), 1251-1262

Przedborski S. (2004) Programmed cell death in amyotrophic lateral sclerosis: a mechanism of pathogenic and therapeutic importance. *Neurologist.* 10, 1-7

Ramirez, D.C., Gomez-Mejiba, S.E., Corbett, J.T., Deterding, L.J., Tomer, K.B. & Mason, R.P. (2009) Cu,Zn-superoxide dismutase-driven free radical modifications: copper- and carbonate radical anion-initiated protein radical chemistry. *Biochem. J.* 417 (1), 341-353

Rolfe, D.F.S. & Brown, G.C. (1997) Cellular energy utilization and molecular origin of standard metabolic rate in mammals. *Physiol. Rev.* 77, 731-758

Rowland, L.P. & Shneider, N.A. (2001) Amyotrophic lateral sclerosis. *N. Engl. J. Med.* 344 (22), 1688-1700

Shook, S.J. & Pioro, E.P. (2009) Racing against the clock: Recognizing differentiating, diagnosing, and referring the amyotrophic lateral sclerosis patient. *Ann. Neurol.*, 65 (suppl.), S10-S16

Starkov, A.A. (2008) The role of mitochondria in reactive oxygen species metabolism and signaling. *Ann. New York Acad. Sci.* 1147, 37-52

Stowe, D.F. & Camara, A.K. (2009) Mitochondrial reactive oxygen species production in excitable cells: Modulators of mitochondrial and cell function. *Antioxidants & Redox Signaling.* 11 (6), 1381-1414

St-Pierre, J., Buckingham, J.A., Roebuck, S.J. & Brand, M.D. (2002) Topology of superoxide production from different sites in the mitochondrial electron transport chain. *J. Biol. Chem.* 277 (47), 44784-44790

Stolzenburg, J.U., Reichenbach, A. & Neumann, M. (1989) Size and density of glial and neuronal cells within the cerebral neocortex of various insectivorian species. *Glia.* 2 (2), 78-84

Sullivan P.G., Rabchevsky, A.G., Keller, J.Y.N., Lovell, M., Sodhi, A., Hart, R.P. & Scheffer, S.W. (2004) Intrinsic differences in brain and spinal cord mitochondria: implication for therapeutic interventions. *J. Comparative Neurol.* 474, 524–534

Suzuki, A., Stern, S.A., Bozdagi, O., Huntley, G.W., Walker, R.H., Magistretti, P.J. & Alberini, C.M. (2011) Astrocyte-neuron lactate transport is required for long-term memory formation. *Cell.* 144 (5), 810-823

Tillakaratne N.J., Medina-Kauwe, L. & Gibson, K.M. (1995) Gamma-aminobutyric acid (gaba) metabolism in mammalian neural and nonneural tissues. *Comp. Biochem. Physiol. A Physiol.* 112 (2), 247-263

Tateno M., Sadakata H., Tanaka M., Itohara S., Shin R.M., Miura M., Masuda M., Aosaki T., Urushitani M., Misawa H. & Takahashi R. (2004) Calcium-permeable AMPA receptors promote misfolding of mutant SOD1 protein and development of amyotrophic lateral sclerosis in a transgenic mouse model. *Hum. Mol. Genet.* 13, 2183-2196

Tretter, L., Takacs, K., Hegedus, V. & Adam-Vizi, V. (2007) Characteristics of alpha-glycerophosphate-evoked H2O2 generation in brain mitochondria. *J. Neurochem.* 100 (3), 650-663

Valentine, J.S., Doucette, P.A. & Potter, S.Z. (2005) Copper-zinc superoxide dismutase and amyotrophic lateral sclerosis. *Annu. Rev. Biochem.* 74, 563-593

Vande Velde, C., Miller, T.M., Cashman, N.R. & Cleveland, D.W. (2008) Selective association of misfolded ALS-linked mutant SOD1 with the cytoplasmic face of mitochondria. *Proc. Natl. Acad. Sci. USA.* 105 (10), 4022-4027

Von Lewinski, F. & B. U. Keller (2005). Ca2+, mitochondria and selective motoneuron vulnerability: implications for ALS. *Trends Neurosci.* 28 (9), 494-500

Votyakova, T.V. & Reynolds, I.J. (2001) $\Delta\Psi$-dependent and independent production of reactive oxygen species by rat brain mitochondria. *J. Neurochem.* 79, 266-277

Waagepetersen, H.S., Sonnewald. U., Larsson, O.M. & Schousboe, A. (1999) Synthesis of vesicular GABA from glutamine involves TCA cycle metabolism in neocortical neurons. *J. Neurosci. Res.* 57 (3), 342-349

Wallace, D.C. (2001) Mouse models for mitochondrial disease. *Am. J. Med. Genet.* 106, 71-93

Wilson, J.M., Khabazian, I., Wong, M.C., Seyedalikhani, A., Bains, J.S., Pasqualotto, B.A., Williams, D.E., Andersen, R.J., Simpson, R.J., Smith, R., Craig, U.K., Kurland, L.T., & Shaw, C.A. (2002) Behavioral and neurological correlates of ALS-parkinsonism dementia complex in adult mice fed washed cycad flour. *Neuromolecular Med.* 1 (3), 207-221

Wong-Riley, M.T. (1989) Cytochrome oxidase: An endogenous metabolic marker for neuronal activity. *Trends Neurosci.* 12 (3), 94-101

Xu, G-P., Dave, K.R., Moraes, C.T., Busto, R., Sick, T.J., Bradley, W.G. & Perez-Pinzon, M.A. (2001) Dysfunctional mitochondrial respiration in the wobbler mouse brain. *Neurosci. Letters.* 300, 141-144

Yudkoff, M., Nelson, D., Daikhin, Y. & Erecinska, M. (1994). Tricarboxylic acid cycle in rat brain synaptosomes. Fluxes and interactions with aspartate aminotransferase and malate/aspartate shuttle. *J. Biol. Chem.* 269 (44), 27414-27420.

Zoccarato, F., Cavallini, L., Bortolami, S. & Alexandre, A. (2007) Succinate modulation of H_2O_2 release at NADH -ubiquinone oxidoreductase (Complex I) in brain mitochondria. *Biochem. J.* 406 (1), 125-129

11

Folding and Aggregation of Cu, Zn-Superoxide Dismutase

Helen R. Broom, Heather A. Primmer, Jessica A.O. Rumfeldt, Peter B. Stathopulos, Kenrick A. Vassall, Young-Mi Hwang and Elizabeth M. Meiering
Guelph-Waterloo Centre for Graduate Work in Chemistry and Biochemistry, University of Waterloo
Canada

1. Introduction

1.1 ALS and SOD1

In 1993, a genetic link was established between amyotrophic lateral sclerosis (ALS) and mutant forms of Cu,Zn superoxide dismutase (SOD1) (Deng et al. 1993; Rosen et al. 1993), an antioxidant enzyme that catalyzes the dismutation of the damaging free radical superoxide anion (O_2^-) to hydrogen peroxide (H_2O_2) and diatomic oxygen (O_2) via cyclic reduction and oxidation of a protein-bound Cu ion (Valentine et al. 2005). Today, over 150, predominantly missense mutations have been identified at ~75 sites spread throughout the protein (http://alsod.iop.kcl.ac.uk/). SOD1 mutations are found in ~15-20% of inherited or familial ALS (fALS) cases and in a small percentage of sporadic ALS (sALS) cases (Rosen et al. 1993; Kato et al. 2000; Liu et al. 2009; Forsberg et al. 2011). fALS accounts for ~10% of all ALS cases and so SOD1 mutations comprise ~1.5-2% of all ALS cases, but nevertheless represent a major known cause of the disease. The clinical symptoms of fALS and sALS are similar, yet fALS patients with SOD1 mutations have an earlier age of disease onset than sALS (by ~10 years) (Wijesekera and Leigh 2009). Furthermore, while the age of disease onset has not been identified as statistically different between different SOD1 mutations, disease duration for each mutation is often different, ranging from shorter (e.g. ~1 year for A4V, the most common mutation in North America) than the typical 3-5 years to longer (e.g. ~18 years for H46R) (Cudkowicz et al. 1997; Valentine et al. 2005; Wang et al. 2008). In humans and murine models of ALS, mutations in the gene encoding SOD1 are typically autosomal dominant and are associated with a toxic gain of function. Despite extensive research, the molecular basis for mutant SOD1 toxicity remains unclear (Valentine et al. 2005; Boillee et al. 2006; Ilieva et al. 2009). Extensive research has been conducted on SOD1-linked fALS, as understanding and treatment of this disease may be relevant to ALS in general. While ALS patients share many clinical symptoms, numerous genes have been linked to ALS, and there is evidence for differences in pathology related to both genetic and environmental factors; hence, ALS is a syndrome and not a single disease with unique pathology (Cozzolino et al. 2008).

Currently, there are two prevailing hypotheses for the toxic gain of SOD1 function that is observed in ALS: 1) new toxic enzymatic activity, and 2) protein misfolding resulting in formation of toxic aggregates (Valentine et al. 2005; Andersen 2006; Pasinelli and Brown 2006; Cozzolino et al. 2008; Turner and Talbot 2008). Since toxic enzymatic activity can damage the protein and cause aggregation, and conversely aggregation may result in toxic activity, these two hypotheses are not mutually exclusive. Theories involving gain of toxic activity involve altered metal binding by SOD1, resulting in the generation of reactive oxygen species, such as damaging hydroxyl and peroxynitrite radicals (Kurahashi et al. 2001; Alvarez et al. 2004). Alternatively, there is extensive evidence that ALS belongs to a growing group of protein misfolding diseases (Valentine et al. 2005; Chiti and Dobson 2006; Turner and Talbot 2008; Chiti and Dobson 2009; Deng et al. 2011). Protein inclusions, or aggregates, observed in the motor neurons and glial cells stain immunopositive for SOD1 in SOD1-linked fALS and some sALS patients (Kato et al. 2000; Liu et al. 2009; Forsberg et al. 2011) and are observed in mutant SOD1 animal models of ALS (Bruijn et al. 1998; Johnston et al. 2000). Thus, a major hypothesis in the field of ALS research is that SOD1 mutations decrease protein stability, alter protein folding and metal binding, and/or cause changes in other biophysical properties of the protein, resulting in an increased propensity of mutant SOD1 to form neurotoxic aggregates (Valentine et al. 2005).

Many reviews have summarized extensive investigations into the role of SOD1 in ALS, including *in vivo* mutant SOD1 models of ALS pathogenesis and their clinical implications (Bruijn et al. 2004; Boillee et al. 2006; Mitchell and Borasio 2007; Cozzolino et al. 2008), the numerous genetic elements and complex disease etiology associated with sALS and fALS (Boillee et al. 2006; Vucic and Kiernan 2009; Bastos et al. 2011), the various ALS rodent models used to study the underlying genetics and cause of motor neuron death in ALS (Van Den Bosch 2011), and the biophysical properties of mutant SOD1 in relation to possible disease mechanisms (Valentine et al. 2005). In this chapter we review recent research characterizing the stability, folding and misfolding, and the physical characteristics and mechanisms governing aggregation of mutant SOD1 *in vitro*. We describe in detail studies that reflect our own research and interests, but also include references to related work, to which we refer the interested reader. We will first review the general principles of protein stability and aggregation, which are pertinent to protein conformational diseases in general. Following this overview, we examine recent research that has characterized folding and aggregation of SOD1 and the relevance of this work to ALS.

1.2 Characteristics of protein aggregation

Protein aggregation is a common phenomenon observed in both normal and abnormal physiological processes, and has been studied extensively for more than 30 years (Chiti and Dobson 2006). While protein association reactions are highly regulated and essential for cellular function, unregulated protein association causes a wide range of diseases, such as sickle-cell anaemia, serpinopathies, and, in particular, many neurodegenerative diseases including prion, Parkinson's, Alzheimer's, and Huntington's diseases (Chiti and Dobson 2006; Eisenberg et al. 2006; Chiti and Dobson 2009). These protein misfolding diseases are characterized by the formation of insoluble proteinacious deposits (aggregates) (Chiti and Dobson 2006), and the mechanisms and biological effects of aggregation in different diseases are an area of active research. In some cases, toxicity may be caused by large protein aggregates; however, smaller oligomeric protein species are generally considered more neurotoxic (Caughey and Lansbury 2003). The harmful nature of these oligomers compared to larger protein aggregates may be due to their lower stability, higher degree of solvent accessible surface area, and an increased tendency to form non-native associations with essential cellular components (Bucciantini et al. 2002; Knowles et al. 2007). For example, aggregates of many disease-associated proteins, including mutant SOD1, have been found to interact with the ubiquitin-proteasome system (Mouradian 2002; Sakamoto 2002; Urushitani et al. 2002; Valentine et al. 2005), folding chaperones (Bruening et al. 1999; Wyttenbach et al. 2000; Shinder et al. 2001; Okado-Matsumoto and Fridovich 2002), and the outer mitochondrial membrane (Vande Velde et al. 2008). These cellular components play central roles in regulating many critical cellular events ranging from cell division to apoptosis, and their impairment may represent common mechanisms by which aggregates of different proteins can cause cellular dysregulation and cell death (Hol and Scheper 2008; Gidalevitz et al. 2010). Many factors are involved in modulating protein aggregation, and are surveyed in the following sections.

1.2.1 Protein folding, stability and aggregation

Globular protein folding begins on the ribosome, as newly synthesized, unstructured polypeptide chains start to make favourable intramolecular contacts (Dobson 2004). As it further folds into its mature, native state, a protein may populate multiple conformational or intermediate states, and undergo various co- and post-translational modifications (refer to Figure 1). The rate determining step of folding involves overcoming the major energetic barrier to folding by forming a transition state complex prior to attaining the native state. In more complex cases, protein folding can involve more than one energetic barrier (Dobson 2004). Other proteins are unable to adopt a stable, well folded structure and exist as an ensemble of fluctuating, poorly structured conformations (Uversky and Dunker 2010). Thermodynamic protein stability is defined as the difference in energy between the denatured, unfolded state and the native, folded state. If there is a large separation in energy between the unfolded and folded states, the protein has high global thermodynamic stability. Stability can also be assessed by the rate of native protein unfolding, which determines how long the polypeptide remains in the folded state. This is referred to as kinetic stability, defined as the difference in energy between the folded conformation and the transition state. The closer these species are in energy, the higher the rate of unfolding and the lower the kinetic stability (Figure 1A).

In general, both thermodynamic and kinetic destabilization of proteins by chemical modifications or by mutations favours global protein unfolding and exposure of the hydrophobic groups that are normally buried in the protein core. This can promote the formation of non-native intermolecular contacts between proteins and the formation of aggregates. However, even subtle decreases in global protein stability are often accompanied by local destabilization and recent investigations have provided evidence for aggregate formation from native-like species (N*, Figure 1) that have undergone much more restricted unfolding (Nelson and Eisenberg 2006; Chiti and Dobson 2009). Examples of aggregate formation from native-like states include various proteins associated with disease such as mutant lysozyme (Chiti and Dobson 2009), β2-microglobulin (Chiti and Dobson 2009), and SOD1 (Hwang et al. 2010). The propensity of a given globular protein to aggregate depends on how energetically feasible it is for the protein to access locally, partially or fully unfolded aggregation-prone state(s). Protein folding generally occurs in a cooperative fashion with minimal formation of partially folded species and this cooperativity generates a sufficiently large energy barrier between the unfolded and folded states, which decreases the likelihood of unfolding and aggregation (Dobson 1999; Dobson 2004; Tartaglia et al. 2008).

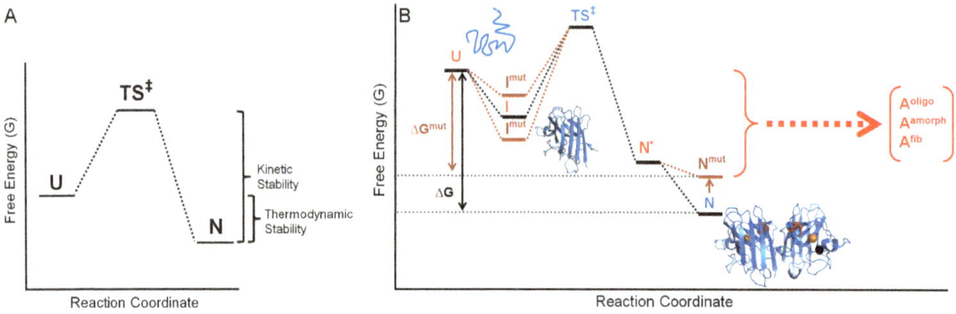

Fig. 1. Protein stability, misfolding and aggregation.
In panel A, the difference between thermodynamic and kinetic stability is shown. U, TS‡, and N refer to the unfolded, transition and native states of the protein, respectively. Refer to the main text for further explanation. In panel B, the effects of native state (N) destabilization by mutation on the population of locally unfolded, native-like (N*), partially folded intermediate (I) and fully unfolded (U) states is shown. Aggregation may occur from N*, I or U, and the morphology of the aggregates formed may depend on the conformation of the protein prior to aggregation. Mutations that destabilize N, decrease the energy difference between the N and the more unfolded states (N*, I or U), and thereby promote aggregation. Note that destabilization of N, does not necessarily imply destabilization of I. Mutations that destabilize N, may stabilize or destabilize I, resulting in a large increase or decrease, respectively, in the population of I compared to levels observed in the native folding pathway. Panel B was adapted from (Chiti and Dobson 2009).

1.2.2 Factors that modulate aggregation of polypeptides

In addition to protein stability and structure, many other factors, such as physicochemical properties of amino acids within a protein sequence and solution conditions, can affect protein aggregation. Hydrophobicity, β-sheet propensity, and charge of a polypeptide sequence have been shown to modulate the formation of amyloid aggregates (refer to section 1.2.3) by unfolded proteins (Chiti et al. 2003). Interestingly, these properties are also important for facilitating correct protein folding, suggesting that while similar forces contribute to both processes, different key residues are involved in forming the initial contacts that drive native protein folding and aggregation (Jahn and Radford 2008). In many cases, the overall aggregation propensity of a protein increases if the primary sequence contains short stretches of amino acids with properties that favour aggregation, for example, low net charge, extensive hydrophobicity, and/or a tendency to form a β-sheet over an α-helix (Tartaglia et al. 2008). Interestingly, many fALS-associated SOD1 mutations decrease the net charge of the protein, which may promote aggregation and explain why certain mutations give rise to a shorter disease duration (Sandelin et al. 2007; Shaw and Valentine 2007; Bystrom et al. 2010). Sequence hydrophobicity also plays a large role in modulating the aggregation propensity of a protein (Chiti et al. 2003). Several studies have suggested that SOD1 mutations promote exposure of hydrophobic regions that can promote aggregation (Tiwari et al. 2009; Munch and Bertolotti 2010). Taken together, these studies indicate that aggregation is at least partially controlled by the physicochemical properties of amino acid residues within a polypeptide sequence (Chiti et al. 2003; Tartaglia et al. 2008). In addition, solution conditions can modulate the stability, conformation, and the intermolecular interactions of a protein in solution, and can thereby influence the rate of protein aggregation and the type of aggregate structure formed (Chi et al. 2003; Mahler et al. 2009). Importantly, variations in solution conditions can cause the same protein to aggregate by fundamentally different mechanisms (Goers et al. 2002; Vetri and Militello 2005; Necula et al. 2007). Temperature, pH, macromolecular crowding, agitation, and ionic strength are all variables that can influence aggregation (Chi et al. 2003; Munishkina et al. 2004; Mahler et al. 2009; Sicorello et al. 2009). A number of studies have used different solution conditions (increased temperature, decreased pH, increased ionic strength, sonication or agitation) to promote the formation of well-structured, fibrillar amyloid aggregates (see 1.2.3) by various forms of SOD1 (Stathopulos et al. 2004; Chattopadhyay et al. 2008; Chattopadhyay and Valentine 2009; Oztug Durer et al. 2009). Other studies have demonstrated soluble oligomer and small aggregate formation by various forms of SOD1 in quiescent, physiologically relevant solution conditions (Vassall, 2011, Hwang, 2010, Banci, 2008). Thus, it is evident that multiple factors can greatly influence protein folding and aggregation and these factors must be considered when investigating the molecular mechanisms of protein aggregation.

1.2.3 Amyloid formation

Protein aggregation is a general term that describes a number of diverse processes that culminate in the formation of non-native, multimeric complexes of varied conformations. These aggregates can range from small, soluble oligomers, to larger amorphous structures, and insoluble, well-structured fibrils (Uversky and Dunker 2010). Amyloid is a common, well characterized, type of aggregate formed by proteins associated with many diseases, including the neurodegenerative prion, Parkinson's, Alzheimer's, and Huntington's diseases (Chiti and Dobson 2006; Chiti and Dobson 2009). Extensive studies of amyloid have resulted in significant advances in understanding the underlying molecular basis of protein aggregation (Sipe and Cohen 2000; Chiti and Dobson 2006; Eisenberg et al. 2006; Chiti and Dobson 2009). Classically defined amyloid is characterized by an unbranched, fibrillar aggregate morphology, which exhibits green-gold birefringence upon binding Congo red (Sipe and Cohen 2000), a dye used in disease diagnosis, and a cross-β x-ray diffraction pattern due to the presence of β-strands oriented perpendicular to the long axis of the fibre (Serpell 2000). These large aggregates can be extremely stable and unaffected by cellular clearance machinery (Dobson 1999; Knowles et al. 2007). There is extensive evidence that most and perhaps all proteins can form amyloid under suitable, typically destabilizing, conditions (Dobson 1999; Munishkina et al. 2004; Stathopulos et al. 2004). Amyloid formation can arise from association of unstructured, partially folded, or native-like species, and can be prevented by factors that favour native folding (Chiti and Dobson 2009). These include such factors as: interactions with molecular chaperones that can stabilize partially folded conformations and increase the folding rate; and post-translational modifications or ligand binding that can stabilize the native state and prevent unfolding (Dobson 2004; Chiti and Dobson 2009). Protein size is also a factor that modulates the propensity of a protein to

form amyloid fibrils, as it is less energetically favourable for large proteins to form an amyloid core, compared to smaller proteins (Baldwin et al. 2011; Ramshini et al. 2011).
It should be noted that ALS is not classified by pathologists as an amyloid disease (Kerman et al. 2010). Recent studies have reported the formation of SOD1 aggregates *in vitro* that exhibit some features of amyloid (Banci et al. 2008; Furukawa et al. 2008; Oztug Durer et al. 2009); however, the relevance of such studies to human disease is not known. Typically, there is considerable structural heterogeneity in amyloid (Platt and Radford 2009) and in other amorphous or ordered aggregate structures formed by many peptides and proteins (Fink 1998; Seshadri et al. 2009) (see 1.2.4). Careful analyses using multiple probes are required to distinguish between these different aggregate structures. Appropriately characterizing mixtures of aggregate structures is a major, ongoing challenge in the study of protein aggregation.

1.2.4 Protein aggregation heterogeneity and disease complexity

Neurodegenerative disorders characterized by protein misfolding and aggregation, including ALS, commonly display phenotypic diversity, such as variation in the age of onset, the rate of neuronal dysregulation, and the area of the nervous system affected (Armstrong et al. 2000; Goedert et al. 2001; Frost and Diamond 2009; Williamson et al. 2009). Although the molecular origins of such phenotypic diversity are complex and may differ between diseases, in recent years it has been shown that protein aggregates, including amyloid fibrils, exhibit extensive structural heterogeneity both *in vivo* and *in vitro* (Berryman et al. 2009; Frost and Diamond 2009). Not only do fibrils formed by different amino acid sequences adopt conformations that differ in length and twist, but the structure of fibrils formed by the *same* sequence can vary depending on solution conditions (Berryman et al. 2009). Fibres can vary in the number of amino acids that participate in forming the amyloid core, the arrangement of β-strands in a parallel or antiparallel conformation within each protofilament, and the alignment of β-sheets along the protofilament axis (Tycko 2006). The structure that a particular protein adopts prior to aggregation influences the structure of the aggregate formed and the conformational plasticity of a native protein may play a large role in determining the number of structurally different aggregates produced (Jones and Surewicz 2005; Natalello et al. 2008). Although aggregate structures formed from the same protein can be quite diverse (ie. amorphous versus amyloid structures), in many cases the formation of such structures is energetically favourable and therefore switching between aggregate conformations can require a large amount of energy. As a result, a particular fibril can become trapped in a single conformation (Berryman et al. 2009).
Structural heterogeneity of protein aggregates has been known for many years for amyloid fibrils derived from prion proteins, infectious protein agents that give rise to a number of neurodegenerative disorders known as spongiform encephalopathies or prionopathies. In these diseases, the infectious agent is a misfolded prion protein (PrP^{Sc}, S referring to Scrapie, the disease caused by this infectious agent), which once introduced into a host cell can bind to the native prion protein (PrP^{c}, c referring to cellular) and induce conversion to the PrP^{Sc} form, inevitably resulting in the spread of the disease phenotype (Tuite and Serio 2010). Because a prion protein can adopt a number of conformations, there is considerable heterogeneity in the structure of the amyloid fibrils that are formed from these proteins. Prion amyloid fibrils can differ in stability, surface charge and degree of polypeptide incorporation into the amyloid core, differences that may play a large role in determining

rate of prion replication and the strength of the disease phenotype (Verges et al. 2011). In recent years, evidence for conformational diversity, or different strains, of protein aggregates has also been described for non-infectious protein conformational disorders such as Alzheimer's, Parkinson's, Frontal Temporal Dementia, and ALS (Frost and Diamond 2009; Furukawa et al. 2010). The proteins linked to many of these diseases are natively disordered, and so can easily sample different conformations, which may facilitate aggregation via multiple pathways. Mutations and/or post-translational modifications can greatly influence the population of different conformations of a protein, and thus can largely influence the aggregation process. This point may be particularly relevant to ALS toxicity, since SOD1, although natively folded, undergoes extensive post-translational modification *in vivo* (Valentine et al. 2005), and is increasingly malleable in its less stable, immature forms (refer to section 3). How different fALS-associated mutations modulate the stability of different forms of SOD1 may largely determine the ALS phenotype (Vassall et al. 2011).

2. Structure and function of Cu, Zn-superoxide dismutase (SOD1)

Before discussing SOD1 folding, misfolding and aggregation, we will give a brief description of the tertiary and quaternary structure of SOD1. Human SOD1 is a 32 kDa homodimeric metalloenzyme, with each subunit consisting of a 153 amino acid chain that is often N-terminally acetylated, contains a highly conserved, intrasubunit disulfide bond, and binds one Cu ion and one Zn ion (Figure 2A, C).

Each monomer folds into a Greek key β-barrel, comprised of two, four-stranded antiparallel β-sheets arranged at an angle with respect to one another. The β-barrel has a non-continuous topology such that strands 1 through 3 together with strand 6 form the first β-sheet, while strands 4, 5, 7 and 8 form the second β-sheet. The β-strands are connected by seven loops that differ greatly in length. Loop IV and loop VII are known as the metal binding and electrostatic loops, respectively, and play important roles in both stability and catalytic function by binding the metals and forming the catalytic site pocket. In addition to forming the Zn-binding site, Loop IV contains residues that are important for dimer interface and intrasubunit disulfide bond formation, which tethers Loop IV to β-strand 8 (Tainer et al. 1982). Thus, Zn binding, disulfide bond formation and dimerization together stabilize the native conformation of this long loop, greatly affecting the overall stability of the protein. Loop VII mainly plays a functional role, containing charged residues that shield the active site. These charged residues are important for guiding the superoxide anion from the surface of the protein into the active site where the redox active Cu ion is bound (Valentine et al. 2005).

SOD1 is abundant and ubiquitously expressed in the cytosol of aerobic organisms (Brown et al. 2004). Maturation of the protein involves a series of post-translational modifications, which are understood to varying extents. When it is initially synthesized in the reducing environment of the cytosol the protein is thought to adopt a marginally stable, folded, monomer structure with a reduced disulfide bond and no bound metals. How the protein acquires Zn is not known; however, Cu can be acquired by interaction with the copper chaperone for SOD1 (CCS) or by a CCS-independent mechanism that may involve glutathione, but that is not well understood (Leitch et al. 2009). CCS also catalyzes intrasubunit disulfide bond formation in the reducing cellular environment (Leitch et al. 2009). Although the most abundant form of SOD1 is usually the native, fully mature, dimeric protein (Valentine et al. 2005), there is also evidence for a significant pool of SOD1 that lacks bound Cu, and is activated in response to oxidative stress (Brown et al. 2004). From here we will refer to the various states of the protein in terms of disulfide and metallation status, with a focus on the disulfide reduced (2SH), disulfide oxidized (S-S), fully metallated (holo) and metal free (apo) states.

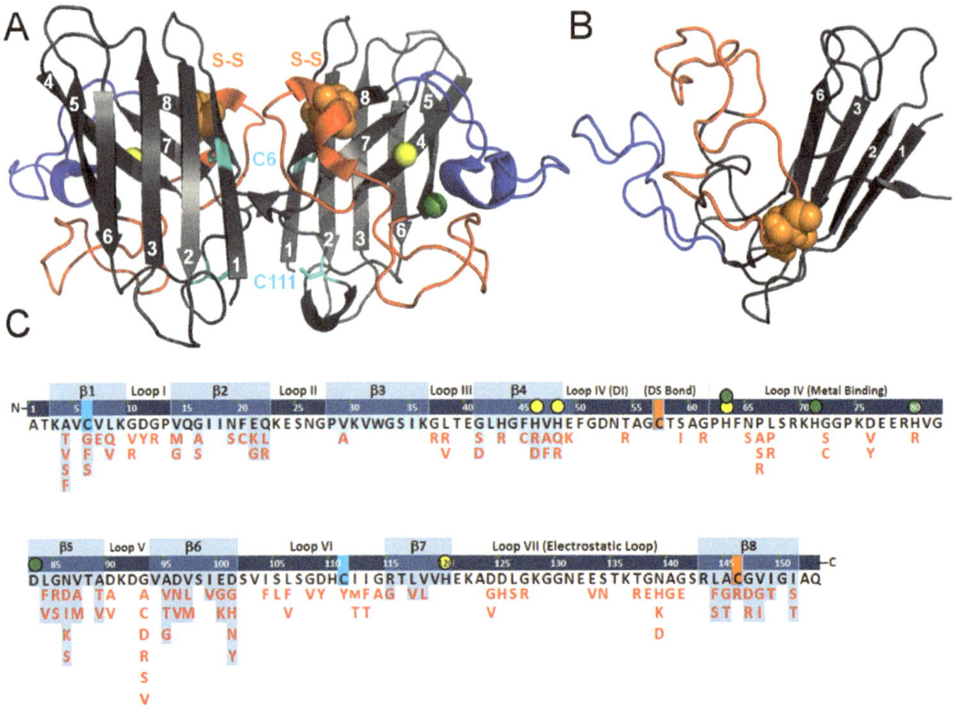

Fig. 2. The structural elements of SOD1.
The crystal structure of fully mature SOD1 is shown in panel A (pdb: 1HL5) (Strange et al. 2003). The β-strands are shown in gray and labelled in white starting from the N-terminus; the functional loops IV and VII are shown in red and blue, respectively; the conserved disulfide bond (S-S) between Cys57 and Cys146 is indicated by orange spheres, the non-conserved free Cys (6 and 111) are shown in cyan; and Cu and Zn are indicated by yellow and green spheres, respectively. The solution structure of the metal free SOD1 monomer variant (pWT*mon*, refer to the introduction of section 3) is shown in panel B (pdb: 1RK7) (Banci et al. 2003). In this structure, only β-strands 1-3 and 6 are well defined. The colour scheme in panel B is identical to panel A. The primary sequence of the SOD1 monomer is shown in panel C. The colours used to depict the secondary structure elements are identical to those used in panels A and B. The positions of known fALS-associated mutations are listed vertically in red below the naturally occurring amino acid in black. The yellow and green spheres indicate the metal binding residues and the secondary structure elements are listed above the primary sequence.

3. Folding, unfolding and misfolding of SOD1

A common and powerful approach to understanding the molecular basis for aggregate formation is to investigate the biophysical properties of mutant proteins in the native and unfolded states, as well as any equilibrium or kinetic intermediates that arise as the protein folds or unfolds (Dobson 2004). Equilibrium species refer to the most stable conformations that are significantly populated under specific steady-state conditions, while kinetic species refer to conformations that are transiently populated as an unfolded protein folds into its native conformation. Typically, kinetic folding intermediates have a relatively low energy barrier of formation, and therefore can form quickly, but they are generally not the most stable conformations. Before protein folding has reached equilibrium (ie. during kinetic conditions), it is not the stability of each state that determines the relative population of each species along the folding/unfolding pathway, but rather how rapidly these states can be accessed on the time scale of protein folding/unfolding. Investigating the molecular characteristics that govern the stability of different states and enable efficient folding of SOD1 can provide key insights into the cause of ALS (Rumfeldt et al. 2006; Stathopulos et al. 2006; Vassall et al. 2006; Rumfeldt et al. 2009; Vassall et al. 2011).

In recent years, systematic analyses of the effects of fALS-associated mutations on the stability and folding of various forms of SOD1, including holoS-S, apoS-S and apoSH, have been reported. Human SOD1 contains two free cysteine residues at amino acid positions 6 and 111 (Figure 2), and these free cysteine residues inhibit reversible unfolding of SOD1 *in vitro* by forming intramolecular and intermolecular non-native disulfide bonds, which promote SOD1 aggregation (Lepock et al. 1990; McRee et al. 1990). Reversible unfolding is a prerequisite for thermodynamic analysis, and so to overcome this limitation pseudo-wild type (pWT) constructs lacking these free cysteines have been used extensively for *in vitro* studies of SOD1. In the most widely used pWT construct, the free cysteines are mutated to alanine and serine at positions 6 and 111, respectively (Lepock et al. 1990; McRee et al. 1990; Stathopulos et al. 2003; Rumfeldt et al. 2006; Stathopulos et al. 2006; Vassall et al. 2006; Kayatekin et al. 2008; Rumfeldt et al. 2009; Vassall et al. 2011); however, other mutations at these positions have also been used (most notably C6A and C111A) (Lindberg et al. 2004; Nordlund and Oliveberg 2006; Nordlund et al. 2009). Not only are these chemically and structurally conservative mutations, a serine at position 111 is found in most other mammalian SOD1, and alanine at position 6 is observed in other non-mammalian organisms (Getzoff et al. 1989). Mutating the free cysteines results in highly reversible unfolding of pWT, while having very minimal effects on structure, function and stability (Lepock et al. 1990; McRee et al. 1990; Hallewell et al. 1991; Parge et al. 1992; Vassall et al. 2011). In addition, an engineered monomer construct (pWT*mon* SOD1) has been used to investigate the effects of ALS mutations on the stability and folding behaviour of individual SOD1 subunits (Nordlund and Oliveberg 2006; Hornberg et al. 2007; Kayatekin et al. 2008; Nordlund et al. 2009; Kayatekin et al. 2010). The monomer construct contains two glutamic acid residues in place of Phe50 and Gly51, and the presence of these charged residues in the dimer interface prevents SOD1 dimerization (Bertini et al. 1994; Banci et al. 1998). The use of both pWT and pWT*mon* SOD1 constructs has provided valuable insights into the mechanism of SOD1 folding and misfolding, which are described in the following sections, starting with the most immature to most mature form of SOD1.

SOD1 Form	t_m pWT (°C)	t_m WT (°C)	ΔG, 37°C pWT (kcal mol^{-1})
HoloS-S	92.0[a] (81.7[b])	80.1[b]	33.0[a,c]
ApoS-S	59.0[a]	52.5[d]	13.2[a,c]
Apo2SH	47.6[e]	46.8[e]	1.8[e,f]

Table 1. Stability parameters obtained from DSC measurements of different forms of wild type (WT) and pWT SOD1
[a](Stathopulos et al. 2006) The parameters were obtained using average fitted values determined using 0.5 mg mL^{-1} protein in 20 mM Hepes pH 7.8.
[b](Lepock et al. 1990) t_m defined as the temperature of half completion of the DSC profiles determined using 2-4 mg mL^{-1} protein in 100 mM phosphate.
[c]ΔG extrapolated to 37°C using methods described in (Stathopulos et al. 2006). Value is in units of per mol dimer.
[d](rodriguiz/valentine,2005,PNAS)determined using 2 mg mL^{-1} protein in 100 mM potassium phosphate pH 7.4.
[e](Vassal,2011,PNAS) parameters obtained using average fitted values determined using 0.5 mg mL^{-1} protein in 20 mM Hepes pH 7.4, 1mM TCEP.
[f]Value is in units of per mol monomer.

3.1 Equilibrium denaturation of apo2SH SOD1

In its most immature form, with no bound metals and reduced disulfide bond, apo2SH SOD1 adopts a marginally stable folded monomer structure. Chemical and thermal equilibrium denaturation of apo2SH SOD1 is well described by a 2-state unfolding transition between folded and unfolded monomers, denoted as M and U, respectively (M ↔ U) (Kayatekin et al. 2010; Vassall et al. 2011). At 37°C and neutral pH, this form of the protein has a low free energy of unfolding, 1.8 kcal mol^{-1} and 1.6 kcal mol^{-1} for pWT and WT, respectively (Vassall et al. 2011), indicating that ~95 % and 93 % of the protein is folded. Furthermore, the corresponding melting temperatures are 48 °C and 47 °C, respectively. This stability is relatively low compared to other globular proteins, which typically have unfolding free energies of ~5-15 kcal mol^{-1} (Jackson 1998) as well as to more mature forms of SOD1 (see sections 3.2-3.4, 3.6, 3.7, Table 1).

Structural investigations by x-ray crystallography and NMR have shown that without the bound metals and disulfide bond, the interface loop (Loop IV) is minimally structured and the dimer interface is disrupted (Arnesano et al. 2004; Hornberg et al. 2007). The NMR solution structure of monomeric (pWT*mon*) with no bound metals but intact disulfide bond, apoS-S (Banci et al. 2003) provides an interesting comparison (Figure 2B). pWT*mon* apoS-S SOD1 adopts an open β-barrel structure due to the flexibility of β-strands 4 and 5, and the inability of the two β-sheets to effectively pack against one another. Furthermore, Loops IV and VII are extensively disordered (Banci et al. 2003; Banci et al. 2010). Disulfide bond reduction promotes further disorder of the marginally stable Loop IV structure by releasing it from its anchor to β-strand 8 (Hornberg et al. 2007). Because Loop IV contains residues required for Zn binding, disulfide bond formation and dimerization, these modifications are thermodynamically coupled. When the disulfide bond is reduced, SOD1 has a much lower affinity for Zn (75 nM *verses* 100 pM for apoS-S SOD1) (Kayatekin et al. 2010), and dimer formation is energetically unfavourable (Arnesano et al. 2004).

Diverse fALS-associated mutations have markedly different effects on the stability and the folding reversibility of apo2SH SOD1 (Kayatekin et al. 2010; Vassall et al. 2011). Wild-type, pWT, and pWT*mon* apo2SH SOD1 are predominantly folded and can undergo reversible chemical and thermal denaturation, and hence resist aggregation from partially or fully unfolded states (Kayatekin et al. 2010; Vassall et al. 2011). Various fALS-associated mutations decrease the unfolding reversibility, which precludes determination of the free energy of unfolding, and suggests that these mutations increase the aggregation propensity of apo2SH SOD1 (Vassall et al. 2011). Interestingly, an increased tendency to aggregate is not observed for all fALS-associated mutants, in particular not for those with compromised metal binding (Kayatekin et al. 2010; Vassall et al. 2011). Although the free energy of unfolding could not be determined for all mutants studied, owing to the limited stability of this form of the protein, the effects of each mutation on stability could be estimated from their apparent melting temperatures. This revealed that fALS-associated mutations generally have the largest effect on the stability of this most immature form of SOD1 (Table 1), often decreasing the melting temperature of apoSH to below 37°C, and so markedly increasing the fraction of protein that is unfolded at physiological temperature (Furukawa and O'Halloran 2005; Kayatekin et al. 2010; Vassall et al. 2011). Of the mutant SOD1s that unfold reversibly, most show decreased thermodynamic stability, but some (e.g. those involved in metal binding) have little or even a stabilizing effect on stability (Valentine et al. 2005; Kayatekin et al. 2010; Vassall et al. 2011). These findings imply that in some cases the key effects of mutations in ALS may be manifested in more mature forms of SOD1.

3.2 Kinetic unfolding and refolding of apo2SH

Relatively little is known about the kinetic folding mechanism of apo2SH SOD1. Initial studies of engineered reduced monomer variants have reported 2-state (U ↔ M) folding kinetics, which resembles the behaviour of monomeric apoS-S SOD1s (Lindberg et al. 2004; Kayatekin et al. 2010) (see section 3.4). A study using a monomeric C6A/C111A/C57A/C146A construct that resembles the apo2SH form, due to its inability to form a disulfide bond and dimerize, showed that disulfide bond formation was not required to facilitate the early contacts made in the monomer folding pathway (Lindberg et al. 2004). Thus, the transition state between unfolded and folded monomers in both the apo2SH and the apoS-S monomer folding pathways may be similar. However, the disulfide bond stabilizes the folded monomer by decreasing the rate of unfolding, thereby increasing the population of folded monomer (Lindberg et al. 2004) (see section 3.4).

3.3 Equilibrium denaturation of apoS-S SOD1

Formation of a disulfide bond between Cys57 and Cys146 greatly diminishes the conformational freedom of Loop IV (Hornberg et al. 2007), and gives rise to energetically favourable dimer formation (Lindberg et al. 2004; Vassall et al. 2006; Ding and Dokholyan 2008; Kayatekin et al. 2010; Vassall et al. 2011). The observed equilibrium folding mechanism of the pWT apoS-S SOD1 dimer depends on the method of inducing denaturation (i.e. chemical denaturant *versus* heat). Spectroscopically-monitored chemical denaturation of pWT apoS-S SOD1 can be described by a 3-state mechanism in which dimer dissociation is followed by monomer unfolding ($N_2 \leftrightarrow 2M \leftrightarrow 2U$) (Vassall et al. 2006). Due to mass action, however, at increased protein concentrations there is little population of the folded monomer and the mechanism appears 2-state ($N_2 \leftrightarrow 2U$) (Lindberg et al. 2004; Svensson et al. 2006; Vassall et al. 2006). Similarly, due to the higher stability of the apoS-S dimer compared to the apoS-S monomer and the high protein concentration requirement, thermal denaturation by differential scanning calorimetry (DSC) of apoS-S pWT SOD1 appears 2-state ($N_2 \leftrightarrow 2U$) and so does not provide direct information about the energetics of dimer dissocation ($N_2 \leftrightarrow 2M$) (Stathopulos et al. 2006; Vassall et al. 2006). Thermal denaturation does reveal, however, that the melting temperatures of wild-type and pWT apoS-S SOD1 are approximately 53°C (Rodriguez et al. 2005) and 60°C (Stathopulos et al. 2006), respectively; therefore, the oxidized form of the protein is predominantly folded at physiological temperature. The differences in the reported melting temperatures may be related to different buffer conditions used as well as the folding irreversibility of wild-type SOD1 (Lepock et al. 1992; Chrunyk and Wetzel 1993; Stathopulos et al. 2003). The changes in melting temperatures caused by fALS mutations generally range from -15°C to +2°C; thus, apoS-S SOD1 mutants are also mainly folded at physiological temperature (Rodriguez et al. 2005; Vassall et al. 2006; Kayatekin et al. 2010).

The stability as well as the conformational dynamics of a protein can be assessed using hydrogen-deuterium (H/D) exchange measurements, which can identify regions of the protein undergoing structural opening (Bai et al. 1995). Interestingly, a number of fALS-associated mutants, in particular those that compromise metal binding, display a similar exchange rate as wild type (Rodriguez et al. 2005). However, others increase the rate of structural fluctuations of apoS-S SOD1 (Rodriguez et al. 2005; Prudencio et al. 2009). In particular, some mutants show pronounced opening of the β-barrel around the edge strands at physiological temperatures (Prudencio et al. 2009). Thus, both equilibrium denaturation and H/D exchange experiments reveal that fALS-associated mutations have diverse effects on the stability of apoS-S SOD1, ranging from destabilizing to stabilizing.

Highly reversible chemical denaturation behaviour has enabled accurate measurements of the energetics of both dimer dissociation and monomer unfolding for pWT and mutant apoS-S. Determining how mutations affect the energy, and thus the population, of each species formed along the (un)folding pathway, provides insight into the mechanisms of apoS-S aggregation. Chemical denaturation experiments have revealed that for structurally and chemically diverse mutations, fALS-associated mutations generally decrease the stability of apoS-S SOD1 by destabilizing both the monomer and the dimer interface, with a larger affect on monomer stability compared to the dimer stability (Vassall et al. 2006). Remarkably, the effects of the mutations appear to propagate extensively through the apoS-S form of the protein, inevitably destabilizing the dimer interface (Vassall, K.A. et al. unpublished data) (Khare et al. 2006; Bystrom et al. 2010). Structurally, the apoS-S SOD1 dimer interface is small compared to the amount of solvent exposed surface area (Tainer et al. 1982; Parge et al. 1992); consequently, the dimer interface may be more easily perturbed in the apoS-S state. Moreover, metal loss induces asymmetry in the dynamics of the apoS-S SOD1 monomers, indicative of a structure that is less compact than the holoS-S dimer (Strange et al. 2007). The conformation of both the β-barrel core, in particular β-strand 5, and the functional Loops IV and VII are less rigid in the absence of bound metal (Banci et al. 2009; Teilum et al. 2009). It has been proposed that metal binding is important for shielding the charged residues in Loops IV and VII, which contain too few hydrophobic residues to facilitate close packing with the β-barrel core in the absence of bound metal (Nordlund et al. 2009). Similarly, metal binding may protect against conformational changes in SOD1 that increase hydrophobic exposure (Tiwari et al. 2009).

Therefore, it seems reasonable that many fALS-associated mutations have a large effect on the global stability of apoS-S SOD1. Structural perturbations in one region of the apoS-S SOD1 structure are likely to result in structural perturbations in another region. However, it is clear that fALS-associated mutations have differing effects on the global stability of apoS-S SOD1. In particular, both the apoS-S and apo2SH forms of the metal-binding mutants appear to possess similar stability compared to the wild-type protein (Rodriguez et al. 2005; Vassall et al. 2011). In fact, some fALS-associated mutations increase the stability of apo2SH and apoS-S forms compared to pWT SOD1 (Vassall et al. unpublished data) (Vassall et al. 2011). For example, the mutation H46R increases the stability of both apo2SH and apoS-S SOD1 and the reason for this increase in stability may be due to the introduction of a positively charged side chain into the metal binding pocket of the protein, effectively mimicking the stabilizing effects of the charged metals.

3.4 Kinetic unfolding and refolding of apoS-S SOD1

The kinetic unfolding mechanism of pWT apoS-S SOD1 can be described by the same 3-state mechanism previously outlined for equilibrium denaturation of the wild-type and pWT apoS-S form, where dimer dissociation is followed by the unfolding of two monomers (Figure 3) (Svensson et al. 2006). The overall observed rate of unfolding depends on four microscopic rate constants: the rate constant for folding (k_f), unfolding (k_u), monomer association (k_a), and dimer dissociation (k_d) (Figure 3B); however, under highly denaturing conditions (ie. high denaturant concentration), the marginally stable monomer unfolds rapidly and the rate of the entire unfolding pathway is determined by the rate of dimer dissociation (k_d) (Lindberg et al. 2004; Svensson et al. 2006). In contrast, the overall rate of the refolding pathway of wild-type and pWT apoS-S is limited only by the rate of monomer folding. Therefore, once the monomer has folded the rate of monomer association is extremely rapid (Lindberg et al. 2004; Svensson et al. 2006). The transition state for monomer association is similar to the native dimer with respect to the amount of buried surface area (Svensson et al. 2006). This is similar to the transition state between unfolded and folded monomer, which represents the major energetic barrier of the unfolding/refolding pathway. It has been observed that ~70% of the structure that is buried in the monomer intermediate is also buried in the transition state between the unfolded and folded monomer, suggesting that considerable structural rearrangements must occur before that transition state can form (Svensson et al. 2006). Interestingly, under both equilibrium and kinetic conditions, the population of monomer intermediate remains below 0.5% at physiologically relevant protein concentrations, suggesting that the folding pathway of SOD1 has evolved to limit accumulation of marginally stable monomer intermediates (Svensson et al. 2006). Equilibrium denaturation analyses of fALS-associated mutant apoS-S SOD1 demonstrate a decreased stability of both the monomer intermediate and the dimer interface, increasing the population of monomeric intermediate as well as the unfolded monomer (Lindberg et al. 2004; Vassall et al. 2006), which enhances the accessibility of partially folded, high energy states that may give rise to aggregation.

Kinetic unfolding/refolding studies of the monomeric apoS-S SOD1 (pWT*mon*) and the apo2SH forms of SOD1 can be compared to gain an understanding of how disulfide bond formation modulates the SOD1 folding pathway. Both the pWT apo2SH and the pWT*mon* apoS-S forms of SOD1 fold via a 2-state mechanism, whereby the unfolded monomer adopts a folded conformation in one step ($U \leftrightarrow M$) (Lindberg et al. 2004; Nordlund and Oliveberg

2006; Kayatekin et al. 2010). Owing to the similar folding/unfolding mechanism of apo2SH and pWT*mon* apoS-S, disulfide bond formation is probably not requisite in the early monomer folding events. Consistent with this notion, the topology of the β-barrel brings Cys57 and Cys146 close in space, promoting disulfide bond formation. Although reduction of the disulfide bond does not prevent formation of the necessary contacts that facilitate monomer folding, the maintenance of the disulfide bond modulates the stability of the SOD1 monomer by decreasing the rate of unfolding and to a smaller extent increasing the rate of folding (Lindberg et al. 2004; Kayatekin et al. 2010).

Removal of Loops IV and VII has little effect on the structure and dynamics of the core apoS-S β-barrel (Nordlund et al. 2009). Additionally, the folding behaviour of pWT*mon* apoS-S SOD1 in the absence of these functional loops remains 2-state; however, this SOD1 construct has a 10-fold increase in the rate of folding, while the rate of unfolding is less affected (Nordlund et al. 2009). Removing the Zn-binding site has little effect on the rate of folding, but decreases the rate of unfolding, stabilizing the folded apoS-S SOD1 monomer (Nordlund et al. 2009). These results suggest that while the β-barrel can fold independently of Loop IV and VII, these critical functional loops endow the protein with a less than optimal folding mechanism and may increase the aggregation propensity of the immature forms of the protein.

The overall rate of both apo2SH and apoS-S SOD1 folding appears to be dictated largely by the structural determinants of the monomer folding nucleus. Furthermore, regions extraneous to this folding nucleus are the more labile regions of the protein that unfold first, and thus have been suggested to play a role in SOD1 aggregation. It has been shown that β-strands 1-3 of the first β-sheet must make contact with β-strands 4 and 7 in the second β-sheet to overcome the monomer folding energy barrier. The other strands (β5, β6 and β8) remain disordered in the transition state between unfolded and folded monomers (Nordlund and Oliveberg 2006). By attaching Loop IV to β-strand 8 and forming the dimer interface the disulfide bond may prevent the structural fluctuations that lead to the unravelling of the more dynamic strands of the β-barrel.

3.5 Are the metal free forms of SOD1 the common denominator in fALS toxicity?

Taken together, equilibrium and kinetic folding studies of apo2SH and apoS-S SOD1 suggest that a number of factors may contribute to an increased tendency to aggregate. Many fALS-associated mutations increase the fraction of partially folded monomers, while a few mutations remain wild-type-like in their folding behaviour and aggregation propensity. Because the β-strands display differences in conformational freedom, the location of each fALS-associated mutation and the physicochemical properties of the amino acid introduced seem to greatly affect SOD1 stability and accessibility to partially folded species that may bridge the gap between productive folding and aggregation pathways. These differences may also change the structural properties of the aggregates formed. In recent years, many studies have focused on characterizing a common underlying cause of toxicity in all SOD1-associated fALS cases. Thus a great deal of attention has been directed towards studying the biophysical properties of the more immature forms of SOD1, since fALS-associated mutations have a greater effect on the stability of these forms compared to the fully mature holoS-S form (Lindberg et al. 2004; Furukawa and O'Halloran 2005; Furukawa and O'Halloran 2006; Khare et al. 2006; Nordlund and Oliveberg 2006; Svensson et al. 2006; Smith et al. 2007; Furukawa et al. 2008; Nordlund et al. 2009; Oztug Durer et al. 2009; Tiwari et al. 2009; Kayatekin et al. 2010; Vassall et al. 2011). Despite this recent focus, the form of SOD1 that is most relevant to ALS pathogenesis remains unknown. It is clear that some fALS-associated mutations minimally affect the stability and folding kinetics of apo2SH and apoS-S SOD1, which suggests that it is necessary to look beyond the immature forms of SOD to uncover the cause of ALS.

3.6 Equilibrium denaturation of holoS-S SOD1

Similar to the equilibrium denaturation pathway of apoS-S SOD1, the observed equilibrium denaturation mechanism of holoS-S SOD1 depends on the mode of denaturation and protein concentration. For pWT SOD1, holoS-S equilibrium denaturation curves fit a reversible 3-state model in which the folded holo native dimer transitions to the unfolded monomer through a folded, metallated, monomeric intermediate (Rumfeldt et al. 2006). The presence of bound metal stabilizes the monomer intermediate far more than the dimer interface. Thus, the dimer is only slightly stronger in holoS-S compared to apoS-S, while the free energy of monomer folding is much higher for holoS-S SOD1 compared to apoS-S SOD1 (Rumfeldt et al. 2006; Vassall et al. 2006). At high protein concentrations, the population of the monomer intermediate is significantly reduced and the equilibrium denaturation mechanism approaches 2-state (Rumfeldt et al. 2006). Similarly, in thermal denaturation by DSC, the monomeric intermediate is not significantly populated and the unfolding appears 2-state (Stathopulos et al. 2006). In both chemical and thermal denaturation of holoS-S SOD1, metals remain bound throughout the transition, although binding is weakened in the monomer intermediate and unfolded state compared to the dimer (Rumfeldt et al. 2006; Stathopulos et al. 2006; Kayatekin et al. 2008). Equilibrium denaturation of holoS-S SOD1 reveals that metal binding significantly increases the free energy of unfolding (Table 1). Consistent with this, the melting temperature of holoS-S SOD1 is ~30°C higher than apoS-S SOD1. Thus, it is likely that the stabilizing effects of metallation as well as disulfide bond formation are intrinsic inhibitors of SOD1 aggregation. Mutations therefore may exert toxicity to the cell by inhibiting SOD1 maturation and/or by promoting metal loss, dimer dissociation and/or disulfide reduction (Tiwari and Hayward 2003; Lindberg et al. 2004; Furukawa and O'Halloran 2005; Furukawa and O'Halloran 2006; Banci et al. 2007; Hornberg et al. 2007; Ding and Dokholyan 2008; Furukawa et al. 2008; Tiwari et al. 2009).

Comparable to apoS-S SOD1, the equilibrium denaturation mechanism of fALS-associated mutant holoS-S SOD1 remains the same as pWT. In a number of cases mutations have been shown to decrease the stability of holoS-S, by decreasing the stability of the monomer, with less effect on dimerization (Rumfeldt et al. 2006; Stathopulos et al. 2006; Vassall et al. 2006). This decreased stability of the holoS-S monomer can often be attributed to weakened metal binding (Hayward et al. 2002), as metal dissociation results in an increased population of the less stable apo state. Thus, in most cases mutations appear to have a more local effect on the stability of holoS-S SOD1 compared to apoS-S SOD1 (Rumfeldt et al. 2006; Vassall et al. 2006); yet, structural perturbations due to mutation may propagate further if metal binding is compromised since loop dynamics and interface stability are greatly affected by the presence of metals (Valentine et al. 2005; Smith et al. 2007; Museth et al. 2009). The overwhelming majority of fALS-associated mutations destabilize the holo state, but because of its extremely high thermodynamic stability the absolute increase in the amount of unfolded species will still be very small, and thus unlikely to affect aggregation. What seems more likely to impact disease is increased local structural fluctuations that can arise from metal loss and/or dimer dissociation, exposing regions of the SOD1 structure that can make favourable contacts with other SOD1 molecules, and thereby give rise to aggregation from native-like states (Elam et al. 2003; Hwang et al. 2010).

3.7 Kinetic unfolding and refolding of holoS-S SOD1

Analyzing the kinetics of holoS-S SOD1 folding and unfolding provides a method for further characterizing the marginally stable intermediates that form along the folding pathway as these are not always detected at equilibrium where only the most stable species are measurably populated. These kinetic intermediates nevertheless may play significant roles in holoS-S SOD1 aggregation. Both pWT and wild-type holoS-S kinetically unfold slowly *in vitro* via a monomeric intermediate species which has somewhat weaker metal binding affinity relative to the native dimer (Rumfeldt et al. 2006; Kayatekin et al. 2008; Mulligan et al. 2008; Rumfeldt et al. 2009). The overall rate of holoS-S unfolding is dependent on the microscopic rate constants that define each equilibrium transition (Figure 3A).

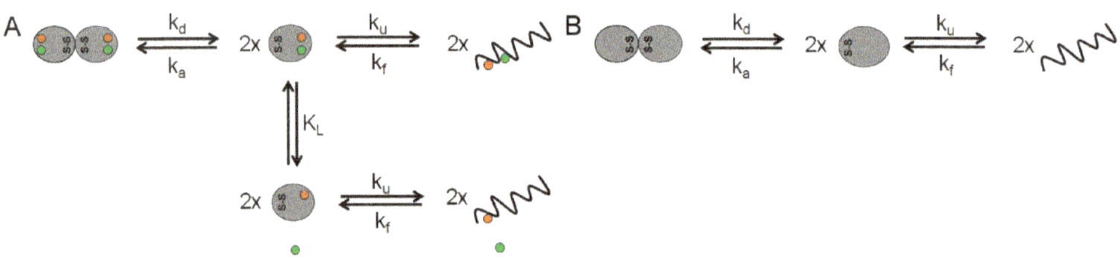

Fig. 3. The kinetic unfolding mechanism of holoS-S and apoS-S SOD1.
In panel A, the kinetic unfolding mechanism of holoS-S SOD1 is shown. The overall rate of unfolding is dependent on the microscopic rate constants k_d, k_a, k_u, k_f, and protein and metal concentration, as well as the equilibrium constant for Zn dissociation from the monomeric intermediate. For a more detailed description refer to (Rumfeldt et al. 2009). In panel B, the simpler kinetic unfolding mechanism of apoS-S SOD1 is shown. The overall rate of unfolding depends only on the microscopic rate constants k_d, k_a, k_u, k_f and protein concentration.

The observed unfolding kinetics therefore depend on the rate of dimer dissociation, which occurs rapidly, and the rate of monomer unfolding, a much slower process (Lynch et al. 2004; Rumfeldt et al. 2009). Under high protein concentration conditions, or in the presence of excess metals, pWT holoS-S SOD1 remains fully metallated as it unfolds, with metals remaining bound to the unfolded state, while at low protein concentrations, Zn can dissociate from both the monomeric intermediate and unfolded monomer (Rumfeldt et al. 2009). Similar results were obtained in kinetic unfolding studies of wild-type holoS-S SOD1 in the presence of a metal chelator, where dimer dissociation and Zn loss were found to occur simultaneously, followed by a conformational change in the β-barrel that precedes and facilitates Cu loss (Mulligan et al. 2008).

The differences in Cu and Zn binding as holoS-S SOD1 unfolds can be rationalized by considering the structural differences in the Cu and Zn binding sites, as follows. While SOD1 binds both metals with extremely high affinity, Cu binds with higher affinity than Zn, with dissociation constants (K_d) estimated as 10^{-18} M and 10^{-14} M (Crow et al. 1997), respectively. In principal, structural differences between the transition state resembling the free energy barrier between the folded and unfolded monomer, compared to the structure of the folded monomer, determine the regions of the protein that, if changed, will have the largest effect on the rate of unfolding. If a particular region is structured in both the monomer and the transition state, then alterations in the stability of that region, either by metal binding or mutation, will affect the free energy of the monomer and its unfolding transition state in a similar way. As a result, the difference in free energy between the folded monomer and transition state and therefore the rate of monomer unfolding will be unaffected. Alternatively, if a particular region of the protein is structured in the folded monomer, but not in the transition state, then changes in the stability of that region will affect the energetics of the folded monomer and transition state differently. In this case the rate of unfolding will be affected. The Cu binding site is formed by residues in β-strands 4 and 7, which are thought to be structured in the transition state, while the Zn binding site is formed mainly by residues in Loop IV and β-strand 5, which are thought to be disordered in the transition state (Nordlund and Oliveberg 2006). Therefore, the rate of unfolding should be affected more by Zn binding than Cu binding and indeed there is some experimental evidence that suggests this to be the case (Rumfeldt et al. 2009).

It has been shown that fALS-associated mutant holoS-S SOD1s increase the unfolding rates of holoS-S SOD1 (Rumfeldt et al. 2009; Ip et al. 2010). Increased unfolding rates and accessibility of either on or off-folding pathway intermediates may increase the accessibility of transient protein species that can initiate aggregation (Dobson 2003; Wang et al. 2008). Furthermore, it has been proposed that fALS-associated mutations, even those far from the metal binding sites, promote increased levels of Cu-deficient intermediates along the holoS-S SOD1 unfolding pathway (Ip et al. 2010). Cu-deficient intermediates are lower in stability and therefore may have a higher tendency to aggregate.

The *in vitro* refolding mechanism of holoS-S SOD1 is more complex than apoS-S SOD1 due to the presence of metal (Figure 3). While the apoS-S form folds via a simple 3-state (2-step) mechanism, with a rate constant that is limited by the rate of monomer folding (see section 3.4), holoS-S refolding occurs through parallel pathways that differ with respect to the fraction of metal bound to the unfolded and transition states (Rumfeldt et al. 2009). However, in the presence of excess Cu and Zn and at high protein concentrations, conditions that favour metal binding to the unfolded state, the refolding kinetics can be described as a simple 2-step process, as each unfolded SOD1 monomer is saturated with metal. Zn coordination in the native binding site stabilizes the monomer intermediate and folded dimer more than the unfolded monomer, accelerating refolding of apoS-S 100 fold (Kayatekin et al. 2008). However, Zn can also bind to non-native sites on the protein (Kayatekin et al. 2008; Nordlund et al. 2009). The Cu-coordinating residues are capable of binding Zn with micromolar affinity in the denatured state after mutation of the native Zn coordinating residues (Nordlund et al. 2009). This non-native coordination of Zn augments the stability of apoS-S SOD1 by increasing the rate of folding and decreasing the rate of unfolding, but forces SOD1 to adopt a non-native conformation. Thus misligation of Zn can cause misfolding and decrease the efficiency of folding (Nordlund et al. 2009). However, with intact Cu and Zn binding sites, Zn may be coordinated by the Cu-binding site first, helping to overcome the main energy barrier of folding, before moving to the Zn-binding site (Nordlund et al. 2009). Other studies have demonstrated that Zn-binding is required to pre-organize the Cu-binding site (Banci et al. 2003). Together these studies show that metal binding significantly modulates the efficiency of the SOD1 folding pathway by stabilizing both the monomer and dimer and decreasing the rate of unfolding. However, non-native metal binding may force the protein to be kinetically trapped in a partially folded, aggregation prone conformation that is more stable than the unfolded state (Nordlund et al. 2009). Together these results show that the kinetic unfolding and refolding mechanism of SOD1 is highly dependent on metal binding.

3.8 fALS mutations and modifications have complex effects on the folding and stability of SOD1

It is evident that fALS-associated mutants have different and complex effects on the stability of SOD1, and these effects depend on the form of SOD1 being studied. For example, mutations that have a large effect on holoS-S SOD1 stability, such as metal binding mutants, tend to have a much smaller effect on the more immature forms of the protein (Valentine et al. 2005). Also, the effects of mutations are more pronounced, but to varying extents for different mutations, with decreasing stability in immature forms of SOD1 (Vassall et al. 2006; Vassall et al. 2011). It is important to understand how both the equilibrium and kinetic folding pathways of all forms of SOD1 are altered by fALS-associated mutations to untangle the complexity of SOD1 aggregation. Certain mutations may have a large effect on the thermodynamic stability of the protein, through weakened metal binding or by decreasing the stability of the dimer interface, while having a smaller effect on the kinetic stability of SOD1. Other mutations may only subtly alter the thermodynamic stability of the native state, exerting their effects by altering the kinetic stability of SOD1 by decreasing the rate of folding, or by increasing the rate of unfolding (Rumfeldt et al. 2006). These effects can increase the equilibrium and/or transient population of folded or unfolded monomeric species that are prone to aggregate (see section 4).

In addition, fALS mutations may alter the susceptibility of SOD1 to post-translational modifications which will tend to decrease protein stability. These include not only enhanced metal loss and disulfide reduction (resulting in higher population of immature species), but also other modifications, in particular ones that are enhanced under oxidizing cellular conditions, which may occur late in disease. Examples include cysteine oxidation (Gruzman et al. 2007; Karch et al. 2009; Bosco et al. 2010), glutathionylation (Proctor et al. 2011), tryptophan oxidation (Elam et al. 2003), and glycation (Meiering 2008). While there is relatively little quantitative data on the effects of these modifications on stability, there is evidence that they can be destabilizing. Such modifications may play different roles at different disease stages; for example, oxidative modifications may become more pronounced as the disease progresses and contribute to rapid disease progression by enhancing formation of toxic aggregates (Karch et al. 2009).

4. SOD1 aggregation

Numerous experimental studies have characterized the aggregation of multiple forms of SOD1. These are described below, focussing mainly on *in vitro* studies, and their implications for disease. It is important to note, however, that it is not yet known what forms of SOD1 are involved in human disease: neither the disulfide bond status nor metal content of SOD1 in aggregates is known. Evidence supports the population of multiple forms of SOD1 *in vivo* (see section 2). Collectively, experimental findings provide support for contributions from many forms of SOD1 to toxic aggregation in ALS.

4.1 Aggregation of Apo2SH SOD1

4.1.1 Evidence of Apo2SH SOD1 aggregation

Aggregation of the marginally stable apoSH form of SOD1 has been suggested in a number of studies to be particularly important in ALS pathogenesis. Studies from multiple groups have reported that wild-type, pWT and fALS-associated mutant apoSH SOD1 are all predisposed to aggregate (Lindberg et al. 2004; Furukawa and O'Halloran 2005; Hornberg et al. 2007; Chattopadhyay et al. 2008; Furukawa et al. 2008; Oztug Durer et al. 2009; Vassall et al. 2011). Additional support for the biological significance of apoSH aggregation is that fALS-associated mutants expressed in insect cells tend to be more metal deficient and disulfide reduced compared to wild type; this finding was proposed to be a consequence of enhanced opening of the mutant SOD1 structures, exposing the disulfide bond to the reducing environment of the cytosol (Tiwari and Hayward 2003). Furthermore, murine models of fALS have revealed the presence of aggregated disulfide reduced SOD1 species (Jonsson et al. 2006; Zetterstrom et al. 2007). Based on what is known about the relationship between protein stability and aggregation propensity (see section 1.2.1), and on the relatively low stability and the expanded, fluctuating structure of apoSH SOD1 (see section 3.1), it appears that aggregation of this form of SOD1 could be significant under cellular conditions (Furukawa et al. 2008). Consistent with this idea, *in vitro* agitation of apo2SH SOD1 results in amyloid fibril formation (Chattopadhyay et al. 2008; Oztug Durer et al. 2009; Furukawa et al. 2010). Although the agitation phenomenon is poorly understood at a molecular level it may favour amyloid fibril formation over pathways to other morphologies. Agitation may enhance aggregation in general by promoting the formation of aggregation-prone species at air-solution or solid-solution interfaces, as well as increase the rate of aggregation by distributing aggregation nuclei more efficiently and causing preformed aggregates to break and create new nucleation sites (Sicorello et al. 2009). Again, it should be noted that since agitation can promote aggregation of many proteins (Rousseau et al. 2008; Mahler et al. 2009; Sicorello et al. 2009), and ALS is not classified as an amyloid disease (Kerman et al. 2010), it is not yet clear how agitation-induced aggregation *in vitro* is related to aggregation in disease.

4.1.2 Mechanisms of Apo2SH SOD1 aggregation

Intriguing structural variations in apoSH amyloid and non-amyloid aggregates have been reported and may be related to the different disease durations for different SOD1 mutants. Structural diversity has been observed in the amyloid fibrils formed by different SOD1 mutants (Furukawa et al. 2010). In addition, *in vitro* aggregation experiments without agitation showed that different apo2SH SOD1 mutants may form different sized, small (~40 nm - 1000 nm), soluble, non-amyloid aggregates (Vassall et al. 2011). These soluble species may be particularly relevant to fALS toxicity, as oligomeric protein aggregates have been implicated as key neurotoxic species in many other neurodegenerative diseases (Caughey and Lansbury 2003; Soto and Estrada 2008). The variations in structural characteristics for apo2SH SOD1s aggregates may indicate that different mutants favour distinct aggregation pathways, depending on the aggregation-prone conformations that mutants may adopt.

Another factor in the heterogeneity of aggregate structures formed may be that apo2SH is appreciably unfolded at physiological temperatures, and therefore may sample multiple aggregation-prone conformations.

4.2 Aggregation of ApoS-S SOD1

4.2.1 Evidence of ApoS-S SOD1 aggregation

Aggregation of the apo S-S form of SOD1 has been studied extensively *in vitro*. This is likely related to the reasonable ease of preparation and aggregation of this quite stable form of the protein (Table 1) (see section 3.3 and 3.4). A role for apoS-S in disease is supported by various *in vitro* and *in vivo* evidence for aggregation of metal-deficient SOD1 as well as evidence that mutations can promote loss of bound metals (Valentine et al. 2005; Molnar et al. 2009; Oztug Durer et al. 2009; Hwang et al. 2010; Lelie et al. 2011). Both wild-type and fALS mutant apoS-S SOD1s are predominantly folded, but mutations can significantly increase the population of folded and unfolded monomeric species (Lindberg et al. 2004; Svensson et al. 2006; Vassall et al. 2006), and increase structural fluctuations (Ding and Dokholyan 2008; Teilum et al. 2009), both of which can promote aggregation. The formation of the disulfide bond decreases the propensity of apoS-S to aggregate compared to apoSH (see section 4.1), while the absence of bound metals in apoS-S SOD1 increases its aggregation propensity compared to holoS-S (see also section 4.3).

Several studies have described the *in vitro* formation of amyloid-like soluble or fibrillar aggregates for wild-type and fALS-associated apoS-S SOD1 mutants (Furukawa and O'Halloran 2005; Banci et al. 2007; Banci et al. 2008; Oztug Durer et al. 2009). Aggregation of mutant SOD1 in these studies was often accelerated by agitation, resulting in the formation of aberrant disulfide bonds between Cys6 and Cys111 (Figure 2) and removal of the free thiol groups by mutation (Banci et al. 2007; Cozzolino et al. 2008) generally diminished aggregation. The role of aberrant disulfide bond formation has been investigated extensively using fALS mutant SOD1 mice models of ALS where it appears that such bonds are observed mainly late in disease (Cozzolino et al. 2008; Karch and Borchelt 2008). These results highlight an important question: does the role of SOD1 differ at different stages of disease? Considerable evidence suggests that the answer is yes; in particular, soluble oligomers may be particularly important early in disease, whereas larger aggregates become prominent after the onset of disease symptoms (Boillee et al. 2006; Cozzolino et al. 2008; Turner and Talbot 2008). Many questions on the roles of different aggregate species and their targets remain unanswered.

A number of studies have reported aggregation of apoS-S SOD1 in the absence of aberrant disulfide bond formation. Formation of such amyloid-like aggregates by pWT and mutant SOD1 can be induced by agitation at neutral pH; however, in these studies the observed ease of aggregation was not correlated with disease duration (Chattopadhyay et al. 2008; Furukawa et al. 2008; Oztug Durer et al. 2009; Furukawa et al. 2010). Also, soluble, reversible aggregates induced by heat were detected by DSC (Vassall et al. unpublished data) (Stathopulos et al. 2006; Vassall et al. 2006). In these studies, mutations in a pWT background generally increased aggregate formation. Furthermore, decreased stability of fALS-associated mutant apoS-S SOD1 was correlated with increased formation of amorphous aggregates that mature into fibril structures that resemble those found in fALS patients (Stathopulos et al. 2003).

4.2.2 Mechanisms of ApoS-S Aggregation

A number of studies have focussed on possible molecular mechanisms of apoS-S SOD1 aggregation, often based on various structural and dynamic data. In the absence of bound metal, there is still extensive disorder in the functional Loops IV and VII, and this disorder may promote exposure of the β-barrel core and deprotection of the β-barrel edge strands (β-strands 5 and 6) (Strange et al. 2007). With these edge strands exposed, H-bonding ligands within the strands are free to interact with the edge strands of other SOD1 molecules and these aberrant contacts can lead to fibril formation (Elam et al. 2003; Nordlund and Oliveberg 2006). As an evolutionary strategy to avoid this fibrillation mechanism, the edge strands of β-proteins often contain charged "gatekeeper" residues, advantageously positioned to disfavour β-sheet extension (Otzen et al. 2000). Protection of the β-barrel edge strands in SOD1 is facilitated both by charged residues in β-strands 5 and 6 and by Loops IV and VII, which block the edge of the β-barrel in the holoS-S form (Nordlund and Oliveberg 2006). The other edge of the β-barrel is buried within the dimer interface. Therefore, the dynamics of Loop IV and VII that cause exposure of either β-strands 5 and 6, or the dimer interface, may lead to fibrillation. Solution NMR experiments of wild-type apoS-S SOD1 suggest that disorder in Loops IV and VII allows stretches of amino acids within these functional loops to form additional β-strands, thereby initiating oligomerization (Banci et al. 2010).

In addition, β-strands 4 and 5 are connected by Loop IV and β-strands 7 and 8 by Loop VII, and the disorder in these long loops appears to propagate to the flanking β-strands. Consequently, the β-sheet formed by strands 4, 5, 7 and 8 is less defined in apoS-S SOD1 compared to the β-sheet formed by strands 1-3 and 6 (Banci et al. 2003; Banci et al. 2010). Thus, metal loss and increased mobility of Loops IV and VII may result in exposure of hydrophobic residues in the β-barrel core (Tiwari et al. 2009). In addition, β-strands 1-3 have been proposed to be a nucleation site for aggregation of apoS-S as they form a continuous patch of hydrophobic residues (Nordlund and Oliveberg 2006). These 3 strands form early in the monomer folding pathway (Lindberg et al. 2004; Nordlund and Oliveberg 2006) and therefore may become exposed by partial unfolding of the apoS-S protein.

The destabilizing effects of fALS-associated mutations appear to propagate significantly in apoS-S SOD1, in particular generally weakening the dimer interface (see section 3.3) (Vassall et al. unpublished data) (Khare et al. 2006; Bystrom et al. 2010). Destabilization of the apoS-S dimer interface can increase the levels of marginally stable, apoS-S monomers. Furthermore, it was demonstrated recently that breathing motions of the wild-type apoS-S monomer result in transient formation of a higher energy species with weakened packing and a partially exposed hydrophobic core (Teilum et al. 2009). fALS-mutations induce further perturbations in this higher energy state that open up the structure of the mutant apoS-S SOD1 monomer more compared to wild type (Teilum et al. 2009) and so may further promote aggregation.

The increased structural dynamics observed for metal-free SOD1 described above, suggests that apoS-S may be predisposed to aggregate compared to the holoS-S state. Several studies have demonstrated that apoS-S SOD1 can aggregate by a variety of different mechanisms that give rise to different aggregate morphologies, including both disulphide cross-linked and non cross-linked species, amyloid-like fibrils and non-amyloid amorphous aggregates.

4.3 Aggregation of SOD1 from the holoS-S state

4.3.1 Evidence of aggregation from the holoS-S state

While the highly stable, native holoS-S form of SOD1 (see section 3.5) generally appears to be much less susceptible to aggregation than other forms of the protein (Stathopulos et al. 2003; Valentine et al. 2005), there is evidence that a number of SOD1 mutants can give rise to aggregation from the holoS-S form. Hwang et al. found that prolonged incubation of both pWT and fALS-associated holoS-S SOD1 mutants at physiological temperature and pH results in changes in metal binding and/or dimerization, diminished specific dismutase activity, and the nucleated formation of low levels of amorphous aggregates (Hwang et al. 2010). Furthermore, these experiments show that, although the aggregated SOD1 demonstrated some metal loss, there was still a significant amount of metal bound, indicating that complete metal loss was not essential for aggregation. Although both pWT and mutant holoS-S SOD1 were observed to aggregate, in general the holoS-S SOD1 mutants lose specific activity quicker, and aggregate more rapidly, and to a greater extent, than pWT. Importantly, the aggregates formed from holoS-S SOD1 in this study exhibited similar structural, dye-binding, and immunological characteristics as the aggregates found in fALS patients (Hwang et al. 2010). In contrast, other studies have reported that SOD1 does not aggregate from the holoS-S form (Chattopadhyay et al. 2008), or requires extremely destabilizing conditions with agitation to promote fibrilization (Oztug Durer et al. 2009). The differences between these findings may be related to the different experimental conditions for studying SOD1 aggregation, such as length of incubation, frequency of sampling, and methods for monitoring aggregation.

4.3.2 Mechanisms of holoS-S aggregation

Immature forms of SOD1 can form amyloid fibrils far more readily than holoS-S (Banci et al. 2007; Furukawa et al. 2008; Oztug Durer et al. 2009), and this difference in aggregation tendency is likely related to the very high stability and rigidity of holoS-S compared to the less mature forms (Stathopulos et al. 2003; Rumfeldt et al. 2006; Stathopulos et al. 2006; Svensson et al. 2006; Vassall et al. 2006; Furukawa et al. 2008; Kayatekin et al. 2008; Kayatekin et al. 2010; Vassall et al. 2011). Highly disordered, predominantly unfolded, proteins tend to favour the formation of amyloid (as may be the case for apo forms of SOD1), whereas more structured proteins favour formation of amorphous aggregates (as for holoS-S) (Munishkina et al. 2004). Measurements of global thermodynamic stability have shown that, owing to the high stability of the holo form, destabilizing mutations will in general cause very small increases in the population of unfolded protein (Rumfeldt et al. 2006; Stathopulos et al. 2006); these increases are unlikely to account for SOD1 aggregation in ALS. Aggregation may alternatively arise from native-like, locally unfolded states (Chiti and Dobson 2009; Hwang et al. 2010) (Figure 1B) which appear to be enhanced in holoS-S SOD1 by some fALS-associated mutations (Shipp et al. 2003; Hough et al. 2004; Banci et al. 2005; Museth et al. 2009). Ultimately, it is likely that some sort of relatively rare/slow structural change is required to bring about aggregation from holoS-S SOD1 (Hwang et al. 2010), in contrast to the apo2SH form, which aggregates readily for some fALS-associated mutant SOD1s (Vassall et al. 2011).

SOD1 aggregation arising from the holoS-S form appears to occur through a nucleation-dependent mechanism that is characterized by a lag phase (i.e. slow nucleation) followed by fast aggregate growth (Hwang et al. 2010). The lag phase corresponds to the time required for holoS-S SOD1 to arrange into an aggregation-prone state and/or form the necessary contacts required for aggregation. It is likely that dimer dissociation and/or metal loss from SOD1 occur during this lag phase and may be important triggers of aggregation (Hwang et al. 2010). Furthermore, various fALS-associated mutations appear to decrease the length of the lag phase, perhaps due to weakened metal binding and/or a weakened dimer interface, (Crow et al. 1997; Khare et al. 2004; Tiwari et al. 2009).

These results suggest that fully mature SOD1 is not devoid of the ability to aggregate, as it could give rise to native-like aggregation-prone species via loss of metal, dimer dissociation, or local structural openings, promoted by mutation. Such aggregation may be highly relevant to fALS toxicity, since holo S-S is generally the most highly abundant form of SOD1 *in vivo* (Valentine et al. 2005).

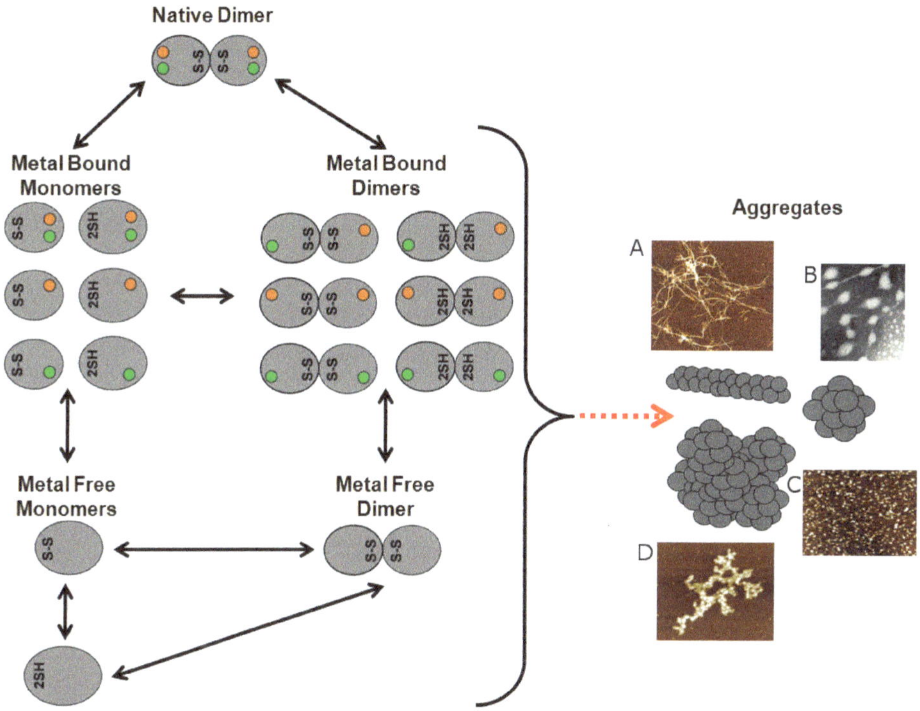

Fig. 4. Many forms of SOD1 may be relevant to ALS toxicity.
SOD1 can exist in many forms *in vivo*, which is illustrated in Figure 4. Each monomer is depicted as a grey sphere that is smaller when metals are bound and/or the disulfide is formed. The presence of Cu and Zn is shown by orange and green spheres, respectively; and S-S and 2SH indicate disulfide oxidized and reduced species, respectively. The difference in SOD1 conformation prior to aggregation may largely influence the morphology of the aggregates formed. Images and schematic representation of possible aggregate morphologies are shown in the centre on the right. Panels A, C and D are Atomic Force Microscopy images of SOD1 aggregates formed *in vitro* (Broom et al, unpublished data) (Hwang et al. 2010) and panel B is an electron microscopy image obtain from of SOD1 aggregates formed *in vitro* (Stathopulos et al. 2003).

5. Conclusion

Numerous studies have revealed that the effects of fALS-associated mutations on the folding, unfolding and aggregation of different forms of SOD1 are highly complex. Mutations can alter both equilibrium stability, in terms of the energetics of dimer dissociation, monomer intermediate stability, and metal binding, and kinetic stability, in terms of the rates of interconversion between various SOD1 species (Section 3). As a consequence, the populations of various aggregation prone species may be increased for different mutations, and this may give rise to different aggregate structures.

There have been a number of attempts to identify the relationships between the effects of the mutations and ALS disease characteristics. In particular, disease duration, which is characteristic for patients carrying a given SOD1 mutation, has been used as a measure of the toxicity of each fALS-associated SOD1 mutation. Early work focused on the loss of superoxide dismutase activity, and increased oxidative stress as the common underlying cause of disease (Valentine et al. 2005). Subsequently, the focus shifted to the toxic gain of function for mutant SOD1, both aberrant enzymatic SOD1 activity, or increased SOD1 aggregation, the latter being the predominant focus of this review. Owing to the high stability and lower aggregation propensity of the holoS-S form, many studies have focused on characterizing the stability and aggregation mechanisms of the more immature, metal deficient SOD1 forms. However, recent work suggests that disease duration does not correlate strongly with the stability of the apoS-S form of mutant SOD1 (Bystrom et al. 2010). This observation was rationalized by considering the role of factors beyond destabilization in modulating aggregation, such as changes in protein net charge and hydrogen bonding. An interesting study by Wang et al. reported that predicted aggregation propensity, based on the physicochemical properties of the polypeptide sequence (Chiti et al. 2003) combined with the stability of mutant apoS-S SOD1 in a summative score and weighted towards mutants with more patient data, correlated fairly well with fALS disease durations (Wang et al. 2008). On the other hand, recent work by Vassall et al. demonstrated that observed aggregation of the apo2SH form is not correlated with disease duration (Vassall et al. 2011). Collectively, these studies demonstrate that multiple factors including protein stability, dynamics, and biophysical characteristics are likely to play a role in modulating SOD1 aggregation, and that fALS phenotypic characteristics are not likely to be fully explained by the aggregation behaviour of any one form of SOD1.

Aggregation studies on holoS-S, apoS-S, and apo2SH SOD1 mutants have identified multiple mechanisms and aggregate morphologies (Section 4 and Figure 4). HoloS-S SOD1, widely thought believed to be much less susceptible to aggregation, has nevertheless been shown to form amorphous aggregates in a nucleation-dependent manner where the lag phase may involve metal loss or monomerization (Hwang et al. 2010). ApoS-S SOD1 may form amyloid- or non-amyloid-like aggregates with or without disulphide cross-linking depending on the solution conditions, and apo2SH SOD1 has been found to adopt the most diverse range of aggregate morphologies, including soluble aggregates under physiologically relevant conditions which may be particularly neurotoxic (Caughey and Lansbury 2003). Considering the influence of SOD1 mutations on the stability, unfolding and folding patterns of all forms of SOD, together with the diverse mechanisms of aggregation, different mutations may be influencing the protein in variable ways, resulting in a wide spectrum of effects. This diversity is likely to play a significant role in the variable disease courses for fALS patients with SOD1 mutations. Ultimately, the role of SOD1 in ALS may be similar to the roles of other globular, oligomeric proteins in misfolding diseases such as: transthyretin in familial amyloidotic polyneuropathy and senile systemic amyloidosis, lysozyme in hereditary non-neuropathic systemic amyloidosis, immunoglobulin light chain in monoclonal protein systemic amyloidosis, prion protein in Kreutzfeld Jakob, and serpins in serpinopathies (Ohnishi and Takano 2004; Harrison et al. 2007). In these diseases mutations are generally destabilizing, but the extent of destabilization of monomer versus subunit interfaces varies widely. The role of SOD1 in disease may be further complicated by the potential aberrant enzymatic activity of misfolded and/or aggregated species which could cause oxidative damage. In addition, it is worth considering the different roles of various types of SOD1 aggregate structures, or contributions of aberrant activity and the effects of these on other cellular components, at different stages throughout the disease course of ALS. For these reasons, it is important that future studies continue to consider the possible roles of multiple forms of SOD1 mutants in modulating the formation of different aggregate structures (Figure 4). A combination of further *in vitro* and *in vivo* studies of folding and aggregation will be critical for untangling the role of toxic aggregation in the syndrome of ALS.

6. Acknowledgements

We thank the ALS Society of Canada, Muscular Dystrophy Canada, and Canadian Institutes of Health Research for their financial support. Furthermore, we would like to express our appreciation to all the members of the Meiering group for their insightful and meaningful discussions, in particular Aron Broom, Martin Smith, Ming Sze Tong and Sarah M. Sullivan.

7. References

Alvarez, B., Demicheli, V., Duran, R., Trujillo, M., Cervenansky, C., Freeman, B. A. and Radi, R. (2004). "Inactivation of human Cu,Zn superoxide dismutase by peroxynitrite and formation of histidinyl radical." *Free Radic Biol Med* 37(6): 813-22.

Andersen, P. M. (2006). "Amyotrophic lateral sclerosis associated with mutations in the CuZn superoxide dismutase gene." *Curr Neurol Neurosci Rep* 6(1): 37-46.

Armstrong, R. A., Nochlin, D. and Bird, T. D. (2000). "Neuropathological heterogeneity in Alzheimer's disease: a study of 80 cases using principal components analysis." *Neuropathology* 20(1): 31-7.

Arnesano, F., Banci, L., Bertini, I., Martinelli, M., Furukawa, Y. and O'Halloran, T. V. (2004). "The unusually stable quaternary structure of human Cu,Zn-superoxide dismutase 1 is controlled by both metal occupancy and disulfide status." *J Biol Chem* 279(46): 47998-8003.

Bai, Y., Englander, J. J., Mayne, L., Milne, J. S. and Englander, S. W. (1995). "Thermodynamic parameters from hydrogen exchange measurements." *Methods Enzymol* 259: 344-56.

Baldwin, A. J., Knowles, T. P., Tartaglia, G., Fitzpatrick, A., Devlin, G., Shammas, S., Waudby, C. A., Mossuto, M. F., Gras, S. L., Christodoulou, J., Anthony-Cahill, S. J., Barker, P. D., Vendruscolo, M. and Dobson, C. M. (2011). "Metastability of Native Proteins and the Phenomenon of Amyloid Formation." *J Am Chem Soc.*

Banci, L., Benedetto, M., Bertini, I., Del Conte, R., Piccioli, M. and Viezzoli, M. S. (1998). "Solution structure of reduced monomeric Q133M2 copper, zinc superoxide dismutase (SOD). Why is SOD a dimeric enzyme?" *Biochemistry* 37(34): 11780-91.

Banci, L., Bertini, I., Blazevits, O., Cantini, F., Lelli, M., Luchinat, C., Mao, J. and Vieru, M. (2010). "NMR Characterization of a "Fibril-Ready" State of Demetalated Wild-Type Superoxide Dismutase." *J Am Chem Soc.*

Banci, L., Bertini, I., Boca, M., Calderone, V., Cantini, F., Girotto, S. and Vieru, M. (2009). "Structural and dynamic aspects related to oligomerization of apo SOD1 and its mutants." *Proc Natl Acad Sci U S A* 106(17): 6980-5.

Banci, L., Bertini, I., Boca, M., Girotto, S., Martinelli, M., Valentine, J. S. and Vieru, M. (2008). "SOD1 and amyotrophic lateral sclerosis: mutations and oligomerization." *PLoS One* 3(2): e1677.

Banci, L., Bertini, I., Cramaro, F., Del Conte, R. and Viezzoli, M. S. (2003). "Solution structure of Apo Cu,Zn superoxide dismutase: role of metal ions in protein folding." *Biochemistry* 42(32): 9543-53.

Banci, L., Bertini, I., D'Amelio, N., Gaggelli, E., Libralesso, E., Matecko, I., Turano, P. and Valentine, J. S. (2005). "Fully metallated S134N Cu,Zn-superoxide dismutase displays abnormal mobility and intermolecular contacts in solution." *J Biol Chem* 280(43): 35815-21.

Banci, L., Bertini, I., Durazo, A., Girotto, S., Gralla, E. B., Martinelli, M., Valentine, J. S., Vieru, M. and Whitelegge, J. P. (2007). "Metal-free superoxide dismutase forms soluble oligomers under physiological conditions: a possible general mechanism for familial ALS." *Proc Natl Acad Sci U S A* 104(27): 11263-7.

Bastos, A. F., Orsini, M., Machado, D., Mello, M. P., Nader, S., Silva, J. G., da Silva Catharino, A. M., de Freitas, M. R., Pereira, A., Pessoa, L. L., Sztajnbok, F. R., Leite, M. A., Nascimento, O. J. and Bastos, V. H. (2011). "Amyotrophic lateral sclerosis: one or multiple causes?" *Neurol Int* 3(1): e4.

Berryman, J. T., Radford, S. E. and Harris, S. A. (2009). "Thermodynamic description of polymorphism in Q- and N-rich peptide aggregates revealed by atomistic simulation." *Biophys J* 97(1): 1-11.

Bertini, I., Piccioli, M., Viezzoli, M. S., Chiu, C. Y. and Mullenbach, G. T. (1994). "A spectroscopic characterization of a monomeric analog of copper, zinc superoxide dismutase." *Eur Biophys J* 23(3): 167-76.

Boillee, S., Vande Velde, C. and Cleveland, D. W. (2006). "ALS: a disease of motor neurons and their nonneuronal neighbors." *Neuron* 52(1): 39-59.

Bosco, D. A., Morfini, G., Karabacak, N. M., Song, Y., Gros-Louis, F., Pasinelli, P., Goolsby, H., Fontaine, B. A., Lemay, N., McKenna-Yasek, D., Frosch, M. P., Agar, J. N., Julien, J. P., Brady, S. T. and Brown, R. H., Jr. (2010). "Wild-type and mutant SOD1 share an aberrant conformation and a common pathogenic pathway in ALS." *Nat Neurosci* 13(11): 1396-403.

Brown, N. M., Torres, A. S., Doan, P. E. and O'Halloran, T. V. (2004). "Oxygen and the copper chaperone CCS regulate posttranslational activation of Cu,Zn superoxide dismutase." *Proc Natl Acad Sci U S A* 101(15): 5518-23.

Bruening, W., Roy, J., Giasson, B., Figlewicz, D. A., Mushynski, W. E. and Durham, H. D. (1999). "Up-regulation of protein chaperones preserves viability of cells expressing toxic Cu/Zn-superoxide dismutase mutants associated with amyotrophic lateral sclerosis." *J Neurochem* 72(2): 693-9.

Bruijn, L. I., Houseweart, M. K., Kato, S., Anderson, K. L., Anderson, S. D., Ohama, E., Reaume, A. G., Scott, R. W. and Cleveland, D. W. (1998). "Aggregation and motor neuron toxicity of an ALS-linked SOD1 mutant independent from wild-type SOD1." *Science* 281(5384): 1851-4.

Bruijn, L. I., Miller, T. M. and Cleveland, D. W. (2004). "Unraveling the mechanisms involved in motor neuron degeneration in ALS." *Annu Rev Neurosci* 27: 723-49.

Bucciantini, M., Giannoni, E., Chiti, F., Baroni, F., Formigli, L., Zurdo, J., Taddei, N., Ramponi, G., Dobson, C. M. and Stefani, M. (2002). "Inherent toxicity of aggregates implies a common mechanism for protein misfolding diseases." *Nature* 416(6880): 507-11.

Bystrom, R., Andersen, P. M., Grobner, G. and Oliveberg, M. (2010). "SOD1 mutations targeting surface hydrogen bonds promote amyotrophic lateral sclerosis without reducing apo-state stability." *J Biol Chem* 285(25): 19544-52.

Caughey, B. and Lansbury, P. T., Jr. (2003). "Protofibrils, Pores, Fibrils, and Neurodegeneration: Separating the Responsibility Protein Aggregates from The Innocent Bystanders." *Annual Review of Neuroscience* 26: 267-298.

Chattopadhyay, M., Durazo, A., Sohn, S. H., Strong, C. D., Gralla, E. B., Whitelegge, J. P. and Valentine, J. S. (2008). "Initiation and elongation in fibrillation of ALS-linked superoxide dismutase." *Proc Natl Acad Sci U S A* 105(48): 18663-8.

Chattopadhyay, M. and Valentine, J. S. (2009). "Aggregation of Copper-Zinc Superoxide Dismutase in Familial and Sporadic ALS." *Antioxid Redox Signal.*

Chi, E. Y., Krishnan, S., Randolph, T. W. and Carpenter, J. F. (2003). "Physical stability of proteins in aqueous solution: mechanism and driving forces in nonnative protein aggregation." *Pharm Res* 20(9): 1325-36.

Chiti, F. and Dobson, C. M. (2006). "Protein misfolding, functional amyloid, and human disease." *Annu Rev Biochem* 75: 333-66.

Chiti, F. and Dobson, C. M. (2009). "Amyloid formation by globular proteins under native conditions." *Nat Chem Biol* 5(1): 15-22.

Chiti, F., Stefani, M., Taddei, N., Ramponi, G. and Dobson, C. M. (2003). "Rationalization of the effects of mutations on peptide and protein aggregation rates." *Nature* 424(6950): 805-8.

Chrunyk, B. A. and Wetzel, R. (1993). "Breakdown in the relationship between thermal and thermodynamic stability in an interleukin-1 beta point mutant modified in a surface loop." *Protein Eng* 6(7): 733-8.

Cozzolino, M., Ferri, A. and Carri, M. T. (2008). "Amyotrophic lateral sclerosis: from current developments in the laboratory to clinical implications." *Antioxid Redox Signal* 10(3): 405-43.

Crow, J. P., Sampson, J. B., Zhuang, Y., Thompson, J. A. and Beckman, J. S. (1997). "Decreased zinc affinity of amyotrophic lateral sclerosis-associated superoxide dismutase mutants leads to enhanced catalysis of tyrosine nitration by peroxynitrite." *J Neurochem* 69(5): 1936-44.

Cudkowicz, M. E., McKenna-Yasek, D., Sapp, P. E., Chin, W., Geller, B., Hayden, D. L., Schoenfeld, D. A., Hosler, B. A., Horvitz, H. R. and Brown, R. H. (1997).

"Epidemiology of mutations in superoxide dismutase in amyotrophic lateral sclerosis." *Ann Neurol* 41(2): 210-21.

Deng, H. X., Chen, W., Hong, S. T., Boycott, K. M., Gorrie, G. H., Siddique, N., Yang, Y., Fecto, F., Shi, Y., Zhai, H., Jiang, H., Hirano, M., Rampersaud, E., Jansen, G. H., Donkervoort, S., Bigio, E. H., Brooks, B. R., Ajroud, K., Sufit, R. L., Haines, J. L., Mugnaini, E., Pericak-Vance, M. A. and Siddique, T. (2011). "Mutations in UBQLN2 cause dominant X-linked juvenile and adult-onset ALS and ALS/dementia." *Nature*.

Deng, H. X., Hentati, A., Tainer, J. A., Iqbal, Z., Cayabyab, A., Hung, W. Y., Getzoff, E. D., Hu, P., Herzfeldt, B., Roos, R. P. and et al. (1993). "Amyotrophic lateral sclerosis and structural defects in Cu,Zn superoxide dismutase." *Science* 261(5124): 1047-51.

Ding, F. and Dokholyan, N. V. (2008). "Dynamical roles of metal ions and the disulfide bond in Cu, Zn superoxide dismutase folding and aggregation." *Proc Natl Acad Sci U S A* 105(50): 19696-701.

Dobson, C. M. (1999). "Protein misfolding, evolution and disease." *Trends Biochem Sci* 24(9): 329-32.

Dobson, C. M. (2003). "Protein folding and misfolding." *Nature* 426(6968): 884-90.

Dobson, C. M. (2004). "Principles of protein folding, misfolding and aggregation." *Semin Cell Dev Biol* 15(1): 3-16.

Eisenberg, D., Nelson, R., Sawaya, M. R., Balbirnie, M., Sambashivan, S., Ivanova, M. I., Madsen, A. O. and Riekel, C. (2006). "The structural biology of protein aggregation diseases: Fundamental questions and some answers." *Acc Chem Res* 39(9): 568-75.

Elam, J. S., Taylor, A. B., Strange, R., Antonyuk, S., Doucette, P. A., Rodriguez, J. A., Hasnain, S. S., Hayward, L. J., Valentine, J. S., Yeates, T. O. and Hart, P. J. (2003). "Amyloid-like filaments and water-filled nanotubes formed by SOD1 mutant proteins linked to familial ALS." *Nat Struct Biol* 10(6): 461-7.

Fink, A. L. (1998). "Protein aggregation: folding aggregates, inclusion bodies and amyloid." *Fold Des* 3(1): R9-23.

Forsberg, K., Andersen, P. M., Marklund, S. L. and Brannstrom, T. (2011). "Glial nuclear aggregates of superoxide dismutase-1 are regularly present in patients with amyotrophic lateral sclerosis." *Acta Neuropathol*.

Frost, B. and Diamond, M. I. (2009). "The expanding realm of prion phenomena in neurodegenerative disease." *Prion* 3(2): 74-7.

Furukawa, Y., Kaneko, K., Yamanaka, K. and Nukina, N. (2010). "Mutation-dependent polymorphism of Cu,Zn-superoxide dismutase aggregates in the familial form of amyotrophic lateral sclerosis." *J Biol Chem* 285(29): 22221-31.

Furukawa, Y., Kaneko, K., Yamanaka, K., O'Halloran, T. V. and Nukina, N. (2008). "Complete loss of post-translational modifications triggers fibrillar aggregation of SOD1 in the familial form of amyotrophic lateral sclerosis." *J Biol Chem* 283(35): 24167-76.

Furukawa, Y. and O'Halloran, T. V. (2005). "Amyotrophic lateral sclerosis mutations have the greatest destabilizing effect on the apo- and reduced form of SOD1, leading to unfolding and oxidative aggregation." *J Biol Chem* 280(17): 17266-74.

Furukawa, Y. and O'Halloran, T. V. (2006). "Posttranslational modifications in Cu,Zn-superoxide dismutase and mutations associated with amyotrophic lateral sclerosis." *Antioxid Redox Signal* 8(5-6): 847-67.

Getzoff, E. D., Tainer, J. A., Stempien, M. M., Bell, G. I. and Hallewell, R. A. (1989). "Evolution of CuZn superoxide dismutase and the Greek key beta-barrel structural motif." *Proteins* 5(4): 322-36.

Gidalevitz, T., Kikis, E. A. and Morimoto, R. I. (2010). "A cellular perspective on conformational disease: the role of genetic background and proteostasis networks." *Curr Opin Struct Biol* 20(1): 23-32.

Goedert, M., Spillantini, M. G., Serpell, L. C., Berriman, J., Smith, M. J., Jakes, R. and Crowther, R. A. (2001). "From genetics to pathology: tau and alpha-synuclein assemblies in neurodegenerative diseases." *Philos Trans R Soc Lond B Biol Sci* 356(1406): 213-27.

Goers, J., Permyakov, S. E., Permyakov, E. A., Uversky, V. N. and Fink, A. L. (2002). "Conformational prerequisites for alpha-lactalbumin fibrillation." *Biochemistry* 41(41): 12546-51.

Gruzman, A., Wood, W. L., Alpert, E., Prasad, M. D., Miller, R. G., Rothstein, J. D., Bowser, R., Hamilton, R., Wood, T. D., Cleveland, D. W., Lingappa, V. R. and Liu, J. (2007). "Common molecular signature in SOD1 for both sporadic and familial amyotrophic lateral sclerosis." *Proc Natl Acad Sci U S A* 104(30): 12524-9.

Hallewell, R. A., Imlay, K. C., Lee, P., Fong, N. M., Gallegos, C., Getzoff, E. D., Tainer, J. A., Cabelli, D. E., Tekamp-Olson, P., Mullenbach, G. T. and et al. (1991). "Thermostabilization of recombinant human and bovine CuZn superoxide dismutases by replacement of free cysteines." *Biochem Biophys Res Commun* 181(1): 474-80.

Harrison, R. S., Sharpe, P. C., Singh, Y. and Fairlie, D. P. (2007). "Amyloid peptides and proteins in review." *Rev Physiol Biochem Pharmacol* 159: 1-77.

Hayward, L. J., Rodriguez, J. A., Kim, J. W., Tiwari, A., Goto, J. J., Cabelli, D. E., Valentine, J. S. and Brown, R. H., Jr. (2002). "Decreased metallation and activity in subsets of mutant superoxide dismutases associated with familial amyotrophic lateral sclerosis." *J Biol Chem* 277(18): 15923-31.

Hol, E. M. and Scheper, W. (2008). "Protein quality control in neurodegeneration: walking the tight rope between health and disease." *J Mol Neurosci* 34(1): 23-33.

Hornberg, A., Logan, D. T., Marklund, S. L. and Oliveberg, M. (2007). "The coupling between disulphide status, metallation and dimer interface strength in Cu/Zn superoxide dismutase." *J Mol Biol* 365(2): 333-42.

Hough, M. A., Grossmann, J. G., Antonyuk, S. V., Strange, R. W., Doucette, P. A., Rodriguez, J. A., Whitson, L. J., Hart, P. J., Hayward, L. J., Valentine, J. S. and Hasnain, S. S. (2004). "Dimer destabilization in superoxide dismutase may result in disease-causing properties: structures of motor neuron disease mutants." *Proc Natl Acad Sci U S A* 101(16): 5976-81.

http://alsod.iop.kcl.ac.uk/.

Hwang, Y. M., Stathopulos, P. B., Dimmick, K., Yang, H., Badiei, H. R., Tong, M. S., Rumfeldt, J. A., Chen, P., Karanassios, V. and Meiering, E. M. (2010). "Nonamyloid aggregates arising from mature copper/zinc superoxide dismutases resemble those observed in amyotrophic lateral sclerosis." *J Biol Chem* 285(53): 41701-11.

Ilieva, H., Polymenidou, M. and Cleveland, D. W. (2009). "Non-cell autonomous toxicity in neurodegenerative disorders: ALS and beyond." *J Cell Biol* 187(6): 761-72.

Ip, P., Mulligan, V. K. and Chakrabartty, A. (2010). "ALS-causing SOD1 mutations promote production of copper-deficient misfolded species." *J Mol Biol* 409(5): 839-52.

Jackson, S. E. (1998). "How do small single-domain proteins fold? ." *Folding and Design* 3(4): R81-R91.

Jahn, T. R. and Radford, S. E. (2008). "Folding versus aggregation: polypeptide conformations on competing pathways." *Arch Biochem Biophys* 469(1): 100-17.

Johnston, J. A., Dalton, M. J., Gurney, M. E. and Kopito, R. R. (2000). "Formation of high molecular weight complexes of mutant Cu, Zn-superoxide dismutase in a mouse model for familial amyotrophic lateral sclerosis." *Proc Natl Acad Sci U S A* 97(23): 12571-6.

Jones, E. M. and Surewicz, W. K. (2005). "Fibril conformation as the basis of species- and strain-dependent seeding specificity of mammalian prion amyloids." *Cell* 121(1): 63-72.

Jonsson, P. A., Graffmo, K. S., Andersen, P. M., Brannstrom, T., Lindberg, M., Oliveberg, M. and Marklund, S. L. (2006). "Disulphide-reduced superoxide dismutase-1 in CNS of transgenic amyotrophic lateral sclerosis models." *Brain* 129(Pt 2): 451-64.

Karch, C. M. and Borchelt, D. R. (2008). "A limited role for disulfide cross-linking in the aggregation of mutant SOD1 linked to familial amyotrophic lateral sclerosis." *J Biol Chem* 283(20): 13528-37.

Karch, C. M., Prudencio, M., Winkler, D. D., Hart, P. J. and Borchelt, D. R. (2009). "Role of mutant SOD1 disulfide oxidation and aggregation in the pathogenesis of familial ALS." *Proc Natl Acad Sci U S A* 106(19): 7774-9.

Kato, S., Horiuchi, S., Liu, J., Cleveland, D. W., Shibata, N., Nakashima, K., Nagai, R., Hirano, A., Takikawa, M., Kato, M., Nakano, I. and Ohama, E. (2000). "Advanced glycation endproduct-modified superoxide dismutase-1 (SOD1)-positive inclusions are common to familial amyotrophic lateral sclerosis patients with SOD1 gene mutations and transgenic mice expressing human SOD1 with a G85R mutation." *Acta Neuropathol* 100(5): 490-505.

Kayatekin, C., Zitzewitz, J. A. and Matthews, C. R. (2008). "Zinc binding modulates the entire folding free energy surface of human Cu,Zn superoxide dismutase." *J Mol Biol* 384(2): 540-55.

Kayatekin, C., Zitzewitz, J. A. and Matthews, C. R. (2010). "Disulfide-reduced ALS variants of Cu, Zn superoxide dismutase exhibit increased populations of unfolded species." *J Mol Biol* 398(2): 320-31.

Kerman, A., Liu, H. N., Croul, S., Bilbao, J., Rogaeva, E., Zinman, L., Robertson, J. and Chakrabartty, A. (2010). "Amyotrophic lateral sclerosis is a non-amyloid disease in which extensive misfolding of SOD1 is unique to the familial form." *Acta Neuropathol* 119(3): 335-344.

Khare, S. D., Caplow, M. and Dokholyan, N. V. (2004). "The rate and equilibrium constants for a multistep reaction sequence for the aggregation of superoxide dismutase in amyotrophic lateral sclerosis." *Proc Natl Acad Sci U S A* 101(42): 15094-9.

Khare, S. D., Caplow, M. and Dokholyan, N. V. (2006). "FALS mutations in Cu, Zn superoxide dismutase destabilize the dimer and increase dimer dissociation propensity: a large-scale thermodynamic analysis." *Amyloid* 13(4): 226-35.

Knowles, T. P., Fitzpatrick, A. W., Meehan, S., Mott, H. R., Vendruscolo, M., Dobson, C. M. and Welland, M. E. (2007). "Role of intermolecular forces in defining material properties of protein nanofibrils." *Science* 318(5858): 1900-3.

Kurahashi, T., Miyazaki, A., Suwan, S. and Isobe, M. (2001). "Extensive investigations on oxidized amino acid residues in H(2)O(2)-treated Cu,Zn-SOd protein with LC-ESI-Q-TOF-MS, MS/MS for the determination of the copper-binding site." *J Am Chem Soc* 123(38): 9268-78.

Leitch, J. M., Yick, P. J. and Culotta, V. C. (2009). "The right to choose: multiple pathways for activating copper,zinc superoxide dismutase." *J Biol Chem* 284(37): 24679-83.

Lelie, H. L., Liba, A., Bourassa, M. W., Chattopadhyay, M., Chan, P. K., Gralla, E. B., Miller, L. M., Borchelt, D. R., Valentine, J. S. and Whitelegge, J. P. (2011). "Copper and zinc metallation status of copper-zinc superoxide dismutase from amyotrophic lateral sclerosis transgenic mice." *J Biol Chem* 286(4): 2795-806.

Lepock, J. R., Frey, H. E. and Hallewell, R. A. (1990). "Contribution of conformational stability and reversibility of unfolding to the increased thermostability of human and bovine superoxide dismutase mutated at free cysteines." *J Biol Chem* 265(35): 21612-8.

Lepock, J. R., Ritchie, K. P., Kolios, M. C., Rodahl, A. M., Heinz, K. A. and Kruuv, J. (1992). "Influence of transition rates and scan rate on kinetic simulations of differential scanning calorimetry profiles of reversible and irreversible protein denaturation." *Biochemistry* 31(50): 12706-12.

Lindberg, M. J., Normark, J., Holmgren, A. and Oliveberg, M. (2004). "Folding of human superoxide dismutase: disulfide reduction prevents dimerization and produces marginally stable monomers." *Proc Natl Acad Sci U S A* 101(45): 15893-8.

Liu, H. N., Sanelli, T., Horne, P., Pioro, E. P., Strong, M. J., Rogaeva, E., Bilbao, J., Zinman, L. and Robertson, J. (2009). "Lack of evidence of monomer/misfolded superoxide dismutase-1 in sporadic amyotrophic lateral sclerosis." *Ann Neurol* 66(1): 75-80.

Lynch, S. M., Boswell, S. A. and Colon, W. (2004). "Kinetic stability of Cu/Zn superoxide dismutase is dependent on its metal ligands: implications for ALS." *Biochemistry* 43(51): 16525-31.

Mahler, H. C., Friess, W., Grauschopf, U. and Kiese, S. (2009). "Protein aggregation: pathways, induction factors and analysis." *J Pharm Sci* 98(9): 2909-34.

McRee, D. E., Redford, S. M., Getzoff, E. D., Lepock, J. R., Hallewell, R. A. and Tainer, J. A. (1990). "Changes in crystallographic structure and thermostability of a Cu,Zn superoxide dismutase mutant resulting from the removal of a buried cysteine." *J Biol Chem* 265(24): 14234-41.

Meiering, E. M. (2008). "The threat of instability: neurodegeneration predicted by protein destabilization and aggregation propensity." *PLoS Biol* 6(7): e193.

Mitchell, J. D. and Borasio, G. D. (2007). "Amyotrophic lateral sclerosis." *Lancet* 369(9578): 2031-41.

Molnar, K. S., Karabacak, N. M., Johnson, J. L., Wang, Q., Tiwari, A., Hayward, L. J., Coales, S. J., Hamuro, Y. and Agar, J. N. (2009). "A common property of amyotrophic lateral sclerosis-associated variants: destabilization of the copper/zinc superoxide dismutase electrostatic loop." *J Biol Chem* 284(45): 30965-73.

Mouradian, M. M. (2002). "Recent advances in the genetics and pathogenesis of Parkinson disease." *Neurology* 58(2): 179-85.

Mulligan, V. K., Kerman, A., Ho, S. and Chakrabartty, A. (2008). "Denaturational stress induces formation of zinc-deficient monomers of Cu,Zn superoxide dismutase: implications for pathogenesis in amyotrophic lateral sclerosis." *J Mol Biol* 383(2): 424-36.

Munch, C. and Bertolotti, A. (2010). "Exposure of hydrophobic surfaces initiates aggregation of diverse ALS-causing superoxide dismutase-1 mutants." *J Mol Biol* 399(3): 512-25.

Munishkina, L. A., Henriques, J., Uversky, V. N. and Fink, A. L. (2004). "Role of protein-water interactions and electrostatics in alpha-synuclein fibril formation." *Biochemistry* 43(11): 3289-300.

Museth, A. K., Brorsson, A. C., Lundqvist, M., Tibell, L. A. and Jonsson, B. H. (2009). "The ALS-associated mutation G93A in human copper-zinc superoxide dismutase selectively destabilizes the remote metal binding region." *Biochemistry* 48(37): 8817-29.

Natalello, A., Prokorov, V. V., Tagliavini, F., Morbin, M., Forloni, G., Beeg, M., Manzoni, C., Colombo, L., Gobbi, M., Salmona, M. and Doglia, S. M. (2008). "Conformational plasticity of the Gerstmann-Straussler-Scheinker disease peptide as indicated by its multiple aggregation pathways." *J Mol Biol* 381(5): 1349-61.

Necula, M., Breydo, L., Milton, S., Kayed, R., van der Veer, W. E., Tone, P. and Glabe, C. G. (2007). "Methylene blue inhibits amyloid Abeta oligomerization by promoting fibrillization." *Biochemistry* 46(30): 8850-60.

Nelson, R. and Eisenberg, D. (2006). "Structural models of amyloid-like fibrils." *Adv Protein Chem* 73: 235-82.

Nordlund, A., Leinartaite, L., Saraboji, K., Aisenbrey, C., Grobner, G., Zetterstrom, P., Danielsson, J., Logan, D. T. and Oliveberg, M. (2009). "Functional features cause misfolding of the ALS-provoking enzyme SOD1." *Proc Natl Acad Sci U S A* 106(24): 9667-72.

Nordlund, A. and Oliveberg, M. (2006). "Folding of Cu/Zn superoxide dismutase suggests structural hotspots for gain of neurotoxic function in ALS: parallels to precursors in amyloid disease." *Proc Natl Acad Sci U S A* 103(27): 10218-23.

Ohnishi, S. and Takano, K. (2004). "Amyloid fibrils from the viewpoint of protein folding." *Cell Mol Life Sci* 61(5): 511-24.

Okado-Matsumoto, A. and Fridovich, I. (2002). "Amyotrophic lateral sclerosis: a proposed mechanism." *Proc Natl Acad Sci U S A* 99(13): 9010-4.

Otzen, D. E., Kristensen, O. and Oliveberg, M. (2000). "Designed protein tetramer zipped together with a hydrophobic Alzheimer homology: a structural clue to amyloid assembly." *Proc Natl Acad Sci U S A* 97(18): 9907-12.

Oztug Durer, Z. A., Cohlberg, J. A., Dinh, P., Padua, S., Ehrenclou, K., Downes, S., Tan, J. K., Nakano, Y., Bowman, C. J., Hoskins, J. L., Kwon, C., Mason, A. Z., Rodriguez, J. A., Doucette, P. A., Shaw, B. F. and Selverstone Valentine, J. (2009). "Loss of metal ions, disulfide reduction and mutations related to familial ALS promote formation of amyloid-like aggregates from superoxide dismutase." *PLoS One* 4(3): e5004.

Parge, H. E., Hallewell, R. A. and Tainer, J. A. (1992). "Atomic structures of wild-type and thermostable mutant recombinant human Cu,Zn superoxide dismutase." *Proc Natl Acad Sci U S A* 89(13): 6109-13.

Pasinelli, P. and Brown, R. H. (2006). "Molecular biology of amyotrophic lateral sclerosis: insights from genetics." *Nat Rev Neurosci* 7(9): 710-23.

Platt, G. W. and Radford, S. E. (2009). "Glimpses of the molecular mechanisms of beta2-microglobulin fibril formation in vitro: aggregation on a complex energy landscape." *FEBS Lett* 583(16): 2623-9.

Proctor, E. A., Ding, F. and Dokholyan, N. V. (2011). "Structural and thermodynamic effects of post-translational modifications in mutant and wild type Cu, Zn superoxide dismutase." *J Mol Biol* 408(3): 555-67.

Prudencio, M., Durazo, A., Whitelegge, J. P. and Borchelt, D. R. (2009). "Modulation of mutant superoxide dismutase 1 aggregation by co-expression of wild-type enzyme." *J Neurochem* 108(4): 1009-18.

Ramshini, H., Parrini, C., Relini, A., Zampagni, M., Mannini, B., Pesce, A., Saboury, A. A., Nemat-Gorgani, M. and Chiti, F. (2011). "Large proteins have a great tendency to aggregate but a low propensity to form amyloid fibrils." *PLoS One* 6(1): e16075.

Rodriguez, J. A., Shaw, B. F., Durazo, A., Sohn, S. H., Doucette, P. A., Nersissian, A. M., Faull, K. F., Eggers, D. K., Tiwari, A., Hayward, L. J. and Valentine, J. S. (2005). "Destabilization of apoprotein is insufficient to explain Cu,Zn-superoxide dismutase-linked ALS pathogenesis." *Proc Natl Acad Sci U S A* 102(30): 10516-21.

Rosen, D. R., Siddique, T., Patterson, D., Figlewicz, D. A., Sapp, P., Hentati, A., Donaldson, D., Goto, J., O'Regan, J. P., Deng, H. X. and et al. (1993). "Mutations in Cu/Zn superoxide dismutase gene are associated with familial amyotrophic lateral sclerosis." *Nature* 362(6415): 59-62.

Rousseau, F., Schymkowitz, J. and Oliveberg, M. (2008). "ALS precursor finally shaken into fibrils." *Proc Natl Acad Sci U S A* 105(48): 18649-50.

Rumfeldt, J. A., Lepock, J. R. and Meiering, E. M. (2009). "Unfolding and folding kinetics of amyotrophic lateral sclerosis-associated mutant Cu,Zn superoxide dismutases." *J Mol Biol* 385(1): 278-98.

Rumfeldt, J. A., Stathopulos, P. B., Chakrabarrty, A., Lepock, J. R. and Meiering, E. M. (2006). "Mechanism and thermodynamics of guanidinium chloride-induced denaturation of ALS-associated mutant Cu,Zn superoxide dismutases." *J Mol Biol* 355(1): 106-23.

Sakamoto, K. M. (2002). "Ubiquitin-dependent proteolysis: its role in human diseases and the design of therapeutic strategies." *Mol Genet Metab* 77(1-2): 44-56.

Sandelin, E., Nordlund, A., Andersen, P. M., Marklund, S. S. and Oliveberg, M. (2007). "Amyotrophic lateral sclerosis-associated copper/zinc superoxide dismutase mutations preferentially reduce the repulsive charge of the proteins." *J Biol Chem* 282(29): 21230-6.

Serpell, L. C. (2000). "Alzheimer's amyloid fibrils: structure and assembly." *Biochim Biophys Acta* 1502(1): 16-30.

Seshadri, S., Oberg, K. A. and Uversky, V. N. (2009). "Mechanisms and consequences of protein aggregation: the role of folding intermediates." *Curr Protein Pept Sci* 10(5): 456-63.

Shaw, B. F. and Valentine, J. S. (2007). "How do ALS-associated mutations in superoxide dismutase 1 promote aggregation of the protein?" *Trends Biochem Sci* 32(2): 78-85.

Shinder, G. A., Lacourse, M. C., Minotti, S. and Durham, H. D. (2001). "Mutant Cu/Zn-superoxide dismutase proteins have altered solubility and interact with heat shock/stress proteins in models of amyotrophic lateral sclerosis." *J Biol Chem* 276(16): 12791-6.

Shipp, E. L., Cantini, F., Bertini, I., Valentine, J. S. and Banci, L. (2003). "Dynamic properties of the G93A mutant of copper-zinc superoxide dismutase as detected by NMR spectroscopy: implications for the pathology of familial amyotrophic lateral sclerosis." *Biochemistry* 42(7): 1890-9.

Sicorello, A., Torrassa, S., Soldi, G., Gianni, S., Travaglini-Allocatelli, C., Taddei, N., Relini, A. and Chiti, F. (2009). "Agitation and high ionic strength induce amyloidogenesis of a folded PDZ domain in native conditions." *Biophys J* 96(6): 2289-98.

Sipe, J. D. and Cohen, A. S. (2000). "Review: history of the amyloid fibril." *J Struct Biol* 130(2-3): 88-98.

Smith, M. I., Sharp, J. S. and Roberts, C. J. (2007). "Nucleation and growth of insulin fibrils in bulk solution and at hydrophobic polystyrene surfaces." *Biophys J* 93(6): 2143-51.

Soto, C. and Estrada, L. D. (2008). "Protein misfolding and neurodegeneration." *Arch Neurol* 65(2): 184-9.

Stathopulos, P. B., Rumfeldt, J. A., Karbassi, F., Siddall, C. A., Lepock, J. R. and Meiering, E. M. (2006). "Calorimetric analysis of thermodynamic stability and aggregation for apo and holo amyotrophic lateral sclerosis-associated Gly-93 mutants of superoxide dismutase." *J Biol Chem* 281(10): 6184-93.

Stathopulos, P. B., Rumfeldt, J. A., Scholz, G. A., Irani, R. A., Frey, H. E., Hallewell, R. A., Lepock, J. R. and Meiering, E. M. (2003). "Cu/Zn superoxide dismutase mutants associated with amyotrophic lateral sclerosis show enhanced formation of aggregates in vitro." *Proc Natl Acad Sci U S A* 100(12): 7021-6.

Stathopulos, P. B., Scholz, G. A., Hwang, Y. M., Rumfeldt, J. A., Lepock, J. R. and Meiering, E. M. (2004). "Sonication of proteins causes formation of aggregates that resemble amyloid." *Protein Sci* 13(11): 3017-27.

Strange, R. W., Antonyuk, S., Hough, M. A., Doucette, P. A., Rodriguez, J. A., Hart, P. J., Hayward, L. J., Valentine, J. S. and Hasnain, S. S. (2003). "The structure of holo and metal-deficient wild-type human Cu, Zn superoxide dismutase and its relevance to familial amyotrophic lateral sclerosis." *J Mol Biol* 328(4): 877-91.

Strange, R. W., Yong, C. W., Smith, W. and Hasnain, S. S. (2007). "Molecular dynamics using atomic-resolution structure reveal structural fluctuations that may lead to polymerization of human Cu-Zn superoxide dismutase." *Proc Natl Acad Sci U S A* 104(24): 10040-4.

Svensson, A. K., Bilsel, O., Kondrashkina, E., Zitzewitz, J. A. and Matthews, C. R. (2006). "Mapping the folding free energy surface for metal-free human Cu,Zn superoxide dismutase." *J Mol Biol* 364(5): 1084-102.

Tainer, J. A., Getzoff, E. D., Beem, K. M., Richardson, J. S. and Richardson, D. C. (1982). "Determination and analysis of the 2 A-structure of copper, zinc superoxide dismutase." *J Mol Biol* 160(2): 181-217.

Tartaglia, G. G., Pawar, A. P., Campioni, S., Dobson, C. M., Chiti, F. and Vendruscolo, M. (2008). "Prediction of aggregation-prone regions in structured proteins." *J Mol Biol* 380(2): 425-36.

Teilum, K., Smith, M. H., Schulz, E., Christensen, L. C., Solomentsev, G., Oliveberg, M. and Akke, M. (2009). "Transient structural distortion of metal-free Cu/Zn superoxide dismutase triggers aberrant oligomerization." *Proc Natl Acad Sci U S A* 106(43): 18273-8.

Tiwari, A. and Hayward, L. J. (2003). "Familial amyotrophic lateral sclerosis mutants of copper/zinc superoxide dismutase are susceptible to disulfide reduction." *J Biol Chem* 278(8): 5984-92.

Tiwari, A., Liba, A., Sohn, S. H., Seetharaman, S. V., Bilsel, O., Matthews, C. R., Hart, P. J., Valentine, J. S. and Hayward, L. J. (2009). "Metal deficiency increases aberrant hydrophobicity of mutant superoxide dismutases that cause amyotrophic lateral sclerosis." *J Biol Chem* 284(40): 27746-58.

Tuite, M. F. and Serio, T. R. (2010). "The prion hypothesis: from biological anomaly to basic regulatory mechanism." *Nat Rev Mol Cell Biol* 11(12): 823-33.

Turner, B. J. and Talbot, K. (2008). "Transgenics, toxicity and therapeutics in rodent models of mutant SOD1-mediated familial ALS." *Prog Neurobiol* 85(1): 94-134.

Tycko, R. (2006). "Solid-state NMR as a probe of amyloid structure." *Protein Pept Lett* 13(3): 229-34.

Urushitani, M., Kurisu, J., Tsukita, K. and Takahashi, R. (2002). "Proteasomal inhibition by misfolded mutant superoxide dismutase 1 induces selective motor neuron death in familial amyotrophic lateral sclerosis." *J Neurochem* 83(5): 1030-42.

Uversky, V. N. and Dunker, A. K. (2010). "Understanding protein non-folding." *Biochim Biophys Acta* 1804(6): 1231-64.

Valentine, J. S., Doucette, P. A. and Zittin Potter, S. (2005). "Copper-zinc superoxide dismutase and amyotrophic lateral sclerosis." *Annu Rev Biochem* 74: 563-93.

Van Den Bosch, L. (2011). "Genetic rodent models of amyotrophic lateral sclerosis." *Journal of biomedicine & biotechnology* 348765.

Vande Velde, C., Miller, T. M., Cashman, N. R. and Cleveland, D. W. (2008). "Selective association of misfolded ALS-linked mutant SOD1 with the cytoplasmic face of mitochondria." *Proc Natl Acad Sci U S A* 105(10): 4022-7.

Vassall, K. A., Stathopulos, P. B., Rumfeldt, J. A., Lepock, J. R. and Meiering, E. M. (2006). "Equilibrium thermodynamic analysis of amyotrophic lateral sclerosis-associated mutant apo Cu,Zn superoxide dismutases." *Biochemistry* 45(23): 7366-79.

Vassall, K. A., Stubbs, H. R., Primmer, H. A., Tong, M. S., Sullivan, S. M., Sobering, R., Srinivasan, S., Briere, L. A., Dunn, S. D., Colon, W. and Meiering, E. M. (2011). "Decreased stability and increased formation of soluble aggregates by immature superoxide dismutase do not account for disease severity in ALS." *Proc Natl Acad Sci U S A* 108(6): 2210-5.

Verges, K. J., Smith, M. H., Toyama, B. H. and Weissman, J. S. (2011). "Strain conformation, primary structure and the propagation of the yeast prion [PSI+]." *Nat Struct Mol Biol* 18(4): 493-9.

Vetri, V. and Militello, V. (2005). "Thermal induced conformational changes involved in the aggregation pathways of beta-lactoglobulin." *Biophys Chem* 113(1): 83-91.

Vucic, S. and Kiernan, M. C. (2009). "Pathophysiology of neurodegeneration in familial amyotrophic lateral sclerosis." *Curr Mol Med* 9(3): 255-72.

Wang, Q., Johnson, J. L., Agar, N. Y. and Agar, J. N. (2008). "Protein aggregation and protein instability govern familial amyotrophic lateral sclerosis patient survival." *PLoS Biol* 6(7): e170.

Wijesekera, L. C. and Leigh, P. N. (2009). "Amyotrophic lateral sclerosis." *Orphanet J Rare Dis* 4: 3.

Williamson, J., Goldman, J. and Marder, K. S. (2009). "Genetic aspects of Alzheimer disease." *Neurologist* 15(2): 80-6.

Wyttenbach, A., Carmichael, J., Swartz, J., Furlong, R. A., Narain, Y., Rankin, J. and Rubinsztein, D. C. (2000). "Effects of heat shock, heat shock protein 40 (HDJ-2), and proteasome inhibition on protein aggregation in cellular models of Huntington's disease." *Proc Natl Acad Sci U S A* 97(6): 2898-903.

Zetterstrom, P., Stewart, H. G., Bergemalm, D., Jonsson, P. A., Graffmo, K. S., Andersen, P. M., Brannstrom, T., Oliveberg, M. and Marklund, S. L. (2007). "Soluble misfolded subfractions of mutant superoxide dismutase-1s are enriched in spinal cords throughout life in murine ALS models." *Proc Natl Acad Sci U S A* 104(35): 14157-62.

12

Oxidative Modifications of Cu, Zn-Superoxide Dismutase (SOD1) – The Relevance to Amyotrophic Lateral Sclerosis (ALS)

Seiichi Nagano
Department of Peripheral Nervous System Research, National Institute of Neuroscience, National Center of Neurology and Psychiatry
Japan

1. Introduction

Amyotrophic lateral sclerosis (ALS) is a fatal degenerative disease of motor neurons. About 10 % of ALS cases are affected in a familial trait, a subset of which is caused by the mutation of *Cu, Zn-superoxide dismutase (SOD1)* gene (Rosen et al., 1993). Since the identification of the gene for familial ALS, research emphasis for ALS has been placed on uncovering the pathogenic mechanism of motor neuronal death by the disease-causing mutant SOD1. So far over 150 different mutations of *SOD1* gene have been found in familial ALS patients, and they are scattered throughout the entire sequence of the gene regardless of specific functional domains. Transgenic mice that express mutant SOD1, but not wild type SOD1 nor SOD1 knockout mice, develop motor neuron disease, often while retaining normal dismutase activity (Gurney et al., 1994; Reaume et al., 1996). It means that mutant SOD1 gains a new aberrant toxic function apart from the primary enzymatic function of the protein, which has remained uncertain to date. Although the nature of mutant SOD1 toxicity has not been fully determined, conformational abnormalities of mutant SOD1 protein are deeply involved in the pathogenesis of familial ALS (Chattopadhyay & Valentine, 2009). Moreover, recent studies suggest that the phenotype of sporadic ALS also might be regulated by the conformational change of wild type SOD1 (Bosco et al., 2010). I review the recent concept of neuronal toxicity by oxidatively-modified SOD1, which is closely related to its conformational change, in ALS pathogenesis.

2. Cu-mediated oxidative toxicity by mutant SOD1

SOD1 is a major metal-binding enzyme expressed constitutively in tissues, and converts pro-oxidant superoxide radicals to hydrogen peroxide and oxygen (Valentine et al., 2005). In a metal-coordinated state, SOD1 forms homodimer to accomplish its full enzymatic activity. Each subunit coordinates one atom each of Cu and Zn. Cu is necessary for the enzymatic activity, whereas Zn mainly works to maintain the stable structure of the protein. Because Cu is catalytically redox-active and has a potential to oxidize proteins including SOD1 itself, inappropriate reactivity of Cu coordinated in SOD1 can underlie the conformational change of mutant SOD1. Inversely, conformational change in mutant SOD1 may increase the accessibility of substrates to Cu in the protein to generate reactive oxygen or nitrogen species. There is direct evidence that mutant SOD1 can promote abnormal pro-oxidant reactions cooperated with Cu. Mutant SOD1, unlike wild type SOD1, has a potential to generate hydroxyl radicals (Wiedau-Pazos et al., 1996; Yim et al., 1996) or peroxynitrite (Estevez et al., 1999) by Cu-dependent reaction *in vitro*, which can be inhibited by Cu chelators in cultured cells (Ghadge et al., 1997). Cu-mediated toxicity in mutant SOD1 is also reinforced with the reports that decreasing intracellular Cu, by treatment with Cu chelators or genetic reduction of Cu uptake, alleviates ALS phenotype in mutant SOD1 transgenic mice (Hottinger et al., 1997; Kiaei et al., 2004 ; Nagano et al., 2003; Tokuda et al., 2008). Moreover, metallothioneins, which bind Cu to prevent it from being pro-oxidant, are increased in the spinal cord of mutant SOD1 mice to attenuate the disease expression (Hashimoto et al., 2011; Nagano et al., 2001; Tokuda et al., 2007). These facts suggest that Cu-mediated oxidative chemistry underlies the pathogenesis of familial ALS linked to mutations of *SOD1* gene.

On the other hand, the phenotype of mutant SOD1 mice was not rescued by genetic removal of the Cu chaperone for SOD1 (CCS), which incorporates Cu into the buried active site of SOD1 (Subramaniam et al., 2002). Furthermore, mutant SOD1 still induces the disease in transgenic mice even when the active copper-binding site is totally disrupted by multiple mutations (Wang et al., 2003). These findings had been taken as evidence against the hypothesis of aberrant Cu chemistry in the toxicity of mutant SOD1. However, the theory implicating Cu toxicity cannot be excluded since ectopic binding of Cu away from the active site, for example, could contribute to the pathogenesis. In fact, H46R mutant SOD1, which disrupts Cu binding at the active site, still has the ectopic binding of Cu (Liu et al., 2000).

3. Increased affinity for Cu in mutant SOD1

To clarify a possible aberrant interaction of mutant SOD1 with Cu outside the active site in the context of familial ALS, we characterized the affinity for Cu of the mutants by immobilized metal affinity chromatography (IMAC), a method that separates proteins based on their affinities with an immobilized metal such as Cu (Watanabe et al., 2007). Mutant SOD1 commonly exhibited an aberrant fraction with **h**igh **a**ffinity for **C**u (SOD1HAC), in addition to that with **l**ow **a**ffinity for **C**u (SOD1LAC) seen in wild type SOD1 as well. SOD1HAC was detected whether the mutants were expressed in yeasts, mammalian cells or spinal cords of transgenic mice, while an unknown cellular factor(s) other than SOD1 was needed for its generation (Nagano, unpublished data). We observed SOD1HAC even in H46R or G85R mutant SOD1, the mutants that do not efficiently incorporate Cu into the active site, and therefore the immobilized Cu is likely to interact with SOD1 outside the active site, on a solvent-facing surface of the protein. Considering that mutant SOD1 is separated into two distinct fractions (SOD1LAC and HAC) and the interaction of proteins on IMAC is determined by topology of metal-coordinating residues on solvent-facing surfaces (Porath et al., 1975), conformational transition from the native to non-native state is implied to be critical for the increased affinity for Cu in SOD1HAC.

4. Monomerization of SOD1 by cysteine oxidation

Then what is the determinant of conformational transition for SOD1HAC in mutant SOD1? Human SOD1 has four cysteine residues—Cys6, Cys57, Cys111 and Cys146—in a subunit.

Two of them (Cys57 and Cys146) form an intramolecular disulfide bond that maintains the rigid structure and enzymatic activity of SOD1 protein, whereas the remaining two (Cys6 and Cys111) are present as cysteines having free sulfhydryl groups. Of the latter, Cys6 is deeply buried in the protein molecule and less accessible by substrates, while Cys111 is located on the surface of the protein near the dimer interface. Substitution of serine for Cys111 (C111S) is known to increase the structural stability and resistance to heat inactivation of wild type SOD1 (Lepock et al., 1990), implying that the mode of Cys111 may regulate the conformational state of mutant SOD1. H46R mutant SOD1, which has an ectopic binding to Cu as mentioned above, has been reported to bind the metal at Cys111 (Liu et al., 2000). We hypothesized that Cys111 might be a candidate site in human SOD1 that could enhance the coordination of the protein with immobilized Cu. Indeed, C111S substitution eliminated the increase of Cu binding in mutant SOD1. Moreover, the protein degradation assay in cell culture indicated that the decrease of SOD1HAC by C111S substitution well correlated with the stability of each mutant protein. That is, the stability was lower, the affinity for Cu was higher in mutant SOD1. In agreement with our findings, a previous report indicated that the decreased stability of mutant SOD1 correlated with its toxicity and the disease progression rate in familial ALS patients (Sato et al., 2005).

Next, to examine whether other cysteine residues play the same role as Cys111 in mutant SOD1, we introduced C57S substitution into the protein. In contrast to the effect of C111S, C57S substitution rather increased Cu binding, and did not rescue the instability of the mutant. C57S substitution prevents the disulfide bond between Cys57 and Cys146, which is supposed to make SOD1 protein difficult to keep its structure and stabilize. Although the function of the disulfide bond in SOD1 is not fully elucidated, it could be related to either the dimerization of SOD1 or the metal binding process at the active site or both. Thus, mutant SOD1 with C57S may become conformationally further destabilized, exposing Cu-interaction sites to enhance Cu affinity of the protein.

We performed further biochemical characterization of SOD1HAC and determined what properties could cause its formation and toxicity. Since mutant SOD1 is known to susceptible to intramolecular disulfide reduction (Tiwari & Hayward, 2003), we employed a cysteine-modifying reagent to estimate the redox status of cysteine residues in SOD1HAC. We found that sulfhydryl groups of free cysteine residues, especially of Cys111, were oxidized in SOD1HAC while the residues remained reduced in SOD1LAC (Kishigami et al., 2010). The intramolecular disulfide bond between Cys57 and Cys146 was unchanged in both components.

The dimeric structure of SOD1 is destabilized in pathogenic SOD1 mutants (Furukawa & O'Halloran, 2005). We therefore investigated the dimer/monomer status of SOD1LAC and SOD1HAC using gel filtration chromatography. SOD1HAC eluted predominantly as a monomer, whereas SOD1LAC consisted of a dimer structure. It means that SOD1HAC formation is concordant with the loss of dimeric stability to form a monomer.

We further employed nitrosoglutathione or hydrogen peroxide, cysteine-oxidizing reagents, in wild type SOD1 to mimic the sulfhydryl oxidation of Cys111 in SOD1HAC. We observed that the reaction actually modified Cys111, and engendered SOD1HAC. Moreover, we saw that Cys111-modified wild type SOD1 lost its dimeric conformation and mainly consisted of a monomer in SOD1HAC. Conversely, intersubunit crosslinking between Cys111 of each subunit prevented mutant SOD1 from monomerizing and developing SOD1HAC. These results mean that Cys111 is labile to be oxidized by endogenous agents such as nitrosoglutathione or hydrogen peroxide in familial ALS-linked mutant SOD1, which is the first step for the substantial monomerization of the protein and increase of the Cu affinity probably by exposing a Cu-accessible interface of the dimer.

5. Oxidative stress by cysteine-oxidized SOD1

In case that SOD1 is monomerized through conformational destabilization mediated by Cys111 oxidation, Cu coordinated at the ectopic binding site can be redox-active. To see whether SOD1HAC causes an aberrant redox reaction, we measured thiol oxidase activity, a Cu-dependent activity that is reported in human SOD1 (Winterbourn et al., 2002). We found that mutant or Cys111-oxidized wild type SOD1 developed the thiol oxidase activity when it was loaded with Cu, and that the activity was decreased by C111S substitution or intermolecular crosslinking of Cys111. Because SOD1 modified at Cys111 possesses the thiol oxidase activity, it is unlikely that Cys111 itself is the direct binding site for Cu. These results indicate that cysteine-oxidized SOD1 may exert the potentially toxic pro-oxidant activity through ectopic binding of Cu to SOD1HAC at a site within the dimer interface, which becomes exposed upon the dissociation of SOD1. The thiol oxidase activity of mutant SOD1 can promote oxidative stress because of the exhaustion of glutathione, the major free thiol and antioxidant. The activity may also oxidize cysteine residues of other proteins, deteriorating various cell functions (Fig. 1).

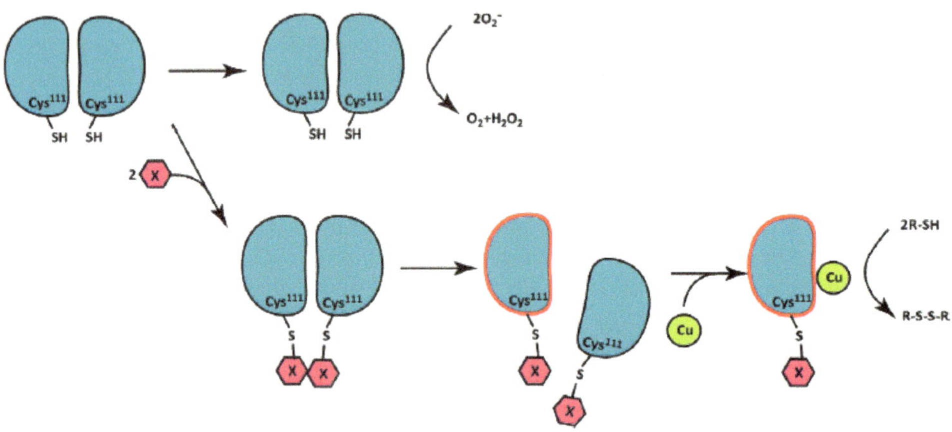

Fig. 1. Proposed model of mutant SOD1 toxicity. Modification of Cys111 leads to dissociation of SOD1 dimers into monomers. Cu, either resulting from rearrangement of the active site or from an external source, becomes ectopically bound to the former dimer interface surface, where it can now catalyze thiol oxidase activity (Kishigami et al., 2010).

6. Role of cysteine-oxidized mutant SOD1 in familial ALS

What is the role of Cys111 modification on the neuronal toxicity by mutant SOD1? In the spinal cords of familial ALS patients and mutant SOD1 transgenic mice, degenerating motor neurons contain SOD1-positive inclusion bodies, suggesting that mutant SOD1 is conformationally misfolded and subject to aggregate (Chattopadhyay & Valentine, 2009). As seen in other neurodegenerative diseases, abnormal protein accumulation in neurons can impair their cellular functions such as axonal transport (Tateno et al., 2009), oxidative phosphorylation in mitochondria and protein degradation machinery.

Various factors can cause conformational rearrangement or misfolding of mutant SOD1, including decreased metallation (Hayward et al., 2002), hydrophobicity (Tiwari et al., 2005) and reduction of repulsive charge (Sandelin et al., 2007). Modification of amino acid residues, especially by oxidative stress, can be a critical factor to enhance the misfolding of mutant SOD1 (Rakhit & Chakrabartty, 2006). Cysteine is in particular susceptible to oxidative modification, since its sulfhydryl moiety is readily attacked by redox active substrates such as glutathione or peroxides to form S-S or S-O covalent modification. Sulfhydryl groups also crosslink each other to form intra- or inter-molecular disulfide bond, which have important roles to maintain or disrupt physiological conformation of proteins. Oxidative reactivity and modification of Cys111, such as glutathionylation (Kajihara et al., 1988; Schinina et al., 1996) and peroxidation (Fujiwara et al., 2007), was documented with human or chick wild type SOD1, although the effect of which on the enzymatic activity or dimer stability had not been determined. Because Cys111 is located on the edge of the dimer interface of each subunit, the modification of Cys111, especially when a large molecule such as glutathione is adducted to the residue, can interrupt the dimer contact at the interface stereochemically and cause the dissociation of SOD1. Molecular dynamics simulations of SOD1 imply that the region including Cys111 is important for the residue interaction network in the protein, and likely to affect the dimer interface through the network and may disrupt their coupled motions (Khare & Dokholyan, 2006). In fact, glutathionylation of Cys111 has been confirmed with native human SOD1 in erythrocytes (Nakanishi et al., 1998; Wilcox et al., 2009), and it was noted that the modification caused SOD1 liable to monomerize and decrease its enzymatic activity (Wilcox et al., 2009). The SOD1 monomer is prone to form aggregates that might be the origin of intracellular inclusions found in motor neurons with SOD1-linked familial ALS. Supporting that, Cys111-peroxidized SOD1 was detected in the neuronal inclusions of mutant SOD1 mice (Fujiwara et al., 2007).

Oxidative modification of cysteine residues, including Cys111, is also possible to be involved in the aggregation process of mutant SOD1. High molecular weight dimers and multimers of mutant SOD1 can be detected in the spinal cords of transgenic mice in parallel to the disease onset (Deng et al., 2006; Furukawa et al., 2006). They are detergent-insoluble and reversed by reductants, supposing that disulfide-mediated crosslinking at cysteine residues is a major factor for mutant SOD1 to form aggregates and ALS phenotype. Cysteines forming the intramolecular disulfide bond (Cys57 and Cys146) are possibly involved in the crosslinking, since the disulfide bond between the residues is labile to be reduced (Tiwari & Hayward, 2003) and cause aberrant oxidation in mutant SOD1. The disulfide-reduced mutant SOD1 is actually enriched in the spinal cord of transgenic mice (Jonsson et al., 2006). The reduced form of mutant SOD1 can also translocate into the intermembrane space of mitochondria cooperated by CCS (Field et al., 2003), which may be components of aggregates in mitochondria (Deng et al., 2006; Ferri et al., 2006) and harmful to the mitochondrial function. However, intermolecular disulfide bonds mediated at free cysteines (Cys6 and Cys111) can also be components of the detergent-insoluble SOD1 aggregates (Banci et al., 2007; Niwa et al., 2007). In either case, apo SOD1 is more prone to the disulfide-linked oxidative aggregation than holo SOD1 (Banci et al., 2007; Furukawa & O'Halloran, 2005). That is in concert with the notion that immature SOD1 is the pathogenic species in familial ALS (Seetharaman et al., 2009).

It is still controversial whether the cysteine-mediated misfolding or aggregation of mutant SOD1 is the origin of the protein's toxicity. Removal of free cysteines, especially of Cys111, strongly reduced the ability of mutant SOD1 to form disulfide crosslinking and aggregates, and improved cell viability in cultured cells (Cozzolino et al., 2008; Niwa et al., 2007). Moreover, glutaredoxins, which specifically catalyze the reduction of protein-SSG-mixed disulfides, significantly increased the solubility of mutant SOD1 and protected neuronal cells (Cozzolino et al., 2008; Ferri et al., 2010). On the other hand, the intermolecular disulfide binding at cysteines is shown to have a limited effect on the aggregation of mutant SOD1 (Karch & Borchelt, 2008). Even in this case, Cys111-modified mutant SOD1 may cause neuronal toxicity independently of the aggregation, by oxidative stress such as thiol oxidase activity we have shown (Kishigami et al., 2010).

7. Role of cysteine-oxidized wild type SOD1 in sporadic ALS

In sporadic ALS, there had been no direct evidence that SOD1 was involved in the pathogenesis of the disease, except that some mutations of *SOD1* gene expressed familial ALS in a low penetration rate with seemingly 'sporadic' cases. The link between SOD1 and sporadic ALS was first introduced by the detection of SOD1 specifically modifiable with a chemical compound commonly in familial and sporadic ALS, although the molecular basis for it has not been determined in detail (Gruzman et al., 2007). It indicates that a similar conformational change in mutant and wild type SOD1 can trigger the phenotype of familial and sporadic ALS in common. In *in vitro* study, wild type SOD1 acquires toxic properties of mutant SOD1 through oxidation by hydrogen peroxide (Ezzi et al., 2007), implying that cysteine-oxidized wild type SOD1 may be a contributor to motor neuronal death in sporadic ALS.

Recently, a conformation-specific antibody generated against misfolded mutant SOD1 has been shown to recognize wild type SOD1 only when the protein was sulfonylated ($-SO_3H$) at Cys111, and the antibody immunostained motor neurons in the spinal cords of sporadic ALS patients, but not of SOD1-unrelated familial ALS patients or controls (Bosco et al., 2010). Chemically oxidized or purified wild type SOD1 from sporadic ALS spinal cords inhibited kinesin-based fast axonal transport as did mutant SOD1, supposing that Cys111-mediated conformational change or misfolding of SOD1 is a shared pathological denominator of familial and sporadic ALS. Interestingly, most of the sporadic ALS-derived toxic SOD1 was soluble and non-aggregated, meaning that misfolding or monomerization is sufficient for SOD1 to gain the toxic property such as oxidative insult we have shown in mutant and wild type SOD1 (Kishigami et al., 2010). Further studies *in vivo* will be required to clarify the detailed mechanism of SOD1 toxicity mediated by oxidation of cysteine residues including Cys111.

8. Conclusion

The findings mentioned above indicate that oxidative modification of SOD1 at cysteine residues is a critical factor to contribute to the oxidative stress, inclusion pathology and degeneration of motor neurons commonly to familial and sporadic ALS. Based on them, steric inhibition of cysteine oxidation, monomerization or exposure of the dimer interface can be the first-line treatment strategy of this incurable disease.

9. References

Banci, L.; Bertini, I.; Durazo, A.; Girotto, S.; Gralla, E.B.; Martinelli, M.; Valentine, J.S.; Vieru, M. & Whitelegge, J.P. (2007). Metal-free superoxide dismutase forms soluble oligomers under physiological conditions: A possible general mechanism for familial ALS. *Proceedings of the National Academy of Sciences of the United States of America,* Vol.104, No.27, pp. 11263-11267

Bosco, D.A.; Morfini, G.; Karabacak, N.M.; Song, Y.; Gros-Louis, F.; Pasinelli, P.; Goolsby, H.; Fontaine, B.A.; Lemay, N.; McKenna-Yasek, D.; Frosch, M.P.; Agar, J.N.; Julien, J.P.; Brady, S.T. & Brown R.H.J. (2010). Wild-type and mutant SOD1 share an aberrant conformation and a common pathogenic pathway in ALS. *Nature Neuroscience,* Vol.13, No.11, pp. 1396–1403

Chattopadhyay, M. & Valentine, J.S. (2009). Aggregation of copper-zinc superoxide dismutase in familial and sporadic ALS. *Antioxidants & Redox Signaling,* Vol.11, No.7, pp. 1603-1614

Deng, H.X.; Shi, Y.; Furukawa, Y.; Zhai, H.; Fu, R.; Liu, E.; Gorrie, G.H.; Khan, M.S.; Hung, W.Y.; Bigio, E.H.; Lukas, T.; Dal Canto, M.C.; O'Halloran, T.V. & Siddique, T. (2006). Conversion to the amyotrophic lateral sclerosis phenotype is associated with intermolecular linked insoluble aggregates of SOD1 in mitochondria. *Proceedings of the National Academy of Sciences of the United States of America,* Vol.103, No.18, pp. 7142-7147

Cozzolino, M.; Amori, I.; Pesaresi, M.G.; Ferri, A.; Nencini, M. & Carri, M.T. (2008). Cysteine 111 affects aggregation and cytotoxicity of mutant Cu,Zn-superoxide dismutase associated with familial amyotrophic lateral sclerosis. *Journal of Biological Chemistry,* Vol.283, No.2, pp. 866–874

Estevez, A.G.; Crow, J.P.; Sampson, J.B.; Reiter, C.; Zhuang, Y.; Richardson, G.J.; Tarpey, M.M.; Barbeito, L. & Beckman, J.S. (1999). Induction of nitric oxide-dependent apoptosis in motor neurons by zinc-deficient superoxide dismutase. *Science,* Vol.286, No.5449, pp. 2498–2500

Ezzi, S.A.; Urushitani, M. & Julien, J.P. (2007). Wild-type superoxide dismutase acquires binding and toxic properties of ALS-linked mutant forms through oxidation. *Journal of Neurochemistry,* Vol.102, No.1, pp. 170–178

Ferri, A.; Cozzolino, M.; Crosio, C.; Nencini, M.; Casciati, A.; Gralla, E.B.; Rotilio, G.; Valentine, J.S. & Carri, M.T. (2006). Familial ALS-superoxide dismutases associate with mitochondria and shift their redox potentials. *Proceedings of the National Academy of Sciences of the United States of America,* Vol.103, No.37, pp. 13860–13865

Ferri, A.; Fiorenzo, P.; Nencini, M.; Cozzolino, M.; Pesaresi, M.G.; Valle, C.; Sepe, S.; Moreno, S. & Carri, M.T. (2010). Glutaredoxin 2 prevents aggregation of mutant SOD1 in mitochondria and abolishes its toxicity. *Human Molecular Genetics,* Vol.19, No.22, pp. 4529-4542

Field, L.S.; Furukawa, Y.; O'Halloran, T.V. & Culotta, V.C. (2003). Factors controlling the uptake of yeast copper/zinc superoxide dismutase into mitochondria. *Journal of Biological Chemistry,* Vol.278, No.30, pp. 28052–28059

Fujiwara, N.; Nakano, M.; Kato, S.; Yoshihara, D.; Ookawara, T.; Eguchi, H.; Taniguchi, N. & Suzuki, K. (2007). Oxidative modification to cysteine sulfonic acid of Cys111 in human copper-zinc superoxide dismutase. *Journal of Biological Chemistry,* Vol.282, No.49, pp. 35933–35944

Furukawa, Y. & O'Halloran, T.V. (2005). Amyotrophic lateral sclerosis mutations have the greatest destabilizing effect on the apo- and reduced form of SOD1, leading to unfolding and oxidative aggregation. *Journal of Biological Chemistry,* Vol.280, No.17, pp. 17266-17274

Furukawa, Y.; Fu, R.; Deng, H.X.; Siddique, T. & O'Halloran, T.V. (2006). Disulfide cross-linked protein represents a significant fraction of ALS-associated Cu, Zn-superoxide dismutase aggregates in spinal cords of model mice. *Proceedings of the National Academy of Sciences of the United States of America,* Vol.103, No.18, pp. 7148-7153

Ghadge, G.D.; Lee, J.P.; Bindokas, V.P.; Jordan, J.; Ma, L.; Miller, R.J. & Roos, R.P. (1997). Mutant superoxide dismutase-1-linked familial amyotrophic lateral sclerosis: molecular mechanisms of neuronal death and protection. *Journal of Neuroscience,* Vol.17, No.22, pp. 8756-8766

Gruzman, A.; Wood, W.L.; Alpert, E.; Prasad, M.D.; Miller, R.G.; Rothstein, J.D.; Bowser, R.; Hamilton, R.; Wood, T.D.; Cleveland, D.W.; Lingappa, V.R. & Liu, J. (2007). Common molecular signature in SOD1 for both sporadic and familial amyotrophic lateral sclerosis. *Proceedings of the National Academy of Sciences of the United States of America,* Vol.104, No.30, pp. 12524-12529

Gurney, M.E.; Pu, H.; Chiu, A.Y.; Dal Canto, M.C.; Polchow, C.Y.; Alexander, D.D.; Caliendo, J.; Hentati, A.; Kwon, Y.W.; Deng, H.X.; Chen, W.; Zhai, P.; Sufit, R.L. & Siddique, T. (1994). Motor neuron degeneration in mice that express a human Cu,Zn superoxide dismutase mutation. *Science,* Vol.264, No.5166, pp. 1772-1775

Hashimoto, K; Hayashi, Y; Watabe, K; Inuzuka, T & Hozumi, I. (2011). Metallothionein-III prevents neuronal death and prolongs life span in amyotrophic lateral sclerosis model mice. *Neuroscience,* Vol.189, No.1, pp. 293-298

Hayward, L.J.; Rodriguez, J.A.; Kim, J.W.; Tiwari, A.; Goto, J.J.; Cabelli, D.E.; Valentine, J.S. & Brown, R.H.J. (2002). Decreased metallation and activity in subsets of mutant superoxide dismutases associated with familial amyotrophic lateral sclerosis. *Journal of Biological Chemistry,* Vol.277, No.18, pp. 15923-15931

Hottinger, A.F.; Fine, E.G.; Gurney, M.E.; Zurn, A.D. & Aebischer, P. (1997). The copper chelator d-penicillamine delays onset of disease and extends survival in a transgenic mouse model of familial amyotrophic lateral sclerosis. *European Journal of Neuroscence,* Vol.9, No.7, pp. 1548-1551

Jonsson, P.A.; Graffmo, K.S.; Andersen, P.M.; Brannstrom, T,; Lindberg, M.; Oliveberg, M. & Marklund, S.L. (2006). Disulphide-reduced superoxide dismutase-1 in CNS of transgenic amyotrophic lateral sclerosis models. *Brain,* Vol.129, No.2, pp. 451–464

Kajihara, J.; Enomoto, M.; Seya, K.; Sukenaga, Y. & Katoh, K. (1988). Physicochemical properties of charge isomers of recombinant human superoxide dismutase. *Journal of Biochemistry,* Vol.104, No.4, pp. 638-642

Karch, C.M. & Borchelt, D.R. (2008). A limited role for disulfide cross-linking in the aggregation of mutant SOD1 linked to familial amyotrophic lateral sclerosis. *Journal of Biological Chemistry,* Vol.283, No.20, pp. 13528–13537

Khare, S.D. & Dokholyan, N.V. (2006). Common dynamical signatures of familial amyotrophic lateral sclerosis-associated structurally diverse Cu, Zn superoxide dismutase mutants. *Proceedings of the National Academy of Sciences of the United States of America,* Vol.103, No.9, pp. 3147-3152

Kiaei, M.; Bush, A.I.; Morrison, B.M.; Morrison, J.H.; Cherny, R.A.; Volitakis, I.; Beal, M.F. & Gordon, J.W. (2004). Genetically decreased spinal cord copper concentration prolongs life in a transgenic mouse model of amyotrophic lateral sclerosis. *Journal of Neuroscience,* Vol.24, No.36, pp. 7945-7950

Kishigami, H.; Nagano, S.; Bush, A.I. & Sakoda, S. (2010). Monomerized Cu,Zn-superoxide dismutase induces oxidative stress through aberrant Cu binding. *Free Radical Biology & Medicine,* Vol.48, No.7, pp. 945–952

Lepock, J.R.; Frey, H.E. & Hallewell, R.A. (1990). Contribution of conformational stability and reversibility of unfolding to the increased thermostability of human and bovine superoxide dismutase mutated at free cysteines. *Journal of Biological Chemistry,* Vol.265, No.35, pp. 21612-21618

Liu, H.; Zhu, H.; Eggers, D.K.; Nersissian, A.M.; Faull, K.F.; Goto, J.J.; Ai, J.; Sanders-Loehr, J.; Gralla, E.B. & Valentine, J.S. (2000). Copper(2+) binding to the surface residue cysteine 111 of His46Arg human copper–zinc superoxide dismutase, a familial amyotrophic lateral sclerosis mutant. *Biochemistry,* Vol.39, No.28, pp. 8125–8132

Nagano, S.; Satoh, M.; Sumi, H.; Fujimura, H.; Tohyama, C.; Yanagihara, T. & Sakoda, S. (2001). Reduction of metallothioneins promotes the disease expression of familial amyotrophic lateral sclerosis mice in a dose-dependent manner. *European Journal of Neuroscience,* Vol.13, No.7, pp. 1363-1370

Nagano, S.; Fujii, Y.; Yamamoto, T.; Taniyama, M.; Fukada, K.; Yanagihara, T. & Sakoda, S. (2003). The efficacy of trientine or ascorbate alone compared to that of the combined treatment with these two agents in familial amyotrophic lateral sclerosis model mice. *Experimental Neurology,* Vol.179, No.2, pp. 176-180

Nakanishi, T.; Kishikawa, M.; Miyazaki, A.; Shimizu, A.; Ogawa, Y.; Sakoda, S.; Ohi, T. & Shoji, H. (1998). Simple and defined method to detect the SOD-1 mutants from patients with familial amyotrophic lateral sclerosis by mass spectrometry. *Journal of Neuroscience Methods,* Vol.81, No.1-2, pp. 41-44

Niwa, J.; Yamada, S.; Ishigaki, S.; Sone, J.; Takahashi, M.; Katsuno, M.; Tanaka, F.; Doyu, M. & Sobue, G. (2007). Disulfide bond mediates aggregation, toxicity, and ubiquitylation of familial amyotrophic lateral sclerosis-linked mutant SOD1. *Journal of Biological Chemistry,* Vol.282, No.38, pp. 28087-28095

Porath, J.; Carlsson, J.; Olsson, I. & Belfrage, G. (1975). Metal chelate affinity chromatography, a new approach to protein fractionation. *Nature,* Vol.258, No.5536, pp. 598–599

Rakhit, R. & Chakrabartty, A. (2006). Structure, folding, and misfolding of Cu,Zn superoxide dismutase in amyotrophic lateral sclerosis. *Biochimica et Biophysica Acta,* Vol.1762, No.11-12, pp. 1025-1037

Reaume, A.G.; Elliott, J.L.; Hoffman, E.K.; Kowall, N.W.; Ferrante, R.J.; Siwek, D.F.; Wilcox, H.M.; Flood, D.G.; Beal, M.F.; Brown R.H.J.; Scott, R.W. & Snider, W.D. (1996). Motor neurons in Cu/Zn superoxide dismutase-deficient mice develop normally but exhibit enhanced cell death after axonal injury. *Nature Genetics,* Vol.13, No.1, pp. 43–47

Rosen, D.R.; Siddique, T.; Patterson, D.; Figlewicz, D.A.; Sapp, P.; Hentati, A.; Donaldson, D.; Goto, J.; O'Regan, J.P.; Deng, H.X.; Rahmani, Z.; Krizus, A.; Mckenna-Yasek, D.; Cayabyab, A.; Gaston, S.M.; Berger, R.; Tanzi, R.E.; Halperin, J.J.; Herzfeldt, B.;Van Den Bergh, R.; Hung, W.Y.; Bird, T.; Deng, G.; Mulder, D.W.; Smyth, C.; Laing, N.G.; Soriano, E.; Pericak-Vance, M.A.; Haines, J.; Rouleau, G.A.; Gusella, J.S.; Horvitz, H.R. & Brown, R.H.J. (1993). Mutations in Cu/Zn superoxide dismutase gene are associated with familial amyotrophic lateral sclerosis. *Nature,* Vol.362, No.6415, pp. 59–62

Sandelin, E.; Nordlund, A.; Andersen, P.M.; Marklund, S.S. & Oliveberg, M. (2007). Amyotrophic lateral sclerosis-associated copper/zinc superoxide dismutase mutations preferentially reduce the repulsive charge of the proteins. *Journal of Biological Chemistry,* Vol.282, No.29, pp. 21230-21236

Seetharaman, S.V.; Prudencio, M.; Karch, C.; Holloway, S.P.; Borchelt, D.R. & Hart, P.J. (2009). Immature copper-zinc superoxide dismutase and familial amyotrophic lateral sclerosis. *Experimental Biology and Medicine,* Vol.234, No.10, pp. 1140–1154

Sato, T.; Nakanishi, T.; Yamamoto, Y.; Andersen, P.M.; Ogawa, Y.; Fukada, K.; Zhou, Z.; Aoike, F.; Sugai, F.; Nagano, S.; Hirata, S.; Ogawa, M.; Nakano, R.; Ohi, T.; Kato, T.; Nakagawa, M.; Hamasaki, T.; Shimizu, A. & Sakoda, S. (2005). Rapid disease progression correlates with instability of mutant SOD1 in familial ALS. *Neurology,* Vol.65, No.12, pp. 1954-1957

Schinina, M.E.; Carlini, P.; Polticelli, F.; Zappacosta, F.; Bossa, F. & Calabrese L. (1996). Amino acid sequence of chicken Cu, Zn-containing superoxide dismutase and identification of glutathionyl adducts at exposed cysteine residues. *European Journal of Biochemistry,* Vol.237, No.2, pp. 433–439

Subramaniam, J.R.; Lyons, W.E.; Liu, J.; Bartnikas, T.B.; Rothstein, J.; Price, D.L.; Cleveland, D.W.; Gitlin, J.D. & Wong, P.C. (2002). Mutant SOD1 causes motor neuron disease independent of copper chaperone-mediated copper loading. *Nature Neuroscience,* Vol.5, No.4, pp. 301–307

Tateno, M.; Kato, S.; Sakurai, T.; Nukina, N.; Takahashi, R. & Araki, T. (2009). Mutant SOD1 impairs axonal transport of choline acetyltransferase and acetylcholine release by sequestering KAP3. *Human Molecular Genetics,* Vol.18, No.5, pp. 942-955

Tiwari, A. & Hayward, L.J. (2003). Familial amyotrophic lateral sclerosis mutants of copper/zinc superoxide dismutase are susceptible to disulfide reduction. *Journal of Biological Chemistry,* Vol.278, No.8, pp. 5984–5992

Tiwari, A.; Xu, Z. & Hayward, L.J. (2005). Aberrantly increased hydrophobicity shared by mutants of Cu,Zn-superoxide dismutase in familial amyotrophic lateral sclerosis. *Journal of Biological Chemistry,* Vol.280, No.33, pp. 29771-29779

Tokuda, E.; Ono, S.; Ishige, K.; Naganuma, A.; Ito, Y. & Suzuki, T. (2007). Metallothionein proteins expression, copper and zinc concentrations, and lipid peroxidation level in a rodent model for amyotrophic lateral sclerosis. *Toxicology,* Vol.229, No.1-2, pp. 33-41

Tokuda, E.; Ono, S.; Ishige, K.; Watanabe, S.; Okawa, E.; Ito, Y. & Suzuki, T. (2008). Ammonium tetrathiomolybdate delays onset, prolongs survival, and slows progression of disease in a mouse model for amyotrophic lateral sclerosis. *Experimental Neurology,* Vol.213, No.1, pp. 122-128.

Valentine, J.S.; Doucette, P.A. & Zittin Potter, S. (2005). Copper-zinc superoxide dismutase and amyotrophic lateral sclerosis. *Annual Review of Biochemistry,* Vol.74, No.1, pp. 563-593

Wang, J.; Slunt, H.; Gonzales, V.; Fromholt, D.; Coonfield, M.; Copeland, N.G.; Jenkins, N.A. & Borchelt, D.R. (2003). Copper-binding-site-null SOD1 causes ALS in transgenic mice: aggregates of non-native SOD1 delineate a common feature. *Human Molecular Genetics,* Vol.12, No.21, pp. 2753-64

Watanabe, S.; Nagano, S.; Duce, J.; Kiaei, M.; Li, Q.X.; Tucker, S.M.; Tiwari, A.; Brown, R.H.J.; Beal, M.F.; Hayward, L.J.; Culotta, V.C.; Yoshihara, S.; Sakoda, S. & Bush, A.I. (2007). Increased affinity for copper mediated by cysteine 111 in forms of mutant superoxide dismutase 1 linked to amyotrophic lateral sclerosis. *Free Radical Biology & Medicine,* Vol.42, No.10, pp. 1534–1542

Wiedau-Pazos, M.; Goto, J.J.; Rabizadeh, S.; Gralla, E.B.; Roe, J.A.; Lee, M.K.; Valentine, J.S. & Bredesen, D.E. (1996). Altered reactivity of superoxide dismutase in familial amyotrophic lateral sclerosis. *Science,* Vol.271, No.5248, pp. 515–518

Wilcox, K.C.; Zhou, L.; Jordon, J.K.; Huang, Y.; Yu, Y.; Redler, R.L.; Chen, X.; Caplow, M. & Dokholyan, N.V. (2009). Modifications of superoxide dismutase (SOD1) in human erythrocytes: a possible role in amyotrophic lateral sclerosis. *Journal of Biological Chemistry,* Vol.284, No.20, pp. 13940-13947

Winterbourn, C.C.; Peskin, A.V. & Parsons-Mair, H.N. (2002). Thiol oxidase activity of copper, zinc superoxide dismutase. *Journal of Biological Chemistry,* Vol.277, No.3, pp. 1906-1911

Yim, M.B.; Kang, J.H.; Yim, H.S.; Kwak, H.S.; Chock, P.B. & Stadtman, E.R. (1996). A gain-of-function of an amyotrophic lateral sclerosis-associated Cu,Zn-superoxide dismutase mutant: an enhancement of free radical formation due to a decrease in Km for hydrogen peroxide. *Proceedings of the National Academy of Sciences of the United States of America*, Vol.93, No.12, pp. 5709–5714

13

Protein Aggregates in Pathological Inclusions of Amyotrophic Lateral Sclerosis

Yoshiaki Furukawa
Department of Chemistry, Keio University
Japan

1. Introduction

Amyotrophic lateral sclerosis (ALS) is a neurodegenerative disorder that is characterized by a progressive loss of upper and/or lower motor neurons (Bruijn et al., 2004). Dysfunction and death of these neurons lead to muscle weakness, atrophy and spasticity. A fatal event for the majority of patients is a failure of the respiratory muscles, which generally occurs within one to five years of disease onset. The typical age of onset is between 50 and 60 years, and the prevalence rate is 5 - 10 cases per 100,000 populations (de Belleroche et al., 1996). No effective cures for this disease are currently available, and the pathomechanism still remains controversial. The majority of ALS cases have no genetic component (sporadic ALS, sALS), while about 10 % are inherited in a dominant manner (familial ALS, fALS).

Historically, ALS has been described by Charcot and Joffroy in 1869 (Charcot & Joffroy, 1869), and linkage analysis of fALS families was performed in 1991, by which the genetic locus was identified to be linked to chromosome 21q (Siddique et al., 1991). In 1993, Rosen et al. (Rosen et al., 1993) and Deng et al. (Deng et al., 1993) have found that mutations in the Cu,Zn-superoxide dismutase (SOD1) gene, which lies on chromosome 21q, are associated with fALS. Because SOD1-related fALS exhibited several clinicopathological similarities to sALS, various animal models including rodents, worms and flies have been constructed, in which mutant forms of SOD1 are expressed. Using these models, furthermore, various drugs have been continuingly tested to cure or alleviate ALS. In 2001, ALS2 (or called alsin) has been also identified as a new gene associated with a rare, recessively inherited and slowly progressed juvenile onset form of ALS, which is, however, significantly different from the disease phenotypes of sALS (Hadano et al., 2001; Yang et al., 2001). Accordingly, studies on mutant SOD1 have served as a "gold standard" for a long time and provided valuable insight into molecular pathomechanisms of ALS.

Recent progress on genetic analysis has fuelled the identification of other genes responsible for fALS: for example, TAR **D**NA-binding **p**rotein-43 (TDP-43) gene reported in 2008 (Gitcho et al., 2008; Kabashi et al., 2008; Sreedharan et al., 2008; Van Deerlin et al., 2008), **Fu**sed in **S**arcoma (FUS) gene in 2009 (Kwiatkowski et al., 2009; Vance et al., 2009). Each of TDP-43 and FUS mutations describes approximately 4 % of total fALS cases, which is a smaller number than that of SOD1 mutations (~20 % of total fALS cases). Unlike SOD1, however, TDP-43 and/or FUS pathologies are observed in many of sALS patients (Deng et al., 2011b; Mackenzie et al., 2007) and also in other neurodegenerative diseases (Lagier-

Tourenne et al., 2010); much attention has thus been increasingly paid on TDP-43/FUS genes. FALS cases with SOD1/TDP-43/FUS mutations exhibit distinct disease phenotypes such as site and age of onset (Millecamps et al., 2010), and the pathomechanism of fALS might be dependent upon which of the genes is mutated. Common to all ALS cases, nonetheless, inclusions can be found in motor neurons of the affected spinal cord; therefore, molecular characterization of such pathological inclusions will be important in understanding the ALS diseases.

2. Protein aggregates in pathological inclusions

Inclusions have been found in many neurodegenerative diseases and are formed by abnormal accumulation of protein aggregates (Ross & Poirier, 2004). Two types of protein aggregates generally constitute pathological inclusions: amorphous and fibrillar aggregates. Amorphous aggregates are assembled from unstructured protein molecules, while well-ordered protein aggregates often exhibit fibrillar morphologies. Among such fibrillar protein aggregates, amyloid constitutes an important structural entity; the amyloid-like aggregate *in vitro* and *in vivo* can be characterized by its fibrillar morphology with widths of approx. 10 nm (Soto, 2003). In a molecular level, amyloid is rich in β-sheet structures, which are maintained by hydrogen-bonding interactions between main chains of constituent proteins; therefore, all proteins seem to possess innate propensities of forming a common amyloid structure (Dobson, 2003). Fibrillar aggregates of amyloid-β peptides, which constitute the senile plaques in the Alzheimer disease patients, are the most famous example of amyloid-like aggregates (Serpell & Smith, 2000). It, however, remains controversial whether the pathological protein aggregates in ALS adopt amyloid-like structures. In all cases of ALS, two types of inclusions characterize the surviving motor neurons in a spinal cord; one is called skein-like inclusions, which are immunostained by anti-ubiquitin antibody, and the other, Bunina body, is eosinophilic but ubiquitin-negative (Piao et al., 2003). Pathogenic proteins such as SOD1, TDP-43 and FUS constitute the skein-like inclusions, while Bunina bodies have been shown to be immunoreactive for cystatin C and transferrin (Okamoto et al., 2008). In this chapter, therefore, I will overview recent studies on the *in vitro* and *in vivo* aggregates of ALS-pathogenic proteins, SOD1, TDP-43 and FUS as follows.

2.1 SOD1-positive inclusions in ALS patients

SOD1 is a copper and zinc-containing protein with 153 amino acids, and its physiological function is to detoxify superoxide radical by its dismutation into oxygen and hydrogen peroxide (McCord & Fridovich, 1969). As of now, approximately 150 pathogenic mutations have been reported (http://alsod.iop.kcl.ac.uk), and any preference is not found for the site and type of mutations.

A subset of these pathogenic mutations affects SOD1 activity, while some mutant SOD1s fully retain the catalytic activity (Hayward et al., 2002). Also, transgenic mice expressing mutant SOD1 reproduce disease-like symptoms (Turner & Talbot, 2008), which are absent in SOD1-knockout mice (Reaume et al., 1996). It has, therefore, been considered that pathogenic mutations in SOD1 cause fALS not through loss of an SOD1 physiological function but by gain of new toxic properties. One of such toxic properties proposed so far includes mutation-induced aggregation of SOD1 proteins, while it remains controversial whether SOD1 aggregation is really toxic or even protective. Neuronal hyaline inclusions in the spinal cord are pathological hallmark of mutant SOD1-linked fALS (Shibata et al., 1996b), and those inclusions are ultrastructurally composed of the granule-coated fibrils with a diameter of 15 - 25 nm that can be labeled by anti-SOD1 antibodies (Kato et al., 2000). Such fibrillar morphologies of protein aggregates are reminiscent of the amyloid formation observed in many neurodegenerative diseases (Ross & Poirier, 2004). Pathological inclusions containing mutant SOD1 seem, however, not fulfill some of the criteria for identification as amyloid; that is, neither Congo Red staining with apple-green birefringence nor Thioflavin T/S staining with significant enhancement of fluorescence has been observed in the fALS patient with $SOD1^{A4V}$ (Kerman et al., 2010). Given that these staining methods for amyloid diagnosis have not been routinely performed in the tissue sections from fALS patients with SOD1 mutations, more investigations will be required on the tissue samples of fALS patients with several different types of SOD1 mutations.

Until recently, involvement of wild-type SOD1 ($SOD1^{WT}$) in pathogenesis of sALS had been considered to be limited (Shibata et al., 1994; Shibata et al., 1996a; Watanabe et al., 2001). Indeed, an antibody called SEDI (**S**OD1-**e**xposed-**d**imer-**i**nterface) that only labels monomer/misfolded forms of SOD1 were failed to immunostain the motor neurons from sALS patients (Liu et al., 2009). Nonetheless, novel antibodies raised against 4 - 20, 57 - 72, and 131 - 153 of an SOD1 amino acid sequence were found to specifically detect unfolded SOD1 and also immunostain inclusions in motor neurons of the spinal cord from all the 29 sporadic and 8 familial ALS patients (Forsberg et al., 2010). Furthermore, motor neurons in the spinal cord of sALS patients (four out of nine cases) are found to be immunoreactive to another monoclonal antibody called C4F6, which specifically recognizes the misfolded conformation of SOD1 (Bosco et al., 2010). The staining patterns of C4F6 in sALS are, however, diffusive, and solubility of $SOD1^{WT}$ is also not different between sALS patients and controls. Pathological $SOD1^{WT}$ in sALS would, therefore, be relatively soluble, compared to mutant SOD1 within the inclusions in fALS patients. Although it appears that SOD1 is not involved in fALS cases without SOD1 mutations (Bosco et al., 2010), more prevailing roles of SOD1 proteins in the pathogenesis of ALS have been recently considered.

2.1.1 SOD1 aggregates in mouse models

Transgenic mice expressing human SOD1 with several fALS-associated mutations have been published, and phenotypes in each model mouse have been concisely summarized in (Turner & Talbot, 2008). These transgenic mice well reproduce the formation of ubiquitin-positive SOD1 inclusions, which is the pathological hallmark of SOD1-related fALS diseases (Watanabe et al., 2001). Biochemical analysis on the inclusions has further suggested the ubiquitination of mutant SOD1, based upon which the molecular pathogenesis of ALS has been proposed to include the inhibition of intracellular ubiquitin-proteasome system clogged by insoluble SOD1 aggregates (Basso et al., 2006). Retardation of proteasomal activity thus decelerates degradation of misfolded mutant SOD1, which further promotes the SOD1 aggregation. Recent mass analysis on inclusions in $SOD1^{G93A}$, $SOD1^{G37R}$, and $SOD1^{H46R/H48Q}$ transgenic mice has, however, not supported any direct modifications on SOD1, and ubiquitinated mutant SOD1 may be a minor constituent of inclusions (Shaw et al., 2008). Immunohistochemical analysis has also shown that the inclusions in transgenic mice are immunostained with antibodies to a copper chaperone for SOD1 (see below) and several heat shock proteins such as Hsp70; however, the results are not always consistent with those in human fALS cases (Watanabe et al., 2001).

It is also important to note that amounts of inclusions in the transgenic mice depend upon the type of mutations in the SOD1 transgene. For example, transgenic mice expressing $SOD1^{G37R}$ and $SOD1^{G93A}$ exhibit prominent vacuolation of mitochondria with less amounts of inclusions; in contrast, significant amounts of inclusions are produced in $SOD1^{G85R}$ and $SOD1^{H46R}$ mice (Turner & Talbot, 2008). While such mutation-dependency of inclusion formation remains to be more characterized, H46R and G85R mutations notably reduce the affinity of SOD1 for copper/zinc ions (Hayward et al., 2002). In contrast, enzymatic activity of SOD1 is almost fully retained by G37R and G93A mutations, suggesting little effects on metal affinity/binding (Hayward et al., 2002). It is thus possible that SOD1 aggregation is facilitated by dissociation of metal ions from SOD1 (*vide infra*).

Ultrastructurally, both filamentous and amorphous aggregates that are immunoreactive to SOD1 and ubiquitin constitute the pathological inclusions in the transgenic mice. Unlike pathological inclusions in human fALS cases ($SOD1^{A4V}$) (Kerman et al., 2010), Thioflavin S does stain inclusions formed in $SOD1^{G37R}$ and $SOD1^{G93A}$ mice, suggesting the formation of amyloid-like protein aggregates (Furukawa et al., 2008; Wang et al., 2002). The apparent discrepancy in Thioflavin S staining between human and mouse needs to be described, but it remains unknown if this is due to the difference in the types of mutations (A4V in human vs. G37R/G93A in mouse). It is notable that SOD1 inclusions in $SOD1^{L126X}$ mice are not stained with Thioflavin S (Wang et al., 2005); therefore, tinctorial properties of SOD1 aggregates in pathological inclusions would depend upon the types of SOD1 mutations.

Disulfide cross-linking between SOD1 molecules is also an important feature of SOD1 aggregates in transgenic mice (Furukawa et al., 2006). A natively folded SOD1 possesses a highly conserved "intra"-molecular disulfide bond, but, in contrast, abnormal disulfide linkages "between" SOD1 molecules are detected in inclusions of the transgenic mice. Accumulation of disulfide-linked SOD1 aggregates occurs primarily in the later stages of the disease, concurrent with the appearance of rapidly progressing symptoms (Karch et al., 2009). Furthermore, the conserved intramolecular disulfide is found to be reduced in most of mutant SOD1 molecules constituting inclusions (Karch et al., 2009). Abnormalities in the thiol-disulfide chemistry of SOD1 would thus facilitate aggregation of mutant SOD1 proteins. These results of SOD1 transgenic mouse models strongly suggest the important roles of post-translational maturation of SOD1 polypeptides in the formation of pathological aggregates, which can be well reproduced by the following *in vitro* experiments.

2.1.2 SOD1 aggregates *in vitro*

Intracellular maturation of SOD1 requires several post-translational processes including copper and zinc binding and formation of an intramolecular disulfide bond (Furukawa & O'Halloran, 2006). These processes confer the significantly high structural stability to an SOD1 protein to the extent that the melting temperature of active SOD1 is around 90 °C (Forman & Fridovich, 1973). Many of ALS mutations have been shown to reduce the melting temperature of copper and/or zinc-bound form of SOD1 (Rodriguez et al., 2002), which is, however, still high enough to retain its structure at the physiological temperature (~37 °C). In general, aggregation associates with drastic conformational changes of protein molecules (Dobson, 2003); therefore, high structural (thermal) stability of fully mature SOD1 even in the presence of ALS mutations might not fit to the general aggregation mechanism. In contrast, immature forms of SOD1 have been shown to exhibit significantly reduced thermostability; the melting temperature of the most immature SOD1 (*i.e.* a metal-unbound (apo) and disulfide-reduced form ($SOD1^{SH}$)) is as low as 43 °C (Furukawa & O'Halloran, 2005). Very interestingly, furthermore, apo-$SOD1^{SH}$ with ALS mutations (A4V and G93A) starts to melt at the temperature below 37 °C, suggesting protein unfolding/misfolding under physiological conditions (Furukawa & O'Halloran, 2005). Although it has been claimed that apo-SOD1s are not universally destabilized by the ALS-causing mutations (Rodriguez et al., 2005), the majority of ALS mutations (18 out of 20 mutations they examined) have been shown to indeed decrease melting temperature of apo-SOD1 to some degrees. It is, therefore, possible that mutation-induced destabilization of SOD1 structures plays critical roles in the formation of pathological inclusions found in SOD1-related fALS.

2.1.3 A key role of a disulfide reduction in SOD1 aggregation

Indeed, I have shown for the first time that the SOD1 polypeptide without any post-translational modifications (*i.e.* apo-$SOD1^{SH}$) exhibits the highest propensities for the formation of amyloid-like fibrillar aggregates *in vitro* (Furukawa et al., 2008). Under physiological solution conditions (such as salt concentration and solution pH), *in vitro* aggregation of SOD1 is completely inhibited by addition of Zn^{2+} ion and/or introduction of an intramolecular disulfide bond. SOD1 is a very rare cytosolic protein that keeps a disulfide bond for its enzymatic activity (Furukawa et al., 2004). As described below, the intramolecular disulfide bond in SOD1 is introduced by its copper chaperone in the cell (Furukawa et al., 2004). Without this disulfide, SOD1 favors a monomeric state; but, once the disulfide forms, SOD1 adopts a dimeric structure (Arnesano et al., 2004). Dimerization of SOD1 appears to protect its disulfide from reduction by burying it in the dimer interface. In most of the mutant SOD1 proteins, however, presumably due to perturbation in the native tertiary structure, the affinity for copper and/or zinc ion is reduced (Hayward et al., 2002), and the susceptibility to a disulfide reduction is increased (Tiwari & Hayward, 2003). Given the reducing environment of the cytosol with high metal-chelating capacity (Rae et al., 1999), therefore, a molecular pathomechanism of SOD1-related fALS would involve increased concentration of aggregation-prone apo-$SOD1^{SH}$ state in neurons. Consistently, insoluble mutant SOD1 purified from inclusions in the transgenic mice appear to have no metal ions bound (Lelie et al., 2011). Although aggregation propensities of apo-$SOD1^{SH}$ were not consistently increased by all pathogenic mutations, the intracellular population of aggregation-prone apo-$SOD1^{SH}$ state is considered to increase by the fALS-causing mutations.

Consistent with these *in vitro* observations, intracellular formation of SOD1 aggregates has been shown to be inhibited by co-expression of a copper chaperone for SOD1 (CCS) in cultured cells (Furukawa et al., 2008). CCS is a metallochaperone that specifically loads a copper ion and introduces a disulfide bond into apo-$SOD1^{SH}$ (Culotta et al., 1997; Furukawa et al., 2004). Intracellular concentration of aggregation-prone apo-$SOD1^{SH}$ will thus be effectively reduced by CCS. Unlike the cultured cells, however, $SOD1^{G93A}$ transgenic mice exhibited accelerated progression of disease-like phenotypes with shortening of mean survival from 242 to 36 days upon overexpression of CCS (Son et al., 2007). In particular, the double transgenic mice presented severe mitochondrial pathologies. CCS has been known to regulate the mitochondrial import of SOD1 (Field et al., 2003; Kawamata & Manfredi, 2008);

therefore, in CCS/SOD1^{G93A} double transgenic mice, CCS overexpression would overload mitochondria with toxic SOD1^{G93A}. Because of such a short survival, it remains unclear whether CCS possesses a preventive role in SOD1 aggregation in rodent models. If CCS effectively protects SOD1 from aggregation by facilitating the post-translational maturation, knockout of the *CCS* gene is expected to increase the population of apo-SOD1^{SH} state and then aggravate the inclusion pathologies in ALS-model mice. Again, however, this is not the case; there are virtually no effects on the disease onset/progression, when the *CCS* gene is knocked out from SOD1^{G37R}, SOD1^{G85R}, and SOD1^{G93A} transgenic mice (Subramaniam et al., 2002). Notably, a significant level of SOD1 activity is confirmed in CCS-knockout mice, and this is in sharp contrast to the observations in *S. cerevisiae*, where SOD1 activity is completely vanished upon genetic removal of the *CCS* gene (Culotta et al., 1997). A CCS-independent pathway(s) of SOD1 activation has, therefore, been recently proposed in mammals, and the presence of a Pro residue in an SOD1 C-terminal region determines the dependency of its enzymatic activation on CCS (Leitch et al., 2009). It, therefore, remains difficult to test the potentially protecting role of CCS in SOD1 aggregation in animal models. Interestingly, *C.elegans* has no *CCS* gene and activates SOD1 in a CCS-independent mechanism (Jensen & Culotta, 2005). Worms may thus be able to use as a model to examine effects of fALS mutations on a CCS-independent pathway of SOD1 activation.

In vitro aggregates prepared from SOD1^{SH} have been recently found to exhibit mutation-dependent structural polymorphism (Furukawa et al., 2010). Three regions in an SOD1 amino acid sequence are resistant to be proteolyzed by proteases in the fibrillar SOD1^{SH} aggregates. These three regions can be regarded as building blocks in an SOD1 aggregate structure, and non-native interactions of these building blocks constitute a core in SOD1 aggregate. FALS-causing mutations are found to modulate non-native interactions of those three building blocks, leading to the formation of discrete core structures among SOD1 aggregates with different mutations. Such a mutation-dependent core structure, furthermore, determines morphological as well as biochemical properties of SOD1 aggregate, which may describe distinct disease phenotypes in patients with different mutations in SOD1 (Wang et al., 2008).

2.1.4 Aggregation of SOD1 with an intact disulfide under destabilizing conditions

Notably, apo-SOD1 with an intramolecular disulfide bond (apo-SOD1^{S-S}) is considered to be partially unfolded under physiological temperature, given the melting temperature of around 40 - 50 ^{o}C (Furukawa & O'Halloran, 2005). While partial unfolding of apo-SOD1^{S-S} could induce misfolding and aggregation, 10 μM apo-SOD1^{S-S} without free cysteines (C6S and C111S mutations) was not aggregated even with agitation in a physiological buffer (100 mM Na-Pi, 100 mM NaCl, 5 mM EDTA, pH 7.0) for at least 72 hours (Furukawa et al., 2008). In the same conditions, I have also confirmed no aggregation of wild-type apo-SOD1^{S-S} (with intact free cysteines, unpublished). Several other groups have nonetheless reported the aggregation of SOD1^{S-S}, which will be summarized below.

One of the conditions for triggering aggregation of non-reduced SOD1 is the addition of a chaotropic agent, guanidine hydrochloride (GdnHCl). Valentine and colleagues have performed agitation of 50 μM apo-SOD1^{S-S} with Teflon balls in a buffer (10 mM K-Pi, pH 7.4) containing 1 M GdnHCl and found the formation of Thioflavin-T (ThT)-positive aggregates after approximately 40 hours (Chattopadhyay et al., 2008; Oztug Durer et al., 2009). These apo-SOD1^{S-S} aggregates possess fibrillar morphologies, and its formation is accelerated when the solution pH becomes acidic (pH 3.0, 4.0, 5.0). Interestingly, aggregation of apo-$SOD1^{S-S}$ was accelerated by addition of sub-stoichiometric amounts of soluble apo-$SOD1^{SH}$, suggesting that apo-$SOD1^{SH}$ can initiate aggregation of apo-$SOD1^{S-S}$ by acting as nuclei. Thus, SOD1 with a disulfide bond would be aggregation-incompetent, but, once the disulfide is somehow reduced in a small fraction of $SOD1^{S-S}$ proteins during the *in vitro* aggregation reaction, the resultant $SOD1^{SH}$ might convert the residual $SOD1^{S-S}$ into aggregation-competent conformations. Chia et al. have also shown that aggregation of 10 μM $SOD1^{S-S}$ in the presence of 0.5 M GdnHCl at pH 4.0 is accelerated by addition of spinal cord homogenates from transgenic mice expressing $SOD1^{G93A}$ (120 days old) (Chia et al., 2010). Such a seeded aggregation was not observed by adding spinal cord homogenates of the non-transgenic littermates. Given that $SOD1^{G93A}$ mice contain pathological inclusions at 120 days of age (Gurney et al., 1994), the *in vitro* $SOD1^{S-S}$ aggregation is seeded by either pathological SOD1 aggregates, soluble $SOD1^{SH}$ or both.

Another aggregation-inducing condition is the addition of trifluoroethanol (TFE). TFE has been considered to stabilize secondary structures but disrupt the native tertiary structure of various intact proteins (Buck, 1998). Consistent with the high thermostability, a holo-form of $SOD1^{S-S}$ remains soluble in the presence of up to 80 % TFE; in contrast, apo-$SOD1^{S-S}$ readily forms visible aggregate in the presence of 15 % TFE (Stathopulos et al., 2003). Stathopulos et al. have further proposed the correlation of the melting temperature with the amount of TFE required for aggregation by using several fALS-causing mutant apo-$SOD1^{S-S}$ proteins (Stathopulos et al., 2003). Morphologies of TFE-induced $SOD1^{S-S}$ aggregates are fibrillar, but those aggregates exhibit 2- to 3-fold ThT fluorescence enhancement and small spectral changes upon addition of Congo Red. These tinctorial changes may be comparable to those in pathological SOD1 aggregates to the extent that inclusions in fALS patients are usually not stained by both Thioflavin S and Congo Red (Kato et al., 2000). Given that the typical amyloid aggregates lead to ~1000-fold increase in the intensity of ThT fluorescence and red-shift a spectrum of Congo Red (Klunk et al., 1999; LeVine, 1999), TFE-induced $SOD1^{S-S}$ aggregates will not be categorized as a typical amyloid.

It is also interesting to note that TFE-induced SOD1 aggregates act as seeds to trigger aggregation of endogenous SOD1 in cultured cells. Münch et al. have prepared the *in vitro* aggregates of $SOD1^{H46R}$ by adding 20 % TFE, although the thiol-disulfide status in the mutant SOD1 was not specified (Munch et al., 2011). These *in vitro* aggregates were found to penetrate inside neuronal cells, *Neuro2a*, by macropinocytosis, rapidly exit the macropinocytic compartment, and then nucleate aggregation of the transiently overexpressed $SOD1^{H46R}$-GFP in the cytosol. Intracellular $SOD1^{WT}$-GFP was not aggregated by exogenously added $SOD1^{H46R}$ aggregates. Importantly, the intracellularly seeded aggregates have been found to transfer from cell to cell; thereby, the phenotypes can be "infected" among cells. Such a seeded infection of protein aggregates is reminiscent of the prion phenomena and has been reported in several other pathogenic proteins for neurodegenerative diseases such as α-synuclein (Luk et al., 2009), Tau (Clavaguera et al., 2009), polyglutamine (Ren et al., 2009), and TDP-43 (Furukawa et al., 2011). Although it has not been confirmed if ALS is infectious, the seeding properties of TFE-induced aggregates may describe the propagation of pathological changes with the progression of diseases.

Metal-catalyzed oxidation of Zn-deficient SOD1 also leads to the protein aggregation (Rakhit et al., 2002; Rakhit et al., 2004). $CuCl_2$ with ascorbic acid generates reactive oxygen species, which then oxidize histidine residues in SOD1. This is consistent with the fact that the aggregation is significantly retarded at pH < 5.5. While SOD1 exists as a dimer, the oxidized SOD1 dissociates into monomers and then forms non-amyloid aggregates with amorphous and fibrillar morphologies. The oxidation-induced aggregation does not occur when SOD1 is in a holo state. Zinc-binding affinity of SOD1 has been known to decrease with fALS mutations (Hayward et al., 2002); therefore, mutant SOD1 is more susceptible to aggregation through the metal-catalyzed oxidation than the wild-type protein.

Incubation time will be another key factor to induce the aggregation of a mature SOD1 (*i.e.* a fully metallated SOD1 with an intramolecular disulfide bond). Usually, the aggregation kinetics of proteins has been monitored for at most 3 - 5 days, where either fully mature or even partially mature SOD1 does not aggregate in a physiological buffer without any chaotropic reagents. Nonetheless, Hwang et al. have extended the incubation time up to more than 300 hours (> 10 days) and found the fibrillar aggregation of fully mature SOD1 (with C6A/C111S mutations) under physiological conditions (~300 μM proteins, pH 7.8, 37 ^{o}C) (Hwang et al., 2010). The SOD1 aggregates after a prolonged incubation did not show apple-green birefringence upon binding Congo Red nor strong enhancement of ThT fluorescence, consistent with properties of inclusions in SOD1-related fALS patients (Kato et al., 2000). It remains unknown if SOD1 retains metal ions even in the aggregated state, it is possible that such a long incubation of SOD1 proteins somehow leads to the partial loss and/or the altered binding geometries of metal ions.

In summary, SOD1 can adopt theoretically 44 types of modified states when metal binding, disulfide formation and dimerization are taken into account (Furukawa & O'Halloran, 2006). Many papers point out the strengths of the SOD1 aggregation model for ALS; however, as mentioned above, there is still no consensus on which state of SOD1 is responsible for aggregation observed in fALS cases. Researchers including myself have thus continuingly pursued a mechanism describing why more than 100 ALS-causing mutations in SOD1 commonly facilitate the SOD1 aggregation process.

2.2 TDP-43-positive inclusions in ALS patients

TDP-43 is a DNA/RNA binding protein with 414 amino acids and contains two RNA recognition motifs (RRM1 and RRM2) and a C-terminal auxiliary region (Ayala et al., 2005). As of now, more than 40 mutations have been identified in the TDP-43 gene as being pathogenic, and most of the mutations are localized in the C-terminal region (http://alsod.iop.kcl.ac.uk). One of physiological functions of TDP-43 is to regulate an alternative splicing of several gene transcripts (Ayala et al., 2008a; Buratti & Baralle, 2001); usually, TDP-43 is localized at the nucleus but is also known to shuttle between nucleus and cytoplasm (Ayala et al., 2008b). Under pathological conditions, in contrast, TDP-43 is cleared from the nucleus and is mislocalized at the cytoplasm, where the ubiquitin- and TDP-43-positive inclusions are observed (Arai et al., 2006; Neumann et al., 2006). Formation of TDP-43 inclusions has been confirmed in sALS and SOD1-negative fALS but not in SOD1-linked fALS (Mackenzie et al., 2007). Actually, before identification of pathogenic mutations in the TDP-43 gene, proteomic analysis of ubiquitin-positive inclusions in sALS patients has revealed TDP-43 as a major component of inclusions (Arai et al., 2006; Neumann et al., 2006). TDP-43 immunoreactive inclusions have also been observed in many other neurodegenerative diseases such as frontotemporal lobar degeneration (FTLD), Huntington disease, and Alzheimer disease, which recently leads to a new disease category called TDP-43 proteinopathies (Geser et al., 2009).

In pathological inclusions, TDP-43 is abnormally hyper-phosphorylated and cleaved to generate C-terminal fragments (Arai et al., 2006; Neumann et al., 2006). Pathological TDP-43 is also distinct from its normal counterpart because it exhibits decreased solubility in a buffer containing a detergent, Sarkosyl. Ultrastructurally, inclusions observed in TDP-43 proteinopathies are characterized by bundles of straight fibrils with 10 - 20 nm diameter that are immunostained by anti-TDP-43 antibodies (Lin & Dickson, 2008). Similar to SOD1-positive inclusions, however, TDP-43 inclusions are also not stained by Thioflavin S and Congo Red (Kerman et al., 2010), implying less amyloid characters. Interestingly, the C-terminal fragments are enriched in the cytoplasmic inclusions in brain of ALS patients, but in the spinal cord, inclusions are composed of full-length TDP-43 (Igaz et al., 2008). Furthermore, Hasegawa et al. have found the immunoblot distinction of TDP-43 among different TDP-43 proteinopathies (Hasegawa et al., 2008); for example, Sarkosyl-insoluble fractions of ALS and FTLD brains exhibit different electrophoretic band patterns of the C-terminal fragments of phosphorylated TDP-43 in the Western blots. Depending upon the clinicopathological subtypes of TDP-43 proteinopathies, multiple pathways can thus be considered for the formation of TDP-43 inclusions; however, molecular mechanisms of truncation and phosphorylation in TDP-43 remain unknown.

2.2.1 TDP-43 aggregates in mouse models

Homozygous disruption of the TDP-43 gene is embryonic lethal in mice (Kraemer et al., 2010), and post-natal deletion of the TDP-43 gene by utilizing a Cre recombinase also produces lethality albeit without any ALS-like symptoms (Chiang et al., 2010). Expression of wild-type human TDP-43 has also been reported to be toxic in mice in a dose-dependent manner; indeed, TDP-43 transgenic mice exhibit a wide variety of motor dysfunctions, which appears to depend upon the promoter regulating the expression of the transgene (Da Cruz & Cleveland, 2011). More toxic effects of ALS-causing mutations (A315T and M337V examined so far) in the TDP-43 transgene has not been established yet. Surprisingly, any of the transgenic mice expressing wild-type and mutant TDP-43 have not reproduced the formation of ubiquitin- and TDP-43-positive inclusions. When human TDP-43 with A315T mutation is expressed in mice under the control of mouse prion promoter (Wegorzewska et al., 2009), the mice develop gait abnormality with an average survival of about 150 days, and ubiquitin-positive inclusions are observed in specific neuronal populations including spinal motor neurons. Despite this, those ubiquitin-positive inclusions are not immunostained with anti-TDP-43 antibodies, and very limited amounts of C-terminally truncated TDP-43 are confirmed. Furthermore, mutant TDP-43 exhibits similar solubility in a Sarkosyl-containing buffer to that of mouse endogenous wild-type TDP-43. Although truncation as well as insolubilization of TDP-43 characterizes the TDP-43 proteinopathies, both of these pathological processes may hence not be required for neurodegeneration.

In contrast, Wils et al. have constructed a mouse expressing wild-type human TDP-43 under the control of a neuronal murine Thy-1 promoter and found a dose-dependent degeneration of cortical and spinal motor neurons (Wils et al., 2010). Immunohistochemical analysis has further confirmed the formation of ubiquitin-positive inclusions, which are stained by an anti-TDP-43 antibody and also an antibody recognizing Ser409/410-phosphorylated TDP-43. Abnormal phosphorylation on TDP-43 is thus reproduced in this model mouse; furthermore, the C-terminal truncation of human TDP-43 is observed albeit much less amounts than that in ALS patients. Despite this, human TDP-43 in the affected mice remains soluble in a Sarkosyl-containing buffer, showing that the pathological processes of TDP-43 are not completely reproduced in the transgenic mouse model.

Transgenic rats expressing human wild-type and mutant (M337V) TDP-43 have also been made (Zhou et al., 2010). Soon after the birth, TDP-43^{M337V} transgenic rats become paralyzed at 20 - 30 days and die at postnatal ages; in contrast, TDP-43^{WT} transgenic rats exhibit no paralysis by the age of 200 days. Mutation-specific toxicity of TDP-43 has thus been reproduced in these rat transgenic models, but TDP-43 inclusions are rarely detected and present only in the cortex of paralyzed TDP-43^{M337V} transgenic rats. A very faint amount of truncated TDP-43 is detected, and phosphorylated TDP-43 is accumulated at the cytoplasm of spinal motor neurons. These molecular changes of TDP-43 are, however, confirmed in both TDP-43^{WT} and TDP-43^{M337V} transgenic rats, implying little roles of truncation and phosphorylation in expressing the mutant-specific toxicity of TDP-43. Accordingly, it still remains to be established in the rodent models how mutant TDP-43 exerts its toxicity and is involved in the inclusion formation under pathological conditions.

2.2.2 TDP-43 aggregates *in vitro*

Bacterially expressed TDP-43 normally forms insoluble inclusion bodies, which hampers biochemical characterization of TDP-43 proteins. Johnson et al. have nonetheless succeeded to obtain soluble full-length 6 x His-tagged TDP-43 by using a cold shock expression system in *E.coli* (Johnson et al., 2009) Agitation of 3 μM full-length TDP-43 in 40 mM HEPES/150 mM KCl/20 mM $MgCl_2$/1 mM DTT, pH 7.4 at 25 °C increases solution turbidity within an hour, supporting the high aggregation propensities of TDP-43. A TDP-43 truncate that is devoid of the C-terminal auxiliary domain does not increase its solution turbidity, suggesting an important role of the C-terminal domain in the aggregation *in vitro*. Aggregates of full-length TDP-43 exhibit both filament-like and thread-like morphologies but did not react with the amyloid-diagnostic dyes, Congo Red and ThT. A subset of fALS-linked mutations (M337V, Q331K) slightly facilitates the aggregation kinetics of full-length TDP-43. A high propensity for fibrillation has been also shown for the synthetic peptide fragment of a TDP-43 C-terminal region (Gly 287- Met 322) (Chen et al., 2010). Fibrillar aggregates of the C-terminal peptide did not increase the intensity of Thioflavin T fluorescence. Interestingly, an ALS-causing mutation, G294A, but not A315T renders the fibrillar aggregates ThT-positive. While fibrils of all C-terminal peptides (wild-type, A315T, G294A) possess β-sheet rich structures, ALS mutations would affect the biochemical/structural properties of TDP-43 aggregates.

I have recently reported that bacterially expressed full-length TDP-43 is resolubilized, purified in the presence of GdnHCl, and then refolded by dilution of GdnHCl (Furukawa et al., 2011). Such refolded TDP-43 proteins retain the physiological DNA binding function but forms fibrillar aggregates by agitation at 37 °C in 100 mM Na-Pi/100 mM NaCl/5 mM EDTA/5 mM DTT/10 % glycerol, pH 8.0. A C-terminal half of TDP-43 assumes a core in the fibrillar aggregates and reproduces the fibrillation propensities of full-length TDP-43 proteins. These *in vitro* TDP-43 fibrils are insoluble in a Sarkosyl-containing buffer, which is a consistent feature with the pathological inclusions. A seeding activity is also a notable feature of TDP-43 fibrils *in vitro*, where pre-formed fibrils (or called "seeds") function as a structural template to facilitate the recruitment of soluble proteins into insoluble fibrils. This seeding reaction has been found to also occur inside the cultured cells by transducing the cells with *in vitro* TDP-43 fibrils; thereby, the formation of Sarkosyl-insoluble and ubiquitinated TDP-43 inclusions is well reproduced in the cell. This is notable because simple overexpression of TDP-43 in the cultured cells has never generated the Sarkosyl-insoluble inclusions. It remains controversial whether the aggregation of TDP-43 is a cause or a result of the disease; however, as recently proposed in the other neurodegenerative diseases (Aguzzi & Rajendran, 2009; Brundin et al., 2010), a seeding activity of TDP-43 proteins may contribute to the propagation of pathological changes with the progression of diseases.

All recent *in vitro* studies on TDP-43 proteins have revealed its high propensities for aggregation, which are provided by the C-terminal auxiliary domain. Given that most of the fALS-causing mutations are located at this domain, the mutational alteration in the aggregation propensities of TDP-43 might be a part of the ALS pathomechanism. More *in vitro* experiments will, however, be required to reveal if the aggregation reactions of TDP-43 are affected by mutation, truncation, and phosphorylation.

2.3 FUS-positive inclusions in ALS patients

FUS was initially identified as the N-terminus of FUS-CHOP (CCAAT/enhancer binding protein homologous protein), a fusion oncoprotein expressed in human myxoid liposarcoma with the t(12;16) chromosomal translocation (Crozat et al., 1993). Like TDP-43, FUS is a DNA/RNA binding protein with 526 amino acids and comprised of multiple domains as follows (from N-terminal to C-terminal); a Q/G/S/Y-rich domain, a G-rich domain, an RNA-recognition motif (RRM), an R/G-rich domain, a Zn-finger motif, and a region containing a nuclear localization signal (NLS) (Dormann et al., 2010; Iko et al., 2004). Under physiological conditions, FUS has been proposed to be involved in transcription regulation (Uranishi et al., 2001), RNA splicing (Yang et al., 1998), and RNA transport including nucleo-cytoplasmic shuttling (Zinszner et al., 1997).

Late in 2007, which was before identification of pathological mutations in the *FUS* gene, FUS protein was found as one of major proteins recruited into neuronal intranuclear inclusions in patients of Huntington disease (Doi et al., 2008). In this neurodegenerative disease, a polyglutamine tract in a protein called huntingtin (HTT) is abnormally expanded, leading to fibrillar aggregation of mutant HTT in affected neurons (Zoghbi & Orr, 2000). FUS is sequestered by fibrillar HTT aggregates and then becomes insoluble and possibly dysfunctional (Doi et al., 2008). Loss of physiological functions of FUS would, therefore, contribute to neuronal cell death in Huntington's disease (Doi et al., 2008) as well as other polyglutamine diseases (Doi et al., 2010).

Then, fALS-causing mutations in the *FUS* gene have been identified in 2009 (Kwiatkowski et al., 2009; Vance et al., 2009), and, as of now, at least 40 mutations have been reported, most of which are localized at a G-rich domain and a C-terminal NLS-containing region (http://alsod.iop.kcl.ac.uk). Although neuropathological analysis of fALS patients with *FUS* mutations has been still limited, cytoplasmic mislocalization of nuclear FUS protein in motor neurons is a major pathological hallmark. Indeed, as shown by a recent study (Dormann et al., 2010), fALS-causing mutations at the C-terminal region of FUS result in the functional impairment of the NLS, facilitating the cytoplasmic mislocalization of mutant FUS. In FUS-related fALS, FUS-immunoreactive cytoplasmic inclusions are observed, which have been recently found to exhibit mutation-dependent heterogeneity (Mackenzie et al., 2011). For example, P525L mutation in FUS associates with a relatively early onset (twenties) of ALS, where round FUS-immunoreactive neuronal cytoplasmic inclusions are found. In contrast, late-onset (forties to sixties) ALS cases are linked to R521C mutation in FUS and have tangle-like FUS-immunoreative neuronal and glial cytoplasmic inclusions. Furthermore, it has been reported that FUS-immunoreactive inclusions are observed in spinall spinal anterior horn neurons in all sporadic and familial ALS cases tested, except for those with SOD1 mutations (Deng et al., 2011b). Although mutations in FUS account for only a small fraction of fALS and sALS cases, FUS proteins may be a common component of cytosolic inclusions in non-SOD1 ALS. In motor neurons of patients with juvenile ALS, FUS has been shown to form filamentous aggregates with a diameter of 15 - 20 nm, which are often associated with small granules (Baumer et al., 2010; Huang et al., 2011). Staining with Thioflavin T/S and Congo Red has not, however, been performed yet on the inclusions of FUS-linked ALS. It also remains unknown if pathological FUS decreases its solubility or is modified/truncated in inclusions.

2.3.1 FUS aggregates in a rat model

As of now, there is no mouse model of FUS-linked ALS, but a transgenic rat expressing wild-type or ALS-causing mutant (R521C) FUS has been published (Huang et al., 2011). Only the mutant FUS transgenic rats developed paralysis at an early age (1 - 2 mo) with a significant loss of neurons in the frontal cortex and dentate gyrus. These pathological changes are not observed in age-matched wild-type FUS transgenic rats, although, at the advanced age (> 1 yr), wild-type FUS transgenic rats display a deficit in spatial learning and memory with a moderate loss of neurons in the frontal cortex and dentate gyrus. Immunohistochemical analysis of the cortex and spinal cord has shown the appearance of ubiquitin-positive inclusions at the paralysis stages of both wild-type and mutant FUS rats; however, the inclusions are not immunostained with anti-FUS antibodies. Given that several different anti-FUS antibodies show distinct immunoreactivities toward FUS-containing inclusions in sALS cases (Deng et al., 2011b), more detailed investigations will be necessary to characterize the possible aggregation of FUS forming pathological inclusions.

2.3.2 FUS aggregates *in vitro*

There is only one paper published on the aggregation reaction of purified FUS proteins (Sun et al., 2011); Sun et al. have prepared GST-fused FUS proteins intervened with a TEV protease site and found that the cleavage of 2.5 - 5 μM GST-FUS with a TEV protease produces full-length FUS in 100 mM Tris/200 mM trehalose/0.5 mM EDTA/20 mM glutathione, pH 8.0, and starts aggregation without a lag-time at 22° C in the absence of agitation. The resultant *in vitro* aggregates of FUS do not increase the intensity of ThT fluorescence and are completely soluble in an SDS-containing buffer. They have further examined the aggregation reactions of several truncated FUS proteins and shown that the N-terminal region of FUS (1 - 422) is enough to reproduce the aggregation behavior of full-length FUS. Aggregates of both full-length FUS and truncated FUS (1 - 422) are fibrillar in the morphologies, which resemble to the FUS inclusions in the ALS patients. No effects of fALS-causing mutations (H517Q, R521H, R521C) are observed on the *in vitro* fibrillation kinetics of full-length FUS proteins.

3. Conclusion

In this chapter, recent progress has been reviewed on aggregation mechanisms of ALS pathogenic proteins, SOD1, TDP-43 and FUS. Common to all these three proteins, structural/biochemical characters of aggregates *in vitro* are much dependent upon experimental conditions, and it remains obscure which of aggregates *in vitro* reproduces the pathological inclusions in patients. In particular, post-translational processes such as metallation, disulfide formation, phosphorylation, and truncation appear to affect the aggregation pathway(s) of the pathogenic proteins. In future, therefore, it will become more important to correlate any abnormalities in these post-translational modifications with pathogenicity of ALS.

Very recently, mutations in another gene, optineurin (OPTN), have been linked to fALS cases, and hyaline inclusions in the anterior horn cells of spinal cord were immunoreactive for OPTN in patients with OPTN mutation (E478G) (Maruyama et al., 2010). Furthermore, albeit controversial, skein-like inclusions in all the sALS and non-SOD1 fALS have been reported to be immunostained with an anti-OPTN antibody (Deng et al., 2011a). Aggregation of an OPTN protein would thus be of relevance to describe the pathomechanism of both sporadic and familial ALS.

In spite of recent efforts to identify the causative genes for fALS, most of the cases are still genetically unidentified (Da Cruz & Cleveland, 2011). Given that the skein-like inclusions in the spinal anterior horn cells are characteristic of ALS, proteomic analysis of those inclusions will help to identify as-yet-unknown proteins pathogenic for ALS. In addition, the component analysis of skein-like inclusions will help to describe the common pathomechanism of sporadic and familial ALS cases.

4. References

Aguzzi, A. & Rajendran, L. (2009). The transcellular spread of cytosolic amyloids, prions, and prionoids. *Neuron*, Vol.64, No.6, pp. 783-790, ISSN 1097-4199

Arai, T.; Hasegawa, M.; Akiyama, H.; Ikeda, K.; Nonaka, T.; Mori, H.; Mann, D.; Tsuchiya, K.; Yoshida, M.; Hashizume, Y. & Oda, T. (2006). TDP-43 is a component of ubiquitin-positive tau-negative inclusions in frontotemporal lobar degeneration and amyotrophic lateral sclerosis. *Biochem Biophys Res Commun*, Vol.351, No.3, pp. 602-611, ISSN 0006-291X

Arnesano, F.; Banci, L.; Bertini, I.; Martinelli, M.; Furukawa, Y. & O'Halloran, T.V. (2004). The unusually stable quaternary structure of human SOD1 is controlled by both metal occupancy and disulfide status. *J Biol Chem*, Vol.279, pp. 47998-48003,

Ayala, Y.M.; Pantano, S.; D'Ambrogio, A.; Buratti, E.; Brindisi, A.; Marchetti, C.; Romano, M. & Baralle, F.E. (2005). Human, Drosophila, and C.elegans TDP43: nucleic acid binding properties and splicing regulatory function. *J Mol Biol*, Vol.348, No.3, pp. 575-588, ISSN 0022-2836

Ayala, Y.M.; Misteli, T. & Baralle, F.E. (2008a). TDP-43 regulates retinoblastoma protein phosphorylation through the repression of cyclin-dependent kinase 6 expression. *Proc Natl Acad Sci U S A*, Vol.105, No.10, pp. 3785-3789, ISSN 1091-6490

Ayala, Y.M.; Zago, P.; D'Ambrogio, A.; Xu, Y.F.; Petrucelli, L.; Buratti, E. & Baralle, F.E. (2008b). Structural determinants of the cellular localization and shuttling of TDP-43. *J Cell Sci*, Vol.121, No.Pt 22, pp. 3778-3785, ISSN 0021-9533

Basso, M.; Massignan, T.; Samengo, G.; Cheroni, C.; De Biasi, S.; Salmona, M.; Bendotti, C. & Bonetto, V. (2006). Insoluble mutant SOD1 is partly oligoubiquitinated in amyotrophic lateral sclerosis mice. *J Biol Chem*, Vol.281, No.44, pp. 33325-33335, ISSN 0021-9258

Baumer, D.; Hilton, D.; Paine, S.M.; Turner, M.R.; Lowe, J.; Talbot, K. & Ansorge, O. (2010). Juvenile ALS with basophilic inclusions is a FUS proteinopathy with FUS mutations. *Neurology*, Vol.75, No.7, pp. 611-618, ISSN 1526-632X

Bosco, D.A.; Morfini, G.; Karabacak, N.M.; Song, Y.; Gros-Louis, F.; Pasinelli, P.; Goolsby, H.; Fontaine, B.A.; Lemay, N.; McKenna-Yasek, D.; Frosch, M.P.; Agar, J.N.; Julien, J.P.; Brady, S.T. & Brown, R.H., Jr. (2010). Wild-type and mutant SOD1 share an aberrant conformation and a common pathogenic pathway in ALS. *Nat Neurosci*, Vol.13, No.11, pp. 1396-1403, ISSN 1546-1726

Bruijn, L.I.; Miller, T.M. & Cleveland, D.W. (2004). Unraveling the Mechanisms Involved in Motor Neuron Degeneration in ALS. *Annu Rev Neurosci*, Vol.27, pp. 723-749,

Brundin, P.; Melki, R. & Kopito, R. (2010). Prion-like transmission of protein aggregates in neurodegenerative diseases. *Nat Rev Mol Cell Biol*, Vol.11, No.4, pp. 301-307, ISSN 1471-0080

Buck, M. (1998). Trifluoroethanol and colleagues: cosolvents come of age. Recent studies with peptides and proteins. *Q Rev Biophys*, Vol.31, No.3, pp. 297-355, ISSN 0033-5835

Buratti, E. & Baralle, F.E. (2001). Characterization and functional implications of the RNA binding properties of nuclear factor TDP-43, a novel splicing regulator of CFTR exon 9. *J Biol Chem*, Vol.276, No.39, pp. 36337-36343, ISSN 0021-9258

Charcot, J.M. & Joffroy, A. (1869). Deux cas d'atrophie musculaire progressive avec lésions de la substance grise et des faisceaux antérolatéraux de la moelle épinière. *Arch. Physiol. Norm. Pathol.*, Vol.6, pp. 744-760,

Chattopadhyay, M.; Durazo, A.; Sohn, S.H.; Strong, C.D.; Gralla, E.B.; Whitelegge, J.P. & Valentine, J.S. (2008). Initiation and elongation in fibrillation of ALS-linked superoxide dismutase. *Proc Natl Acad Sci U S A*, Vol.105, No.48, pp. 18663-18668, ISSN 1091-6490

Chen, A.K.; Lin, R.Y.; Hsieh, E.Z.; Tu, P.H.; Chen, R.P.; Liao, T.Y.; Chen, W.; Wang, C.H. & Huang, J.J. (2010). Induction of amyloid fibrils by the C-terminal fragments of TDP-43 in amyotrophic lateral sclerosis. *J Am Chem Soc*, Vol.132, No.4, pp. 1186-1187, ISSN 1520-5126

Chia, R.; Tattum, M.H.; Jones, S.; Collinge, J.; Fisher, E.M. & Jackson, G.S. (2010). Superoxide dismutase 1 and tgSOD1 mouse spinal cord seed fibrils, suggesting a propagative cell death mechanism in amyotrophic lateral sclerosis. *PLoS One*, Vol.5, No.5, pp. e10627, ISSN 1932-6203

Chiang, P.M.; Ling, J.; Jeong, Y.H.; Price, D.L.; Aja, S.M. & Wong, P.C. (2010). Deletion of TDP-43 down-regulates Tbc1d1, a gene linked to obesity, and alters body fat metabolism. *Proc Natl Acad Sci U S A*, Vol.107, No.37, pp. 16320-16324, ISSN 1091-6490

Clavaguera, F.; Bolmont, T.; Crowther, R.A.; Abramowski, D.; Frank, S.; Probst, A.; Fraser, G.; Stalder, A.K.; Beibel, M.; Staufenbiel, M.; Jucker, M.; Goedert, M. & Tolnay, M. (2009). Transmission and spreading of tauopathy in transgenic mouse brain. *Nat Cell Biol*, Vol.11, No.7, pp. 909-913, ISSN 1476-4679

Crozat, A.; Aman, P.; Mandahl, N. & Ron, D. (1993). Fusion of CHOP to a novel RNA-binding protein in human myxoid liposarcoma. *Nature*, Vol.363, No.6430, pp. 640-644, ISSN 0028-0836

Culotta, V.C.; Klomp, L.W.J.; Strain, J.; Casareno, R.L.B.; Krems, B. & Gitlin, J.D. (1997). The copper chaperone for superoxide dismutase. *J Biol Chem*, Vol.272, No.38, pp. 23469-23472,

Da Cruz, S. & Cleveland, D.W. (2011). Understanding the role of TDP-43 and FUS/TLS in ALS and beyond. *Curr Opin Neurobiol*, pp. ISSN 1873-6882

de Belleroche, J.; Orrell, R.W. & Virgo, L. (1996). Amyotrophic lateral sclerosis: recent advances in understanding disease mechanisms. *J Neuropathol Exp Neurol*, Vol.55, No.7, pp. 747-757, ISSN 0022-3069

Deng, H.X.; Hentati, A.; Tainer, J.A.; Iqbal, Z.; Cayabyab, A.; Hung, W.Y.; Getzoff, E.D.; Hu, P.; Herzfeldt, B.; Roos, R.P. & et al. (1993). Amyotrophic lateral sclerosis and structural defects in Cu,Zn superoxide dismutase. *Science*, Vol.261, No.5124, pp. 1047-1051,

Deng, H.X.; Bigio, E.H.; Zhai, H.; Fecto, F.; Ajroud, K.; Shi, Y.; Yan, J.; Mishra, M.; Ajroud-Driss, S.; Heller, S.; Sufit, R.; Siddique, N.; Mugnaini, E. & Siddique, T. (2011a). Differential Involvement of Optineurin in Amyotrophic Lateral Sclerosis With or Without SOD1 Mutations. *Arch Neurol*, Vol.68, No.8, pp. 1057-1061, ISSN 1538-3687

Deng, H.X.; Zhai, H.; Bigio, E.H.; Yan, J.; Fecto, F.; Ajroud, K.; Mishra, M.; Ajroud-Driss, S.; Heller, S.; Sufit, R.; Siddique, N.; Mugnaini, E. & Siddique, T. (2011b). FUS-immunoreactive inclusions are a common feature in sporadic and non-SOD1 familial amyotrophic lateral sclerosis. *Ann Neurol*, Vol.67, No.6, pp. 739-748, ISSN 1531-8249

Dobson, C.M. (2003). Protein folding and misfolding. *Nature*, Vol.426, No.6968, pp. 884-890,

Doi, H.; Okamura, K.; Bauer, P.O.; Furukawa, Y.; Shimizu, H.; Kurosawa, M.; Machida, Y.; Miyazaki, H.; Mitsui, K.; Kuroiwa, Y. & Nukina, N. (2008). RNA-binding protein TLS is a major nuclear aggregate-interacting protein in huntingtin exon 1 with expanded polyglutamine-expressing cells. *J Biol Chem*, Vol.283, No.10, pp. 6489-6500, ISSN 0021-9258

Doi, H.; Koyano, S.; Suzuki, Y.; Nukina, N. & Kuroiwa, Y. (2010). The RNA-binding protein FUS/TLS is a common aggregate-interacting protein in polyglutamine diseases. *Neurosci Res*, Vol.66, No.1, pp. 131-133, ISSN 1872-8111

Dormann, D.; Rodde, R.; Edbauer, D.; Bentmann, E.; Fischer, I.; Hruscha, A.; Than, M.E.; Mackenzie, I.R.; Capell, A.; Schmid, B.; Neumann, M. & Haass, C. (2010). ALS-associated fused in sarcoma (FUS) mutations disrupt Transportin-mediated nuclear import. *EMBO J*, Vol.29, No.16, pp. 2841-2857, ISSN 1460-2075

Field, L.S.; Furukawa, Y.; O'Halloran, T.V. & Culotta, V.C. (2003). Factors controlling the uptake of yeast copper/zinc superoxide dismutase into mitochondria. *J Biol Chem*, Vol.278, pp. 28052-28059,

Forman, H.J. & Fridovich, I. (1973). On the stability of bovine superoxide dismutase. The effects of metals. *J Biol Chem*, Vol.248, No.8, pp. 2645-2649,

Forsberg, K.; Jonsson, P.A.; Andersen, P.M.; Bergemalm, D.; Graffmo, K.S.; Hultdin, M.; Jacobsson, J.; Rosquist, R.; Marklund, S.L. & Brannstrom, T. (2010). Novel antibodies reveal inclusions containing non-native SOD1 in sporadic ALS patients. *PLoS One*, Vol.5, No.7, pp. e11552, ISSN 1932-6203

Furukawa, Y.; Torres, A.S. & O'Halloran, T.V. (2004). Oxygen-induced maturation of SOD1: a key role for disulfide formation by the copper chaperone CCS. *EMBO J*, Vol.23, pp. 2872-2881,

Furukawa, Y. & O'Halloran, T.V. (2005). ALS mutations have the greatest destabilizing effect on the apo, reduced form of SOD1, leading to unfolding and oxidative aggregation. *J Biol Chem*, Vol.280, pp. 17266-17274,

Furukawa, Y.; Fu, R.; Deng, H.X.; Siddique, T. & O'Halloran, T.V. (2006). Disulfide cross-linked protein represents a significant fraction of ALS-associated Cu, Zn-superoxide dismutase aggregates in spinal cords of model mice. *Proc Natl Acad Sci U S A*, Vol.103, No.18, pp. 7148-7153, ISSN 0027-8424

Furukawa, Y. & O'Halloran, T.V. (2006). Posttranslational modifications in Cu,Zn-superoxide dismutase and mutations associated with amyotrophic lateral sclerosis. *Antioxid Redox Signal*, Vol.8, No.5-6, pp. 847-867, ISSN 1523-0864

Furukawa, Y.; Kaneko, K.; Yamanaka, K.; O'Halloran, T.V. & Nukina, N. (2008). Complete loss of post-translational modifications triggers fibrillar aggregation of SOD1 in familial form of ALS. *J Biol Chem*, Vol.283, No.35, pp. 24167-24176, ISSN 0021-9258

Furukawa, Y.; Kaneko, K.; Yamanaka, K. & Nukina, N. (2010). Mutation-dependent polymorphism of Cu,Zn-superoxide dismutase aggregates in the familial form of amyotrophic lateral sclerosis. *J Biol Chem*, Vol.285, No.29, pp. 22221-22231, ISSN 1083-351X

Furukawa, Y.; Kaneko, K.; Watanabe, S.; Yamanaka, K. & Nukina, N. (2011). A seeding reaction recapitulates intracellular formation of Sarkosyl-insoluble transactivation response element (TAR) DNA-binding protein-43 inclusions. *J Biol Chem*, Vol.286, No.21, pp. 18664-18672, ISSN 1083-351X

Geser, F.; Martinez-Lage, M.; Kwong, L.K.; Lee, V.M. & Trojanowski, J.Q. (2009). Amyotrophic lateral sclerosis, frontotemporal dementia and beyond: the TDP-43 diseases. *J Neurol*, Vol.256, No.8, pp. 1205-1214, ISSN 1432-1459

Gitcho, M.A.; Baloh, R.H.; Chakraverty, S.; Mayo, K.; Norton, J.B.; Levitch, D.; Hatanpaa, K.J.; White, C.L., 3rd; Bigio, E.H.; Caselli, R.; Baker, M.; Al-Lozi, M.T.; Morris, J.C.; Pestronk, A.; Rademakers, R.; Goate, A.M. & Cairns, N.J. (2008). TDP-43 A315T mutation in familial motor neuron disease. *Ann Neurol*, Vol.63, No.4, pp. 535-538, ISSN 1531-8249

Gurney, M.E.; Pu, H.; Chiu, A.Y.; Dal Canto, M.C.; Polchow, C.Y.; Alexander, D.D.; Caliendo, J.; Hentati, A.; Kwon, Y.W.; Deng, H.X. & et al. (1994). Motor neuron degeneration in mice that express a human Cu,Zn superoxide dismutase mutation. *Science*, Vol.264, No.5166, pp. 1772-1775,

Hadano, S.; Hand, C.K.; Osuga, H.; Yanagisawa, Y.; Otomo, A.; Devon, R.S.; Miyamoto, N.; Showguchi-Miyata, J.; Okada, Y.; Singaraja, R.; Figlewicz, D.A.; Kwiatkowski, T.; Hosler, B.A.; Sagie, T.; Skaug, J.; Nasir, J.; Brown, R.H., Jr.; Scherer, S.W.; Rouleau, G.A.; Hayden, M.R. & Ikeda, J.E. (2001). A gene encoding a putative GTPase regulator is mutated in familial amyotrophic lateral sclerosis 2. *Nat Genet*, Vol.29, No.2, pp. 166-173, ISSN 1061-4036

Hasegawa, M.; Arai, T.; Nonaka, T.; Kametani, F.; Yoshida, M.; Hashizume, Y.; Beach, T.G.; Buratti, E.; Baralle, F.; Morita, M.; Nakano, I.; Oda, T.; Tsuchiya, K. & Akiyama, H. (2008). Phosphorylated TDP-43 in frontotemporal lobar degeneration and amyotrophic lateral sclerosis. *Ann Neurol*, Vol.64, No.1, pp. 60-70, ISSN 1531-8249

Hayward, L.J.; Rodriguez, J.A.; Kim, J.W.; Tiwari, A.; Goto, J.J.; Cabelli, D.E.; Valentine, J.S. & Brown, R.H., Jr. (2002). Decreased metallation and activity in subsets of mutant superoxide dismutases associated with familial amyotrophic lateral sclerosis. *J Biol Chem*, Vol.277, No.18, pp. 15923-15931,

Huang, C.; Zhou, H.; Tong, J.; Chen, H.; Liu, Y.J.; Wang, D.; Wei, X. & Xia, X.G. (2011). FUS transgenic rats develop the phenotypes of amyotrophic lateral sclerosis and frontotemporal lobar degeneration. *PLoS Genet*, Vol.7, No.3, pp. e1002011, ISSN 1553-7404

Hwang, Y.M.; Stathopulos, P.B.; Dimmick, K.; Yang, H.; Badiei, H.R.; Tong, M.S.; Rumfeldt, J.A.; Chen, P.; Karanassios, V. & Meiering, E.M. (2010). Nonamyloid aggregates arising from mature copper/zinc superoxide dismutases resemble those observed in amyotrophic lateral sclerosis. *J Biol Chem*, Vol.285, No.53, pp. 41701-41711, ISSN 1083-351X

Igaz, L.M.; Kwong, L.K.; Xu, Y.; Truax, A.C.; Uryu, K.; Neumann, M.; Clark, C.M.; Elman, L.B.; Miller, B.L.; Grossman, M.; McCluskey, L.F.; Trojanowski, J.Q. & Lee, V.M. (2008). Enrichment of C-terminal fragments in TAR DNA-binding protein-43 cytoplasmic inclusions in brain but not in spinal cord of frontotemporal lobar degeneration and amyotrophic lateral sclerosis. *Am J Pathol*, Vol.173, No.1, pp. 182-194, ISSN 1525-2191

Iko, Y.; Kodama, T.S.; Kasai, N.; Oyama, T.; Morita, E.H.; Muto, T.; Okumura, M.; Fujii, R.; Takumi, T.; Tate, S. & Morikawa, K. (2004). Domain architectures and characterization of an RNA-binding protein, TLS. *J Biol Chem*, Vol.279, No.43, pp. 44834-44840, ISSN 0021-9258

Jensen, L.T. & Culotta, V.C. (2005). Activation of CuZn superoxide dismutases from Caenorhabditis elegans does not require the copper chaperone CCS. *J Biol Chem*, Vol.280, No.50, pp. 41373-41379, ISSN 0021-9258

Johnson, B.S.; Snead, D.; Lee, J.J.; McCaffery, J.M.; Shorter, J. & Gitler, A.D. (2009). TDP-43 is intrinsically aggregation-prone, and amyotrophic lateral sclerosis-linked mutations accelerate aggregation and increase toxicity. *J Biol Chem*, Vol.284, No.30, pp. 20329-20339, ISSN 0021-9258

Kabashi, E.; Valdmanis, P.N.; Dion, P.; Spiegelman, D.; McConkey, B.J.; Vande Velde, C.; Bouchard, J.P.; Lacomblez, L.; Pochigaeva, K.; Salachas, F.; Pradat, P.F.; Camu, W.; Meininger, V.; Dupre, N. & Rouleau, G.A. (2008). TARDBP mutations in individuals with sporadic and familial amyotrophic lateral sclerosis. *Nat Genet*, Vol.40, No.5, pp. 572-4, ISSN 1546-1718

Karch, C.M.; Prudencio, M.; Winkler, D.D.; Hart, P.J. & Borchelt, D.R. (2009). Role of mutant SOD1 disulfide oxidation and aggregation in the pathogenesis of familial ALS. *Proc Natl Acad Sci U S A*, Vol.106, No.19, pp. 7774-7779, ISSN 1091-6490

Kato, S.; Takikawa, M.; Nakashima, K.; Hirano, A.; Cleveland, D.W.; Kusaka, H.; Shibata, N.; Kato, M.; Nakano, I. & Ohama, E. (2000). New consensus research on neuropathological aspects of familial amyotrophic lateral sclerosis with superoxide dismutase 1 (SOD1) gene mutations: inclusions containing SOD1 in neurons and astrocytes. *Amyotroph Lateral Scler Other Motor Neuron Disord*, Vol.1, No.3, pp. 163-184, ISSN 1466-0822

Kawamata, H. & Manfredi, G. (2008). Different regulation of wild-type and mutant Cu,Zn superoxide dismutase localization in mammalian mitochondria. *Hum Mol Genet*, Vol.17, No.21, pp. 3303-3317, ISSN 1460-2083

Kerman, A.; Liu, H.N.; Croul, S.; Bilbao, J.; Rogaeva, E.; Zinman, L.; Robertson, J. & Chakrabartty, A. (2010). Amyotrophic lateral sclerosis is a non-amyloid disease in which extensive misfolding of SOD1 is unique to the familial form. *Acta Neuropathol*, Vol.119, No.3, pp. 335-344, ISSN 1432-0533

Klunk, W.E.; Jacob, R.F. & Mason, R.P. (1999). Quantifying amyloid by congo red spectral shift assay. *Methods Enzymol*, Vol.309, pp. 285-305, ISSN 0076-6879

Kraemer, B.C.; Schuck, T.; Wheeler, J.M.; Robinson, L.C.; Trojanowski, J.Q.; Lee, V.M. & Schellenberg, G.D. (2010). Loss of murine TDP-43 disrupts motor function and plays an essential role in embryogenesis. *Acta Neuropathol*, Vol.119, No.4, pp. 409-419, ISSN 1432-0533

Kwiatkowski, T.J., Jr.; Bosco, D.A.; Leclerc, A.L.; Tamrazian, E.; Vanderburg, C.R.; Russ, C.; Davis, A.; Gilchrist, J.; Kasarskis, E.J.; Munsat, T.; Valdmanis, P.; Rouleau, G.A.; Hosler, B.A.; Cortelli, P.; de Jong, P.J.; Yoshinaga, Y.; Haines, J.L.; Pericak-Vance, M.A.; Yan, J.; Ticozzi, N.; Siddique, T.; McKenna-Yasek, D.; Sapp, P.C.; Horvitz, H.R.; Landers, J.E. & Brown, R.H., Jr. (2009). Mutations in the FUS/TLS gene on chromosome 16 cause familial amyotrophic lateral sclerosis. *Science*, Vol.323, No.5918, pp. 1205-1208, ISSN 1095-9203

Lagier-Tourenne, C.; Polymenidou, M. & Cleveland, D.W. (2010). TDP-43 and FUS/TLS: emerging roles in RNA processing and neurodegeneration. *Hum Mol Genet*, Vol.19, pp. R46-R64, ISSN 1460-2083

Leitch, J.M.; Jensen, L.T.; Bouldin, S.D.; Outten, C.E.; Hart, P.J. & Culotta, V.C. (2009). Activation of Cu,Zn-superoxide dismutase in the absence of oxygen and the copper chaperone CCS. *J Biol Chem*, Vol.284, No.33, pp. 21863-21871, 0021-9258

Lelie, H.L.; Liba, A.; Bourassa, M.W.; Chattopadhyay, M.; Chan, P.K.; Gralla, E.B.; Miller, L.M.; Borchelt, D.R.; Valentine, J.S. & Whitelegge, J.P. (2011). Copper and zinc metallation status of copper-zinc superoxide dismutase from amyotrophic lateral sclerosis transgenic mice. *J Biol Chem*, Vol.286, No.4, pp. 2795-2806, ISSN 1083-351X

LeVine, H., 3rd (1999). Quantification of beta-sheet amyloid fibril structures with thioflavin T. *Methods Enzymol*, Vol.309, pp. 274-284, ISSN 0076-6879

Lin, W.L. & Dickson, D.W. (2008). Ultrastructural localization of TDP-43 in filamentous neuronal inclusions in various neurodegenerative diseases. *Acta Neuropathol*, Vol.116, No.2, pp. 205-213, ISSN 0001-6322

Liu, H.N.; Sanelli, T.; Horne, P.; Pioro, E.P.; Strong, M.J.; Rogaeva, E.; Bilbao, J.; Zinman, L. & Robertson, J. (2009). Lack of evidence of monomer/misfolded superoxide dismutase-1 in sporadic amyotrophic lateral sclerosis. *Ann Neurol*, Vol.66, No.1, pp. 75-80, ISSN 1531-8249

Luk, K.C.; Song, C.; O'Brien, P.; Stieber, A.; Branch, J.R.; Brunden, K.R.; Trojanowski, J.Q. & Lee, V.M. (2009). Exogenous alpha-synuclein fibrils seed the formation of Lewy body-like intracellular inclusions in cultured cells. *Proc Natl Acad Sci U S A*, Vol.106, No.47, pp. 20051-20056, ISSN 1091-6490

Mackenzie, I.R.; Bigio, E.H.; Ince, P.G.; Geser, F.; Neumann, M.; Cairns, N.J.; Kwong, L.K.; Forman, M.S.; Ravits, J.; Stewart, H.; Eisen, A.; McClusky, L.; Kretzschmar, H.A.; Monoranu, C.M.; Highley, J.R.; Kirby, J.; Siddique, T.; Shaw, P.J.; Lee, V.M. & Trojanowski, J.Q. (2007). Pathological TDP-43 distinguishes sporadic amyotrophic lateral sclerosis from amyotrophic lateral sclerosis with SOD1 mutations. *Ann Neurol*, Vol.61, No.5, pp. 427-434, ISSN 0364-5134

Mackenzie, I.R.; Ansorge, O.; Strong, M.; Bilbao, J.; Zinman, L.; Ang, L.C.; Baker, M.; Stewart, H.; Eisen, A.; Rademakers, R. & Neumann, M. (2011). Pathological heterogeneity in amyotrophic lateral sclerosis with FUS mutations: two distinct patterns correlating with disease severity and mutation. *Acta Neuropathol*, Vol.122, No.1, pp. 87-98, ISSN 1432-0533

Maruyama, H.; Morino, H.; Ito, H.; Izumi, Y.; Kato, H.; Watanabe, Y.; Kinoshita, Y.; Kamada, M.; Nodera, H.; Suzuki, H.; Komure, O.; Matsuura, S.; Kobatake, K.; Morimoto, N.; Abe, K.; Suzuki, N.; Aoki, M.; Kawata, A.; Hirai, T.; Kato, T.; Ogasawara, K.; Hirano, A.; Takumi, T.; Kusaka, H.; Hagiwara, K.; Kaji, R. & Kawakami, H. (2010). Mutations of optineurin in amyotrophic lateral sclerosis. *Nature*, Vol.465, No.7295, pp. 223-226, ISSN 1476-4687

McCord, J.M. & Fridovich, I. (1969). Superoxide dismutase. An enzymic function for erythrocuprein (hemocuprein). *J Biol Chem*, Vol.244, No.22, pp. 6049-6055,

Millecamps, S.; Salachas, F.; Cazeneuve, C.; Gordon, P.; Bricka, B.; Camuzat, A.; Guillot-Noel, L.; Russaouen, O.; Bruneteau, G.; Pradat, P.F.; Le Forestier, N.; Vandenberghe, N.; Danel-Brunaud, V.; Guy, N.; Thauvin-Robinet, C.; Lacomblez, L.; Couratier, P.; Hannequin, D.; Seilhean, D.; Le Ber, I.; Corcia, P.; Camu, W.; Brice, A.; Rouleau, G.; LeGuern, E. & Meininger, V. (2010). SOD1, ANG, VAPB, TARDBP, and FUS mutations in familial amyotrophic lateral sclerosis: genotype-phenotype correlations. *J Med Genet*, Vol.47, No.8, pp. 554-560, ISSN 1468-6244

Munch, C.; O'Brien, J. & Bertolotti, A. (2011). Prion-like propagation of mutant superoxide dismutase-1 misfolding in neuronal cells. *Proc Natl Acad Sci U S A*, Vol.108, No.9, pp. 3548-3553, ISSN 1091-6490

Neumann, M.; Sampathu, D.M.; Kwong, L.K.; Truax, A.C.; Micsenyi, M.C.; Chou, T.T.; Bruce, J.; Schuck, T.; Grossman, M.; Clark, C.M.; McCluskey, L.F.; Miller, B.L.; Masliah, E.; Mackenzie, I.R.; Feldman, H.; Feiden, W.; Kretzschmar, H.A.; Trojanowski, J.Q. & Lee, V.M. (2006). Ubiquitinated TDP-43 in frontotemporal lobar degeneration and amyotrophic lateral sclerosis. *Science*, Vol.314, No.5796, pp. 130-133, ISSN 1095-9203

Okamoto, K.; Mizuno, Y. & Fujita, Y. (2008). Bunina bodies in amyotrophic lateral sclerosis. *Neuropathology*, Vol.28, No.2, pp. 109-115, ISSN 0919-6544

Oztug Durer, Z.A.; Cohlberg, J.A.; Dinh, P.; Padua, S.; Ehrenclou, K.; Downes, S.; Tan, J.K.; Nakano, Y.; Bowman, C.J.; Hoskins, J.L.; Kwon, C.; Mason, A.Z.; Rodriguez, J.A.; Doucette, P.A.; Shaw, B.F. & Selverstone Valentine, J. (2009). Loss of metal ions, disulfide reduction and mutations related to familial ALS promote formation of amyloid-like aggregates from superoxide dismutase. *PLoS One*, Vol.4, No.3, pp. e5004, ISSN 1932-6203

Piao, Y.S.; Wakabayashi, K.; Kakita, A.; Yamada, M.; Hayashi, S.; Morita, T.; Ikuta, F.; Oyanagi, K. & Takahashi, H. (2003). Neuropathology with clinical correlations of sporadic amyotrophic lateral sclerosis: 102 autopsy cases examined between 1962 and 2000. *Brain Pathol*, Vol.13, No.1, pp. 10-22, ISSN 1015-6305

Rae, T.D.; Schmidt, P.J.; Pufahl, R.A.; Culotta, V.C. & O'Halloran, T.V. (1999). Undetectable intracellular free copper: The requirement of a copper chaperone for superoxide dismutase. *Science*, Vol.284, No.5415, pp. 805-808,

Rakhit, R.; Cunningham, P.; Furtos-Matei, A.; Dahan, S.; Qi, X.F.; Crow, J.P.; Cashman, N.R.; Kondejewski, L.H. & Chakrabartty, A. (2002). Oxidation-induced misfolding and aggregation of superoxide dismutase and its implications for amyotrophic lateral sclerosis. *J Biol Chem*, Vol.277, No.49, pp. 47551-47556,

Rakhit, R.; Crow, J.P.; Lepock, J.R.; Kondejewski, L.H.; Cashman, N.R. & Chakrabartty, A. (2004). Monomeric Cu,Zn-superoxide dismutase is a common misfolding intermediate in the oxidation models of sporadic and familial amyotrophic lateral sclerosis. *J. Biol. Chem.*, Vol.279, No.15, pp. 15499-15504,

Reaume, A.G.; Elliott, J.L.; Hoffman, E.K.; Kowall, N.W.; Ferrante, R.J.; Siwek, D.F.; Wilcox, H.M.; Flood, D.G.; Beal, M.F.; Brown, R.H., Jr.; Scott, R.W. & Snider, W.D. (1996). Motor neurons in Cu/Zn superoxide dismutase-deficient mice develop normally but exhibit enhanced cell death after axonal injury. *Nat Genet*, Vol.13, No.1, pp. 43-47,

Ren, P.H.; Lauckner, J.E.; Kachirskaia, I.; Heuser, J.E.; Melki, R. & Kopito, R.R. (2009). Cytoplasmic penetration and persistent infection of mammalian cells by polyglutamine aggregates. *Nat Cell Biol*, Vol.11, No.2, pp. 219-225, ISSN 1476-4679

Rodriguez, J.A.; Valentine, J.S.; Eggers, D.K.; Roe, J.A.; Tiwari, A.; Brown, R.H. & Hayward, L.J. (2002). Familial amyotrophic lateral sclerosis-associated mutations decrease the thermal stability of distinctly metallated species of human copper/zinc superoxide dismutase. *J Biol Chem*, Vol.277, No.18, pp. 15932-15937,

Rodriguez, J.A.; Shaw, B.F.; Durazo, A.; Sohn, S.H.; Doucette, P.A.; Nersissian, A.M.; Faull, K.F.; Eggers, D.K.; Tiwari, A.; Hayward, L.J. & Valentine, J.S. (2005). Destabilization of apoprotein is insufficient to explain Cu,Zn-superoxide dismutase-linked ALS pathogenesis. *Proc Natl Acad Sci U S A*, Vol.102, No.30, pp. 10516-10521,

Rosen, D.R.; Siddique, T.; Patterson, D.; Figlewicz, D.A.; Sapp, P.; Hentati, A.; Donaldson, D.; Goto, J.; O'Regan, J.P.; Deng, H.X. & et al. (1993). Mutations in Cu/Zn superoxide dismutase gene are associated with familial amyotrophic lateral sclerosis. *Nature*, Vol.362, No.6415, pp. 59-62,

Ross, C.A. & Poirier, M.A. (2004). Protein aggregation and neurodegenerative disease. *Nat Med*, Vol.10 Suppl, pp. S10-S17, ISSN 1078-8956

Serpell, L.C. & Smith, J.M. (2000). Direct visualisation of the beta-sheet structure of synthetic Alzheimer's amyloid. *J Mol Biol*, Vol.299, No.1, pp. 225-231, ISSN 0022-2836

Shaw, B.F.; Lelie, H.L.; Durazo, A.; Nersissian, A.M.; Xu, G.; Chan, P.K.; Gralla, E.B.; Tiwari, A.; Hayward, L.J.; Borchelt, D.R.; Valentine, J.S. & Whitelegge, J.P. (2008). Detergent-insoluble aggregates associated with amyotrophic lateral sclerosis in transgenic mice contain primarily full-length, unmodified superoxide dismutase-1. *J Biol Chem*, Vol.283, No.13, pp. 8340-8350, ISSN 0021-9258

Shibata, N.; Hirano, A.; Kobayashi, M.; Sasaki, S.; Kato, T.; Matsumoto, S.; Shiozawa, Z.; Komori, T.; Ikemoto, A.; Umahara, T. & et al. (1994). Cu/Zn superoxide dismutase-like immunoreactivity in Lewy body-like inclusions of sporadic amyotrophic lateral sclerosis. *Neurosci Lett*, Vol.179, No.1-2, pp. 149-152,

Shibata, N.; Asayama, K.; Hirano, A. & Kobayashi, M. (1996a). Immunohistochemical study on superoxide dismutases in spinal cords from autopsied patients with amyotrophic lateral sclerosis. *Dev Neurosci*, Vol.18, No.5-6, pp. 492-498, ISSN 0378-5866

Shibata, N.; Hirano, A.; Kobayashi, M.; Siddique, T.; Deng, H.X.; Hung, W.Y.; Kato, T. & Asayama, K. (1996b). Intense superoxide dismutase-1 immunoreactivity in intracytoplasmic hyaline inclusions of familial amyotrophic lateral sclerosis with posterior column involvement. *J Neuropathol Exp Neurol*, Vol.55, No.4, pp. 481-490, ISSN 0022-3069

Siddique, T.; Figlewicz, D.A.; Pericak-Vance, M.A.; Haines, J.L.; Rouleau, G.; Jeffers, A.J.; Sapp, P.; Hung, W.Y.; Bebout, J.; McKenna-Yasek, D. & et al. (1991). Linkage of a gene causing familial amyotrophic lateral sclerosis to chromosome 21 and evidence of genetic-locus heterogeneity. *N Engl J Med*, Vol.324, No.20, pp. 1381-1384, ISSN 0028-4793

Son, M.; Puttaparthi, K.; Kawamata, H.; Rajendran, B.; Boyer, P.J.; Manfredi, G. & Elliott, J.L. (2007). Overexpression of CCS in G93A-SOD1 mice leads to accelerated neurological deficits with severe mitochondrial pathology. *Proc Natl Acad Sci U S A*, Vol.104, No.14, pp. 6072-6077, ISSN 0027-8424

Soto, C. (2003). Unfolding the role of protein misfolding in neurodegenerative diseases. *Nat Rev Neurosci*, Vol.4, No.1, pp. 49-60, ISSN 1471-003X

Sreedharan, J.; Blair, I.P.; Tripathi, V.B.; Hu, X.; Vance, C.; Rogelj, B.; Ackerley, S.; Durnall, J.C.; Williams, K.L.; Buratti, E.; Baralle, F.; de Belleroche, J.; Mitchell, J.D.; Leigh, P.N.; Al-Chalabi, A.; Miller, C.C.; Nicholson, G. & Shaw, C.E. (2008). TDP-43 mutations in familial and sporadic amyotrophic lateral sclerosis. *Science*, Vol.319, No.5870, pp. 1668-1672, ISSN 1095-9203

Stathopulos, P.B.; Rumfeldt, J.A.; Scholz, G.A.; Irani, R.A.; Frey, H.E.; Hallewell, R.A.; Lepock, J.R. & Meiering, E.M. (2003). Cu/Zn superoxide dismutase mutants associated with amyotrophic lateral sclerosis show enhanced formation of aggregates in vitro. *Proc Natl Acad Sci USA*, Vol.100, No.12, pp. 7021-7026,

Subramaniam, J.R.; Lyons, W.E.; Liu, J.; Bartnikas, T.B.; Rothstein, J.; Price, D.L.; Cleveland, D.W.; Gitlin, J.D. & Wong, P.C. (2002). Mutant SOD1 causes motor neuron disease independent of copper chaperone-mediated copper loading. *Nat Neurosci*, Vol.5, No.4, pp. 301-307,

Sun, Z.; Diaz, Z.; Fang, X.; Hart, M.P.; Chesi, A.; Shorter, J. & Gitler, A.D. (2011). Molecular determinants and genetic modifiers of aggregation and toxicity for the ALS disease protein FUS/TLS. *PLoS Biol*, Vol.9, No.4, pp. e1000614, ISSN 1545-7885

Tiwari, A. & Hayward, L.J. (2003). Familial amyotrophic lateral sclerosis mutants of copper/zinc superoxide dismutase are susceptible to disulfide reduction. *J Biol Chem*, Vol.278, No.8, pp. 5984-5992, ISSN 0021-9258

Turner, B.J. & Talbot, K. (2008). Transgenics, toxicity and therapeutics in rodent models of mutant SOD1-mediated familial ALS. *Prog Neurobiol*, Vol.85, No.1, pp. 94-134, ISSN 0301-0082

Uranishi, H.; Tetsuka, T.; Yamashita, M.; Asamitsu, K.; Shimizu, M.; Itoh, M. & Okamoto, T. (2001). Involvement of the pro-oncoprotein TLS (translocated in liposarcoma) in nuclear factor-kappa B p65-mediated transcription as a coactivator. *J Biol Chem*, Vol.276, No.16, pp. 13395-13401, ISSN 0021-9258

Van Deerlin, V.M.; Leverenz, J.B.; Bekris, L.M.; Bird, T.D.; Yuan, W.; Elman, L.B.; Clay, D.; Wood, E.M.; Chen-Plotkin, A.S.; Martinez-Lage, M.; Steinbart, E.; McCluskey, L.; Grossman, M.; Neumann, M.; Wu, I.L.; Yang, W.S.; Kalb, R.; Galasko, D.R.; Montine, T.J.; Trojanowski, J.Q.; Lee, V.M.; Schellenberg, G.D. & Yu, C.E. (2008). TARDBP mutations in amyotrophic lateral sclerosis with TDP-43 neuropathology: a genetic and histopathological analysis. *Lancet Neurol*, Vol.7, No.5, pp. 409-416, ISSN 1474-4422

Vance, C.; Rogelj, B.; Hortobagyi, T.; De Vos, K.J.; Nishimura, A.L.; Sreedharan, J.; Hu, X.; Smith, B.; Ruddy, D.; Wright, P.; Ganesalingam, J.; Williams, K.L.; Tripathi, V.; Al-Saraj, S.; Al-Chalabi, A.; Leigh, P.N.; Blair, I.P.; Nicholson, G.; de Belleroche, J.; Gallo, J.M.; Miller, C.C. & Shaw, C.E. (2009). Mutations in FUS, an RNA processing protein, cause familial amyotrophic lateral sclerosis type 6. *Science*, Vol.323, No.5918, pp. 1208-1211, ISSN 1095-9203

Wang, J.; Xu, G.; Gonzales, V.; Coonfield, M.; Fromholt, D.; Copeland, N.G.; Jenkins, N.A. & Borchelt, D.R. (2002). Fibrillar inclusions and motor neuron degeneration in transgenic mice expressing superoxide dismutase 1 with a disrupted copper-binding site. *Neurobiol Dis*, Vol.10, No.2, pp. 128-38, 0969-9961 (Print)

Wang, J.; Xu, G.; Li, H.; Gonzales, V.; Fromholt, D.; Karch, C.; Copeland, N.G.; Jenkins, N.A. & Borchelt, D.R. (2005). Somatodendritic accumulation of misfolded SOD1-L126Z in motor neurons mediates degeneration: alphaB-crystallin modulates aggregation. *Hum Mol Genet*, Vol.14, No.16, pp. 2335-2347, 0964-6906 (Print)

Wang, Q.; Johnson, J.L.; Agar, N.Y. & Agar, J.N. (2008). Protein aggregation and protein instability govern familial amyotrophic lateral sclerosis patient survival. *PLoS Biol*, Vol.6, No.7, pp. e170, ISSN 1545-7885

Watanabe, M.; Dykes-Hoberg, M.; Culotta, V.C.; Price, D.L.; Wong, P.C. & Rothstein, J.D. (2001). Histological evidence of protein aggregation in mutant SOD1 transgenic mice and in amyotrophic lateral sclerosis neural tissues. *Neurobiol Dis*, Vol.8, No.6, pp. 933-941,

Wegorzewska, I.; Bell, S.; Cairns, N.J.; Miller, T.M. & Baloh, R.H. (2009). TDP-43 mutant transgenic mice develop features of ALS and frontotemporal lobar degeneration. *Proc Natl Acad Sci U S A*, Vol.106, No.44, pp. 18809-18814, ISSN 1091-6490

Wils, H.; Kleinberger, G.; Janssens, J.; Pereson, S.; Joris, G.; Cuijt, I.; Smits, V.; Ceuterick-de Groote, C.; Van Broeckhoven, C. & Kumar-Singh, S. (2010). TDP-43 transgenic mice develop spastic paralysis and neuronal inclusions characteristic of ALS and frontotemporal lobar degeneration. *Proc Natl Acad Sci U S A*, Vol.107, No.8, pp. 3858-3863, ISSN 1091-6490

Yang, L.; Embree, L.J.; Tsai, S. & Hickstein, D.D. (1998). Oncoprotein TLS interacts with serine-arginine proteins involved in RNA splicing. *J Biol Chem*, Vol.273, No.43, pp. 27761-27764, ISSN 0021-9258

Yang, Y.; Hentati, A.; Deng, H.X.; Dabbagh, O.; Sasaki, T.; Hirano, M.; Hung, W.Y.; Ouahchi, K.; Yan, J.; Azim, A.C.; Cole, N.; Gascon, G.; Yagmour, A.; Ben-Hamida, M.; Pericak-Vance, M.; Hentati, F. & Siddique, T. (2001). The gene encoding alsin, a protein with three guanine-nucleotide exchange factor domains, is mutated in a form of recessive amyotrophic lateral sclerosis. *Nat Genet*, Vol.29, No.2, pp. 160-165, ISSN 1061-4036

Zhou, H.; Huang, C.; Chen, H.; Wang, D.; Landel, C.P.; Xia, P.Y.; Bowser, R.; Liu, Y.J. & Xia, X.G. (2010). Transgenic rat model of neurodegeneration caused by mutation in the TDP gene. *PLoS Genet*, Vol.6, No.3, pp. e1000887, ISSN 1553-7404

Zinszner, H.; Sok, J.; Immanuel, D.; Yin, Y. & Ron, D. (1997). TLS (FUS) binds RNA in vivo and engages in nucleo-cytoplasmic shuttling. *J Cell Sci*, Vol.110 (Pt 15), pp. 1741-1750, ISSN 0021-9533

Zoghbi, H.Y. & Orr, H.T. (2000). Glutamine repeats and neurodegeneration. *Annu Rev Neurosci*, Vol.23, pp. 217-247, ISSN 0147-006X

14

Reactive Nitrogen Species in Motor Neuron Apoptosis

María Clara Franco and Alvaro G. Estévez
Burnett School of Biomedical Sciences, College of Medicine, University of Central Florida, Orlando, USA

1. Introduction

Nitric oxide is a cellular messenger produced by different cell types in an organism, both in physiological and pathological conditions (Snyder 1993; Beckman and Koppenol 1996; Beckman and Koppenol 1996; Beckman 1996; Colasanti and Suzuki 2000; Pacher, Beckman, and Liaudet 2007). Nitric oxide was first described in biology as the endothelium-derived relaxation factor for its effects on vasodilatation (Ignarro 1990), but soon become evident it have other important physiological functions such as a retrograde messenger in the nervous systems, and during the immune response (Moncada, Palmer, and Higgins 1991). Nitric oxide can also regulate mitochondria respiration (Carreras and Poderoso 2007; Ramachandran et al. 2002), and reacts with oxygen and reactive oxygen species to form reactive nitrogen species, which in turn can damage the cells. The reactivity of nitric oxide and the metabolic state of the cell or tissue are determining factors on the specific actions mediated by nitric oxide. It is not our intention to examine the biochemistry and physiology of nitric oxide, which has been cover in several excellent reviews (Beckman and Crow 1993; Beckman 1996; Pacher, Beckman, and Liaudet 2007), but to concentrate in those nitric oxide-derivate species relevant to the regulation of motor neuron apoptosis. However, some relevant aspects of the biochemistry of nitric oxide will be reviewed as the necessary background to understand the biology of reactive nitrogen species in motor neurons.

2. Peroxynitrite

One important reaction of nitric oxide is with superoxide (another free radical) to produce the strong oxidant peroxynitrite (Beckman et al. 1990). The importance of this reaction is highlighted by its diffusion-limited rate (between $6.7x10^9$ and $2x10^{10}$ $M^{-1}s^{-1}$)(Padmaja and Huie 1993; Nauser and Koppenol 2002), meaning that every collision of a molecule of nitric oxide with a molecule of superoxide results in the formation of peroxynitrite (Fig 1). In other words, peroxynitrite will be formed when superoxide and nitric oxide are formed simultaneously. The reason peroxynitrite is not formed in large amounts in normal metabolic conditions is the high intracellular concentration of the enzyme superoxide dismutase (SOD)(Rae et al. 1999), which competes for the superoxide with a rate of $2x10^9$ $M^{-1}s^{-1}$ (Pacher, Beckman, and Liaudet 2007) (Fig 1). Briefly, when the concentration of nitric oxide is 5 times lower than the concentration of SOD, approximately 50% of the superoxide produced would react with nitric oxide to form peroxynitrite. In normal conditions, the intracellular concentration of SOD is in large excess of the concentrations of nitric oxide (Beckman and Koppenol 1996). However, the prediction from the rates is that a small amount of peroxynitrite will always be formed, allowing the speculation that the oxidant may have a physiological function (Go et al. 1999), or otherwise it is efficiently scavenged by small molecular weight antioxidants such as glutathione with rates in the order of 10^3-10^4 $M^{-1}s^{-1}$ (Radi et al. 1991; Alvarez et al. 1999). Other important aspect of the competition between SOD and nitric oxide for superoxide is the presence of membrane cellular compartments, which limit the diffusion of SOD and superoxide but not nitric oxide. SOD can only compete with nitric oxide when the enzyme is in the same compartment than superoxide is being produced, indicating that peroxynitrite can be formed with relatively high efficiency even at low nitric oxide concentrations if superoxide is formed in a compartment SOD cannot access or where the enzyme has been inactivated (Fig 1).

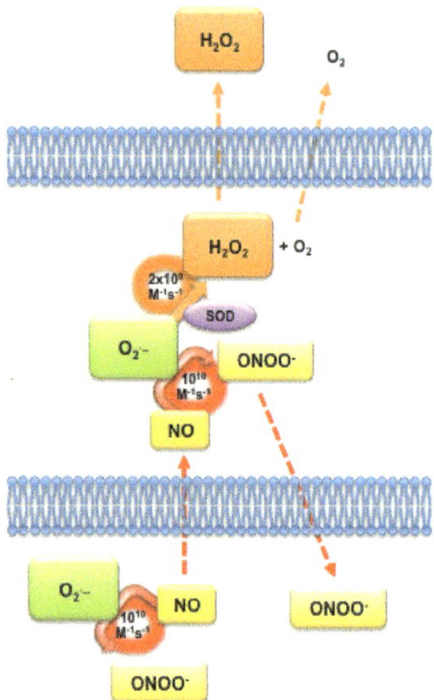

Fig. 1. In the cells, peroxynitrite formation depends on the levels of SOD that competes with nitric oxide for superoxide. Because cellular membranes (in blue) limit the diffusion of SOD and superoxide but not nitric oxide, peroxynitrite formation is also limited by the subcellular localization of the superoxide sources.

In pathological conditions, not only low micromolar concentrations of nitric oxide can be produced, but production of superoxide can also be boosted, increasing the probability for peroxynitrite formation at levels that may overwhelm the intracellular antioxidant defenses (Beckman and Crow 1993; Beckman and Koppenol 1996). Peroxynitrite affects normal cell metabolism by inducing lipid peroxidation (Radi et al. 1991), damage of the DNA (Groves and Marla 1995), and alteration of the mitochondrial function (Radi et al. 2002). In addition, it has been shown that peroxynitrite inhibits the activity in some proteins such as the tyrosine hydroxylase (Ara et al. 1998), mitochondrial manganese SOD, and tyrosine phosphatases (Takakura et al. 1999), activates src kinase (MacMillan-Crow et al. 2000) and alters the functionality of structural proteins such as neurofilament L, synuclein, actin, and tubulin (Aslan et al. 2003; Cappelletti et al. 2003; Eiserich et al. 1999; Chang et al. 2002; Crow et al. 1997; Paxinou et al. 2001). Changes in protein function are caused by oxidative modifications of amino acid residues by peroxynitrite (Alvarez et al. 1999). In the case of phosphatases and zinc-thiolate-containing proteins the oxidation of methionine and cysteine residues is critical for the loss of function of the enzymes (Takakura et al. 1999; Crow, Beckman, and McCord 1995). One particular modification of amino acids by peroxynitrite that has driven much attention is the nitration of tyrosine residues (Beckman et al. 1992). The interest is driven by the fact that nitrotyrosine seems to be a universal marker for inflammation and has been detected in a large number of pathological conditions (Ischiropoulos 1998; Greenacre and Ischiropoulos 2001; Ischiropoulos and Beckman 2003; Schopfer, Baker, and Freeman 2003; Radi 2004). It is accepted that nitration by the formation of the decomposition products of peroxynitrite is a major source of biological nitration, in spite that other mechanisms for tyrosine nitration have been described (Ischiropoulos 1998; Radi 2004; Schopfer, Baker, and Freeman 2003) (Fig 2).

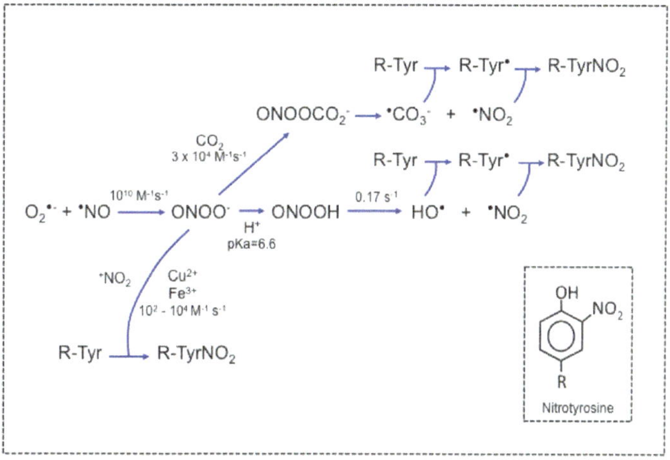

Fig. 2. Mechanisms for tyrosine nitration by the nitrative products of decomposition of peroxynitrite in the cells.

3. Peroxynitrite and apoptosis

Unsurprisingly, peroxynitrite induces apoptosis or necrosis depending on the concentration of the oxidant (Bonfoco et al. 1995; Estévez et al. 1995), and it has become the accepted mechanism for the toxic effects of nitric oxide in biological systems (Dawson and Dawson 1996; Dawson and Dawson 1996; Dawson and Dawson 1996; Beckman and Koppenol 1996). Although growing evidence suggests that peroxynitrite induces apoptosis by interacting with specific cellular signaling pathways (Estévez et al. 1995; Shin et al. 1996; Spear, Estévez, Barbeito, et al. 1997; Spear, Estévez, Radi, et al. 1997; Shacka et al. 2006; Ye et al. 2007) (Fig 3), the cellular targets responsible for peroxynitrite-induced apoptosis remain unknown. In addition, most studies were performed using exogenously applied stock solutions of pure peroxynitrite or peroxynitrite donors (Bonfoco et al. 1995; Estévez et al. 1995).

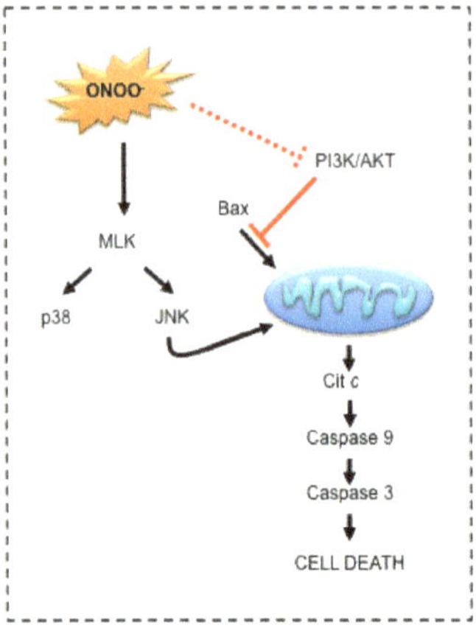

Fig. 3. Cell death-pathway induced by peroxynitrite in PC12 cells.

4. Motor neuron death and peroxynitrite *in vivo*

More recently, cultured motor neurons have become one of the best-described models for apoptosis induced by endogenous peroxynitrite (Estévez, Spear, Manuel, Radi, et al. 1998; Estévez, Spear, Manuel, Barbeito, et al. 1998; Estévez et al. 2000; Sendtner et al. 2000; Raoul et al. 2002; Raoul, Pettmann, and Henderson 2000; Kaal et al. 2000; Bar 2000). Motor neurons are large neurons located in the ventral spinal cord and brain stem responsible for the stimulation of muscle contraction. Motor neuron survival is highly dependent on trophic factors (Oppenheim 1991; Oppenheim 1996; Sendtner et al. 2000). Chronic administration of trophic factors prevents avian and mammalian motor neurons death during the period of programmed cell death (Neff et al. 1993) and motor neuron apoptosis induced by axon injury in mammals (Yan, Elliott, and Snider 1992; Li et al. 1994; Novikov, Novikova, and Kellerth 1995; Pennica et al. 1996). Remarkably, motor neurons induce the expression of neuronal NOS and the p75 neurotrophin receptor after injury (Wu 1993). Trophic factors such as BDNF, and nerve grafts prevent the induction of neuronal NOS and motor neuron death (Wu et al. 1994; Novikov, Novikova, and Kellerth 1995). Furthermore, inhibition of NOS activity prevents motor neuron death induced by axonal injury (Wu and Li 1993; Casanovas et al. 1996), suggesting that induction of motor neuron death after axonal injury may result from trophic factor deprivation leading to the induction of neuronal NOS as well as nitric oxide and peroxynitrite production, evidenced by the increase levels of nitrotyrosine in motor neurons after axotomy (Martin, Kaiser, and Price 1999).

5. Motor neuron apoptosis *in vitro*

Motor neuron survival in culture can be supported by a large number of trophic factors (Oppenheim 1996; Hughes, Sendtner, and Thoenen 1993), which also induce the extension of long and branched neurites. As many other cells in culture, trophic factor-deprived motor neurons undergo protein synthesis and caspase-dependent apoptosis (Milligan, Oppenheim, and Schwartz 1994; Milligan et al. 1995; Estévez, Spear, Manuel, Radi, et al. 1998; Estévez et al. 2000) (Fig 4).

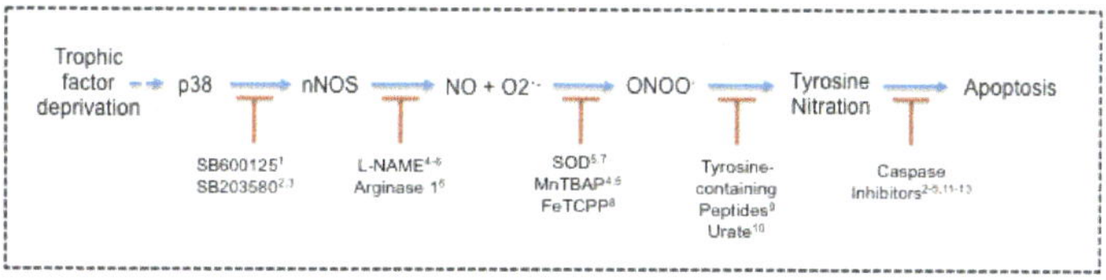

Fig. 4. Motor neuron apoptosis induced by trophic factor deprivation. Induction of motor neuron apoptosis by trophic factor deprivation is prevented by inhibition of JNK and p38 MAP kinases. The induction of neuronal NOS (nNOS) is regulated by the activation of p38 and responsible for the production of nitric oxide. Nitric oxide reacts with superoxide to form peroxynitrite. Inhbition of tyrosine nitration by peroxynitrite using tyrosine-containing peptides is enough to prevent apoptosis induced by trophic factor deprivation. Caspase inhbitors also prevented apoptosis mediated by trophic factors deprivation. [1](Ricart et al., 2006); [2](Raoul et al., 1999b); [3](Raoul et al., 2002); [4](Estévez et al., 1998); [5](Estévez et al., 2000); [6](Estevez et al., 2006); [7](Estévez et al., 1999); [8](Peluffo et al., 2004); [9](Ye et al., 2007); [10](Cassina et al., 2002); [11](Milligan et al., 1995); [12](Li et al., 1998); [13](Li et al., 2001)

Apoptosis induced by trophic factor deprivation is preceded by the induction of Fas ligand expression and prevented, at least in part, by inhibition of Fas and caspase 8 (Raoul, Henderson, and Pettmann 1999). In the presence of trophic factors, Fas activates two parallel pathways leading to motor neuron apoptosis by a mechanism similar to trophic factor deprivation (Raoul et al. 2002)(Fig 5).

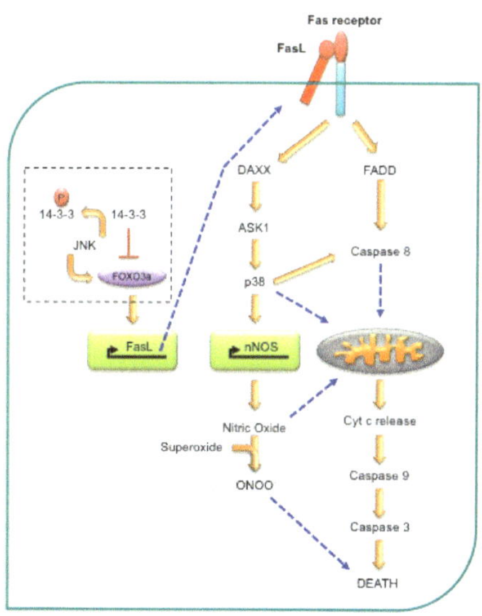

Fig. 5. In motor neurons, the activation of the Fas pathway leads to the simultaneous activation of the FADD and DAXX components of the pathway. Downstream of DAXX, p38 induces the expression of nNOS leading to the formation of peroxynitrite while activation of FADD leads to activation of caspases. Upon activation of Fas, both pathways participate simoultaneously in the induction of cell death. Inhibition of JNK may be upstream of the Fas pathway through activation of the transcription factor FOXO3a and transcription of FasL.

Motor neuron apoptosis induced by trophic factor deprivation is also dependent on the expression of neuronal NOS and the production of nitric oxide (Estévez, Spear, Manuel, Radi, et al. 1998; Estévez, Spear, Manuel, Barbeito, et al. 1998; Estévez et al. 2000; Raoul et al. 2002; Raoul et al. 2005). Either inhibition of nitric oxide production or scavenging of superoxide with Cu,Zn SOD prevents motor neuron apoptosis induced by trophic factor deprivation up to seven days after plating (Estévez et al. 2000). The protective effects of NOS inhibition are reverted by steady state concentrations of exogenous nitric oxide as low as 80 nM (Estévez et al. 2000). Remarkably, 7 days old motor neuron cultures undergo apoptosis when deprived of trophic factors by a mechanism indistinguishably from the cell death induced by plating motor neurons in the absence of trophic factors (Estévez et al. 2000). These results reveal that production of nitric oxide or superoxide alone is not sufficient for the induction of motor neuron apoptosis by trophic factor deprivation (Estévez et al. 2000; Estévez, Spear, Manuel, Radi, et al. 1998; Raoul et al. 2002; Raoul et al. 2005). In addition, an increase in nitrotyrosine immunoreactivity is detected in motor neurons deprived of trophic factors suggesting peroxynitrite formation (Estévez, Spear, Manuel, Radi, et al. 1998; Raoul et al. 2002)(Fig 4).

Inhibition of the JNK MAP kinase activity blocks trophic factor deprivation-induced apoptosis, but has not effect on motor neuron apoptosis induced by Fas activation (Raoul et al. 2002; Ricart et al. 2006; Li, Oppenheim, and Milligan 2001; Newbern et al. 2007). Activation of JNK leads to the phosphorylation of transcription factors and the induction of protein synthesis and might induce the expression of Fas ligand (Le-Niculescu et al. 1999; Morishima et al. 2001), suggesting that JNK activation may be upstream of Fas activation (Barthelemy, Henderson, and Pettmann 2004). JNK phosphorylation of 14-3-3 proteins can stimulate the translocation of Bad to the mitochondria and the activation of FOXO3a (Sunayama et al. 2005; Vogt, Jiang, and Aoki 2005). In turn, FOXO3a regulates the expression of Fas ligand in motor neurons (Barthelemy, Henderson, and Pettmann 2004), which suggests a pathway integrating the dependence of both JNK and FOXO3a in the induction of motor neuron apoptosis.

Inhibition of p38 MAP kinase prevents apoptosis induced by Fas pathway activation but has no effect on trophic factor deprivation-induced apoptosis, further suggesting the activation of more than one apoptotic pathway by trophic factor deprivation. In fact, motor neuron apoptosis induced by Fas activation occurs by an atypical mechanism involving the two parallel pathways (Raoul et al. 2002; Raoul et al. 2006)(Fig 5). One of the pathways is the classical caspase 8-mediated mitochondrial apoptotic pathway. The other pathway is responsible for the induction of neuronal NOS by a mechanism involving sequential activation of DAXX, ASK1 and p38 MAP kinase (Raoul et al. 2002). Activation of either pathway seems to be able to induce apoptosis by itself, but when activated together the process occurs faster. The original discussion on a possible mechanism for peroxynitrite and nitric oxide to enhance the caspase 8-mitochondria apoptotic pathway was based in the literature indicating that both peroxynitrite and nitric oxide affect the mitochondrial function. On the other hand, activation of caspase 8 by Fas occurs by means of the DISC complex recruitment (Medema et al. 1997). Another possible explanation is that peroxynitrite may be able to induce the activation of caspase 8 by interacting with some of the components of the DISC, which also could make the Fas activation of this complex easier, resulting in a faster induction of motor neuron apoptosis.

On the other hand, although formation of nitrotyrosine can be catalyzed from nitrite and hydrogen peroxide by peroxidases and transition metals (van der Vliet et al. 1997; Eiserich et al. 1998; Schopfer, Baker, and Freeman 2003), incubation of motor neurons with micromolar concentrations of nitrite and/or hydrogen peroxide has no effect on the survival of motor neurons in culture (Estévez et al. 2000) or tyrosine nitration (Ye et al. 2007), further supporting peroxynitrite formation. Together these results suggest that peroxynitrite formation is necessary for the induction of motor neuron apoptosis by trophic factor deprivation and after Fas pathway activation. In addition, scavenging the nitrating radical products of peroxynitrite by tyrosine-containing peptides does not affect thiol oxidation but prevents nitrotyrosine formation and motor neuron death (Ye et al. 2007)(Fig 6). These results suggest that tyrosine nitration has a causal role in the induction of motor neurons apoptosis by peroxynitrite and it is not only a marker for the formation of reactive nitrogen species.

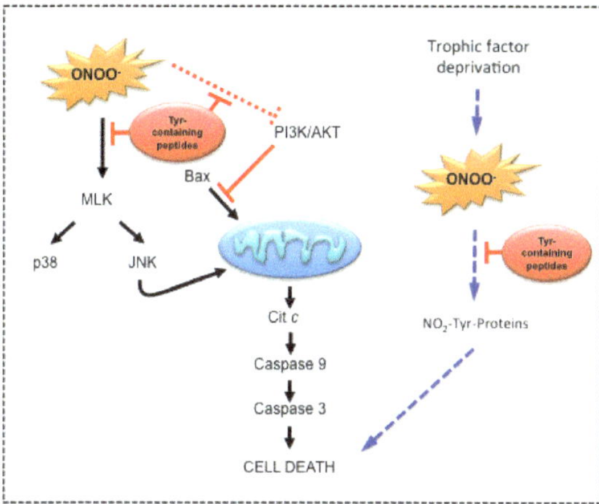

Fig. 6. Peptides that scavenge the nitrating products derived from peroxynitrite decomposition prevent cell death induced by the pure oxidant or endogenously produced peroxynitrite.

6. Extrinsic apoptotic pathway and motor neuron apoptosis *in vivo*

The relevance of the Fas pathways in the regulation of motor neurons death *in vivo* was shown in studies on the effects of axonal injury in mice knockout for Fas and transgenic mice expressing a dominant negative form of FADD, where axotomy-induced motor neuron degeneration was blocked (Ugolini et al. 2003; Martin, Chen, and Liu 2005). Axonal injury is also associated with increased nitrotyrosine immunoreactivity (Martin, Kaiser, and Price 1999; Martin, Chen, and Liu 2005), reveling that in addition to the activation of the classical Fas pathway, peroxynitrite is also produced. These observations suggest that the atypical pathways involved in the induction of motor neuron apoptosis by Fas activation are also active *in vivo* and play a role in the degeneration of adult motor neurons. In addition, SOD deficiency increases motor neuron vulnerability to axotomy (Reaume et al. 1996), indicating that production of superoxide plays an important role in motor neuron degeneration *in vivo*. Even when the source of superoxide for the formation of peroxynitrite *in vivo* and in cultured motor neurons remains unknown, evidence from other neuronal types suggest that the induction and activation of NADPH oxidase might be responsible for the production of superoxide that makes nitric oxide toxic to motor neurons (Noh and Koh 2000; Tammariello, Quinn, and Estus 2000). In motor neurons, activation of the p75 neurotrophic receptor results in apoptosis in different conditions (Ricart et al. 2006; Pehar et al. 2004; Pehar et al. 2007; Wiese et al. 1999). At least in part this toxicity is mediated by induction of superoxide production by mitochondria (Pehar et al. 2007). In summary, inhibition of nitric oxide production blocks motor neuron death induced by ventral root avulsion, and deletion of SOD increases the sensitivity of motor neurons to the same noxious stimulus. Moreover, motor neuron degeneration after ventral root avulsion is preceded by increased tyrosine nitration and the activation of the death receptor pathways. In aggregate these results reveal that motor neuron death *in vitro* and *in vivo* occurs largely by the same mechanisms and through the activation of the same signaling pathways.

7. ALS and reactive nitrogen species

A pathological condition associated with an increased expression of neuronal NOS and nitrotyrosine in motor neurons is amyotrophic lateral sclerosis (ALS)(Abe et al. 1995; Beal et al. 1997; Chou, Wang, and Komai 1996; Chou, Wang, and Taniguchi 1996, , Barber, 2010 #1694). As for today more than 25 reports have found increased levels of nitrotyrosine immunoreactivity or free nitrotyrosine in tissue from patients and animal models of ALS. The definitive evidence for the presence of nitrotyrosine, at least in a transgenic mouse model of ALS, was provided by mass spectrometry studies identifying some of the nitrated proteins and the nitrated residues. Other studies confirmed the identity of the nitrated proteins showing that motor neurons in pre-symptomatic mutant SOD1 mice generate superoxide, NO and ONOO- at higher levels than control motor neurons. In addition, nitration of Cox-I, SOD2 and α-synuclein occurs in pre-symptomatic mutant SOD1 mice suggesting a role for peroxynitrite in the pathogenesis of the disease (Martin et al. 2007).

ALS is a neurodegenerative disease characterized by the death of pyramidal neurons in the motor cortex and motor neurons in the brain stem and ventral spinal cord. About 2% of all ALS cases are due to the presence of one of more than 100 mutations in the gene encoding Cu,Zn SOD (Cleveland and Rothstein 2001; Traub, Mitsumoto, and Rowland 2011). When expressed in mice and rats, some of the human ALS-linked SOD mutations produce a motor neuron disease reminiscent of ALS (Gurney et al. 1994; Dal Canto and Gurney 1995; Wong et al. 1995; Bruijn et al. 1997); these are currently the most widely accepted models for the disease. It is generally accepted that the toxic effect of the mutations is due to a gain-of-function (Cleveland and Rothstein 2001). Growing evidence implicates apoptosis as the mechanism of motor neuron death in the ALS. The fact that the morphological and biochemical characteristics of apoptosis only last upwards of 24 hours in conjunction with the slow progression of the disease, which implicate that only a few motor neurons are dying at a time, make the definitive detection of apoptosis in post mortem tissue from ALS patients challenging (Sathasivam, Ince, and Shaw 2001). However, a comprehensive analysis of degenerating motor neurons in ALS patients revealed their apoptotic morphology in the ventral horn of the spinal cord and motor cortex, combined with an increase in DNA fragmentation and caspase 3 activation (Martin 1999). Further analysis of the post mortem human tissue showed increased formation of Bax-Bax homodimers and a decrease in Bcl-2-Bax heterodimers in motor neurons, suggestive of an increased pro-apoptotic tone in the disease (Martin 1999).

Further evidence for the participation of apoptosis in ALS was provided by the use of transgenic models of the disease (Shibata 2001). Histological analysis of motor neurons from transgenic mice carrying G93A SOD mutant shows decreased expression of the anti-apoptotic proteins Bcl-2 and Bcl-xl and increased expression of the pro-apoptotic Bcl-2 family members Bax and Bad, which expression was attenuated following over-expression of Bcl-2 (Vukosavic et al. 1999; Vukosavic et al. 2000). Genetic deletion of Bax in transgenic mice for the G93A ALS-linked mutant SOD delays onset and extends the lifespan of the animals, but it does not prevent the disease in spite of preventing motor neuron death (Gould et al. 2006). These results are a clear testimony to the complexity of the disease process. Although motor neurons are protected against apoptosis, other abnormalities such as neuromuscular denervation and mitochondrial vacuolization are still occurring (Gould et al. 2006). Other studies suggest that alterations of the neuromuscular junction are between the first symptoms of the disease both in humans and animals models of the disease (Fischer et al. 2004). However, it is important to remember that in the human disease motor neurons do die. The artificial deletion of a gene that regulates apoptosis may just inhibit the final step in the death process, without affecting upstream pathways responsible for the death of the cells. In addition, these results suggest that reactive oxygen and nitrogen species formed during the disease process are not final effectors of cell death, but rather upstream triggers of the activation of signaling pathways resulting in motor neuron death.

Further evidence for the role of apoptosis in the pathogenesis of ALS comes from the delay in onset and progression of the disease due to over-expression of the anti-apoptotic protein Bcl-2 in a transgenic mouse model of ALS (Vukosavic et al. 2000). More recently it was reported that Bcl-2 binds both wild-type and mutant SOD1 *in vitro* and *in vivo*. Because Bcl-2 associated with mutant SOD1 is present in protein aggregates located in mitochondria from the spinal cord of ALS patient and animal models of the disease, it was suggested that entrapment of Bcl-2 by SOD1 leads to the depletion of the anti-apoptotic protein in motor neurons, increasing the vulnerability of these cells (Pasinelli et al. 2004). However, no evidence for the aggregates selectively located in motor neuron mitochondria has been reported. Conversely, BIM, a member of the pro-apoptotic family of Bcl-2 proteins, is upregulated in the $SOD1^{G93A}$ familial ALS mouse model during the symptomatic stage of the disease, and its expression is required to trigger cell death induced by SOD1 mutants *in vitro*. Genetic deletion of BIM in an animal model of ALS results in reduced cellular apoptosis in the spinal cord ventral horn and increases lifespan (Hetz et al. 2007).

The role of caspases in ALS is more controversial. While several authors have reported activation of caspases and a functional role for these activated proteases in animal models of the disease (Friedlander et al. 1997; Li et al. 2000; Pasinelli et al. 1998; Nagai et al. 2001; Pasinelli et al. 2000), others were unable to find a functional role for the enzymes and report that motor neuron death in the G93A mouse model is independent of caspase activation (Martin et al. 2007).

To study the role of mutant SOD1 in different cell types involved in the pathology of ALS, chimeric mice were developed with mixtures of normal and SOD1 mutant-expressing cells. Normal motor neurons in SOD1 mutant chimeras develop features of ALS pathology. However, non-neuronal cells that do not express mutant SOD1 delay degeneration and significantly extend survival of mutant expressing motor neurons (Clement et al. 2003). When primary mouse spinal motor neurons express mutant human SOD1, the cells are not triggered to degenerate, however when rodent astrocytes express mutated SOD1, they kill spinal primary and embryonic mouse stem cell-derived motor neurons (Nagai et al. 2007). In addition, when G93A mutant embryonic stem cells are cultured as motor neurons through *in vitro* differentiation, co-cultures with G93A mutant glial cells lead to a decrease in survival of the motor neurons (Di Giorgio et al. 2007). Using conditional knockout to delete the mutant SOD in specific cell types it was found that the expression of mutant SOD in motor neurons plays a key role on the onset of the disease and the early phases of disease progression. When the levels of mutant SOD were reduced in microglia, the onset and early phases of the disease were not affected, but the later stage of the disease was slowed down. Therefore, onset and progression of ALS are dependent on distinct cell types, indicating the occurrence of a non-cell-autonomous death of motor neurons (Boillee et al. 2006; Boillee, Vande Velde, and Cleveland 2006).

8. SOD1 toxicity

In spite of all the studies done to date on mutant SOD1 in ALS, the mechanism of SOD toxicity remains elusive and highly controversial. The devolpment of an antibody that recognizes the monomer misfolded forms of SOD1 showed the presence of the misfolded monomer in three ALS mouse models with G37R, G85R and G93A SOD1 mutations as well as in a human individual with an A4V SOD1 mutation (Rakhit et al. 2007). One of the hypotheses for mutant SOD toxicity proposes that an aberrant SOD chemistry, which allows small molecules such us peroxynitrite or hydrogen peroxide to produce damaging free radicals, is responsible for the toxic gain-of-function (Beckman and Crow 1993; Lyons et al. 1996). This aberrant chemistry could be the result of a reversal in SOD function caused by the loss of the structural zinc atom (Estévez et al. 1999; Beckman et al. 2001), since the mutant enzymes show a lower affinity for zinc than the wild type SOD, thus increasing the probability for the formation of Zn-deficient SOD (Lyons et al. 1996). There is great controversy about whether this proposed mechanism can take place and its relevance in the pathogenesis of ALS (Subramaniam et al. 2002), but the hypothesis also has its supporters (Liochev and Fridovich 2003).

The Zn-deficient hypothesis was tested using cultured motor neurons and liposomes for the intracellular release of the enzyme (Estévez et al. 1999). These experiments revealed that Zn-deficient human SOD, either mutant or wild type are equally toxic to motor neurons in culture by a mechanism requiring copper and the production of peroxynitrite (Estévez et al. 1999). On the other hand, Cu,Zn mutant and wild type SOD are equally protective for trophic factor deprived motor neurons (Estévez et al. 1999). Based on these results and the characteristics of the altered chemistry of the Zn-deficient SOD, the conclusion was that Zn-deficient SOD produces superoxide using intracellular reducing activities leading to the formation of peroxynitrite (Fig 7).

Further confirmation of an altered mutant SOD chemistry was found using cultured motor neurons isolated from a transgenic mice model of human ALS in conjunction with wild type SOD (Raoul et al. 2002). Nitric oxide is not toxic to non-transgenic mouse and rat motor neurons (Estévez, Spear, Manuel, Radi, et al. 1998; Estévez et al. 2000; Raoul et al. 2002). In contrast, motor neurons isolated from transgenic rats and mice carrying human ALS-linked SOD G85R and G93A die after exposure to nanomolar steady state concentrations of nitric oxide (Raoul et al. 2002; Sahawneh et al. 2010). Transgenic motor neurons carrying mutant SOD are also ten times more sensitive to Fas-induced apoptosis, while transgenic motor neurons carrying human wild type SOD are 100 times more resistant than non-transgenic motor neurons to Fas-mediated apoptosis (Raoul et al. 2002; Raoul et al. 2006). Nitric oxide toxicity in transgenic motor neurons can be reversed by copper chelators and scavenging of superoxide and peroxynitrite (Sahawneh et al. 2010), suggesting production of superoxide in transgenic motor neurons.

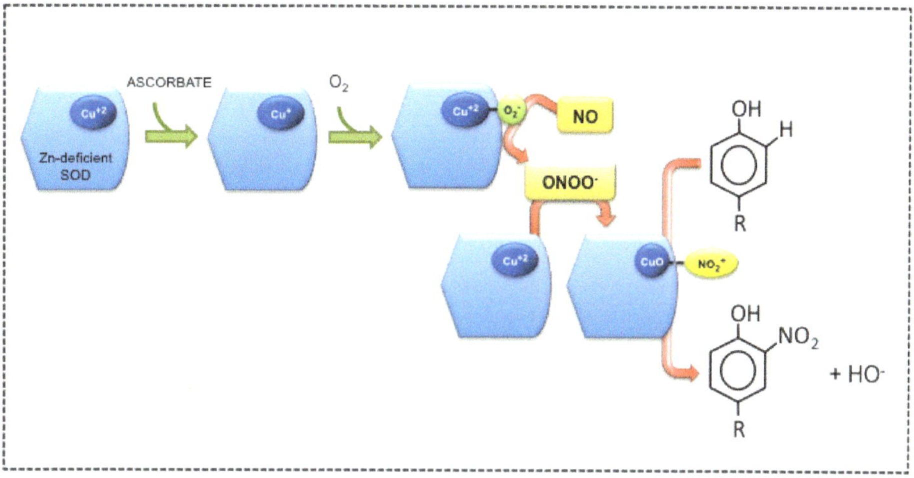

Fig. 7. Zn-deficient SOD as a catalyst for peroxynitrite formation and tyrosine nitration.

Intracellular delivery of wild type Cu,Zn-containing human SOD (Cu,Zn SOD) to motor neurons isolated from transgenic rats overexpressing G93A mutant SOD, has no effect on survival whether the cells are cultured in the presence or absence of trophic factors. However, these motor neurons carrying both, mutant and Cu,Zn-containing SOD are more sensitive to nitric oxide toxicity than transgenic motor neurons without intracellular delivered Cu,Zn SOD (Sahawneh et al. 2010). These *in vitro* results closely mimic the *in vivo* observations of acceleration of death when transgenic mice for mutant SOD are crossbreed with mice transgenic for wild type SOD (Jaarsma et al. 2000; Fukada et al. 2001; Deng et al. 2006). There is some controversy over the effects of wild type SOD on the survival of mice carrying the SOD^{G85R} were one group reported acceleration of disease (Wang et al. 2009) and other claims no effect in a different SOD^{G85R} line (Bruijn et al. 1998). The mechanism through which coexpression of Cu,Zn SOD wild type increases the toxicity of mutant SOD is controversial, with some groups arguing that aggregation plays a role (Deng et al. 2006; Furukawa et al. 2006), while others conclude that increased solubility of the enzyme contributes to the enhanced toxicity (Fig 8) (Fukada et al. 2001; Witan et al. 2008; Witan et al. 2009; Sahawneh et al. 2010).

The mechanisms of mutant SOD-induced motor neuron death in the presence of nitric oxide and Zn-deficient SOD stimulation of motor neuron apoptosis in culture seem identical (Estévez et al. 1999; Raoul et al. 2002; Sahawneh et al. 2010). The dependence on copper and the production of superoxide and peroxynitrite in both conditions indicate that nitrative stress plays a key role in the induction of cell death. In addition, Zn-deficient SOD toxicity is prevented by peptides that inhibit nitration (Ye et al. 2007; Sahawneh et al. 2010), as is the increased toxicity after the addition of Cu,Zn SOD (Sahawneh et al. 2010). Biochemical and biophysical studies indicate that the formation of a dimer between Zn-deficient SOD and Cu,Zn SOD increases the stability of the Zn-deficient SOD monomer (Beckman 1996; Roberts et al. 2007), in agreement with the *in vivo* and *in vitro* studies showing that wild type

SOD increases the stability and solubility of the mutant protein (Fukada et al. 2001; Witan et al. 2008; Witan et al. 2009).

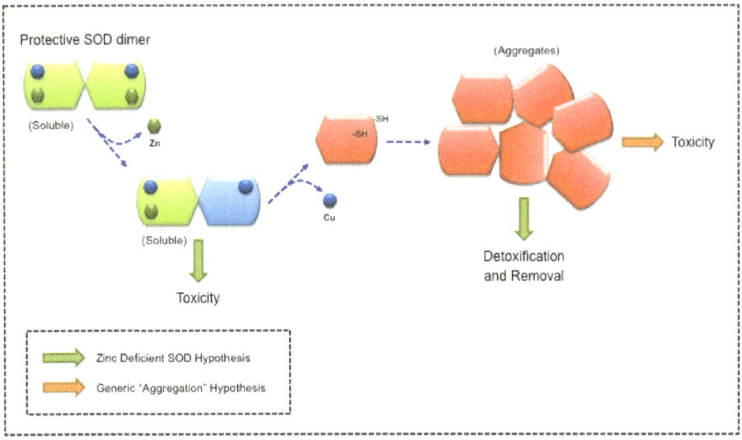

Fig. 8. Proposed mechanisms for the toxicity induced by mutant SOD.

Moreover, in spite of Cu,Zn SOD being a very stable enzyme, the half-life for exchange between this enzyme and Zn-deficient SOD at 37°C is surprisingly fast at 13-17 min when determined using differential mobility gel electrophoresis and 14 min by FRET (Roberts et al. 2007; Sahawneh et al. 2010). An important observation is that the reassociation of Cu,Zn SOD monomers is approximately 10,000 times slower than the reassociation of apoSOD monomers (Lindberg et al. 2004; Svensson et al. 2006), suggesting that the alterations of the dimer interface in the apoSOD are responsibly for the faster association of the monomers even though the stability of the dimer is diminished when compared with Cu,Zn SOD. It is possible that a similar mechanism occurs in the formation of the dimers between Cu,Zn and Zn-deficient SOD, which will explain the increased toxicity by a nitrative mechanism.

In addition, supporting the hypothesis that the increase in stability of Zn-deficient SOD is key in enhancing its toxicity, the substitution of the cysteine residues in positions 6 and 111 by alanine and serine in the human SOD increases its thermostability, and also increases the toxicity of the wild type SOD and $SOD1^{A4V}$ when they are Zn-deficient, but has no effect when the enzymes have the full content of metals (Sahawneh et al. 2010). Other studies reveal that mutation of these two cysteines decreases the stability of the SOD protein but prevents its aggregation (Lindberg et al. 2004; Svensson et al. 2006; Lepock, Frey, and Hallewell 1990). Zn-deficient enzyme with the double cysteine mutation shows more toxicity than the equivalent Zn-deficient SOD with the cysteine residues. In this model, the increased stability of the Zn-deficient form of the SOD is also responsible for the toxicity by a mechanism requiring the production of nitric oxide, superoxide and peroxynitrite followed by tyrosine nitration (Sahawneh et al. 2010).

In summary, reactive nitrogen species and some of their products, such as nitrotyrosine play a causal role in the activation of motor neuron death pathways rather than just having an effector activity. In addition, the abundant evidence indicating the formation of reactive nitrogen species and nitrotyrosine in pathological conditions also suggests that nitrotyrosine is more than a footprint in these conditions. In ALS is well documented the formation of reactive nitrogen species and tyrosine nitration. Most evidence indicates that the source of the toxic nitric oxide is the neuronal isoform of NOS. However, the knockdown of the exon 1 in neuronal NOS, which greatly decreases the enzyme levels, has no effect on the survival of transgenic mouse models of ALS (Facchinetti et al. 1999). On the other hand, inhibitors of neuronal NOS are equally protective to motor neurons isolated from wild type and mice deficient for neuronal NOS (Ricart and Estevez, unpublished observations). These results suggest that the beta isoform of the neuronal NOS, which lacks exon 1, is the responsible for the production of the toxic nitric oxide in motor neurons. If this is the case, then these results may explain why the partial neuronal NOS deficiency is not protective in ALS. The multiple controversies in the role of reactive nitrogen species in ALS are not likely to end soon and will stimulate much needed research to found a cure for this devastating disease.

9. Acknowledgements

This work was supported by the NIH/NIDNS (NS36761). We thanks the constructive criticism of Thong Ma and Mary Ann Sahawneh during the preparation of this manuscript.

10. References

Abe, K, L H Pan, M Watanabe, T Kato, and Y Itoyama. 1995. Induction of nitrotyrosine-like immunoreactivity in the lower motor neuron of amyotrophic lateral sclerosis. *Neurosci. Lett.* 199:152-154.

Alvarez, B, G Ferrer-Sueta, B A Freeman, and R Radi. 1999. Kinetics of peroxynitrite reaction with amino acids and human serum albumin. *J. Biol. Chem.* 274 (2):842-848.

Ara, J, S Przedborski, A B Naini, V Jackson-Lewis, R R Trifiletti, J Horwitz, and H Ischiropoulos. 1998. Inactivation of tyrosine hydroxylase by nitration following exposure to peroxynitrite and 1-methyl-4-phenyl-1,2,3,6-tetrahydropyridine(MPTP). *Proc Natl Acad Sci USA* 95 (13):7659-63.

Aslan, M., T. M. Ryan, T. M. Townes, L. Coward, M. C. Kirk, S. Barnes, C. B. Alexander, S. S. Rosenfeld, and B. A. Freeman. 2003. Nitric oxide-dependent generation of reactive species in sickle cell disease. Actin tyrosine induces defective cytoskeletal polymerization. *J Biol Chem* 278 (6):4194-204.

Bar, P. R. 2000. Motor neuron disease in vitro: the use of cultured motor neurons to study amyotrophic lateral sclerosis. *Eur J Pharmacol* 405 (1-3):285-95.

Barthelemy, C. Catherine, Christopher E. Henderson, and B. Brigitte Pettmann. 2004. Foxo3a induces motoneuron death through the Fas pathway in cooperation with JNK. *BMC neuroscience* 5 (1):48.

Beal, M F, L J Ferrante, S E Browne, R T Matthews, N W Kowall, and R H Brown. 1997. Increased 3-nitrotyrosine in both sporadic and familial amyotrophic lateral sclerosis. *Ann Neurol* 42:644-654.

Beckman, J S. 1996. Nitric oxide: Principles and actions. In *The Physiological and Pathological Chemistry of Nitric Oxide*, edited by J. R. Lanacaster. New York: Academic Press.

Repeated Author. 1996. The Physiological and Pathological Chemistry of Nitric Oxide. In *Nitric Oxide: Principles and Actions*, edited by J. L. Jr: Academic Press Inc.

Beckman, J S, T W Beckman, J Chen, P M Marshall, and B A Freeman. 1990. Apparent hydroxyl radical production by peroxynitrite: Implications for endothelial injury by nitric oxide and superoxide. *Proc. Natl. Acad. Sci. (USA)* 87 (4):1620-1624.

Beckman, J S, and J P Crow. 1993. Pathological implications of nitric oxide, superoxide and peroxynitrite formation. *Biochem. Soc. Trans.* 21 (2):330-334.

Beckman, J S, A G Estévez, J P Crow, and L Barbeito. 2001. Superoxide dismutase and the death of motoneurons in ALS. *TINS* 24 (11):S15-S20.

Beckman, J S, and W H Koppenol. 1996. Nitric oxide, superoxide, and peroxynitrite -- the good, the bad, and the ugly. *Am. J. Physiol.* 271 (Cell Physiol. 40):C1424-C1437.

Beckman, J. S., H. Ischiropoulos, L. Zhu, M. van der Woerd, C. Smith, J. Chen, J. Harrison, J. C. Martin, and M. Tsai. 1992. Kinetics of superoxide dismutase and iron- catalyzed nitration of phenolics by peroxynitrite. *Arch Biochem Biophys* 298 (2):438-445.

Beckman, J. S., and W. H. Koppenol. 1996. Nitric oxide, superoxide, and peroxynitrite: the good, the bad, and ugly. *Am J Physiol* 271 (5 Pt 1):C1424-37.

Boillee, Severine, Christine Vande Velde, and DonW Cleveland. 2006. ALS: A Disease of Motor Neurons and Their Nonneuronal Neighbors. *Neuron* 52 (1):39-59.

Boillee, Severine, Koji Yamanaka, Christian S. Lobsiger, Neal G. Copeland, Nancy A. Jenkins, George Kassiotis, George Kollias, and Don W. Cleveland. 2006. Onset and Progression in Inherited ALS Determined by Motor Neurons and Microglia. *Science* 312 (5778):1389-1392.

Bonfoco, E, D Krainc, M Ankarcrona, P Nicotera, and S A Lipton. 1995. Apoptosis and necrosis: Two distinct events induced, respectively, by mild and intense insults with *N*-methyl-D-aspartate or nitric oxide/superoxide in cortical cell cultures. *Proc. Natl. Acad. Sci. U.S.A.* 92 (16):7162-7166.

Bruijn, L I, M W Becher, M K Lee, K L Anderson, N A Jenkins, N G Copeland, S S Sisodia, J D Rothstein, D R Borchelt, D L Price, and D W Cleveland. 1997. ALS-Linked SOD1 Mutant G85R Mediates Damage to Astrocytes and Promotes Rapidly Progressive Disease with SOD1-Containing Inclusions. *Neuron* 18 (2):327-338.

Bruijn, L I, M K Houseweart, S Kato, K L Anderson, S D Anderson, E Ohama, A G Reaume, R W Scott, and D W Cleveland. 1998. Aggregation and Motor Neuron Toxicity of an ALS-Linked SOD1 Mutant Independent from Wild-Type SOD1. *Science* 281:1851-1854.

Cappelletti, G., M. G. Maggioni, G. Tedeschi, and R. Maci. 2003. Protein tyrosine nitration is triggered by nerve growth factor during neuronal differentiation of PC12 cells. *Exp Cell Res* 288 (1):9-20.

Carreras, Maria Cecilia, and Juan Jose Poderoso. 2007. Mitochondrial nitric oxide in the signaling of cell integrated responses. *Am J Physiol Cell Physiol* 292 (5):C1569-1580.

Casanovas, A., J. Ribera, M. Hukkanen, V. Riveros-Moreno, and J. E. Esquerda. 1996. Prevention by lamotrigine, MK-801 and N omega-nitro-L-arginine methyl ester of motoneuron cell death after neonatal axotomy. *Neuroscience* 71 (2):313-25.

Chang, W., D. R. Webster, A. A. Salam, D. Gruber, A. Prasad, J. P. Eiserich, and J. C. Bulinski. 2002. Alteration of the C-terminal amino acid of tubulin specifically inhibits myogenic differentiation. *Journal of Biological Chemistry* 277 (34):30690-30698.

Chou, S. M., H. S. Wang, and K. Komai. 1996. Colocalization of NOS and SOD1 in neurofilament accumulation within motor neurons of amyotrophic lateral sclerosis: an immunohistochemical study. *J Chem Neuroanat* 10 (3-4):249-58.

Chou, S. M., H. S. Wang, and A. Taniguchi. 1996. Role of SOD-1 and nitric oxide/cyclic GMP cascade on neurofilament aggregation in ALS/MND. *J Neurol Sci* 139 Suppl:16-26.

Clement, A. M., M. D. Nguyen, E. A. Roberts, M. L. Garcia, S. Boillee, M. Rule, A. P. McMahon, W. Doucette, D. Siwek, R. J. Ferrante, R. H. Brown, Jr., J. P. Julien, L. S. Goldstein, and D. W. Cleveland. 2003. Wild-type nonneuronal cells extend survival of SOD1 mutant motor neurons in ALS mice. *Science* 302 (5642):113-7.

Cleveland, D W, and J D Rothstein. 2001. From Charcot to Lou Gehrig: Deciphering Selective Motor Neuron Death in ALS. *Nature Neuroscience Review* 2 (11):806-819.

Colasanti, M., and H. Suzuki. 2000. The dual personality of NO. *Trends Pharmacol Sci* 21 (7):249-52.

Crow, J P, M J Strong, Y Zhuang, Y Ye, and J S Beckman 1997. Superoxide dimutase catalyzes nitration of tyrosines by peroxinitrite in the rod and head domains of neurofilament L. *J Neurochem* 69 (5):1945-1953.

Crow, J. P., J. S. Beckman, and J. M. McCord. 1995. Sensitivity of the essential zinc-thiolate moiety of yeast alcohol dehydrogenase to hypochlorite and peroxynitrite. *Biochemistry* 34 (11):3544-52.

Dal Canto, M.C. , and M.E. Gurney. 1995. Neuropathological changes in two lines of mice carrying a transgene for mutant human Cu, Zn SOD, and in mice overexpressing wild type human SOD: a model of familial amyotrophic lateral sclerosis (FALS). *Brain Res.* 676:25-40.

Dawson, V L, and T M Dawson. 1996. Nitric Oxide Toxicity in Central Nervous System Cultures. *Methods in Neurosciences* 30:26-43.

Dawson, V. L., and T. M. Dawson. 1996. Nitric oxide in neuronal degeneration. *Proc Soc Exp Biol Med* 211 (1):33-40.

Dawson, V.L., and T.M. Dawson. 1996. Nitric oxide neurotoxicity. *J Chem. Neuroanat* 10:179-190.

Deng, Han-Xiang, Yong Shi, Yoshiaki Furukawa, Hong Zhai, Ronggen Fu, Erdong Liu, George H. Gorrie, Mohammad S. Khan, Wu-Yen Hung, Eileen H. Bigio, Thomas Lukas, Mauro C. Dal Canto, Thomas V. O'Halloran, and Teepu Siddique. 2006. Conversion to the amyotrophic lateral sclerosis phenotype is associated with intermolecular linked insoluble aggregates of SOD1 in mitochondria. *PNAS* 103 (18):7142-7147.

Di Giorgio, Francesco Paolo, Monica A. Carrasco, Michelle C. Siao, Tom Maniatis, and Kevin Eggan. 2007. Non-cell autonomous effect of glia on motor neurons in an embryonic stem cell-based ALS model. *Nat Neurosci* 10 (5):608-614.

Eiserich, J P, A G Estévez, T V Bamberg, Y Z Ye, P H Chumley, J S Beckman, and B A Freeman. 1999. Microtubule dysfunction by posttranslational nitrotyrosination of a-tubulin: a nitric oxide-dependent mechanism of cellular injury. *Proc. Natl. Acad. Sci. USA* 96:6365-6370.

Eiserich, J. P., M. Hristova, C. E. Cross, A. D. Jones, B. A. Freeman, B. Halliwell, and A. van der Vliet. 1998. Formation of nitric oxide-derived inflammatory oxidants by myeloperoxidase in neutrophils. *Nature* 391 (6665):393-7.

Estévez, A G, J P Crow, J B Sampson, C Reiter, Y-X Zhuang, G J Richardson, M M Tarpey, L Barbeito, and J S Beckman. 1999. Induction of nitric oxide-dependent apoptosis in motor neurons by zinc-deficient superoxide dismutase. *Science* 286:2498-2500.

Estévez, A G, R Radi, L Barbeito, J T Shin, J A Thompson, and J S Beckman. 1995. Peroxynitrite-induced cytotoxicity in PC12 cells: evidence for an apoptotic mechanism differentially modulated by neurotrophic factors. *J. Neurochem.* 65 (4):1543-1550.

Estévez, A G, J B Sampson, Y-X Zhuang, N Spear, G J Richardson, J P Crow, M M Tarpey, L Barbeito, and J S Beckman. 2000. Liposome-delivered superoxide dismutase prevents nitric oxide-dependent motor neuron death induced by trophic factor withdrawal. *Free Rad. Biol. Med.* 28 (3):437-446.

Estévez, A G, N Spear, S Machelle Manuel, R Radi, C E Henderson, L Barbeito, and J S Beckman. 1998. Nitric oxide and superoxide contribute to motor neuron apoptosis induced by trophic factor deprivation. *J. Neurosci.* 18 (3):923-931.

Estévez, A. G. , N. Spear, S. Machelle Manuel, L. Barbeito, R. Radi, and J. S. Beckman. 1998. Role of endogenous nitric oxide and peroxinitrite formation in the survival and death of motor neurons in culture. *Progress in Brain Research* 118:269-280.

Facchinetti, F., M. Sasaki, F. B. Cutting, P. Zhai, J. E. MacDonald, D. Reif, M. F. Beal, P. L. Huang, T. M. Dawson, M. E. Gurney, and V. L. Dawson. 1999. Lack of involvement of neuronal nitric oxide synthase in the pathogenesis of a transgenic mouse model of familial amyotrophic lateral sclerosis. *Neuroscience* 90 (4):1483-92.

Fischer, Lindsey R., Deborah G. Culver, Philip Tennant, Albert A. Davis, Minsheng Wang, Amilcar Castellano-Sanchez, Jaffar Khan, Meraida A. Polak, and Jonathan D. Glass. 2004. Amyotrophic lateral sclerosis is a distal axonopathy: evidence in mice and man. *Experimental Neurology* 185 (2):232-240.

Friedlander, R M, J Wang, V Gagliardini, R H Jr Brown, and J Yuan. 1997. Inhibition of ICE slows ALS in mice. *Nature* 388:31.

Fukada, K., S. Nagano, M. Satoh, C. Tohyama, T. Nakanishi, A. Shimizu, T. Yanagihara, and S. Sakoda. 2001. Stabilization of mutant Cu/Zn superoxide dismutase (SOD1) protein by coexpressed wild SOD1 protein accelerates the disease progression in familial amyotrophic lateral sclerosis mice. *Eur J Neurosci* 14 (12):2032-6.

Furukawa, Yoshiaki, Ronggen Fu, Han-Xiang Deng, Teepu Siddique, and Thomas V. O'Halloran. 2006. From the Cover: Disulfide cross-linked protein represents a significant fraction of ALS-associated Cu, Zn-superoxide dismutase aggregates in spinal cords of model mice. *PNAS* 103 (18):7148-7153.

Go, Y. M., R. P. Patel, M. C. Maland, H. Park, J. S. Beckman, V. M. Darley-Usmar, and H. Jo. 1999. Evidence for peroxynitrite as a signaling molecule in flow-dependent activation of c-Jun NH(2)-terminal kinase. *Am J Physiol* 277 (4 Pt 2):H1647-53.

Gould, Thomas W., Robert R. Buss, Sharon Vinsant, David Prevette, Woong Sun, C. Michael Knudson, Carol E. Milligan, and Ronald W. Oppenheim. 2006. Complete Dissociation of Motor Neuron Death from Motor Dysfunction by Bax Deletion in a Mouse Model of ALS. *J. Neurosci.* 26 (34):8774-8786.

Greenacre, S A, and H Ischiropoulos. 2001. Tyrosine nitration: localisation, quantification, consequences for protein function and signal transduction. *Free Radical Research* 34 (6):541-581.

Groves, J T, and S S Marla. 1995. Peroxynitrite-induced DNA strand scission mediated by a manganese porphyrin. *J. Am. Chem. Soc.* 117:9578-9579.

Gurney, M E, H Pu, A Y Chiu, M C Dal Canto, C Y Polchow, D D Alexander, J Caliendo, A Hentati, Y W Kwon, H-X Deng, W Chen, P Zhai, R L Sufit, and T Siddique. 1994.

Motor neuron degeneration in mice that express a human Cu,Zn superoxide dismutase mutation. *Science* 264 (5166):1772-1775.

Hetz, C., P. Thielen, J. Fisher, P. Pasinelli, R. H. Brown, S. Korsmeyer, and L. Glimcher. 2007. The proapoptotic BCL-2 family member BIM mediates motoneuron loss in a model of amyotrophic lateral sclerosis. *Cell Death Differ* 14 (7):1386-1389.

Hughes, R A, M Sendtner, and H Thoenen. 1993. Members of several gene families influence survival of rat motoneurons *in vitro* and *in vivo*. *J. Neurosci. Res.* 36:663-671.

Ignarro, L. J. 1990. Biosynthesis and metabolism of endothelium-derived nitric oxide. *Annu Rev Pharmacol Toxicol* 30:535-60.

Ischiropoulos, H. 1998. Biological tyrosine nitration: A pathophysiological function of nitric oxide and reactive oxygen species. *Arch Biochem Biophys* 356:1-11.

Ischiropoulos, H., and J. S. Beckman. 2003. Oxidative stress and nitration in neurodegeneration: Cause, effect, or association? *Journal of Clinical Investigation* 111 (2):163-169.

Jaarsma, Dick, Elize D Haasdijk, J A C Grashorn, Richard Hawkins, Wim van Duijn, Hein W Verspaget, Jacqueline London, and Jan C Holstege. 2000. Human Cu/Zn superoxide dismutase (SOD1) overexpression in mice causes mitochondial vacuolization, axonal degeneration, and premature motor neuron death and accelerates motor neuron disease in mice expressing a familial amyotrophic lateral sclerosis mutant SOD1. *Neurobiol Disease* 7:623-643.

Kaal, E. C., A. S. Vlug, M. W. Versleijen, M. Kuilman, E. A. Joosten, and P. R. Bar. 2000. Chronic mitochondrial inhibition induces selective motoneuron death in vitro: a new model for amyotrophic lateral sclerosis. *J Neurochem* 74 (3):1158-65.

Le-Niculescu, H., E. Bonfoco, Y. Kasuya, F. X. Claret, D. R. Green, and M. Karin. 1999. Withdrawal of survival factors results in activation of the JNK pathway in neuronal cells leading to Fas ligand induction and cell death. *Mol Cell Biol* 19 (1):751-63.

Lepock, J. R., H. E. Frey, and R. A. Hallewell. 1990. Contribution of conformational stability and reversibility of unfolding to the increased thermostability of human and bovine superoxide dismutase mutated at free cysteines. *J Biol Chem* 265 (35):21612-8.

Li, L., R. W. Oppenheim, M. Lei, and L. J. Houenou. 1994. Neurotrophic agents prevent motoneuron death following sciatic nerve section in the neonatal mouse. *J Neurobiol* 25 (7):759-66.

Li, L., R. W. Oppenheim, and C. E. Milligan. 2001. Characterization of the execution pathway of developing motoneurons deprived of trophic support. *J Neurobiol* 46 (4):249-64.

Li, M., V. O. Ona, C. Guegan, M. Chen, V. Jackson-Lewis, L. J. Andrews, A. J. Olszewski, P. E. Stieg, J. P. Lee, S. Przedborski, and R. M. Friedlander. 2000. Functional role of caspase-1 and caspase-3 in an ALS transgenic mouse model. *Science* 288 (5464):335-9.

Lindberg, M. J., J. Normark, A. Holmgren, and M. Oliveberg. 2004. Folding of human superoxide dismutase: disulfide reduction prevents dimerization and produces marginally stable monomers. *Proc Natl Acad Sci U S A* 101 (45):15893-8.

Liochev, S. I., and I. Fridovich. 2003. Mutant Cu,Zn superoxide dismutases and familial amyotrophic lateral sclerosis: evaluation of oxidative hypotheses. *Free Radic Biol Med* 34 (11):1383-9.

Lyons, T J, H Liu, J J Goto, A Nersissian, J A Roe, J A Graden, C Café, L M Ellerby, D E Bredesen, E B Gralla, and J S Valentine. 1996. Mutations in copper-zinc superoxide dismutase that cause amyotrophic lateral sclerosis alter the zinc binding site and the redox behavior of the protein. *Proc. Natl. Acad. Sci. U.S.A.* 93:12240-12244.

MacMillan-Crow, L A, J S Greendorfer, S M Vickers, and J A Thompson. 2000. Tyrosine nitration of c-SRC tyrosine kinase in human pancreatic ductal adenocarcinoma. *Arch. Biochem. Biophys.* 377 (2):350-356.

Martin, L. J. 1999. Neuronal death in amyotrophic lateral sclerosis is apoptosis: possible contribution of a programmed cell death mechanism. *J Neuropathol Exp Neurol* 58 (5):459-71.

Martin, L. J., K. Chen, and Z. Liu. 2005. Adult motor neuron apoptosis is mediated by nitric oxide and Fas death receptor linked by DNA damage and p53 activation. *J Neurosci* 25 (27):6449-59.

Martin, L. J., A. Kaiser, and A. C. Price. 1999. Motor neuron degeneration after sciatic nerve avulsion in adult rat evolves with oxidative stress and is apoptosis. *J Neurobiol* 40 (2):185-201.

Martin, Lee J. , Zhiping Liu, Kevin Chen, Ann C. Price, Pan. Yan, Jason A. Swaby, and W. Christopher Golden. 2007. Motor neuron degeneration in amyotrophic lateral sclerosis mutant superoxide dismutase-1 transgenic mice: Mechanisms of mitochondriopathy and cell death. *The Journal of Comparative Neurology* 500 (1):20-46.

Medema, J. P., C. Scaffidi, F. C. Kischkel, A. Shevchenko, M. Mann, P. H. Krammer, and M. E. Peter. 1997. FLICE is activated by association with the CD95 death-inducing signaling complex (DISC). *Embo J* 16 (10):2794-804.

Milligan, C. E., R. W. Oppenheim, and L. M. Schwartz. 1994. Motoneurons deprived of trophic support in vitro require new gene expression to undergo programmed cell death. *J Neurobiol* 25 (8):1005-16.

Milligan, C. E., D. Prevette, H. Yaginuma, S. Homma, C. Cardwell, L. C. Fritz, K. J. Tomaselli, R. W. Oppenheim, and L. M. Schwartz. 1995. Peptide inhibitors of the ICE protease family arrest programmed cell death of motoneurons in vivo and in vitro. *Neuron* 15 (2):385-93.

Moncada, S , R M J Palmer, and E A Higgins. 1991. Nitric oxide: physiology, pathophysiology, phamacology. *Pharmacol Rev* 43 (2):109-142.

Morishima, Y., Y. Gotoh, J. Zieg, T. Barrett, H. Takano, R. Flavell, R. J. Davis, Y. Shirasaki, and M. E. Greenberg. 2001. Beta-amyloid induces neuronal apoptosis via a mechanism that involves the c-Jun N-terminal kinase pathway and the induction of Fas ligand. *J Neurosci* 21 (19):7551-60.

Nagai, M, M Aoki, I Miyoshi, M Kato, P Pasinelli, N Kasai, R H Jr. Brown, and Y Itoyama. 2001. Rats expressing human cytosolic copper-zinc superoxide dismutase transgenes with amyotrophic lateral sclerosis: associated mutations develop motor neuron disease. *J Neurosci* 21 (21):9246-9254.

Nagai, Makiko, Diane B. Re, Tetsuya Nagata, Alcmene Chalazonitis, Thomas M. Jessell, Hynek Wichterle, and Serge Przedborski. 2007. Astrocytes expressing ALS-linked mutated SOD1 release factors selectively toxic to motor neurons. *Nat Neurosci* 10 (5):615-622.

Nauser, T., and W. H. Koppenol. 2002. The rate constant of the reaction of superoxide with nitrogen monoxide: Approaching the diffusion limit. *Journal of Physical Chemistry A* 106 (16):4084-4086.

Neff, N. T., D. Prevette, L. J. Houenou, M. E. Lewis, M. A. Glicksman, Q. W. Yin, and R. W. Oppenheim. 1993. Insulin-like growth factors: putative muscle-derived trophic agents that promote motoneuron survival. *J Neurobiol* 24 (12):1578-88.

Newbern, J., A. Taylor, M. Robinson, M. O. Lively, and C. E. Milligan. 2007. c-Jun N-terminal kinase signaling regulates events associated with both health and degeneration in motoneurons. *Neuroscience* 147 (3):680-692.

Noh, K. M., and J. Y. Koh. 2000. Induction and activation by zinc of NADPH oxidase in cultured cortical neurons and astrocytes. *J Neurosci* 20 (23):RC111.

Novikov, L, L Novikova, and J-O Kellerth. 1995. Brain-derived neurotrophic factor promotes survival and blocks nitric oxide synthase expression in adult rat spinal motoneurons after ventral root avulsion. *Neurosci. Lett.* 200 (1):45-48.

Oppenheim, R W. 1996. Neurotrophic survival molecules for motoneurons: an embarrassment of riches. *Neuron* 17 (2):195-197.

Oppenheim, R. W. 1991. Cell death during development of the nervous system. *Annu Rev Neurosci* 14:453-501.

Pacher, Pal, Joseph S. Beckman, and Lucas Liaudet. 2007. Nitric Oxide and Peroxynitrite in Health and Disease. *Physiol. Rev.* 87 (1):315-424.

Padmaja, S, and R E Huie. 1993. The reaction of nitric oxide with organic peroxyl radicals. *Biochem. Biophys. Res. Commun.* 195:539-544.

Pasinelli, P , D R Borchelt, M K Houseweart, D W Cleveland, and R H Brown Jr. 1998. Caspase-1 is activated in neural cells and tissue with amyotrophic lateral sclerosis-associated mutations in copper-zinc superoxide dismutase. *Proc Natl Acad Sci USA* 95 (26):15763-8.

Pasinelli, P., M. E. Belford, N. Lennon, B. J. Bacskai, B. T. Hyman, D. Trotti, and R. H. Brown, Jr. 2004. Amyotrophic lateral sclerosis-associated SOD1 mutant proteins bind and aggregate with Bcl-2 in spinal cord mitochondria. *Neuron* 43 (1):19-30.

Pasinelli, P., M. K. Houseweart, R. H. Brown, and D. W. Cleveland. 2000. Caspase-1 and-3 are sequentially activated in motor neuron death in Cu,Zn superoxide dismutase-mediated familial amyotrophic lateral sclerosis. *Proceedings of the National Academy of Sciences of the United States of America* 97 (25):13901-13906.

Paxinou, E., Q. Chen, M. Weisse, B. I. Giasson, E. H. Norris, S. M. Rueter, J. Q. Trojanowski, V. M. Lee, and H. Ischiropoulos. 2001. Induction of alpha-synuclein aggregation by intracellular nitrative insult. *J Neurosci* 21 (20):8053-61.

Pehar, M., P. Cassina, M. R. Vargas, R. Castellanos, L. Viera, J. S. Beckman, A. G. Estevez, and L. Barbeito. 2004. Astrocytic production of nerve growth factor in motor neuron apoptosis: implications for amyotrophic lateral sclerosis. *J Neurochem* 89 (2):464-73.

Pehar, Mariana, Marcelo R. Vargas, Kristine M. Robinson, Patricia Cassina, Pablo J. Diaz-Amarilla, Tory M. Hagen, Rafael Radi, Luis Barbeito, and Joseph S. Beckman. 2007. Mitochondrial Superoxide Production and Nuclear Factor Erythroid 2-Related Factor 2 Activation in p75 Neurotrophin Receptor-Induced Motor Neuron Apoptosis. *J. Neurosci.* 27 (29):7777-7785.

Pennica, D, V Arce, T A Swanson, R Vejsada, R A Pollock, M Armanini, K Dudley, H S Phillips, A Rosenthal, A C Kato, and C E Henderson. 1996. Cardiotrophin-1, a cytokine present in embryonic muscle, supports long-term survival of spinal motoneurons. *Neuron* 17 (1):63-74.

Radi, R, J S Beckman, K M Bush, and B A Freeman. 1991. Peroxynitrite oxidation of sulfhydryls. The cytotoxic potential of superoxide and nitric oxide. *J. Biol. Chem.* 266 (7):4244-4250.

Repeated Author. 1991. Peroxynitrite-induced membrane lipid peroxidation: The cytotoxic potential of superoxide and nitric oxide. *Arch. Biochem. Biophys.* 288 (2):481-487.

Radi, R. 2004. Nitric oxide, oxidants, and protein tyrosine nitration. *Proc Natl Acad Sci U S A* 101 (12):4003-4008.

Radi, R., A. Cassina, R. Hodara, C. Quijano, and L. Castro. 2002. Peroxynitrite reactions and formation in mitochondria. *Free Radic Biol Med* 33 (11):1451-64.

Rae, T. D., P. J. Schmidt, R. A. Pufahl, V. C. Culotta, and T. V. O'Halloran. 1999. Undetectable intracellular free copper: the requirement of a copper chaperone for superoxide dismutase. *Science* 284 (5415):805-8.

Rakhit, R., J. Robertson, C. Vande Velde, P. Horne, D. M. Ruth, J. Griffin, D. W. Cleveland, N. R. Cashman, and A. Chakrabartty. 2007. An immunological epitope selective for pathological monomer-misfolded SOD1 in ALS. *Nature medicine* 13 (6):754-9.

Ramachandran, Anup, Anna-Liisa Levonen, Paul S. Brookes, Erin Ceaser, Sruti Shiva, Maria Cecilia Barone, and Victor Darley-Usmar. 2002. Mitochondria, nitric oxide, and cardiovascular dysfunction. *Free Radical Biology and Medicine* 33 (11):1465-1474.

Raoul, C, C E Henderson, and B Pettmann. 1999. Programmed cell death of embryonic motoneurons triggered though the Fas death receptor. *J Cell Biol* 147 (5):1049-1062.

Raoul, C, B Pettmann, and C E Henderson. 2000. Active killing of neurons during development and following stress: a role for $p75^{NTR}$ and Fas? *Curr Op Neurobiol* 10 (1):111-117.

Raoul, C., E. Buhler, C. Sadeghi, A. Jacquier, P. Aebischer, B. Pettmann, C. E. Henderson, and G. Haase. 2006. Chronic activation in presymptomatic amyotrophic lateral sclerosis (ALS) mice of a feedback loop involving Fas, Daxx, and FasL. *PNAS* 103 (15):6007-6012.

Raoul, Cedric, Catherine Barthelemy, Arnaud Couzinet, David Hancock, Brigitte Pettmann, and Anne-Odile Hueber. 2005. Expression of a dominant negative form of Daxx <I>in vivo</I> rescues motoneurons from Fas (CD95)-induced cell death. *Journal of Neurobiology* 62 (2):178-188.

Raoul, Cédric, Alvaro G Estévez, Hiroshi Nishimune, Don W Cleveland, Odile deLapeyrière, Chistopher E Henderson, Georg Haase, and Brigitte Pettmann. 2002. Motoneuron death triggered by a specific pathway downstream of Fas: potentiation by ALS-linked SOD1 mutations. *Neuron* 35:1067-1083.

Reaume, A G, J L Elliott, E K Hoffman, N W Kowall, R J Ferrante, D F Siwek, H M Wilcox, D G Flood, M F Beal, R H Jr Brown, R W Scott, and W D Snider. 1996. Motor neurons in Cu/Zn superoxide dimutase-deficient mice develop normally but exhibit enhanced cell death after axonal injury. *Nature Genetics* 13:43-47.

Ricart, Karina C., Richard J. Pearson, Liliana Viera, Patricia Cassina, Andrés Kamaid, Steven L Carroll, and Alvaro G Estévez. 2006. Interactions between b-neuregulin and neurotrophins in motor neuron apoptosis. *Journal of Neurochemistry* 97 (1):222-233.

Roberts, Blaine R., John A. Tainer, Elizabeth D. Getzoff, Dean A. Malencik, Sonia R. Anderson, Valerie C. Bomben, Kathrin R. Meyers, P. Andrew Karplus, and Joseph S. Beckman. 2007. Structural Characterization of Zinc-deficient Human Superoxide Dismutase and Implications for ALS. *Journal of Molecular Biology* 373 (4):877-890.

Sahawneh, M. A., K. C. Ricart, B. R. Roberts, V. C. Bomben, M. Basso, Y. Ye, J. Sahawneh, M. C. Franco, J. S. Beckman, and A. G. Estevez. 2010. Cu,Zn superoxide dismutase (SOD) increases toxicity of mutant and Zn-deficient superoxide dismutase by enhancing protein stability. *J Biol Chem* 285 (44):33885-97.

Sathasivam, S., P. G. Ince, and P. J. Shaw. 2001. Apoptosis in amyotrophic lateral sclerosis: a review of the evidence. *Neuropathology and Applied Neurobiology* 27 (4):257-274.

Schopfer, F. J., P. R. Baker, and B. A. Freeman. 2003. NO-dependent protein nitration: a cell signaling event or an oxidative inflammatory response? *Trends Biochem Sci* 28 (12):646-54.

Sendtner, M., G. Pei, M. Beck, U. Schweizer, and S. Wiese. 2000. Developmental motoneuron cell death and neurotrophic factors. *Cell Tissue Res* 301 (1):71-84.

Shacka, J. J., M. A. Sahawneh, J. D. Gonzalez, Y. Z. Ye, T. L. D'Alessandro, and A. G. Estévez. 2006. Two distinct signaling pathways regulate peroxynitrite-induced apoptosis in PC12 cells. *Cell Death Differ* 13:1506-1514.

Shibata, Noriyuki. 2001. Transgenic mouse model for familial amyotrophic lateral sclerosis with superoxide dismutase-1 mutation. *Neuropathology* 21 (1):82-92.

Shin, J T, L Barbeito, L A MacMillan-Crow, J S Beckman, and J A Thompson. 1996. Acidic fibroblast growth factor enhances peroxynitrite-induced apoptosis in primary murine fibroblasts. *Arch. Biochem. Biophys.* 335 (1):32-41.

Snyder, S. H. 1993. Janus faces of nitric oxide. *Nature* 364 (6438):577.

Spear, N, A G Estévez, L Barbeito, J S Beckman, and G V W Johnson. 1997. Nerve growth factor protects PC12 cells against peroxynitrite-induced apoptosis via a mechanism dependent on phosphatidylinositol-3 kinase. *J. Neurochem.* 69 (1):53-59.

Spear, N, A G Estévez, R Radi, and J S Beckman. 1997. Peroxynitrite and Cell signalling. In *Oxidative Stress and Signal Transduction*, edited by H. J. Forman and E. Cadenas. New york: Chapman&Hall.

Subramaniam, J R, W E Lyons, J Liu, T B Bartnikas, J Rothstein, D L Price, D W Cleveland, J D Gitlin, and P C Wong. 2002. Mutant SOD1 causes motor neuron disease independent of copper chaperone-mediated copper loading. *Nature Neurosci* 5 (4):301-307.

Sunayama, J., F. Tsuruta, N. Masuyama, and Y. Gotoh. 2005. JNK antagonizes Akt-mediated survival signals by phosphorylating 14-3-3. *The Journal of cell biology* 170 (2):295-304.

Svensson, A. K., O. Bilsel, E. Kondrashkina, J. A. Zitzewitz, and C. R. Matthews. 2006. Mapping the folding free energy surface for metal-free human Cu,Zn superoxide dismutase. *J Mol Biol* 364 (5):1084-102.

Takakura, K., J. S. Beckman, L. A. MacMillan-Crow, and J. P. Crow. 1999. Rapid and irreversible inactivation of protein tyrosine phosphatases PTP1B, CD45, and LAR by peroxynitrite. *Arch Biochem Biophys* 369 (2):197-207.

Tammariello, S. P., M. T. Quinn, and S. Estus. 2000. NADPH oxidase contributes directly to oxidative stress and apoptosis in nerve growth factor-deprived sympathetic neurons. *J Neurosci* 20 (1):RC53.

Traub, R., H. Mitsumoto, and L. P. Rowland. 2011. Research advances in amyotrophic lateral sclerosis, 2009 to 2010. *Current neurology and neuroscience reports* 11 (1):67-77.

Ugolini, G., C. Raoul, A. Ferri, C. Haenggeli, Y. Yamamoto, D. Salaun, C. E. Henderson, A. C. Kato, B. Pettmann, and A. O. Hueber. 2003. Fas/tumor necrosis factor receptor death signaling is required for axotomy-induced death of motoneurons in vivo. *J Neurosci* 23 (24):8526-31.

van der Vliet, A., J. P. Eiserich, B. Halliwell, and C. E. Cross. 1997. Formation of reactive nitrogen species during peroxidase-catalyzed oxidation of nitrite. A potential additional mechanism of nitric oxide-dependent toxicity. *J Biol Chem* 272 (12):7617-25.

Vogt, P. K., H. Jiang, and M. Aoki. 2005. Triple layer control: phosphorylation, acetylation and ubiquitination of FOXO proteins. *Cell cycle* 4 (7):908-13.

Vukosavic, S, M Dubois-Dauphin, N Romero, and S Przedborski. 1999. Bax and Bcl-2 interaction in a transgenic mouse model of familial amyotrophic lateral sclerosis. *J Neurochem* 73:2460-2468.

Vukosavic, S., L. Stefanis, V. Jackson-Lewis, C. Guegan, N. Romero, C. Chen, M. Dubois-Dauphin, and S. Przedborski. 2000. Delaying caspase activation by Bcl-2: A clue to disease retardation in a transgenic mouse model of amyotrophic lateral sclerosis. *J Neurosci* 20 (24):9119-25.

Wang, L., H. X. Deng, G. Grisotti, H. Zhai, T. Siddique, and R. P. Roos. 2009. Wild-type SOD1 overexpression accelerates disease onset of a G85R SOD1 mouse. *Hum Mol Genet* 18 (9):1642-51.

Wiese, S, F Metzger, B Holtmann, and M Sendtner. 1999. The role of $p75^{NTR}$ in modulating neurotrophin survival effects in developing motoneurons. *Eur. J. Neurosci.* 11 (5):1668-1676.

Witan, H., P. Gorlovoy, A. M. Kaya, I. Koziollek-Drechsler, H. Neumann, C. Behl, and A. M. Clement. 2009. Wild-type Cu/Zn superoxide dismutase (SOD1) does not facilitate, but impedes the formation of protein aggregates of amyotrophic lateral sclerosis causing mutant SOD1. *Neurobiol Dis* 36 (2):331-42.

Witan, Heidrun, Andreas Kern, Ingrid Koziollek-Drechsler, Rebecca Wade, Christian Behl, and Albrecht M. Clement. 2008. Heterodimer formation of wild-type and amyotrophic lateral sclerosis-causing mutant Cu/Zn-Superoxide dismutase induces toxicity independent of protein aggregation. *Hum. Mol. Genet.* 17 (10):1373-85.

Wong, P C, C A Pardo, D R Borchelt, M K Lee, N G Copeland, N A Jenkins, S S Sisodia, D W Cleveland, and D L Price. 1995. An adverse property of a familial ALS-Linked SOD1 mutation causes motor neuron disease characterised by vacuolar degeneration of mitochondria. *Neuron* 14:1105-1116.

Wu, W. 1993. Expression of nitric-oxide synthase (NOS) in injured CNS neurons as shown by NADPH diaphorase histochemistry. *Exp Neurol* 120 (2):153-9.

Wu, W., K. Han, L. Li, and F. P. Schinco. 1994. Implantation of PNS graft inhibits the induction of neuronal nitric oxide synthase and enhances the survival of spinal motoneurons following root avulsion. *Exp Neurol* 129 (2):335-9.

Wu, W., and L. Li. 1993. Inhibition of nitric oxide synthase reduces motoneuron death due to spinal root avulsion. *Neurosci Lett* 153 (2):121-4.

Yan, Q., J. Elliott, and W. D. Snider. 1992. Brain-derived neurotrophic factor rescues spinal motor neurons from axotomy-induced cell death. *Nature* 360 (6406):753-5.

Ye, Yaozu, Celia Quijano, Kristine M. Robinson, Karina C. Ricart, Amy L. Strayer, Mary Anne Sahawneh, John J. Shacka, Marion Kirk, Stephen Barnes, Mary Ann Accavitti-Loper, Rafael Radi, Joseph S. Beckman, and Alvaro G. Estevez. 2007. Prevention of peroxynitrite-induced apoptosis of motor neurons and PC12 cells by tyrosine-containing peptides. *J. Biol. Chem.* 282:6324-6337.

The Kynurenine Pathway

Yiquan Chen[1] and Gilles Guillemin[1,2]
[1]*Department of Pharmacology, School of Medical Sciences, University of New South Wales, Sydney,*
[2]*St Vincent's Centre for Applied Medical Research, St Vincent's Hospital, Sydney, Australia*

1. Introduction

The kynurenine pathway represents a major route for the catabolism of tryptophan (TRP). In the body, TRP is transported around the periphery either bound to albumin (90%) or in free form (10%), the two states existing in equilibrium (McMenamy 1965). However, only free form TRP can be transported across the blood-brain barrier (BBB) by the competitive and non-specific L-type amino acid transporter (Hargreaves and Pardridge 1988). Once in the central nervous system (CNS), TRP acts as a precursor to several metabolic pathways, such as for the synthesis of kynurenine (KYN), serotonin, melatonin and protein (Fig. 1) (Ruddick *et al.* 2006).

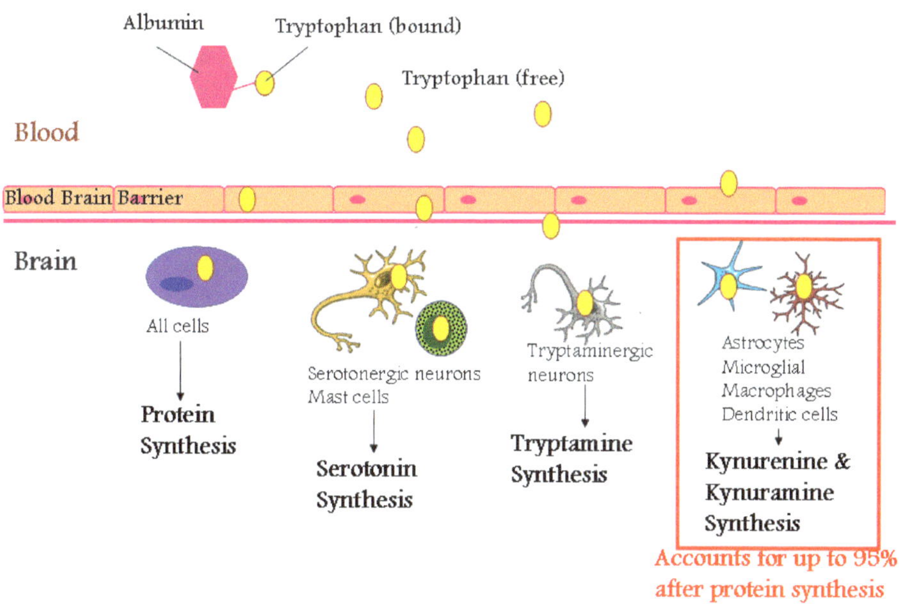

Fig. 1. TRP in the CNS. Only free TRP can cross the BBB and act as precursor for protein, serotonin, tryptamine, and kynurenine and kynuramine synthesis. The kynurenine pathway is a major pathway for TRP catabolism. Adapted from (Ruddick *et al.* 2006).

In the CNS, the kynurenine pathway is present to varying extents in most cell types, including astrocytes (Guillemin *et al.* 2000), neurons (Guillemin *et al.* 2007), infiltrating macrophages and microglia (Guillemin *et al.* 2003), oligodendrocytes (Lim *et al.* 2007), and endothelial cells (Owe-Young *et al.* 2008). Infiltrating macrophages, activated microglia and neurons have the complete repertoire of kynurenine pathway enzymes. On the other hand, neuroprotective astrocytes and oligodendrocytes lack the enzyme, kynurenine 3-monooxygenase (KMO) and indoleamine 2,3-dioxygenase 1 (IDO-1) respectively, and are incapable of synthesizing the excitotoxin, quinolinic acid (QUIN) (Guillemin *et al.* 2000; Lim *et al.* 2007).
The oxidation of TRP, initiating the kynurenine pathway (Fig. 2), may be catalyzed by one of three enzymes - TRP 2,3-dioxygenase (TDO), IDO-1 or IDO-2, a newly discovered IDO related enzyme (Salter and Pogson 1985; Takikawa *et al.* 1986; Ball *et al.* 2007; Metz *et al.* 2007). TDO resides primarily in the liver, although it is also expressed in low quantities in the brain, and is induced by TRP or corticosteroids (Salter and Pogson 1985; Miller *et al.* 2004). In contrast, IDO-1 is the predominant enzyme extra-hepatically and is found in numerous cells, including macrophages, microglia, neurons and astrocytes (Guillemin *et al.* 2001; Guillemin *et al.* 2003; Guillemin *et al.* 2005; Guillemin *et al.* 2007). IDO-1 is up regulated by certain cytokines and inflammatory molecules, such as lipopolysaccharides, amyloid peptides and human immunodeficiency virus (HIV) proteins (Fujigaki *et al.* 1998; Guillemin *et al.* 2003; Takikawa 2005), and its most potent stimulant is interferon gamma (IFN-γ) (Hayaishi and Yoshida 1978; Werner-Felmayer *et al.* 1989). IFN-γ induces both the gene expression and enzymatic activity of IDO-1 (Yasui *et al.* 1986; Dai and Gupta 1990). IDO-2 possesses similar structural and enzymatic activities as IDO-1. However, the two enzymes differ in their expression pattern and signalling pathway, and IDO-2 is preferentially inhibited by D-1-methyl-tryptophan (D-1-MT) (Ball *et al.* 2007; Metz *et al.* 2007).
The first stable intermediate from the kynurenine pathway is KYN. Subsequently, several neuroactive intermediates are generated. They include the free-radical generator, 3-hydroxyanthranilic acid (3HAA) (Goldstein *et al.* 2000), the excitotoxin and *N*-methyl *D*-aspartate (NMDA) receptor agonist, QUIN (Stone and Perkins 1981), the NMDA antagonist, kynurenic acid (KYNA) (Perkins and Stone 1982), and the neuroprotectant, picolinic acid (PIC) (Jhamandas *et al.* 1990).
The kynurenine pathway first aroused great interest when it was observed that an accelerated and sustained degradation of TRP occurred when activated T cells released IFN-γ during an immune response (Pfefferkorn 1984). The significance was speculated to be a defence mechanism that starved tumour cells, pathogens and parasites of TRP (Pfefferkorn 1984; Brown *et al.* 1991). Further research soon discovered that IDO-1 activity was necessary for the preservation of allogeneic foetuses in mice, and that TRP depletion had an anti-proliferative and apoptotic effect on T cells (Munn *et al.* 1998; Munn *et al.* 1999; Lee *et al.* 2002). Hence, the kynurenine pathway appeared to exert an immuno-regulatory effect. In particular, the general control non-derepressible-2 kinase (GCN2) was identified as a key mediator in IDO-1 induced TRP depletion immunosuppression (Munn *et al.* 2005). The activation of GCN2 triggered a stress-response program that resulted in cell-cycle arrest, differentiation, adaptation or apoptosis (de Haro *et al.* 1996; Rao *et al.* 2004; Bi *et al.* 2005). Furthermore, some of the kynurenines, such as QUIN and 3HAA, can selectively target immune cells undergoing activation, thus suppressing T cell proliferation (Frumento *et al.* 2002; Fallarino *et al.* 2003). They can also act in concert to produce an additive effect (Terness *et al.* 2002). Lastly, the production of the excitotoxic QUIN was often significantly increased following inflammation and resulting immune activation (Moffett *et al.* 1997).

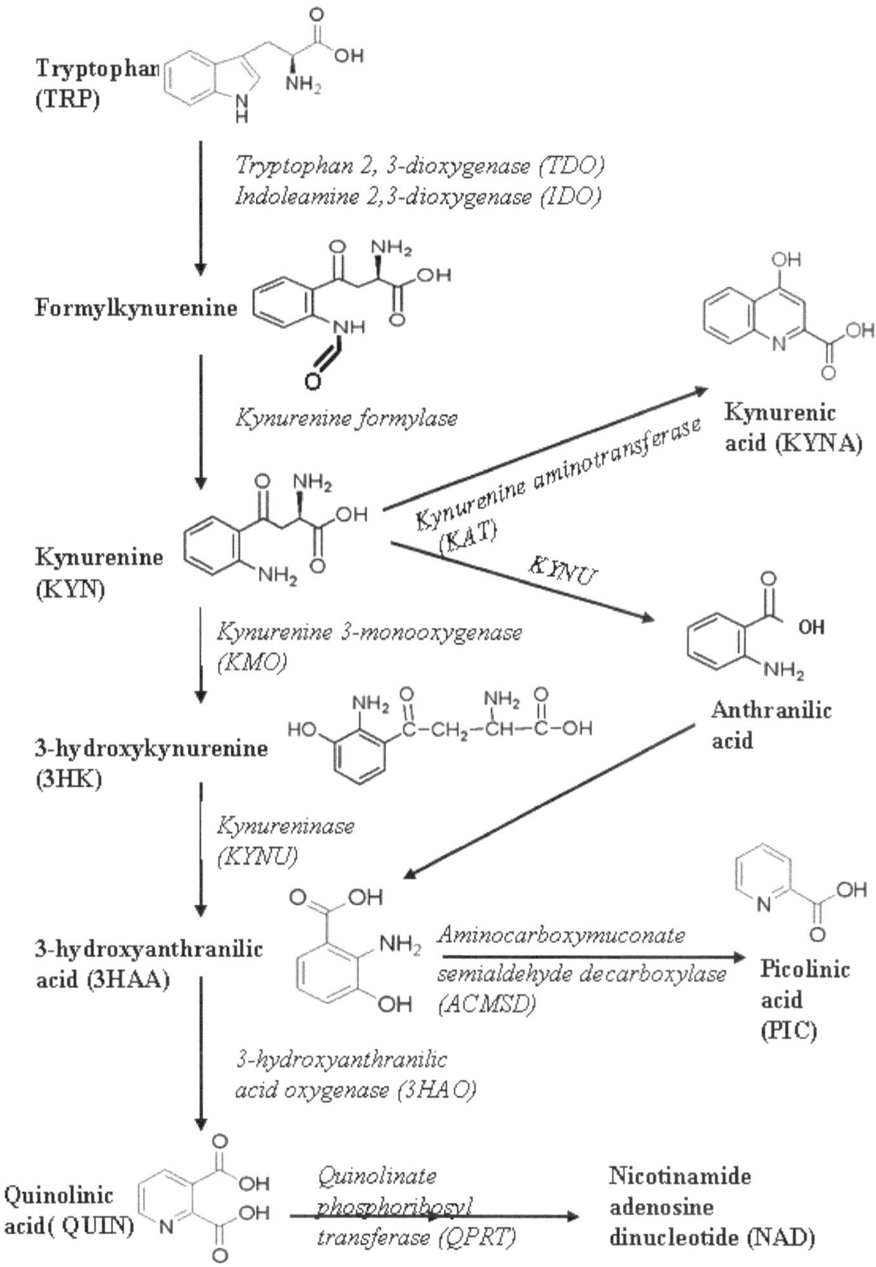

Fig. 2. The kynurenine pathway. Via the kynurenine pathway, TRP is converted to nicotinamide adenine dinucleotide (NAD) in a series of biochemical steps. In the process, neuroactive intermediates are produced. The neuroprotectants include kynurenic acid and picolinic, and the neurotoxin, QUIN.

To date, the kynurenine pathway has been implicated in a wide range of diseases and disorders, including infectious diseases (e.g. HIV), neurological disorders (e.g. Alzheimer's disease (AD), Huntington's disease (HD) and ALS), affective disorders (e.g. schizophrenia, depression and anxiety), autoimmune diseases (e.g. multiple sclerosis and rheumatoid arthritis), peripheral conditions (e.g. cardiovascular disease) and malignancy, and a key indicator is often the up-regulation in IDO-1 resulting in an accelerated and sustained degradation in TRP.

2. The kynurenine pathway and QUIN in ALS

The interest in the kynurenine pathway in the pathogenesis of ALS is relatively new. However, a number of studies have provided relevant results demonstrating the involvement of the kynurenine pathway in ALS.

For the kynurenine pathway to be involved in the pathogenesis and progression of ALS, a key prerequisite has to be met - the activation of the immune response, particularly the presence of: (1) IFN-γ, which is the most potent stimulator of IDO-1 (Takikawa *et al.* 1999); and (2) activated microglia and/or infiltrating macrophages, which are the main producers of QUIN in the CNS (Brew *et al.* 1995; Heyes *et al.* 1996). Figure 3 summarizes the main adverse events exerted by QUIN leading to motor neuron injury and death.

A few studies have provided direct evidence between TRP metabolism and ALS. Patients with severe clinical status had significantly higher cerebrospinal fluid (CSF) KYNA levels compared to controls; however, serum KYNA levels were significantly lower in patients with severe clinical status compared to either controls or patients with mild clinical status (Ilzecka *et al.* 2003). This increase in CSF KYNA in patients was conjectured to be associated with the neuroprotective effect of KYNA, produced mainly by activated astrocytes (Guillemin *et al.* 2001). ALS samples have also been found to have significantly higher levels of CSF and serum KYN and QUIN and decreased levels of serum PIC (Chen *et al.* 2010).

Another study looked at Trp-32 in superoxide dismutase 1 (SOD1) protein. The aggregation of SOD1 is one of the hallmarks of familial ALS. Trp-32 is the only aromatic residue in SOD1 protein and is found on the SOD1 protein surface (Zhang *et al.* 2003). The oxidation of Trp-32 to KYN is responsible for bicarbonate mediated peroxidase activity induced SOD1 aggregation (Zhang *et al.* 2003). By substituting Trp-32 with phenylalanine, which oxidizes more slowly, mutant SOD-1 motor neurons survived longer and were less likely to form cytoplasmic inclusions (Taylor *et al.* 2007).

3. Indirect evidence for the role of QUIN in ALS

In addition to the direct evidence demonstrating the link between the kynurenine pathway and ALS, numerous other studies have provided indirect evidence supporting the role of QUIN, in particular, in ALS.

3.1 QUIN and SOD1 expression

Mutations in SOD1 constitute about 20% of familial ALS cases. In rat brain, intracerebral injection of QUIN resulted in significant neuronal loss and a markedly increased level of SOD1 expression in a time-dependent manner (Noack *et al.* 1998). This increase in SOD1 expression was thought to be a neuroprotective response to limit the oxidative damage caused by QUIN. Presumably, QUIN could have a similar effect on mutant SOD1, which would amplify the deleterious effects associated with mutant SOD1 pathology in ALS.

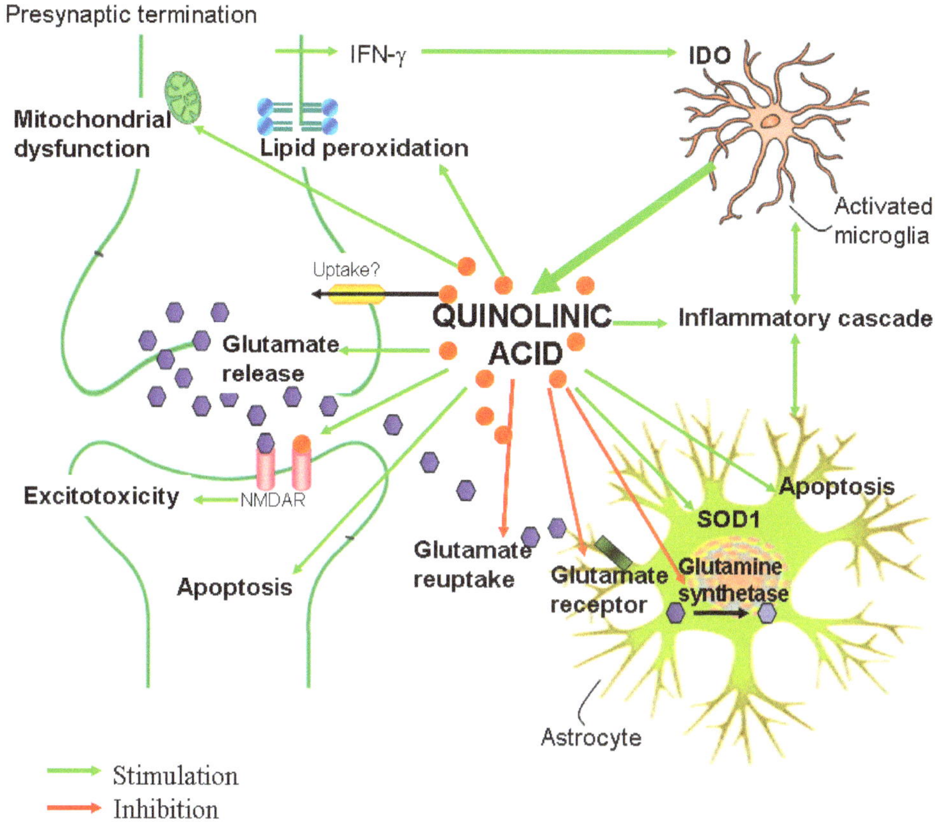

Fig. 3. Hypothetical model of the involvement of QUIN in the pathogenesis of ALS. QUIN, released from activated microglia, can induce various effects in astrocytes and motor neurons, including excitotoxicity, oxidative stress, apoptosis, mitochondrial dysfunction and the inflammatory cascade, all putatively thought to contribute to ALS disease pathogenesis and progression. Adapted from (Guillemin *et al.* 2005).

3.2 QUIN and excitotoxicity

QUIN is an excitotoxin and can be linked to excitotoxicity in ALS in two ways: (1) through the activation of the NMDA receptor; and (2) its effect on glutamate levels. The heteromeric NMDA receptor (NR) has three families of subunits: NR1 (A and B), NR2 (A to D) and NR3 (A and B). In the ventral and dorsal horns of ALS spinal cord, up to 78% loss of NR2A has been detected (Samarasinghe *et al.* 1996). Interestingly, QUIN acts on the NR subtypes, NR1+NR2A and NR1+NR2B (Priestley *et al.* 1995), and the loss of NR2A in ALS patients may possibly reflect an excitotoxic mechanism involving QUIN.

Glutamate induced toxicity has been implicated in the selective neuronal damage seen in ALS and counteracting glutamatergic toxicity, thus far, is the only treatment available for ALS. QUIN can potentiate its own toxicity and that of other excitatory amino acids, such as glutamate, under energy deprived conditions (Schurr and Rigor 1993). Moreover, QUIN contributes to excessive microenvironment glutamate concentrations and neurotoxicity via at least three mechanisms: (1) stimulation of synaptosomal glutamate release by neurons (Tavares *et al.* 2002); (2) inhibition of glutamate uptake into synaptic vesicle by astrocytes (Tavares *et al.* 2000); and (3) limiting glutamate to glutamine recycling in astrocytes by decreasing glutamine synthetase activity (Baverel *et al.* 1990).

3.3 QUIN and oxidative stress

One of the putative causes of ALS is the increased production and accumulation of reactive oxygen species (ROS) leading to oxidative stress and lipid peroxidation. Toxicity induced by QUIN has been related to increase ROS and oxidative stress. Intracerebral injection of QUIN shows neuronal damage and increase in ROS content occurring as early as 4 hrs after administration (Ganzella *et al.* 2006).

The lipid peroxidative effect of QUIN has also been demonstrated *in vivo* in adult rat brain (Rios and Santamaria 1991), and in rat brain synaptosomes *in vitro* (Santamaria *et al.* 2001). Similarly, in sheep foetal brain infused with QUIN, 4-hydroxynonenal (4-HNE), a toxic product of lipid peroxidation, immunoreactivity was observed in Purkinje cells and in the cytoplasm of cell bodies and dendrites, reaching into the molecular layer of the cerebellum (Yan *et al.* 2005). A sub-lethal dose of 4-HNE will also lead to the loss of spinal motor neurons in mice (Vigh *et al.* 2005). This may be a consequence of microglia activation, as 4-HNE is a potent activator of microglia, which will further contribute to neuroinflammation and oxidative stress in ALS (Hall *et al.* 1998).

In sporadic ALS patients, 4-HNE was enhanced in motor neurons and glia cells in the spinal cord (Shibata *et al.* 2001), and significantly elevated in the serum and CSF, correlating positively with the stage of disease (Simpson *et al.* 2004). CSF 4-HNE levels from sporadic ALS patients were also sufficient to cause the demise of motor neurons *in vitro* (Smith *et al.* 1998).

3.4 QUIN and mitochondrial dysfunction

Mitochondrial dysfunction is a prominent feature of ALS and predisposes motor neurons to ionotropic glutamate receptor-mediated excitotoxicity (Kanki *et al.* 2004). Excitotoxicity may lead to the activation of mitochondrial permeability transition pore, resulting in mitochondrial swelling and progressive motor neuron death (Bendotti *et al.* 2001). Intracerebral injection of QUIN, in addition to being excitotoxic, also produces progressive mitochondrial dysfunction leading to time-dependent energetic dysfunction, which may be a common and critical event in the cell death cascade seen in ALS (Bordelon *et al.* 1997).

3.5 QUIN and the inflammatory cascade

The presence of neuroinflammation is a pathological hallmark of ALS. Activated astrocytes and microglia are often seen in the degenerating areas surrounding injured motor neurons (McGeer and McGeer 2002). Elevated levels of chemokines and cytokines, such as monocyte chemoattractant protein 1 (MCP-1), macrophage inflammatory protein (MIP)1-α, chemokine ligand 5, interleukin (IL)-1 to IL-12, TNF-α and IFN-γ, have been detected in both G93A SOD1 mice and ALS patients (Hensley *et al.* 2003; Wilms *et al.* 2003; Henkel *et al.* 2004). It has been demonstrated that QUIN can induce astrocyte proliferation and the production of chemokines, particularly MCP-1 (Croitoru-Lamoury *et al.* 2003; Guillemin *et al.* 2003; Ting 2008), and IL-1β messenger ribonucleic acid (mRNA) expression (Guillemin *et al.* 2003) in human astrocytes and macrophages.

3.6 QUIN and apoptosis

In ALS, apoptosis is evident from the increased expression of pro-apoptotic proto-oncogenes, BCl-2 and c-jun, and caspases 1 and 3 in tissue, and from the morphological features of apoptosis displayed by dying motor neurons. QUIN has been demonstrated to induce neuronal and astrocytic apoptosis involving the activation of caspase 3 (Macaya *et al.* 1994; Jeon *et al.* 1999; Guillemin *et al.* 2005). Astrocytes are essential for the homeostasis of the CNS and so, the well-being of neurons. Hence, the loss of normal astrocytes in ALS would be detrimental to motor neurons and could exacerbate disease progression in ALS (Yamanaka *et al.* 2008).

4. Potential therapeutics targeted at the kynurenine pawthay for ALS

In 1995, riluzole became the first drug, and remains the only drug, approved by the FDA (USA) for treatment of ALS. The approval was based on two large placebo controlled clinical studies where riluzole decreased the rate of muscle deterioration and modestly improved the survival rate of ALS patients (Bensimon *et al.* 1994; Lacomblez *et al.* 1996). Though the precise mechanism of riluzole remains unclear, it appears to interfere with excitatory amino acid signalling, perhaps through the inhibition of glutamate release (Mizoule *et al.* 1985; Cheramy *et al.* 1992; Martin *et al.* 1993), blockade of inactivated sodium channels (Benoit and Escande 1991) and interaction with guanosine triphosphate (GTP)-binding proteins (Doble *et al.* 1992). 16 years on, there is still a lack of effective treatment available and an intense search is on going to discover better treatments for ALS.

In developing therapeutic agents aimed at modulating the kynurenine pathway, two approaches may be taken: (1) to develop analogues of the neuroprotective kynurenines; (2) to inhibit the synthesis of the neurotoxic QUIN. Figure 4 summarizes the drugs targeting the kynurenine pathway that could be potential candidates for ALS.

4.1 IDO inhibitors

As the first enzyme in the kynurenine pathway, suppression of IDO would lead to decrease QUIN production. Although it has not been specifically tested in neurodegenerative disorders, it is a novel therapeutic target in cancer research and the results have been positive. Using transgenic mouse model of breast cancer, IDO-1 inhibitors, 1-MT and methyl-thiohydantoin-tryptophan, were able to potentiate the efficacy of chemotherapy drugs, promoting tumour regression without increasing the side effects (Muller *et al.* 2005).

4.2 4-chlorokynurenine

QUIN neurotoxicity can be prevented by blocking the glycine modulatory site of the NMDA receptor (Foster *et al.* 1990; Hartley *et al.* 1990). 7-chlorokynurenate, a synthetic derivative of KYNA, is such an NMDA receptor antagonist (Kemp *et al.* 1988) but has difficulty crossing the BBB (Rao *et al.* 1993). On the other hand, its precursor, 4-chlorokynurenine, is rapidly transported across the BBB (Hokari *et al.* 1996). Intracerebral and intraperitoneal administration of 4-chlorokynurenine with QUIN showed successful enzymatic transamination of 4-chlorokynurenine into the neuroprotective 7-chlorokynurenate (Wu *et al.* 1997; Wu *et al.* 2000).

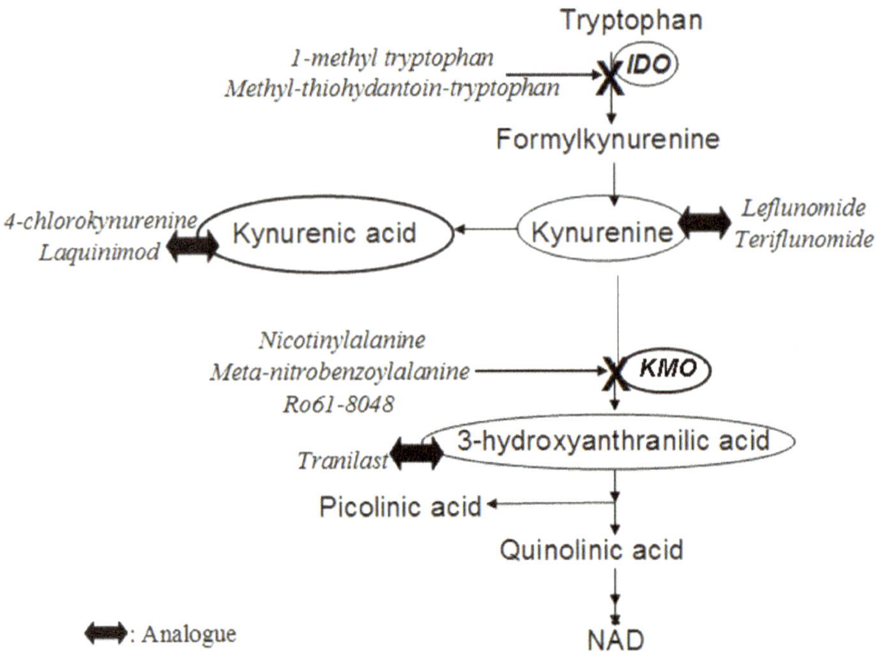

Fig. 4. Potential drug candidates targeting the kynurenine pathway for ALS. 1-MT, methyl-thiohydantoin-tryptophan, nicotinylalanine, meta-nitrobenzoylalanine and Ro61-8048 are kynurenine pathway inhibitors, while 4-chlorokynurenine, laquinimod, leflunomide, teriflunomide and tranilast are analogues of kynurenines.

4.3 Laquinimod

Laquinimod (ABR-215062) is a novel synthetic quinoline with high oral bioavailability. In preclinical trials, the compound exhibited immunomodulatory properties without immunosuppression (Brunmark *et al.* 2002; Zou *et al.* 2002; Yang *et al.* 2004). In rats with experimental autoimmune encephalomyelitis (EAE), a widely used animal model for MS, laquinimod inhibited disease progression and infiltration of CD4+ T cells and macrophages into the CNS (Yang *et al.* 2004). It also shifted the cytokine profile towards Th2/Th3 cytokines IL-4, IL-10 and transforming growth factor β (TGF-β) (Yang *et al.* 2004). Furthermore, laquinimod is able to act synergistically with IFN-β, though the mechanism of action is currently unknown but is independent of IFN-β (Runstrom *et al.* 2006). In addition, laquinimod has also successfully reduced the development of active lesions in patients with relapsing MS (Polman *et al.* 2005).

4.4 Leflunomide

Leflunomide (Avara®) is an immunosuppressive and anti-inflammatory pro-drug, which is converted *in vivo* to its active open-ring metabolite, teriflunomide (A771726), an inhibitor of mitochondrial dihydroorotate dehydrogenase, an essential enzyme for *de novo* pyrimidine synthesis (Williamson *et al.* 1995). Leflunomide is a potent inhibitor of the nuclear factor *kappa*-light-chain-enhancer of activated B cells (NF-κB) activation (Manna and Aggarwal

1999) and prevents Th1 cell activation while promoting Th2 cell differentiation (Dimitrova *et al.* 2002). The exact mechanism of action is still unclear though it has been shown to attenuate EAE independent of pyrimidine depletion (Korn *et al.* 2004).

In 1998, leflunomide was approved by the FDA (USA) for the treatment of rheumatoid arthritis. Leflunomide has also been successful in inhibiting disease progression in animal models of autoimmune diseases, such as experimental autoimmune neuritis (Ogawa *et al.* 1990), EAE (Bartlett *et al.* 1993) and experimental myasthenia gravis (Vidic-Dankovic *et al.* 1995). In a phase II trial recently, teriflunomide proved to be well tolerated and effective in reducing active lesions in patients with relapsing MS (O'Connor *et al.* 2006).

4.5 Tranilast

Tranilast (Rizaben®) is a synthetic anthranilic acid derivative drug with several inhibitory actions. It has the ability to inhibit the release of chemical mediators, such as histamine, during hypersensitivity reactions and from mast cells and also suppresses the release of TGF-β and inhibits angiogenesis (Suzawa *et al.* 1992; Isaji *et al.* 1997). Thus, it is effective against many diseases, including allergic rhinitis, atopic dermatitis, bronchial asthma, hypertrophic scar formation and keloid. Recently, tranilast showed promising results against EAE, shifting the cytokine profile towards favouring Th2 cells, inhibiting the actions of Th1 cells and promoting the generation of IL-10 producing Th2 cells, an effect similar to that of natural TRP catabolites (Platten *et al.* 2005).

4.6 Alanine derivatives

The synthesis of QUIN can also be blocked by inhibiting either KYNU or KMO activity, thus diverting the kynurenine pathway towards the synthesis of KYNA. Nicotinylalanine is one such agent (Decker *et al.* 1963). When administered together with probenecid (to allow for the accumulation of KYNA by inhibiting the organic acid transport system), nicotinylalanine increased the amount of KYNA produced in the brain and protected the brain from induced seizures (Connick *et al.* 1992; Russi *et al.* 1992) and QUIN induced striatal damage (Harris *et al.* 1998).

Another alanine derivative capable of inhibiting KMO is meta-nitrobenzoylalanine (Pellicciari *et al.* 1994). The inhibition of KMO results in an increase in brain KYN and KYNA, which is associated with sedation and anticonvulsant effects (Chiarugi and Moroni 1999) and reduction in neuronal loss from brain ischemia (Cozzi *et al.* 1999). In immune activated mice, meta-nitrobenzoylalanine also significantly reduced the formation of QUIN in the periphery and CNS (Chiarugi and Moroni 1999).

4.7 Ro61-8048

Ro61-8048 (3,4-dimethoxy-N-[4-(3-nitrophenyl)thiazol-2-yl] benzenesulfon-amide) is another potent KMO inhibitor (Rover *et al.* 1997). In addition to raising brain KYNA level, Ro61-8048 also reduces glutamate concentration in the extracellular spaces of the basal ganglia in rats without impairing the learning or memory process typically associated with glutamate receptor antagonists (Moroni *et al.* 2005). In rats with EAE, administration of Ro61-8048 significantly reduces the neurotoxic levels of 3-hydroxykynurenine and QUIN in the CNS (Chiarugi *et al.* 2001). Like meta-nitrobenzoylalanine, Ro61-8048 also decreases neuronal loss due to brain ischemia (Cozzi *et al.* 1999).

4.8 Clioquinol

Clioquinol (5-chloro-7-iodo-8-hydroxyquinoline) is a quinoline metal chelator that binds selectively to zinc and copper ions (Cherny *et al.* 2001). Having a hydrophobic nature, it crosses the BBB easily. Recent research with clioquinol in neurological disorders contributed by an imbalance in metal ions has led to promising results, presenting the possibility of a new therapeutic strategy. In AD transgenic mice, treatment with clioquinol resulted in the dissolution of aberrant neocortex beta amyloid (Aβ) aggregates, which are enriched with copper and zinc ions (Cherny *et al.* 2001). In a pilot phase II clinical trial, the drug was well tolerated and led to a significant decrease in Aβ plasma levels in AD patients, providing support for future trials (Ritchie *et al.* 2003). In PD, elevated levels of iron in the substantia nigra, the brain region affected in PD, has been reported. In mice, oral administration of clioquinol antagonized the action of the Parkinson's inducing agent 1-methyl-4-phenyl-1,2,3,6-tetra-pyridine (MPTP) (Kaur *et al.* 2003). In HD, where iron, copper and zinc have been implicated, clioquinol improved the symptoms and lifespan of transgenic HD mice (Nguyen *et al.* 2005).

A second generation 8-hydroxyquinoline, PBT2, has been developed to improve the safety and efficacy of clioquinol and also its pharmaceutical properties, such as solubility and bioavailability. In preclinical *in vivo* and *in vitro* trials on transgenic AD mice, PBT2 was more effective in lowering plaque formation and reducing plaque toxicity. More importantly, it may also improve cognition.

5. Conclusion

The current consensus is that ALS is a multifactorial disease. However, an explanation for the initiation of the putative causative mechanism of ALS remains elusive, and there lacks a hypothesis that can link all the mechanisms together. In recent years, the implication of the kynurenine pathway in multiple diseases, particularly neurodegenerative diseases, has led to an increase in assessing the efficacy of drugs targeting the kynurenine pathway in ameliorating disease symptoms and/or retarding disease progression.

The kynurenine pathway has been demonstrated to be involved in ALS and this provides an important link that ties together some of the major hypotheses underlying the pathogenesis of ALS, namely glutamate excitotoxicity, oxidative stress, non-cell-autonomous mechanism and apoptosis, which are also the major mechanisms via which QUIN exerts its neurotoxicity effects. Due to the multiple pathways involved in the pathogenesis and progression of ALS, it may be speculated that a combination therapy could be more efficacious. Hence, by targeting the kynurenine pathway, it is hoped that more effective therapeutic agents, acting in synergy with other agents, may uncover a better treatment for ALS.

6. Appendix

3HAA3-hydroxyanthranilic acid
4-HNE4-hydroxynonenal
Aβ Beta amyloid
ADAlzheimer's disease
ALSAmyotrophic lateral sclerosis
BBBBlood-brain barrier

CNSCentral nervous system
CSFCerebrospinal fluid
D-1-MTD-1-methyl-tryptophan
EAEExperimental autoimmune encephalomyelitis
GCN2General control non-derepressible-2 kinase
GTPGuanosine triphosphate
HDHuntington's disease
HIVHuman immunodeficiency virus
IDOIndoleamine 2,3-dioxygenase
IFN-γInterferon gamma
ILInterleukin
KMOKynurenine 3-monooxygenase
KYNKynurenine
KYNAKynurenic acid
MCPMonocyte chemoattractant protein
MIPMacrophage inflammatory protein
MPTPMethyl-4-phenyl-1,2,3,6-tetra-pyridine
mRNAMessenger ribonucleic acid
NF-κBNuclear factor *kappa*-light-chain-enhancer of activated *B* cells
NMDA*N*-methyl *D*-aspartate
NRNMDA receptor
PICPicolinic acid
QUINQuinolinic acid
ROSReactive oxygen species
SOD1Superoxide dismutase 1
TDOTryptophan 2,3-dioxygenase
TGF-βtransforming growth factor β
TRPTryptophan

7. References

Ball, H. J., A. Sanchez-Perez, *et al.* (2007). Characterization of an indoleamine 2,3-dioxygenase-like protein found in humans and mice. *Gene* 396(1): 203-13.
Bartlett, R. R., H. Anagnostopulos, *et al.* (1993). Effects of leflunomide on immune responses and models of inflammation. *Springer Semin Immunopathol* 14(4): 381-94.
Baverel, G., G. Martin, *et al.* (1990). Glutamine synthesis from aspartate in guinea-pig renal cortex. *Biochem J* 268(2): 437-42.
Bendotti, C., N. Calvaresi, *et al.* (2001). Early vacuolization and mitochondrial damage in motor neurons of FALS mice are not associated with apoptosis or with changes in cytochrome oxidase histochemical reactivity. *J Neurol Sci* 191(1-2): 25-33.
Benoit, E. and D. Escande (1991). Riluzole specifically blocks inactivated Na channels in myelinated nerve fibre. *Pflugers Arch* 419(6): 603-9.
Bensimon, G., L. Lacomblez, *et al.* (1994). A controlled trial of riluzole in amyotrophic lateral sclerosis. ALS/Riluzole Study Group. *N Engl J Med* 330(9): 585-91.
Bi, M., C. Naczki, *et al.* (2005). ER stress-regulated translation increases tolerance to extreme hypoxia and promotes tumor growth. *Embo J* 24(19): 3470-81.

Bordelon, Y. M., M. F. Chesselet, *et al.* (1997). Energetic dysfunction in quinolinic acid-lesioned rat striatum. *J Neurochem* 69(4): 1629-39.

Brew, B. J., J. Corbeil, *et al.* (1995). Quinolinic acid production is related to macrophage tropic isolates of HIV-1. *J Neurovirol* 1(5-6): 369-74.

Brown, R. R., Y. Ozaki, *et al.* (1991). Implications of interferon-induced tryptophan catabolism in cancer, auto-immune diseases and AIDS. *Adv Exp Med Biol* 294: 425-35.

Brunmark, C., A. Runstrom, *et al.* (2002). The new orally active immunoregulator laquinimod (ABR-215062) effectively inhibits development and relapses of experimental autoimmune encephalomyelitis. *J Neuroimmunol* 130(1-2): 163-72.

Chen, Y. and G. J. Guillemin (2009). Kynurenine pathway metabolites in humans: disease and healthy states. *International Journal of Tryptophan Research* 2: 1-19.

Cheramy, A., L. Barbeito, *et al.* (1992). Riluzole inhibits the release of glutamate in the caudate nucleus of the cat in vivo. *Neurosci Lett* 147(2): 209-12.

Cherny, R. A., C. S. Atwood, *et al.* (2001). Treatment with a copper-zinc chelator markedly and rapidly inhibits beta-amyloid accumulation in Alzheimer's disease transgenic mice. *Neuron* 30(3): 665-76.

Chiarugi, A., A. Cozzi, *et al.* (2001). Kynurenine 3-mono-oxygenase activity and neurotoxic kynurenine metabolites increase in the spinal cord of rats with experimental allergic encephalomyelitis. *Neuroscience* 102(3): 687-95.

Chiarugi, A. and F. Moroni (1999). Quinolinic acid formation in immune-activated mice: studies with (m-nitrobenzoyl)-alanine (mNBA) and 3,4-dimethoxy-[-N-4-(-3-nitrophenyl)thiazol-2yl]-benzenesul fonamide (Ro 61-8048), two potent and selective inhibitors of kynurenine hydroxylase. *Neuropharmacology* 38(8): 1225-33.

Connick, J. H., G. C. Heywood, *et al.* (1992). Nicotinylalanine increases cerebral kynurenic acid content and has anticonvulsant activity. *Gen Pharmacol* 23(2): 235-9.

Cozzi, A., R. Carpenedo, *et al.* (1999). Kynurenine hydroxylase inhibitors reduce ischemic brain damage: studies with (m-nitrobenzoyl)-alanine (mNBA) and 3,4-dimethoxy-[-N-4-(nitrophenyl)thiazol-2yl]-benzenesulfonamide (Ro 61-8048) in models of focal or global brain ischemia. *J Cereb Blood Flow Metab* 19(7): 771-7.

Croitoru-Lamoury, J., G. J. Guillemin, *et al.* (2003). Expression of chemokines and their receptors in human and simian astrocytes: evidence for a central role of TNF alpha and IFN gamma in CXCR4 and CCR5 modulation. *Glia* 41(4): 354-70.

Dai, W. and S. L. Gupta (1990). Regulation of indoleamine 2,3-dioxygenase gene expression in human fibroblasts by interferon-gamma. Upstream control

Decker, R. H., R. R. Brown, *et al.* (1963). Studies on the biological activity of nicotinylalanine, an analogue of kynurenine. *J Biol Chem* 238: 1049-53.

region discriminates between interferon-gamma and interferon-alpha. *J Biol Chem* 265(32): 19871-7.

de Haro, C., R. Mendez, *et al.* (1996). The eIF-2alpha kinases and the control of protein synthesis. *Faseb J* 10(12): 1378-87.

Dimitrova, P., A. Skapenko, *et al.* (2002). Restriction of de novo pyrimidine biosynthesis inhibits Th1 cell activation and promotes Th2 cell differentiation. *J Immunol* 169(6): 3392-9.

Doble, A., J. P. Hubert, *et al.* (1992). Pertussis toxin pretreatment abolishes the inhibitory effect of riluzole and carbachol on D-[3H]aspartate release from cultured cerebellar granule cells. *Neurosci Lett* 140(2): 251-4.

Fallarino, F., U. Grohmann, *et al.* (2003). T cell apoptosis by kynurenines. *Adv Exp Med Biol* 527: 183-90.

Foster, A. C., C. L. Willis, *et al.* (1990). Protection Against N-methyl-D-aspartate Receptor-Mediated Neuronal Degeneration In Rat Brain by 7-chlorokynurenate and 3-amino-1-hydroxypyrrolid-2-one, Antagonists at The Allosteric Site for Glycine. *Eur J Neurosci* 2(3): 270-277.

Frumento, G., R. Rotondo, *et al.* (2002). Tryptophan-derived catabolites are responsible for inhibition of T and natural killer cell proliferation induced by indoleamine 2,3-dioxygenase. *J Exp Med* 196(4): 459-68.

Fujigaki, S., K. Saito, *et al.* (1998). Species differences in L-tryptophan-kynurenine pathway metabolism: quantification of anthranilic acid and its related enzymes. *Arch Biochem Biophys* 358(2): 329-35.

Ganzella, M., F. M. Jardim, *et al.* (2006). Time course of oxidative events in the hippocampus following intracerebroventricular infusion of quinolinic acid in mice. *Neurosci Res* 55(4): 397-402.

Goldstein, L. E., M. C. Leopold, *et al.* (2000). 3-Hydroxykynurenine and 3-hydroxyanthranilic acid generate hydrogen peroxide and promote alpha-crystallin cross-linking by metal ion reduction. *Biochemistry* 39(24): 7266-75.

Guillemin, G. J., B. J. Brew, *et al.* (2005). Indoleamine 2,3 dioxygenase and quinolinic acid immunoreactivity in Alzheimer's disease hippocampus. *Neuropathol Appl Neurobiol* 31: 395-404.

Guillemin, G. J., J. Croitoru-Lamoury, *et al.* (2003). Quinolinic acid upregulates chemokine production and chemokine receptor expression in astrocytes. *Glia* 41: 371-381.

Guillemin, G. J., K. M. Cullen, *et al.* (2007). Characterization of the kynurenine pathway in human neurons. *J Neurosci* 27(47): 12884-12892.

Guillemin, G. J., S. J. Kerr, *et al.* (2004). Involvement of quinolinic acid in AIDS dementia complex. *Neurotox Res* 7: 103-124.

Guillemin, G. J., S. J. Kerr, *et al.* (2001). IFN-beta 1b induces kynurenine pathway metabolism in human macrophages: potential implications for multiple sclerosis treatment. *J Intereron Cytokine Res* 21(12): 1097-101.

Guillemin, G. J., S. J. Kerr, *et al.* (2001). Kynurenine pathway metabolism in human astrocytes: a paradox for neuronal protection. *Journal of Neurochemistry* 78: 842-853.

Guillemin, G. J., V. Meininger, *et al.* (2005). Implications for the kynurenine pathway and quinolinic acid in amyotrophic lateral sclerosis. *Neurodegener Dis.* 2(3-4): 166-76.

Guillemin, G. J., D. G. Smith, *et al.* (2000). Characterisation of kynurenine pathway metabolism in human astrocytes and implications in neuropathogenesis. *Redox Report* 5(2/3): 108-111.

Guillemin, G. J., D. G. Smith, *et al.* (2003). Expression of the kynurenine pathway enzymes in human microglia and macrophages. *Adv Exp Med Biol* 527: 105-12.

Guillemin, G. J., G. Smythe, *et al.* (2004). Expression of indoleamine 2,3-dioxygenase and production of quinolinic acid by human microglia, astrocytes, and neurons. *Glia* 49(1): 15-23.

Guillemin, G. J., G. A. Smythe, *et al.* (2003). A beta 1-42 induces production of quinolinic acid by human macrophages and microglia. *Neuroreport* 14(18): 2311-5.

Guillemin, G. J., L. Wang, *et al.* (2005). Quinolinic acid selectively induces apoptosis of human astrocytes: potential role in AIDS dementia complex. *J Neuroinflammation* 2: 16.

Guillemin, G. J., K. R. Williams, *et al.* (2003). Quinolinic acid in the pathogenesis of Alzheimer's disease. *Adv Exp Med Biol* 527: 167-76.

Hall, E. D., P. K. Andrus, *et al.* (1998). Relationship of oxygen radical-induced lipid peroxidative damage to disease onset and progression in a transgenic model of familial ALS. *J Neurosci Res* 53(1): 66-77.

Hargreaves, K. M. and W. M. Pardridge (1988). Neutral amino acid transport at the human blood-brain barrier. *J Biol Chem* 263(36): 19392-7.

Harris, C. A., A. F. Miranda, *et al.* (1998). Modulation of striatal quinolinate neurotoxicity by elevation of endogenous brain kynurenic acid. *Br J Pharmacol* 124(2): 391-9.

Hartley, D. M., H. Monyer, *et al.* (1990). 7-Chlorokynurenate Blocks NMDA Receptor-Mediated Neurotoxicity in Murine Cortical Culture. *Eur J Neurosci* 2(4): 291-295.

Hayaishi, O. and R. Yoshida (1978). Specific induction of pulmonary indoleamine 2,3-dioxygenase by bacterial lipopolysaccharide. *Ciba Found Symp*(65): 199-203.

Henkel, J. S., J. I. Engelhardt, *et al.* (2004). Presence of dendritic cells, MCP-1, and activated microglia/macrophages in amyotrophic lateral sclerosis spinal cord tissue. *Ann Neurol* 55(2): 221-35.

Hensley, K., J. Fedynyshyn, *et al.* (2003). Message and protein-level elevation of tumor necrosis factor alpha (TNF alpha) and TNF alpha-modulating cytokines in spinal cords of the G93A-SOD1 mouse model for amyotrophic lateral sclerosis. *Neurobiol Dis* 14(1): 74-80.

Heyes, M. P., C. L. Achim, *et al.* (1996). Human microglia convert l-tryptophan into the neurotoxin quinolinic acid. *Biochem J* 320 (Pt 2): 595-7.

Hokari, M., H. Q. Wu, *et al.* (1996). Facilitated brain uptake of 4-chlorokynurenine and conversion to 7-chlorokynurenic acid. *Neuroreport* 8(1): 15-8.

Ilzecka, J., T. Kocki, *et al.* (2003). Endogenous protectant kynurenic acid in amyotrophic lateral sclerosis. *Acta Neurol Scand* 107(6): 412-8.

Isaji, M., H. Miyata, *et al.* (1997). Tranilast inhibits the proliferation, chemotaxis and tube formation of human microvascular endothelial cells in vitro and angiogenesis in vivo. *Br J Pharmacol* 122(6): 1061-6.

Jeon, B. S., N. G. Kholodilov, *et al.* (1999). Activation of caspase-3 in developmental models of programmed cell death in neurons of the substantia nigra. *J Neurochem* 73(1): 322-33.

Jhamandas, K., R. J. Boegman, *et al.* (1990). Quinolinate-induced cortical cholinergic damage: modulation by tryptophan metabolites. *Brain Res* 529(1-2): 185-91.

Kanki, R., T. Nakamizo, *et al.* (2004). Effects of mitochondrial dysfunction on glutamate receptor-mediated neurotoxicity in cultured rat spinal motor neurons. *Brain Res* 1015(1-2): 73-81.

Kaur, D., F. Yantiri, *et al.* (2003). Genetic or pharmacological iron chelation prevents MPTP-induced neurotoxicity in vivo: a novel therapy for Parkinson's disease. *Neuron* 37(6): 899-909.

Kemp, J. A., A. C. Foster, *et al.* (1988). 7-Chlorokynurenic acid is a selective antagonist at the glycine modulatory site of the N-methyl-D-aspartate receptor complex. *Proc Natl Acad Sci U S A* 85(17): 6547-50.

Korn, T., T. Magnus, *et al.* (2004). Modulation of effector cell functions in experimental autoimmune encephalomyelitis by leflunomide--mechanisms independent of pyrimidine depletion. *J Leukoc Biol* 76(5): 950-60.

Lacomblez, L., G. Bensimon, *et al.* (1996). Dose-ranging study of riluzole in amyotrophic lateral sclerosis. Amyotrophic Lateral Sclerosis/Riluzole Study Group II. *Lancet* 347(9013): 1425-31.

Lee, G. K., H. J. Park, *et al.* (2002). Tryptophan deprivation sensitizes activated T cells to apoptosis prior to cell division. *Immunology* 107(4): 452-60.

Lim, C. K., G. A. Symthe, *et al.* (2007). Characterization of the kynurenine pathway in human oligodendrocytes. *International Congress Series* 1304: 213-217.

Ogawa, T., M. Inazu, *et al.* (1990). Effects of leflunomide on glomerulonephritis induced by antibasement membrane antibody in rats. *Agents Actions* 31(3-4): 321-8.

Macaya, A., F. Munell, *et al.* (1994). Apoptosis in substantia nigra following developmental striatal excitotoxic injury. *Proc Natl Acad Sci U S A* 91(17): 8117-21.

Manna, S. K. and B. B. Aggarwal (1999). Immunosuppressive leflunomide metabolite (A77 1726) blocks TNF-dependent nuclear factor-kappa B activation and gene expression. *J Immunol* 162(4): 2095-102.

Martin, D., M. A. Thompson, *et al.* (1993). The neuroprotective agent riluzole inhibits release of glutamate and aspartate from slices of hippocampal area CA1. *Eur J Pharmacol* 250(3): 473-6.

McGeer, P. L. and E. G. McGeer (2002). Inflammatory processes in amyotrophic lateral sclerosis. *Muscle Nerve* 26(4): 459-70.

McMenamy, R. H. (1965). Binding of indole analogues to human serum albumin. Effects of fatty acids. *J Biol Chem* 240(11): 4235-43.

Metz, R., J. B. Duhadaway, *et al.* (2007). Novel tryptophan catabolic enzyme IDO2 is the preferred biochemical target of the antitumor indoleamine 2,3-dioxygenase inhibitory compound D-1-methyl-tryptophan. *Cancer Res* 67(15): 7082-7.

Miller, C. L., I. C. Llenos, *et al.* (2004). Expression of the kynurenine pathway enzyme tryptophan 2,3-dioxygenase is increased in the frontal cortex of individuals with schizophrenia. *Neurobiol Dis* 15(3): 618-29.

Mizoule, J., B. Meldrum, *et al.* (1985). 2-Amino-6-trifluoromethoxy benzothiazole, a possible antagonist of excitatory amino acid neurotransmission--I. Anticonvulsant properties. *Neuropharmacology* 24(8): 767-73.

Moffett, J. R., T. Els, *et al.* (1997). Quinolinate immunoreactivity in experimental rat brain tumors is present in macrophages but not in astrocytes. *Exp Neurol* 144(2): 287-301.

Moroni, F., A. Cozzi, *et al.* (2005). Kynurenine 3-mono-oxygenase inhibitors reduce glutamate concentration in the extracellular spaces of the basal ganglia but not in those of the cortex or hippocampus. *Neuropharmacology* 48(6): 788-95.

Muller, A. J., J. B. DuHadaway, *et al.* (2005). Inhibition of indoleamine 2,3-dioxygenase, an immunoregulatory target of the cancer suppression gene Bin1, potentiates cancer chemotherapy. *Nat Med* 11(3): 312-9.

Munn, D. H., E. Shafizadeh, *et al.* (1999). Inhibition of T cell proliferation by macrophage tryptophan catabolism. *J Exp Med* 189(9): 1363-72.

Munn, D. H., M. D. Sharma, *et al.* (2005). GCN2 kinase in T cells mediates proliferative arrest and anergy induction in response to indoleamine 2,3-dioxygenase. *Immunity* 22(5): 633-42.

Munn, D. H., M. Zhou, *et al.* (1998). Prevention of allogeneic fetal rejection by tryptophan catabolism. *Science* 281(5380): 1191-3.

Nguyen, T., A. Hamby, *et al.* (2005). Clioquinol down-regulates mutant huntingtin expression in vitro and mitigates pathology in a Huntington's disease mouse model. *Proc Natl Acad Sci U S A* 102(33): 11840-5.

Noack, H., J. Lindenau, *et al.* (1998). Differential expression of superoxide dismutase isoforms in neuronal and glial compartments in the course of excitotoxically mediated neurodegeneration: relation to oxidative and nitrergic stress. *Glia* 23(4): 285-97.

O'Connor, P. W., D. Li, *et al.* (2006). A Phase II study of the safety and efficacy of teriflunomide in multiple sclerosis with relapses. *Neurology* 66(6): 894-900.

Owe-Young, R., N. L. Webster, *et al.* (2008). Kynurenine Pathway Metabolism in Human Blood-Brain Barrier Cells: Implications for Immune Tolerance & Neurotoxicity. *J Neurochem.*

Pellicciari, R., B. Natalini, *et al.* (1994). Modulation of the kynurenine pathway in search for new neuroprotective agents. Synthesis and preliminary evaluation of (m-nitrobenzoyl)alanine, a potent inhibitor of kynurenine-3-hydroxylase. *J Med Chem* 37(5): 647-55.

Perkins, M. N. and T. W. Stone (1982). An iontophoretic investigation of the actions of convulsant kynurenines and their interaction with the endogenous excitant quinolinic acid. *Brain Res* 247(1): 184-7.

Pfefferkorn, E. R. (1984). Interferon gamma blocks the growth of Toxoplasma gondii in human fibroblasts by inducing the host cells to degrade tryptophan. *Proc Natl Acad Sci U S A* 81(3): 908-12.

Platten, M., P. P. Ho, *et al.* (2005). Treatment of autoimmune neuroinflammation with a synthetic tryptophan metabolite. *Science* 310(5749): 850-5.

Polman, C., F. Barkhof, *et al.* (2005). Treatment with laquinimod reduces development of active MRI lesions in relapsing MS. *Neurology* 64(6): 987-91.

Priestley, T., P. Laughton, *et al.* (1995). Pharmacological properties of recombinant human N-methyl-D-aspartate receptors comprising NR1a/NR2A and NR1a/NR2B subunit assemblies expressed in permanently transfected mouse fibroblast cells. *Mol Pharmacol* 48(5): 841-8.

Rao, R. V., H. M. Ellerby, *et al.* (2004). Coupling endoplasmic reticulum stress to the cell death program. *Cell Death Differ* 11(4): 372-80.

Rao, T. S., N. M. Gray, *et al.* (1993). Indole-2-carboxylates, novel antagonists of the N-methyl-D-aspartate (NMDA)-associated glycine recognition sites: in vivo characterization. *Neuropharmacology* 32(2): 139-47.

Ritchie, C. W., A. I. Bush, *et al.* (2003). Metal-protein attenuation with iodochlorhydroxyquin (clioquinol) targeting Abeta amyloid deposition and toxicity in Alzheimer disease: a pilot phase 2 clinical trial. *Arch Neurol* 60(12): 1685-91.

Rover, S., A. M. Cesura, *et al.* (1997). Synthesis and biochemical evaluation of N-(4-phenylthiazol-2-yl)benzenesulfonamides as high-affinity inhibitors of kynurenine 3-hydroxylase. *J Med Chem* 40(26): 4378-85.

Ruddick, J. P., A. K. Evans, *et al.* (2006). Tryptophan metabolism in the central nervous system: medical implications. *Expert Rev Mol Med* 8(20): 1-27.

Runstrom, A., T. Leanderson, *et al.* (2006). Inhibition of the development of chronic experimental autoimmune encephalomyelitis by laquinimod (ABR-215062) in IFN-beta k.o. and wild type mice. *J Neuroimmunol* 173(1-2): 69-78.

Russi, P., M. Alesiani, *et al.* (1992). Nicotinylalanine increases the formation of kynurenic acid in the brain and antagonizes convulsions. *J Neurochem* 59(6): 2076-80.

Salter, M. and C. I. Pogson (1985). The role of tryptophan 2,3-dioxygenase in the hormonal control of tryptophan metabolism in isolated rat liver cells. Effects of glucocorticoids and experimental diabetes. *Biochem J* 229(2): 499-504.

Samarasinghe, S., L. Virgo, *et al.* (1996). Distribution of the N-methyl-D-aspartate glutamate receptor subunit NR2A in control and amyotrophic lateral sclerosis spinal cord. *Brain Res* 727(1-2): 233-7.

Santamaria, A., S. Galvan-Arzate, *et al.* (2001). Quinolinic acid induces oxidative stress in rat brain synaptosomes. *Neuroreport* 12(4): 871-4.

Schurr, A. and B. M. Rigor (1993). Quinolinate potentiates the neurotoxicity of excitatory amino acids in hypoxic neuronal tissue in vitro. *Brain Res* 617(1): 76-80.

Shibata, N., R. Nagai, *et al.* (2001). Morphological evidence for lipid peroxidation and protein glycoxidation in spinal cords from sporadic amyotrophic lateral sclerosis patients. *Brain Res* 917(1): 97-104.

Simpson, E. P., Y. K. Henry, *et al.* (2004). Increased lipid peroxidation in sera of ALS patients: a potential biomarker of disease burden. *Neurology* 62(10): 1758-65.

Smith, R. G., Y. K. Henry, *et al.* (1998). Presence of 4-hydroxynonenal in cerebrospinal fluid of patients with sporadic amyotrophic lateral sclerosis. *Ann Neurol* 44(4): 696-9.

Stone, T. W. and M. N. Perkins (1981). Quinolinic acid: a potent endogenous excitant at amino acid receptors in CNS. *Eur J Pharmacol* 72(4): 411-2.

Suzawa, H., S. Kikuchi, *et al.* (1992). The mechanism involved in the inhibitory action of tranilast on collagen biosynthesis of keloid fibroblasts. *Jpn J Pharmacol* 60(2): 91-6.

Takikawa, O. (2005). Biochemical and medical aspects of the indoleamine 2,3-dioxygenase-initiated L-tryptophan metabolism. *Biochem Biophys Res Commun* 338(1): 12-9.

Takikawa, O., Y. Tagawa, *et al.* (1999). Interferon-gamma-dependent/independent expression of indoleamine 2,3-dioxygenase. Studies with interferon-gamma-knockout mice. *Adv Exp Med Biol* 467: 553-7.

Takikawa, O., R. Yoshida, *et al.* (1986). Tryptophan degradation in mice initiated by indoleamine 2,3-dioxygenase. *J Biol Chem* 261(8): 3648-53.

Tavares, R. G., C. I. Tasca, *et al.* (2002). Quinolinic acid stimulates synaptosomal glutamate release and inhibits glutamate uptake into astrocytes. *Neurochem Int* 40(7): 621-7.

Tavares, R. G., C. I. Tasca, *et al.* (2000). Quinolinic acid inhibits glutamate uptake into synaptic vesicles from rat brain. *Neuroreport* 11(2): 249-53.

Taylor, D. M., B. F. Gibbs, *et al.* (2007). Tryptophan 32 potentiates aggregation and cytotoxicity of a copper/zinc superoxide dismutase mutant associated with familial amyotrophic lateral sclerosis. *J Biol Chem* 282(22): 16329-35.

Terness, P., T. M. Bauer, *et al.* (2002). Inhibition of allogeneic T cell proliferation by indoleamine 2,3-dioxygenase-expressing dendritic cells: mediation of suppression by tryptophan metabolites. *J Exp Med* 196(4): 447-57.

Ting, K. K. (2008). Quinolinic acid and its effect on the astrocyte with relevance to the pathogenesis of Alzheimer's disease [Thesis].

Vidic-Dankovic, B., D. Kosec, *et al.* (1995). Leflunomide prevents the development of experimentally induced myasthenia gravis. *Int J Immunopharmacol* 17(4): 273-81.

Vigh, L., R. G. Smith, *et al.* (2005). Sublethal dose of 4-hydroxynonenal reduces intracellular calcium in surviving motor neurons in vivo. *Acta Neuropathol* 109(6): 567-75.

Werner-Felmayer, G., E. R. Werner, *et al.* (1989). Characteristics of interferon induced tryptophan metabolism in human cells in vitro. *Biochim Biophys Acta* 1012(2): 140-7.

Williamson, R. A., C. M. Yea, *et al.* (1995). Dihydroorotate dehydrogenase is a high affinity binding protein for A77 1726 and mediator of a range of biological effects of the immunomodulatory compound. *J Biol Chem* 270(38): 22467-72.

Wilms, H., J. Sievers, *et al.* (2003). Intrathecal synthesis of monocyte chemoattractant protein-1 (MCP-1) in amyotrophic lateral sclerosis: further evidence for microglial activation in neurodegeneration. *J Neuroimmunol* 144(1-2): 139-42.

Wu, H. Q., S. C. Lee, *et al.* (2000). Systemic administration of 4-chlorokynurenine prevents quinolinate neurotoxicity in the rat hippocampus. *Eur J Pharmacol* 390(3): 267-74.

Wu, H. Q., F. G. Salituro, *et al.* (1997). Enzyme-catalyzed production of the neuroprotective NMDA receptor antagonist 7-chlorokynurenic acid in the rat brain in vivo. *Eur J Pharmacol* 319(1): 13-20.

Yamanaka, K., S. J. Chun, *et al.* (2008). Astrocytes as determinants of disease progression in inherited amyotrophic lateral sclerosis. *Nat Neurosci* 11(3): 251-3.

Yan, E., M. Castillo-Melendez, *et al.* (2005). Quinolinic acid promotes albumin deposition in Purkinje cell, astrocytic activation and lipid peroxidation in fetal brain. *Neuroscience* 134(3): 867-75.

Yang, J. S., L. Y. Xu, *et al.* (2004). Laquinimod (ABR-215062) suppresses the development of experimental autoimmune encephalomyelitis, modulates the Th1/Th2 balance and induces the Th3 cytokine TGF-beta in Lewis rats. *J Neuroimmunol* 156(1-2): 3-9.

Yasui, H., K. Takai, *et al.* (1986). Interferon enhances tryptophan metabolism by inducing pulmonary indoleamine 2,3-dioxygenase: its possible occurrence in cancer patients. *Proc Natl Acad Sci U S A* 83(17): 6622-6.

Zhang, H., C. Andrekopoulos, *et al.* (2003). Bicarbonate-dependent peroxidase activity of human Cu,Zn-superoxide dismutase induces covalent aggregation of protein: intermediacy of tryptophan-derived oxidation products. *J Biol Chem* 278(26): 24078-89.

Zou, L. P., N. Abbas, *et al.* (2002). Suppression of experimental autoimmune neuritis by ABR-215062 is associated with altered Th1/Th2 balance and inhibited migration of inflammatory cells into the peripheral nerve tissue. *Neuropharmacology* 42(5): 731-9.

Permissions

The contributors of this book come from diverse backgrounds, making this book a truly international effort. This book will bring forth new frontiers with its revolutionizing research information and detailed analysis of the nascent developments around the world.

We would like to thank Martin H. Maurer, for lending his expertise to make the book truly unique. He has played a crucial role in the development of this book. Without his invaluable contribution this book wouldn't have been possible. He has made vital efforts to compile up to date information on the varied aspects of this subject to make this book a valuable addition to the collection of many professionals and students.

This book was conceptualized with the vision of imparting up-to-date information and advanced data in this field. To ensure the same, a matchless editorial board was set up. Every individual on the board went through rigorous rounds of assessment to prove their worth. After which they invested a large part of their time researching and compiling the most relevant data for our readers. Conferences and sessions were held from time to time between the editorial board and the contributing authors to present the data in the most comprehensible form. The editorial team has worked tirelessly to provide valuable and valid information to help people across the globe.

Every chapter published in this book has been scrutinized by our experts. Their significance has been extensively debated. The topics covered herein carry significant findings which will fuel the growth of the discipline. They may even be implemented as practical applications or may be referred to as a beginning point for another development. Chapters in this book were first published by InTech; hereby published with permission under the Creative Commons Attribution License or equivalent.

The editorial board has been involved in producing this book since its inception. They have spent rigorous hours researching and exploring the diverse topics which have resulted in the successful publishing of this book. They have passed on their knowledge of decades through this book. To expedite this challenging task, the publisher supported the team at every step. A small team of assistant editors was also appointed to further simplify the editing procedure and attain best results for the readers.

Our editorial team has been hand-picked from every corner of the world. Their multi-ethnicity adds dynamic inputs to the discussions which result in innovative outcomes. These outcomes are then further discussed with the researchers and contributors who give their valuable feedback and opinion regarding the same. The feedback is then collaborated with the researches and they are edited in a comprehensive manner to aid the understanding of the subject.

Apart from the editorial board, the designing team has also invested a significant amount of their time in understanding the subject and creating the most relevant covers. They scrutinized every image to scout for the most suitable representation of the subject and create an appropriate cover for the book.

The publishing team has been involved in this book since its early stages. They were actively engaged in every process, be it collecting the data, connecting with the contributors or procuring relevant information. The team has been an ardent support to the editorial, designing and production team. Their endless efforts to recruit the best for this project, has resulted in the accomplishment of this book. They are a veteran in the field of academics and their pool of knowledge is as vast as their experience in printing. Their expertise and guidance has proved useful at every step. Their uncompromising quality standards have made this book an exceptional effort. Their encouragement from time to time has been an inspiration for everyone.

The publisher and the editorial board hope that this book will prove to be a valuable piece of knowledge for researchers, students, practitioners and scholars across the globe.

List of Contributors

Martin H. Maurer
Dept. of Physiology and Pathophysiology, University of Heidelberg, Germany

Cassie S. Mitchell and Robert H. Lee
Georgia Institute of Technology and Emory University, Atlanta, Georgia, United States

Johnathan Cooper-Knock, Joanna J. Bury, Laura Ferraiuolo, Emily F. Goodall, Pamela J. Shaw and Janine Kirby
Sheffield Institute for Translational Neuroscience, University of Sheffield, Sheffield, United Kingdom

François Berthod and François Gros-Louis
Centre LOEX de l'Université Laval,Centre de recherche FRSQ du Centre hospitalier affilié universitaire de Québec, Canada Département de Chirurgie, Faculté de Médecine, Université Laval, Québec, Canada

Sherif M. Elbasiouny and Katharina A. Quinlan
Departments of Physiology, Northwestern University, USA

Charles J. Heckman
Departments of Physiology, Northwestern University, USA Physical Medicine and Rehabilitation, Northwestern University, USA Physical Therapy and Human Movement Sciences, Northwestern University, USA

Tahra L. Eissa
Department of Biological and Environmental Engineering, Cornell University, USA

C.J. Heckman
Department of Physiology, Northwestern University Feinberg School of Medicine, USA Department of Physical Medicine and Rehabilitation, Northwestern University Feinberg School of Medicine, USA Department of Physical Therapy and Human Movement Sciences, Northwestern University Feinberg School of Medicine, USA

Katharina A. Quinlan and Sherif M. Elbasiouny
Department of Physiology, Northwestern University Feinberg School of Medicine, USA

Marina Boido, Elisa Buschini, Antonio Piras, Giada Spigolon, Valeria Valsecchi and Alessandro Vercelli
Neuroscience Institute of the Cavalieri Ottolenghi Foundation, University of Turin, Italy

Letizia Mazzini
ALS Centre, Department of Neurology, Eastern Piedmont University, "Maggiore della Carità" Hospital, Novara, Italy

Jari Koistinaho and Gundars Goldsteins
A.I.Virtanen Institute for Molecular Sciences, University of Eastern Finland, Finland

Luz Diana Santa-Cruz, Uri Nimrod Ramírez-Jarquín and Ricardo Tapia
División de Neurociencias, Instituto de Fisiología Celular, Universidad Nacional Autónoma de México, México, D.F., México

Nury Steuerwald and Herbert L. Bonkovsky
Cannon Research Center, Carolinas Medical Center, Charlotte, NC, USA

Valentin Vavilin
Institute of Molecular Biology and Biophysics, Novosibirsk, Russia

Svetlana Dambinova and Alexander Panov
Laboratory of Brain Biomarkers, WellStar College of Health & Human Services, Kennesaw State University, Kennesaw, GA, USA

Helen R. Broom, Heather A. Primmer, Jessica A.O. Rumfeldt, Peter B. Stathopulos, Kenrick A. Vassall, Young-Mi Hwang and Elizabeth M. Meiering
Guelph-Waterloo Centre for Graduate Work in Chemistry and Biochemistry, University of Waterloo, Canada

Seiichi Nagano
Department of Peripheral Nervous System Research, National Institute of Neuroscience, National Center of Neurology and Psychiatry, Japan

Yoshiaki Furukawa
Department of Chemistry, Keio University, Japan

María Clara Franco and Alvaro G. Estévez
Burnett School of Biomedical Sciences, College of Medicine, University of Central Florida, Orlando, USA

Gilles Guillemin
Department of Pharmacology, School of Medical Sciences, University of New South Wales, Sydney, Australia St Vincent's Centre for Applied Medical Research, St Vincent's Hospital, Sydney, Australia

Yiquan Chen
Department of Pharmacology, School of Medical Sciences, University of New South Wales, Sydney, Australia